Current Therapy in Critical Care Medicine

Second Edition

Medical Titles in the Current Therapy Series

Bardin:
   Current Therapy in Endocrinology and Metabolism
Bayless:
   Current Management of Inflammatory Bowel Disease
Bayless:
   Current Therapy in Gastroenterology and Liver Disease
Brain, Carbone:
   Current Therapy in Hematology–Oncology
Callaham:
   Current Therapy in Emergency Medicine
Charles, Glover:
   Current Therapy in Obstetrics
Cherniack:
   Current Therapy of Respiratory Disease
Dubovsky, Shore:
   Current Therapy in Psychiatry
Dzau and Cooke:
   Current Management of Hypertension
Eichenwald, Ströder:
   Current Therapy in Pediatrics
Foley, Payne:
   Current Therapy of Pain
Garcia, Mastroianni, Amelar, Dubin:
   Current Therapy of Infertility
Glassock:
   Current Therapy in Nephrology and Hypertension
Horowitz:
   Current Management of Arrhythmias
Hurst:
   Current Therapy in Cardiovascular Disease
Jeejeebhoy:
   Current Therapy in Nutrition
Johnson:
   Current Therapy in Neurologic Disease
Kacmarek, Stoller:
   Current Respiratory Care
Kass, Platt:
   Current Therapy in Infectious Disease
Kassirer:
   Current Therapy in Internal Medicine
Lichtenstein, Fauci:
   Current Therapy in Allergy, Immunology, and Rheumatology
Nelson:
   Current Therapy in Neonatal–Perinatal Medicine
Nelson:
   Current Therapy in Pediatric Infectious Disease
Parrillo:
   Current Therapy in Critical Care Medicine
Provost, Farmer:
   Current Therapy in Dermatology
Rogers:
   Current Practice in Anesthesiology

CURRENT THERAPY IN CRITICAL CARE MEDICINE

Second Edition

JOSEPH E. PARRILLO, M.D.
James B. Herrick Professor of Medicine
Chief, Section of Cardiology
Chief, Section of Critical Care Medicine
Medical Director, Rush Heart Institute
Rush-Presbyterian-St. Luke's Medical Center
Chicago, Illinois

B. C. Decker Inc. • Philadelphia • Hamilton

Publisher	**B.C. Decker Inc** One James Street South 11th Floor Hamilton, Ontario L8P 4R5	**B.C. Decker Inc** 320 Walnut Street Suite 400 Philadelphia, Pennsylvania 19106

Sales and Distribution

United States and Puerto Rico
Mosby-Year Book Inc.
11830 Westline Industrial Drive
Saint Louis, Missouri 63146

Canada
Mosby-Year Book Limited
5240 Finch Avenue E., Unit 1
Scarborough, Ontario M1S 5A2

Australia
McGraw-Hill Book Company Australia Pty. Ltd.
4 Barcoo Street
Roseville East 2069
New South Wales, Australia

Brazil
Editora McGraw-Hill do Brasil, Ltda.
rua Tabapua, 1.105, Itaim-Bibi
Sao Paulo, S.P. Brasil

Colombia
Interamericana/McGraw-Hill de Colombia, S.A.
Apartado Aereo 81078
Bogota, D.E., Colombia

Europe, United Kingdom, Middle East and Africa
Wolfe Publishing Limited
Brook House
2-16 Torrington Place
London WC1E 7LT
England

Hong Kong and China
McGraw-Hill Book Company
Suite 618, Ocean Centre
5 Canton Road
Tsimshatsui, Kowloon
Hong Kong

India
Tata McGraw-Hill Publishing Company, Ltd.
12/4 Asaf Ali Road, 3rd Floor
New Delhi 110002, India

Indonesia
Mr. Wong Fin Fah
P.O. Box 122/JAT
Jakarta, 1300 Indonesia

Japan
Igaku-Shoin Ltd.
Tokyo International P.O. Box 5063
1-28-36 Hongo, Bunkyo-ku,
Tokyo 113, Japan

Korea
Mr. Don-Gap Choi
C.P.O. Box 10583
Seoul, Korea

Malaysia
Mr. Lim Tao Slong
No. 8 Jalan SS 7/6B
Kelana Jaya
47301 Petaling Jaya
Selangor, Malaysia

Mexico
Interamericana/McGraw-Hill de Mexico, S.A. de C.V.
Cedro 512, Colonia Atlampa
(Apartado Postal 26370)
06450 Mexico, D.F., Mexico

New Zealand
McGraw-Hill Book Co. New Zealand Ltd.
5 Joval Place, Wiri
Manukau City, New Zealand

Portugal
Editora McGraw-Hill de Portugal, Ltda.
Rua Rosa Damasceno 11A–B
1900 Lisboa, Portugal

South Africa
Libriger Book Distributors
Warehouse Number 8
"Die Ou Looiery"
Tannery Road
Hamilton, Bloemfontein 9300

Singapore and Southeast Asia
McGraw-Hill Book Co.
21 Neythal Road
Jurong, Singapore 2262

Spain
McGraw-Hill/Interamericana de Espana, S.A.
Manuel Ferrero, 13
28020 Madrid, Spain

Taiwan
Mr. George Lim
P.O. Box 87-601
Taipei, Taiwan

Thailand
Mr. Vitit Lim
632/5 Phaholyothin Road
Sapan Kwai
Bangkok 10400
Thailand

Venezuela
Editorial Interamericana de Venezuela, C.A.
2da. calle Bello Monte
Local G-2
Caracas, Venezuela

NOTICE

The authors and publisher have made every effort to ensure that the patient care recommended herein, including choice of drugs and drug dosages, is in accord with the accepted standards and practice at the time of publication. However, since research and regulation constantly change clinical standards, the reader is urged to check the product information sheet included in the package of each drug, which includes recommended doses, warnings, and contraindications. This is particularly important with new or infrequently used drugs.

Current Therapy in Critical Care Medicine–Second Edition

ISBN 1-55664-268-7
ISSN 0899-3904

© 1991 by B.C. Decker Incorporated under the International Copyright Union. All rights reserved. No part of this publication may be reused or republished in any form without written permission of the publisher.

CONTRIBUTORS

JOHANE P. ALLARD, M.D.

Assistant Professor of Medicine, University of Toronto Faculty of Medicine; Staff Physician, Toronto General Hospital, Toronto, Ontario, Canada
Nutrition in the Critically Ill

DAVID BALDWIN, Jr., M.D.

Assistant Professor of Medicine, Rush Medical College of Rush University; Director, Clinical Endocrinology, Rush-Presbyterian-St. Luke's Medical Center, Chicago, Illinois
Diabetes and Diabetic Coma

ROBERT A. BALK, M.D.

Associate Professor of Medicine, Rush Medical College of Rush University; Director, Medical Intensive Care Unit and Respiratory Therapy, Rush-Presbyterian-St. Luke's Medical Center, Chicago, Illinois
Mechanical Ventilation
Obstructive Lung Disease
Weaning From Mechanical Ventilation

ALAN J. BANK, M.D.

Cardiology Fellow, University of Minnesota Medical School–Minneapolis, Minneapolis, Minnesota
Congestive Heart Failure: Inotropic Agents

DAVID A. BARON, M.S.Ed., D.O.

Clinical Associate Professor of Psychiatry, University of Southern California School of Medicine, Los Angeles, California; Deputy Clinical Director, National Institutes of Mental Health, Bethesda, Maryland
Psychiatric Problems

JOHN T. BARRON, M.D., Ph.D

Assistant Professor, Section of Cardiology, Rush Medical College of Rush University; Assistant Attending Physician, Department of Medicine, Rush-Presbyterian-St. Luke's Medical Center, Chicago, Illinois
Congestive Heart Failure: Vasodilator Therapy
Severe Aortic or Mitral Valvular Regurgitation

WILLIAM BAUMGARTNER, M.D.

Associate Professor of Surgery, The Johns Hopkins University School of Medicine, Baltimore, Maryland
Heart and Great Vessel Trauma

MARGARET JOHNSON BIA, M.D.

Associate Professor of Medicine, and Director of Transplant Neurology, Renal Section, Department of Medicine, Yale University School of Medicine, New Haven, Connecticut
Acute Renal Failure
Life-Threatening Electrolyte and Metabolic Disorders

THOMAS P. BLECK, M.D.

Associate Professor of Neurology, University of Virginia School of Medicine; Director, Nerancy Neuroscience Intensive Care Unit, University of Virginia Medical Center, Charlottesville, Virginia
Seizures in the Intensive Care Unit
Increased Intracranial Pressure

ROGER C. BONE, M.D.

The Ralph C. Brown Professor and Chairman, Department of Medicine, Rush Medical College of Rush University; Chief, Pulmonary and Critical Care Medicine, Rush-Presbyterian-St. Luke's Medical Center, Chicago, Illinois
Adult Respiratory Distress Syndrome
Acute Respiratory Failure

THOMAS A. BUCKINGHAM, M.D.

Associate Professor, Rush Medical College of Rush University; Director, Arrhythmia Services, Rush-Presbyterian-St. Luke's Medical Center, Chicago, Illinois
Ventricular Arrhythmia
Atrioventricular Block in the Critically Ill

RANDALL L. BUSCH, M.D., D.D.S.

Resident, Department of Internal Medicine, Rush-Presbyterian-St. Luke's Medical Center, Chicago, Illinois
Acute Respiratory Failure

ALFRED S. CASALE, M.D.

Assistant Professor of Surgery, The Johns Hopkins University School of Medicine, Baltimore, Maryland
Heart and Great Vessel Trauma

NISHA C. CHANDRA, M.D.

Associate Professor of Medicine, Johns Hopkins University School of Medicine; Director, Coronary Care Unit, Francis Scott Key Medical Center, Baltimore, Maryland
Cardiopulmonary Resuscitation

vi / Contributors

ROBERT J. CODY, M.D.
James Hay and Ruth Jansson Wilson Professor of Medicine, Ohio State University College of Medicine; Research Director, Division of Cardiology, Ohio State University Hospitals, Columbus, Ohio
Hypertensive Emergency and Aortic Dissection

JOHN MICHAEL CRILEY, M.D.
Professor of Medicine and Radiological Sciences, University of California, Los Angeles, School of Medicine, Los Angeles; Medical Director, Saint John's Heart Institute, Santa Monica, California
Hypertrophic Cardiomyopathy

ROBERT E. CUNNION, M.D.
Senior Investigator and Chief, Cardiology Section, Critical Care Medicine Department, National Institutes of Health, Bethesda, Maryland
Acute Myopericarditis
Dilated Cardiomyopathy

RICHARD J. DAVEY, M.D.
Deputy Chief, Department of Transfusion Medicine, National Institutes of Health, Bethesda, Maryland
Blood Product Therapy

BENNETT P. deBOISBLANC, M.D., F.C.C.P.
Assistant Professor of Medicine and Director of Clinical Research, Pulmonary/Critical Care, Louisiana State University Medical School in New Orleans, New Orleans, Louisiana
Alveolar Hypoventilation and Respiratory Muscle Fatigue
Bedside Hemodynamic Monitoring

ROBERT DEMLING, M.D.
Professor of Surgery, Harvard Medical School; Director, Longwood Area Trauma Center, Boston, Massachusetts
Burn Management

KATHLEEN MARIE DIXON, Ph.D.
Assistant Professor of Philosophy, Bowling Green State University, Bowling Green, Ohio
Ethical Issues

PAUL M. DORINSKY, M.D.
Associate Professor of Medicine, Division of Pulmonary and Critical Care, Ohio State University College of Medicine; Attending Physician, Ohio State University Hospital, Columbus, Ohio
Oxygen Toxicity

J. CHRISTOPHER FARMER, M.D.
Assistant Professor of Medicine, Uniformed Services University of the Health Sciences, F. Edward Hébert School of Medicine, Bethesda, Maryland; Deputy Director, Critical Care, Wilford Hall USAF Medical Center, Lackland AFB, Texas
Hypothermia and Hyperthermia

ANN MARIE FLANNERY, M.D.
Assistant Professor of Surgery and Pediatrics, Medical College of Georgia, Augusta, Georgia
Head Trauma

ALAN D. GUERCI, M.D.
Associate Professor of Medicine, The Johns Hopkins University School of Medicine; Director, Coronary Care Unit, The Johns Hopkins Hospital, Baltimore, Maryland
Cardiopulmonary Resuscitation

PAUL K. HANASHIRO, M.D.
Associate Professor of Medicine, Rush Medical College of Rush University; Medical Director, Emergency Services, Rush-Presbyterian-St. Luke's Medical Center, Chicago, Illinois
Approach to Toxicology

ERNEST WILLIAM HANCOCK, M.D.
Professor of Medicine, Stanford University School of Medicine, Stanford, California
Restrictive Cardiomyopathy
Cardiac Tamponade

MARILYN T. HAUPT, M.D.
Associate Professor of Medicine, Wayne State University School of Medicine; Director, Medical Intensive Care Unit, Detroit Receiving Hospital, Detroit, Michigan
Anaphylaxis and Anaphylactic Shock

WILLIAM D. HOFFMAN, M.D.
Senior Investigator, Critical Care Medicine Department, National Institutes of Health, Bethesda, Maryland
Endotracheal Intubation
Septic Shock and Other Forms of Distributive Shock

CYRUS C. HOPKINS, M.D.
Associate Professor of Medicine, Harvard Medical School; Physician and Hospital Epidemiologist, Massachusetts General Hospital, Boston, Massachusetts
Pneumonitis

KHURSHEED N. JEEJEEBHOY, M.D., Ph.D.
Professor of Medicine, University of Toronto Faculty of Medicine; Staff Physician, St. Michael's Hospital, Toronto, Ontario, Canada
Nutrition in the Critically Ill

DONALD M. JENSEN, M.D., F.A.C.P.
Associate Professor of Medicine, Section of Digestive Diseases, Rush Medical College of Rush University; Chief, Hepatology Unit, Rush-Presbyterian-St. Luke's Medical Center, Chicago, Illinois
Acute Pancreatitis

ROBERT A. KAPLAN, M.D.
   Assistant Clinical Professor of Medicine, University of California College of Medicine, Irvine; Staff Physician, Long Beach Veterans Administration Medical Center, Long Beach, California
   Pneumonitis

MARK A. KELLEY, M.D.
   Vice Dean for Clinical Affairs, University of Pennsylvania School of Medicine; Pulmonary Specialist, Hospital of the University of Pennsylvania, Philadelphia, Pennsylvania
   Airflow Obstruction Caused by Bronchospasm

LLOYD W. KLEIN, M.D.
   Associate Professor of Medicine, Rush Medical College of Rush University; Co-Director, Cardiac Catheterization Laboratories, and Director, Interventional Cardiology, Rush-Presbyterian-St. Luke's Medical Center, Chicago, Illinois
   The Postoperative Surgical Patient

JOSEPH A. KOVACS, M.D.
   Head, AIDS Section, National Institutes of Health, Bethesda, Maryland
   The Immunosuppressed Host

SPENCER H. KUBO, M.D.
   Assistant Professor of Medicine, University of Minnesota Medical School–Minneapolis; Medical Director, Heart Failure–Heart Transplantation Program, University of Minnesota Hospital, Minneapolis, Minnesota
   Congestive Heart Failure: Inotropic Agents

ROBERT S. LEBOVICS, M.D., F.A.C.S.
   Chief, Otolaryngology/Head and Neck Surgery, National Institute on Deafness and Other Communication Disorders, National Institutes of Health, Bethesda, Maryland
   Upper Airway Obstruction

CARL V. LEIER, M.D.
   James W. Overstreet Professor of Medicine and Pharmacology, and Director, Division of Cardiology, Ohio State University College of Medicine, Columbus, Ohio
   Cardiogenic Shock

JERROLD B. LEIKIN, M.D., F.A.C.P., F.A.C.E.P.
   Assistant Professor of Medicine, Rush Medical College of Rush University; Associate Medical Director, Emergency Services/Poison Control Center, Rush-Presbyterian-St. Luke's Medical Center, Chicago, Illinois
   Approach to Toxicology

DAVID E. LEVY, M.D.
   Associate Professor of Neurology and Neuroscience, Cornell University Medical College; Associate Attending Neurologist and Executive Vice Chair, Department of Neurology, The New York Hospital, New York, New York
   Coma

RICHARD P. LEWIS, M.D.
   Professor of Medicine, Ohio State University College of Medicine, Columbus, Ohio
   Congestive Heart Failure: Digitalis Therapy
   Supraventricular Arrhythmia

PHILIP R. LIEBSON, M.D.
   Professor of Medicine, Rush Medical College of Rush University; Director, Cardiac Graphics Laboratory and Preventative Cardiology Program, Rush-Presbyterian-St. Luke's Medical Center, Chicago, Illinois
   Congestive Heart Failure: Diuretic Therapy
   Echocardiography

DAN L. LONGO, M.D.
   Director, Biological Response Modifiers Program, Division of Cancer Treatment, National Cancer Institute–Frederick Cancer Research and Development Center, Frederick, Maryland
   The Cancer Patient

D. LYNN LORIAUX, M.D., Ph.D.
   Clinical Director, National Institute of Child Health and Human Development, National Institutes of Health, Bethesda, Maryland
   Adrenal Insufficiency

DENNIS G. MAKI, M.D.
   Ovid O. Meyer Professor of Medicine, University of Wisconsin Medical School; Head, Section of Infectious Diseases, and Attending Physician, Center for Trauma and Life Support, University of Wisconsin Hospitals and Clinics, Madison, Wisconsin
   Nosocomial Infection

DOUGLAS L. MALLORY, M.D.
   Assistant Clinical Professor of Medicine, Saint Louis University School of Medicine; Director, Critical Care Research, Saint John's Mercy Medical Center, St. Louis, Missouri
   The Near-Drowning Victim

HENRY MASUR, M.D.
   Professor of Clinical Medicine, George Washington University School of Medicine and Health Sciences, Washington, D.C.; Chief, Critical Care Medicine Department, National Institutes of Health Clinical Center, Bethesda, Maryland
   Antibiotic Usage in the Intensive Care Unit

viii / Contributors

PAUL MISKOVITZ, M.D.
Associate Professor of Clinical Medicine, Cornell University Medical College; Associate Attending Physician, The New York Hospital, New York, New York
Hepatic Failure

CHARLES NATANSON, M.D.
Senior Investigator, Critical Care Medicine Department, National Institutes of Health, Bethesda, Maryland
Endotracheal Intubation
Septic Shock and Other Forms of Distributive Shock

FREDERICK P. OGNIBENE, M.D.
Assistant Clinical Professor of Medicine, George Washington University School of Medicine and Health Sciences, Washington, D.C.; Senior Investigator, Critical Care Medicine Department, National Institutes of Health, Bethesda, Maryland
Bronchoscopy in the Intensive Care Unit
Arterial Blood Gases

ERIC R. PACHT, M.D.
Assistant Professor of Medicine, Division of Pulmonary and Critical Care, Ohio State University College of Medicine; Attending Physician, Ohio State University Hospital, Columbus, Ohio
Oxygen Toxicity

REYNOLD A. PANETTIERI, Jr., M.D.
Assistant Professor, University of Pennsylvania School of Medicine; Staff Pulmonologist, Hospital of the University of Pennsylvania, Philadelphia, Pennsylvania
Airflow Obstruction Caused by Bronchospasm

MARGARET M. PARKER, M.D.
Associate Clinical Professor of Medicine, George Washington University School of Medicine, Washington, D.C.; Head, Critical Care Section, Critical Care Medicine Department, National Institutes of Health, Bethesda, Maryland
Nuclear Scanning

JOSEPH E. PARRILLO, M.D.
James B. Herrick Professor of Medicine, Rush Medical College of Rush University; Chief, Section of Cardiology and Section of Critical Care Medicine, and Medical Director, Rush Heart Institute, Rush-Presbyterian-St. Luke's Medical Center, Chicago, Illinois
Congestive Heart Failure: Vasodilator Therapy
Ventricular Arrhythmia

EDWARD L. PASSEN, M.D.
Assistant Professor of Medicine, Rush Medical College of Rush University; Assistant Attending Surgeon, Rush-Presbyterian-St. Luke's Medical Center, Chicago, Illinois
Ischemic Heart Disease
Acute Myocardial Infarction

JOHN PHELAN, M.D.
Instructor, Rush Medical College of Rush University; Chief Cardiology Fellow, Rush-Presbyterian-St. Luke's Medical Center, Chicago, Illinois
The Postoperative Cardiac Surgical Patient

PHILIP A. PIZZO, M.D.
Professor of Pediatrics, Uniformed Services University of the Health Sciences; Chief, Pediatrics Branch, and Head, Infectious Diseases Section, National Cancer Institute, Bethesda, Maryland
Antifungal Therapy

EAMONN M. M. QUIGLEY, M.D., M.R.C.P.
Associate Professor, University of Nebraska College of Medicine; Gastroenterologist, University of Nebraska Hospital and Veterans Administration Medical Center, Omaha, Nebraska
Upper Gastrointestinal Hemorrhage
Lower Gastrointestinal Hemorrhage

H. DAVID REINES, M.D., F.A.C.S., F.C.C.M.
Associate Professor of Surgery and Anesthesia, and Director, Critical Care and Trauma, Medical College of Virginia, Richmond, Virginia
Initial Trauma Management

MARGARET E. RICK, M.D.
Assistant Chief, Hematology Section, Clinical Center, National Institutes of Health, Bethesda, Maryland
Hemorrhagic and Thrombotic Disorders

R. DWAINE RIEVES, M.D.
Fellow, Department of Critical Care Medicine, National Institutes of Health, Bethesda, Maryland
Radiation Pneumonitis and Fibrosis

MICHAEL RUBIN, M.D., FRCP(C)
Assistant Professor of Neurology, Cornell University Medical College; Director, Neuromuscular Service, The New York Hospital, New York, New York
Ascending Polyneuritis (Guillain-Barré Syndrome)

ROBERT H. RUBIN, M.D., F.A.C.P., F.C.C.P.
Associate Professor of Medicine, Harvard Medical School; Director, Clinical Investigation Program, and Chief, Infectious Disease for Transplantation, Massachusetts General Hospital, Boston, Massachusetts
Pneumonitis

RONALD H. RUBIN, M.D.
Associate Professor, Temple University School of Medicine; Deputy Chairman, Internal Medicine, Temple University Hospital, Philadelphia, Pennsylvania
Pulmonary Embolism
Pneumonitis

DAVID R. RUBINOW, M.D.

Clinical Director, National Institute of Mental Health, and Chief, Section on Behavioral Endocrinology, Biological Psychiatry Branch, National Institute of Mental Health, Bethesda, Maryland
Psychiatric Problems

SEYMOUR M. SABESIN, M.D., F.A.C.P.

Dyrenforth Professor of Medicine, Rush Medical College of Rush University; Director, Section of Digestive Diseases, Rush-Presbyterian-St. Luke's Medical Center, Chicago, Illinois
Acute Pancreatitis

SUSUMU SATO, M.D.

Chief, EEG Laboratory, National Institutes of Neurologic Diseases and Stroke, Bethesda, Maryland
Neurologic Criteria for Death

GARY L. SCHAER, M.D.

Associate Professor of Medicine, Rush Medical College of Rush University; Director, Cardiac Catheterization Laboratories, Rush-Presbyterian-St. Luke's Medical Center, Chicago, Illinois
Unstable Angina Pectoris
Acute Myocardial Infarction

DANIEL P. SCHUSTER, M.D.

Associate Professor of Medicine, Washington University School of Medicine; Medical Director, Medical Intensive Care Unit, Barnes Hospital, Saint Louis, Missouri
Bedside Evaluation of Respiratory Function

JAMES H. SHELHAMER, M.D.

Deputy Chief, Critical Care Medicine Department, National Institutes of Health, Bethesda, Maryland
Radiation Pneumonitis and Fibrosis

SOL SHERRY, M.D.

Distinguished Professor of Medicine Emeritus, Temple University School of Medicine, Philadelphia, Pennsylvania
Pulmonary Embolism

ROBERT J. SIEGEL, M.D.

Associate Professor of Medicine, University of California, Los Angeles, School of Medicine; Staff Cardiologist, Cedars-Sinai Medical Center, Los Angeles, California
Hypertrophic Cardiomyopathy

MICHAEL R. SILVER, M.D.

Assistant Professor of Medicine, Rush Medical College of Rush University; Director, Noninvasive Respiratory Care Unit, and Director of Clinical Services, Section of Pulmonary Medicine, Rush-Presbyterian-St. Luke's Medical Center, Chicago, Illinois
Weaning from Mechanical Ventilation

JOHN W. SMITH II, M.D.

Senior Investigator, Biological Response Modifiers Program, Division of Cancer Treatment, National Cancer Institute, Frederick Memorial Hospital Cancer Treatment Center, Frederick, Maryland
The Cancer Patient

ANTHONY F. SUFFREDINI, M.D.

Senior Investigator, and Senior Staff Physician, Critical Care Medicine Department, National Institutes of Health, Bethesda, Maryland
Hemorrhagic and Hypervolemic Shock

WARREN R. SUMMER, M.D., F.C.C.P.

Howard A. Buechner Professor of Medicine and Section Chief, Pulmonary Critical Care Medicine, Louisiana State University School of Medicine in New Orleans, New Orleans, Louisiana
Bedside Hemodynamic Monitoring
Alveolar Hypoventilation and Respiratory Muscle Fatigue

PETER SZIDON, M.D.

Professor of Medicine, Rush Medical College of Rush University, Chicago, Illinois
Syndromes Caused by Aspiration of Stomach Contents

THOMAS J. WALSH, M.D.

Medical Officer, National Cancer Institute, Bethesda, Maryland
Antifungal Therapy

ALISON WICHMAN, M.D.

Chief, Bioethics Program, National Institutes of Health, and Consultant Neurologist, National Institutes of Neurological Diseases and Stroke, Bethesda, Maryland
Neurologic Criteria for Death
Ethical Issues

To Gale

PREFACE

Few specialties in medicine are more suited to the Current Therapy concept than is critical care medicine. The Current Therapy series has been successful because physicians have recognized the enormous clinical utility of a volume devoted completely to the treatment of patients within a specialty. In most reference textbooks, discussions of clinical presentation, pathophysiology, clinical course, and prognosis heavily outweigh discussions of therapy. Such texts usually present general principles of therapy or a nonspecific approach to the disease in question. Since large textbooks are written for broad audiences of medical students, house officers, and general staff physicians, they do not explore specific approaches to therapy or the possible alternatives if the first-line agent is ineffective or results in a serious complication. Yet active physicians, especially critical care physicians, spend much of their time administering therapy and attempting to make it as effective as possible. Thus, a volume devoted to therapy should provide information uniquely applicable to critical care.

Critical care medicine has certain characteristics that render a therapy-oriented volume particularly useful. First, the specialty of intensive care medicine is relatively new and lacks the voluminous literature of other specialities. Therefore, a therapy-oriented volume, written by their peers and teachers, serves to keep critical care physicians in touch with current practices outside their own institutions. The chapters in this book, *Current Therapy in Critical Care Medicine*, though emphasizing therapy, do not ignore underlying clinical findings and pathophysiology, which are so essential to therapeutic decision.

Another characteristic of critical care medicine that favors the present format is that critical care is "action oriented." Patients are selected to enter an ICU because they are critically ill or at high risk of developing a critical illness. Thus, critical care physicians spend most of their time providing or monitoring therapy, the latter by invasive and noninvasive methods. How to institute therapy and when to alter or change a therapeutic approach represent some of the most common problems facing the ICU physician. This book is intended to provide a concise but comprehensive review of the therapeutic options in specific critical illnesses as practiced by our author-experts.

As with the first edition, the chapter authors for this second edition have been carefully chosen. Each is an authority and practicing physician in his or her subspecialty. Only by serving in the front lines and by caring for patients can the critical care physician continue to be informed and to bring authority to the evaluation of therapeutic options. This balance between authoritative knowledge and ongoing experience was my criterion for matching authors with topics.

In compiling this volume, I received assistance from many sources, and I would like to thank those people for their invaluable support. Geri Byrd, Katherine Swanigan, and Sandy Montgomery provided the much needed editorial assistance to assure each chapter was ready for publication. Ms. Mary Mansor of B.C. Decker provided valuable guidance and editorial advice. Brian Decker, the publisher, developed the concept behind Current Therapy and provided his characteristic enthusiasm and support.

Joseph E. Parrillo, M.D.

CONTENTS

DIAGNOSTIC AND THERAPEUTIC TECHNIQUES

Cardiopulmonary Resuscitation 1
Alan D. Guerci
Nisha C. Chandra

Endotracheal Intubation 5
William D. Hoffman
Charles Natanson

Bronchoscopy in the Intensive Care Unit . . 16
Frederick P. Ognibene

Arterial Blood Gases 20
Frederick P. Ognibene

Mechanical Ventilation 24
Robert A. Balk

Bedside Evaluation of Respiratory Function 30
Daniel P. Schuster

Echocardiography 35
Philip R. Liebson

Nuclear Scanning 45
Margaret M. Parker

Bedside Hemodynamic Monitoring 47
Warren R. Summer
Bennett P. deBoisblanc

CARDIOVASCULAR THERAPEUTICS

Cardiogenic Shock 54
Carl V. Leier

Anaphylaxis and Anaphylactic Shock 58
Marilyn T. Haupt

Septic Shock and Other Forms
of Distributive Shock 62
Charles Natanson
William D. Hoffman

Hemorrhagic and Hypovolemic Shock 70
Anthony F. Suffredini

Cardiac Tamponade 74
Ernest William Hancock

Congestive Heart Failure: Digitalis Therapy 78
Richard P. Lewis

Congestive Heart Failure: Diuretic Therapy . 81
Philip R. Liebson

Congestive Heart Failure:
Vasodilator Therapy 87
John T. Barron
Joseph E. Parrillo

Congestive Heart Failure: Inotropic Agents . 92
Alan J. Bank
Spencer H. Kubo

Supraventricular Arrhythmia 97
Richard P. Lewis

Ventricular Arrhythmia 102
Thomas A. Buckingham
Joseph E. Parrillo

Atrioventricular Block in the Critically Ill . 108
Thomas A. Buckingham

Unstable Angina Pectoris 112
Gary L. Schaer

Acute Myocardial Infarction 115
Edward L. Passen
Gary L. Schaer

Pulmonary Embolism 123
  Ronald N. Rubin
  Sol Sherry

Acute Myopericarditis 126
  Robert E. Cunnion

Dilated Cardiomyopathy 131
  Robert E. Cunnion

Hypertrophic Cardiomyopathy 136
  John Michael Criley
  Robert J. Siegel

Restrictive Cardiomyopathy 139
  Ernest William Hancock

Severe Aortic or Mitral
Valvular Regurgitation 142
  John T. Barron

The Postoperative Cardiac Surgical Patient 147
  John Phelan
  Lloyd W. Klein

Hypertensive Emergency and
Aortic Dissection 155
  Robert J. Cody

Heart and Great Vessel Trauma 158
  Alfred S. Casale
  William A. Baumgartner

PULMONARY THERAPEUTICS

Acute Respiratory Failure 162
  Roger C. Bone
  Randall L. Busch

Adult Respiratory Distress Syndrome 165
  Roger C. Bone

Pneumonitis 170
  Robert A. Kaplan
  Cyrus C. Hopkins
  Robert H. Rubin

Obstructive Lung Disease 176
  Robert A. Balk

Airflow Obstruction Caused
by Bronchospasm 180
  Reynold A. Panettieri, Jr.
  Mark A. Kelley

Syndromes Caused by Aspiration of
Stomach Contents 185
  Peter Szidon

Alveolar Hypoventilation and
Respiratory Muscle Fatigue 188
  Bennett P. deBoisblanc
  Warren R. Summer

Upper Airway Obstruction 193
  Robert S. Lebovics

Oxygen Toxicity 198
  Eric R. Pacht
  Paul M. Dorinsky

Radiation Pneumonitis and Fibrosis 201
  R. Dwaine Rieves
  James H. Shelhamer

Weaning From Mechanical Ventilation ... 203
  Michael R. Silver
  Robert A. Balk

THERAPEUTICS FOR INFECTIOUS DISEASES

Nosocomial Infection 208
  Dennis G. Maki

The Immunosuppressed Host 215
  Joseph A. Kovacs

Antibiotic Usage in the Intensive
Care Unit 219
  Henry Masur

Antifungal Therapy 224
  Thomas J. Walsh
  Philip A. Pizzo

NEUROLOGIC THERAPEUTICS

Head Trauma 233
  Ann Marie Flannery

Coma 236
David E. Levy

Neurologic Criteria for Death 240
Alison Wichman
Susumu Sato

Ascending Polyneuritis
(Guillain-Barré Syndrome) 243
Michael Rubin

Seizures in the Intensive Care Unit 246
Thomas P. Bleck

Increased Intracranial Pressure 249
Thomas P. Bleck

RENAL, GASTROINTESTINAL, HEMATOLOGIC, AND METABOLIC THERAPEUTICS

Acute Renal Failure 253
Margaret Johnson Bia

Life-Threatening Electrolyte and
Metabolic Disorders 256
Margaret Johnson Bia

Nutrition in the Critically Ill 262
Johane P. Allard
Khursheed N. Jeejeebhoy

Hepatic Failure 271
Paul Miskovitz

Acute Pancreatitis 275
Donald M. Jensen
Seymour M. Sabesin

Upper Gastrointestinal Hemorrhage 279
Eamonn M. M. Quigley

Lower Gastrointestinal Hemorrhage 284
Eamonn M. M. Quigley

Hemorrhagic and Thrombotic Disorders .. 288
Margaret E. Rick

Blood Product Therapy 292
Richard J. Davey

The Cancer Patient 296
John W. Smith II
Dan L. Longo

Diabetes and Diabetic Coma 302
David Baldwin Jr.

Adrenal Insufficiency 305
D. Lynn Loriaux

THERAPEUTICS FOR PHYSICAL INJURY

Initial Trauma Management 307
H. David Reines

Burn Management 311
Robert Demling

The Near-Drowning Victim 317
Douglas L. Mallory

Approach to Toxicology 320
Jerrold B. Leikin
Paul K. Hanashiro

Hypothermia and Hyperthermia 328
J. Christopher Farmer

PSYCHIATRIC AND ETHICAL ISSUES

Psychiatric Problems 333
David A. Baron
David R. Rubinow

Ethical Issues 338
Alison Wichman
Kathleen Marie Dixon

Index 343

DIAGNOSTIC AND THERAPEUTIC TECHNIQUES

CARDIOPULMONARY RESUSCITATION

ALAN D. GUERCI, M.D.
NISHA C. CHANDRA, M.D.

Cardiopulmonary resuscitation (CPR) comprises a set of procedures and pharmacologic treatments designed to maximize oxygen delivery to the heart and brain during cardiac arrest and, ultimately, to restore spontaneous and effective cardiac and respiratory activity. This chapter focuses on the treatment of adult cardiac arrest.

PATIENT IDENTIFICATION

Respiratory arrest may exist without cardiac arrest, and several of the initial procedures in cardiopulmonary resuscitation, such as chest compression and defibrillation, are extremely painful. Confirmation of cardiac and/or respiratory arrest is therefore a critical first step in the management of any apparent arrest situation. If the patient is unarousable and does not have a pulse, defibrillation should be performed as soon as possible.

DEFIBRILLATION

Defibrillation occupies a central position in the treatment of cardiac arrest. It is the only treatment that routinely terminates ventricular fibrillation and ventricular tachycardia, and it presents little if any danger to patients with bradycardiac arrests. For these reasons and because ventricular tachyarrhythmias account for most arrests, defibrillation is the treatment of first choice for all unmonitored cardiac arrests. After "thump version," it is also the treatment of choice for monitored arrests caused by ventricular tachyarrhythmias. Defibrillation should be performed in rapid sequence at 200, 300, and 400 J (corresponding to delivered energy levels of 180, 270, and 360 J). In these situations, CPR should be performed only for as long as is necessary to obtain and charge a defibrillator. Similarly, initial attempts at defibrillation should not be delayed by efforts to establish an electrocardiographic diagnosis. Because CPR does not generate normal levels of myocardial perfusion, any delay in defibrillation will cause the heart to be more ischemic and more acidotic when defibrillation is finally attempted.

ESTABLISHING AN AIRWAY

If the patient is unarousable, one must determine whether he or she is breathing. If breathing is absent or inadequate, the head and neck must be positioned to eliminate the possibility of upper airway obstruction by the tongue. In the absence of evidence of neck trauma, one hand is placed on the forehead and the chin is grasped with the fingers of the other hand. By pushing on the forehead and pulling vigorously on the chin, the neck is extended and the base of the tongue may be lifted off the oropharynx. In cases in which neck trauma is suspected, the mandible must be extended while the neck is stabilized. Two deep ventilations should be delivered. If resistance to ventilation is encountered, the airway must be repositioned and, if necessary, any obstructing foreign objects or food must be removed. Removal of foreign objects begins with maneuvers that raise intrathoracic pressure and, at least in theory, propel obstructing materials from the trachea or glottis into the oropharynx. A modification of the Heimlich maneuver, in which the heel of one hand, supported by the other hand, is placed under the xiphoid process and driven cephalad and posteriorly is recommended for this purpose. Sternal compression may also be effective. If material is propelled into the oropharynx, it should be swept to the side and then pulled out.

CHEST COMPRESSION

Once the airway is established, the arrest victim should be given two deep breaths every 10 seconds. If the arrest victim does not have a pulse, chest compression must be initiated immediately. The lower sternum (not the xiphoid) should be compressed vigorously 15 times at a rate of 80 to 100 compressions per minute, interrupted for two ventilations, and then resumed. The depth and duration of chest compression are probably more important than compression rate. Compression duration, which is 50 percent of each compression-release cycle, appears to maximize coronary and cerebral perfusion pressure in humans; this duration is achieved naturally by most rescuers at compression rates of 80 to 100 per minute. Proper depth of compression is critical. Too much compression force may cause life-threatening chest wall trauma; too little results in negligible vital organ perfusion and death. The sternum must therefore be displaced to the limits of its stress tolerance, and carotid pulsations should be palpable.

Chest compression and ventilation should be interrupted every few minutes to check for a return of spontaneous pulse.

DRUG THERAPY

Effective drug therapy for cardiac arrest requires consideration of the route of administration as well as the specifics of drug selection and dosage regimens. Dye dilution studies have shown that indicators reach maximal concentration in the femoral artery within 1 to 2 minutes when given into central veins, whereas high concentrations are not attained even within 5 minutes when indicators are given into the dorsal veins of the hand or the femoral vein. Thus, whenever possible, drugs should be given via a central venous line. Injection into an antecubital vein, flushed by 10 to 30 ml of normal saline, may be an effective alternative, but little is known about this approach.

Epinephrine

Current knowledge indicates that epinephrine should be administered to all arrest victims who fail to respond to initial attempts at defibrillation. The positive chronotropic and inotropic properties of this drug make it suitable for asystole, bradycardiac arrests, and electromechanical dissociation, conditions in which increased heart rate and/or contractility are needed. In addition, at high doses, epinephrine is a potent vasoconstrictor. Intense peripheral vasoconstriction induced by epinephrine raises aortic pressure, increases cerebral and myocardial perfusion, and increases the likelihood of successful resuscitation from experimental asystolic and fibrillatory arrest. Thus, above and beyond its direct cardiac effects, high-dose epinephrine maximizes myocardial perfusion during CPR.

The major question with regard to epinephrine administration during CPR is the optimal dose. The current American Heart Association recommendation, 1 mg every 5 to 10 minutes, is the same dose that was found to be effective 25 years ago in 10- to 12-kg dogs. More recent animal studies indicate that a minimum of 5 μg per kilogram per minute of epinephrine is required to maintain coronary perfusion pressure at maximal levels. Converted to bolus dosing, these data suggest that the average-sized adult needs at least 1 mg of epinephrine every 2.8 minutes. Limited human data are consistent with these calculations and support the use of a dose of 2 to 5 mg every 5 minutes after prolonged arrest. Until such time as additional studies and randomized trials clarify this issue, 1 mg of epinephrine should probably be given as a first dose and a minimum of 1 mg should be given every 5 minutes thereafter. The uncertainty surrounding the questions of proper dose, inhibition of catecholamines by acidosis, and the fact that the likelihood of successful resuscitation declines with time justifies the use of 2 or 3 mg of epinephrine for subsequent doses.

Sodium Bicarbonate

No evidence exists that sodium bicarbonate promotes resuscitation from cardiac arrest in humans, and most animal studies indicate no effect on outcome. Extreme metabolic acidosis (arterial pH < 7.10) has not been studied, however, and it is conceivable that the use of sodium bicarbonate is beneficial in such cases. With regard to the use of sodium bicarbonate, the urge to correct reversible abnormalities should be tempered by consideration of its potential toxicity. The carbon dioxide generated in serum by the reaction of sodium bicarbonate with organic acids crosses cell membranes rapidly, causing a paradoxic intracellular acidosis. Contractility actually decreases transiently. Thus, the administration of sodium bicarbonate may temporarily further burden an ischemic and already acidotic heart. The repeated use of sodium bicarbonate can also cause hyperosmolality and intravascular volume overload. Therefore sodium bicarbonate should be used judiciously, if at all, in cases complicated by extreme acidosis and should be accompanied by hyperventilation. Complete correction of calculated base deficits is neither practical nor desirable.

SPECIFIC ARRHYTHMIAS CAUSING CARDIAC ARREST

Ventricular Fibrillation

Ventricular fibrillation refractory to initial countershock requires a systematic effort to maintain adequate gas exchange, maximize coronary perfusion pressure, deliver rapidly acting antiarrhythmics, and repeat defibrillation at points in time when drug therapy is likely to have favorably affected the metabolic and arrhythmogenic milieu. This means that epinephrine should be administered as outlined above, and that 400-J countershocks should be delivered every 3 to 5 minutes. Lidocaine administered intravenously in a dose of 1 mg per kilogram should be given immediately to patients not responding to initial countershock. Repeat doses of 0.5 mg per kilogram may be given every 8 minutes until a total dose of 3 mg per kilogram. It should be understood that this lidocaine regimen establishes therapeutic serum levels as soon as the drug reaches the systemic arterial circulation and maintains therapeutic levels for the duration of the arrest. Since hepatic blood flow is negligible during CPR and because lidocaine is metabolized exclusively by the liver, degradation of lidocaine may be ignored for as long as CPR is necessary. This means that lidocaine infusions are not necessary after the full loading dose (3 mg per kilogram) is given to patients who remain in full cardiac arrest.

Because external chest compression is associated with low levels of myocardial perfusion and progressive myocardial metabolic deterioration, in any patient who is adequately oxygenated but cannot be defibrillated 3 to 5 minutes after lidocaine administration, treatment with lidocaine as a single antiarrhythmic agent should be considered as having failed. The use of lidocaine should probably be continued, but a second agent—usually bretylium tosylate—should be added.

Bretylium tosylate has a short serum distribution half-life (several minutes), slow myocardial uptake (several hours), and a long elimination half-life (approximately 10 hours). Its effectiveness in animals is directly related to intramyocardial levels. Therefore, to be effective, it should be given early and in high doses. The American Heart Association's recommendation of 5 mg per kilogram initially and 10 mg per kilogram twice thereafter at 10-minute intervals is reasonable but may be replaced by regimens in which higher doses (either 500 mg or 10 mg per kilogram) are used earlier.

Intravenous amiodarone, currently restricted to investigational use, appears to have remarkable efficacy for refractory ventricular tachyarrhythmias when given as a 1-g intravenous bolus.

Short-acting beta-blockers may also be of value in refractory or recurrent ventricular fibrillation, particularly in cases in which ischemia is believed to have precipitated the arrhythmia.

Ventricular Tachycardia

Ventricular tachycardia is approached on the basis of whether the patient is conscious ("nonhypotensive") or unconscious ("hypotensive"). Hypotensive ventricular tachycardia should be treated as ventricular fibrillation. Nonhypotensive ventricular tachycardia is usually treated with lidocaine, 3 mg per kilogram over 20 to 30 minutes followed by an infusion at a rate of 20 to 40 μg per kilogram per minute. If the loading dose of lidocaine does not suppress the tachycardia, procainamide, 100 mg over 2 to 3 minutes, may be given. Additional 100-mg doses of procainamide may be given every 5 minutes until any one of the following endpoints is reached: hypotension, widening of the QRS complex by 50 percent, or administration of a total dose of 1 g. Once the patient has received a loading dose of procainamide, an infusion is usually started at 20 to 40 μg per kilogram per minute. Lidocaine is usually also continued. If lidocaine and procainamide fail to terminate the arrhythmia, the patient may be treated with either bretylium tosylate or sedation and electrical cardioversion. The disadvantage of bretylium tosylate is that it often aggravates the relative hypotension that typically accompanies most cases of "nonhypotensive" ventricular tachycardia. With the assistance of a skilled anesthesiologist or low doses of the short-acting benzodiazepine midazolam (1 to 2 mg every 3 minutes titrated to effect), cardioversion can almost always be accomplished with a single 100-J synchronized discharge.

If at any time in the medical therapy of "nonhypotensive" ventricular tachycardia the patient loses consciousness, the patient should be defibrillated immediately.

A diagnosis of catheter-induced ventricular tachycardia should be considered in any patient with sustained or recurrent ventricular tachycardia and right heart lines. Temporary transvenous pacemakers are probably the most common cause of this problem, but right atrial and pulmonary artery catheters may also migrate into arrhythmogenic positions in the right ventricle. When in doubt, one should pull back and reposition right heart lines.

Hypokalemia and hypomagnesemia can also cause refractory ventricular tachyarrhythmias. Hypokalemia and hypomagnesemia are not uncommon in patients taking diuretics. Intravenous potassium replacement should be guided by serum potassium determinations; magnesium can be given as an intravenous bolus of 2 g of magnesium sulfate.

Verapamil is not effective in the treatment of nonhypotensive ventricular tachycardia; indeed, it causes cardiac arrest in this circumstance more often than it converts the tachycardia to sinus rhythm. Wide complex, regular tachycardias, even those with QRS durations of 120 to 140 msec or visible P waves (retrograde conduction is not uncommon during ventricular tachycardia) should be treated as ventricular tachycardia until proven to be otherwise.

Electromechanical Dissociation

Electromechanical dissociation is defined as a relatively normal heart rate with little or no contractile activity. Electromechanical dissociation caused by intrinsic myocardial disease is almost always fatal, whereas electromechanical dissociation resulting from hypovolemia, pericardial, thoracic, or metabolic disease may be treatable. Thus the diagnosis of electromechanical dissociation should always stimulate a search for bleeding, pericardial tamponade, tension pneumothorax, severe acidosis, or electrolyte imbalance.

Treatment of electromechanical dissociation is based on correction of the above abnormalities, ventilation and oxygenation, and epinephrine to stimulate contractility. With the exception of patients known to have severe lung congestion immediately before the arrest, patients who have electromechanical dissociation should also be given 1 to 2 L of normal saline over 5 to 10 minutes. This volume infusion can be stopped as soon as hypovolemia is excluded as a cause of the arrest.

Asystole and Pulseless Idioventricular Rhythms

Asystole and pulseless idioventricular rhythms are usually the result of end-stage heart disease, overwhelming multisystem disease, or severe hypoxemia. Epinephrine is the mainstay of therapy, as the doses used clinically provide sufficient chronotropic as well as inotropic stimulation.

Isoproterenol, once recommended for the treatment of asystolic arrest because of its chronotropic potency, is now understood to be contraindicated in any patient requiring chest compression for circulatory support. Through its beta$_2$ effects, isoproterenol lowers aortic pressure during CPR and can actually abolish coronary perfusion.

Temporary external or transvenous pacing may be of value in the treatment of asystolic arrests, particularly when it is initiated early. Pacing is generally of no value in the treatment of pulseless idioventricular rhythms, as a heart that is too weak to generate a pulse at a rate of 15 or 20 beats per minute is likely too weak to generate a pulse at a rate of 60 to 80 beats per minute.

POSTRESUSCITATION CARE

Transient tachycardia and hypertension are common during the first few minutes after successful resuscitation. These hemodynamic abnormalities are the result of high levels of exogenous and endogenous catecholamines. The latter may persist until the acidosis of the arrest is cleared by hyperventilation (restoration of spontaneous circulation washes large quantities of carbon dioxide and lactic acid out of hypoperfused tissues) and conversion of lactate to pyruvate by the liver. Tachycardia and hypertension are therefore an appropriate physiologic response during the first few minutes after resuscitation and should not be treated with beta-blockers or vasodilators.

Antiarrhythmics should be administered after successful defibrillation. The general rule is to give the patient one more antiarrhythmic than he or she was receiving at the time of the arrest. Lidocaine is ordinarily used for this purpose. If other antiarrhythmics are believed to have been instrumental in the conversion of a ventricular tachyarrhythmia, they should be continued too. Antiarrhythmic therapy is usually continued until diagnostic insight into the genesis of the arrhythmia has been obtained.

OPEN CHEST MASSAGE

Available evidence indicates that cardiac output is only 10 to 20 percent of normal during external chest compression. This amount of blood flow is not sufficient to prevent progression of myocardial ischemia. It is therefore appropriate to consider performing open chest massage, a technique that permits the generation of normal or nearly normal vital organ perfusion, in selected patients who fail to respond to conventional resuscitative measures. Such patients should be young and previously healthy. In the absence of extreme hypothermia or known sedative hypnotic overdose, open chest massage should also be reserved for cases in which time from arrest to initiation of CPR is compatible with full neurologic recovery.

PEDIATRIC RESUSCITATION

A full discussion of pediatric resuscitation is beyond the scope of this chapter. Two rules of thumb may be useful. First, the overwhelming majority of pediatric cardiac arrests are caused by hypoxemia-induced bradyarrhythmias. Treatment with ventilation, oxygenation, and epinephrine is usually sufficient in these cases. Second, in cases in which drugs or defibrillation are necessary, appropriate doses or energy levels can be calculated by dividing standard adult levels by 70 and multiplying by the child's weight in kilograms.

SUGGESTED READING

Textbook of advanced cardiac life support. Dallas: American Heart Association, 1987.
Pearson JW, Redding JS. Influence of peripheral vascular tone on cardiac resuscitation. Anesth Analg 1965; 44:746.
Michael JR, Guerci AD, Koehler RC, et al. Mechanisms by which epinephrine augments cerebral and myocardial perfusion during cardiopulmonary resuscitation in dogs. Circulation 1984; 69:822.
Halperin H, Tsitlik JE, Guerci AD, et al. Determinants of blood flow to vital organs during cardiopulmonary resuscitation in dogs. Circulation 1986; 73:539.
Gonzalez ER, Ornato JP, Levine RL. Vasopressor effect of epinephrine with and without dopamine during cardiopulmonary resuscitation. Drug Intell Clin Pharm 1988; 22:868.

ENDOTRACHEAL INTUBATION

WILLIAM D. HOFFMAN, M.D.
CHARLES NATANSON, M.D.

The critical care physician is commonly required to perform endotracheal intubation for patients with diverse illnesses. This lifesaving procedure, although conceptually simple, often causes considerable anxiety among physicians and nurses. Multiple complications are associated with tracheal intubation, including patient discomfort, aspiration of stomach contents, esophageal intubation, systemic hypotension or hypertension, cardiac arrhythmias, myocardial ischemia, hypoxemia, hypercapnia, oropharyngeal trauma, bleeding, loss of a patent airway, and cardiac arrest. Complications and anxiety can be minimized if the physician is familiar with the procedure, monitors the patient appropriately, and is prepared to handle any problems that may occur.

This chapter provides general background information on the anatomy of the airway, the equipment and pharmacologic agents required for intubation, the various techniques available, and the strategies used to intubate critically ill patients. Knowledge of these areas is essential for critical care physicians who perform endotracheal intubation. For inexperienced physicians, we strongly recommend that endotracheal intubation be supervised by experienced laryngoscopists until proficiency is attained. The critical care physician can often arrange to practice the procedure on elective surgical patients while being supervised by an anesthesiologist.

ANATOMY FOR LARYNGOSCOPY

Figures 1 and 2 show the anatomy of the larynx, vallecula, epiglottis, cricoid, and arytenoids.

Larynx

This structure, which is superior and anterior to the trachea, contains the true and false vocal cords. These structures can be seen directly with a laryngoscope. Ideally, during intubation, the physician can see the endotracheal tube passing between the vocal cords.

Vallecula

Situated between the base of the tongue and the epiglottis, this space serves as a landmark for proper placement of the tip of curved laryngoscope blades (Fig. 3). When the curved blade exerts pressure on this structure, the hyoepiglottic ligament stretches, raising the epiglottis out of view.

Epiglottis

This large cartilaginous organ sits between the base of the tongue and the larynx. It serves as a landmark for proper placement of the tip of straight laryngoscope blades (Fig. 4).

Cricoid

This circle of cartilage sits above the first tracheal ring and below the arytenoids. When compressed posteriorly toward the vertebral bodies (Fig. 5), the cricoid can occlude the esophagus (minimizing gastric content reflux into the airway). During laryngoscopy, this maneuver frequently helps bring the larynx into view.

Arytenoids

These tissues are the posterior cartilaginous attachments of the true vocal cords. In some patients, the arytenoids may be the only structures seen during laryngoscopy and may therefore guide placement of the endotracheal tube (anterior to the arytenoids).

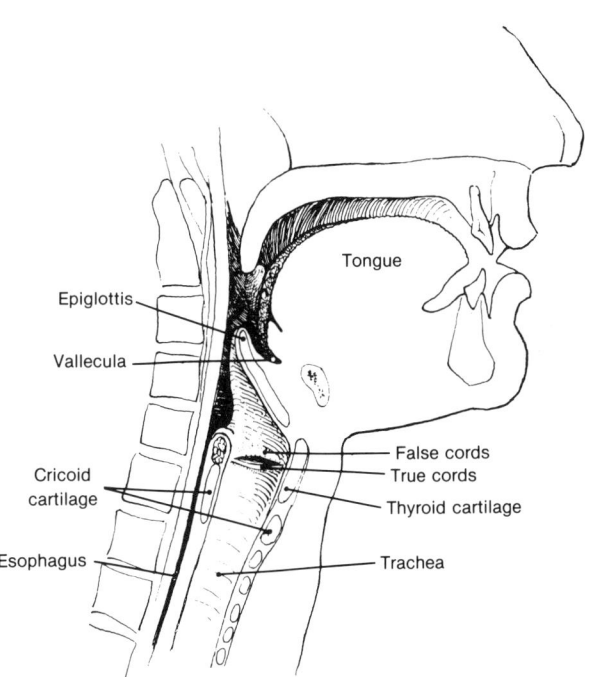

Figure 1 This sagittal view of the head shows the anatomy of the upper airway. Note the anatomic relationship between the epiglottis, vallecula, cricoid cartilage, and vocal cords. (Republished with permission from Natanson C, Shelhamer J, Parrillo J. JAMA 1985; 253:1160–1165.)

INTUBATION EQUIPMENT

Clinicians should be familiar with the proper function of laryngoscopes and endotracheal tubes. Different types of laryngoscope blades have comparative advantages

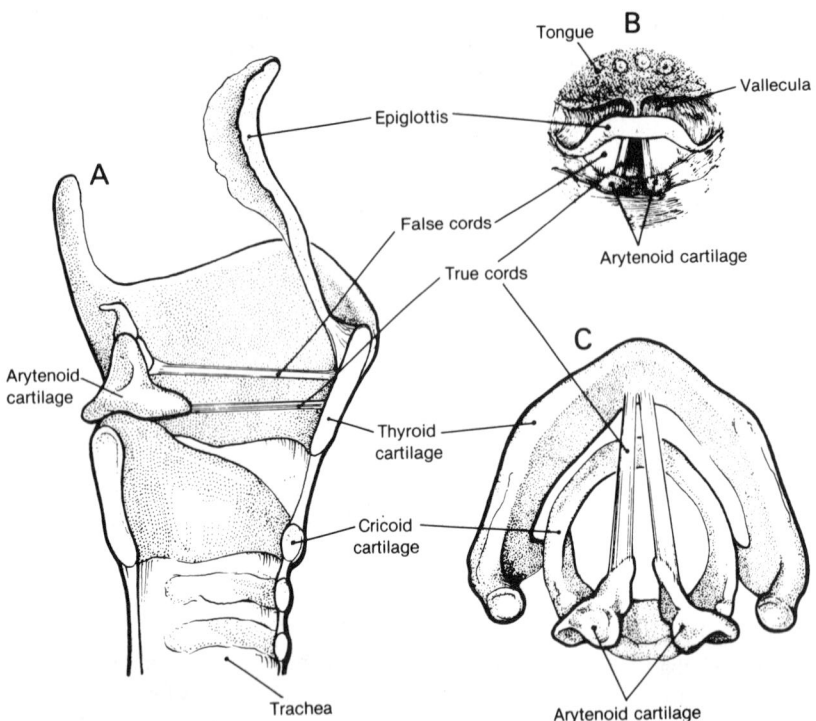

Figure 2 *A*, Sagittal view of the upper airway. *B*, View of the larynx during laryngoscopy. *C*, Laryngoscopist's view of the larynx, with soft tissues removed. (Republished with permission from Natanson C, Shelhamer J, Parrillo J. JAMA 1985; 253:1160–1165.)

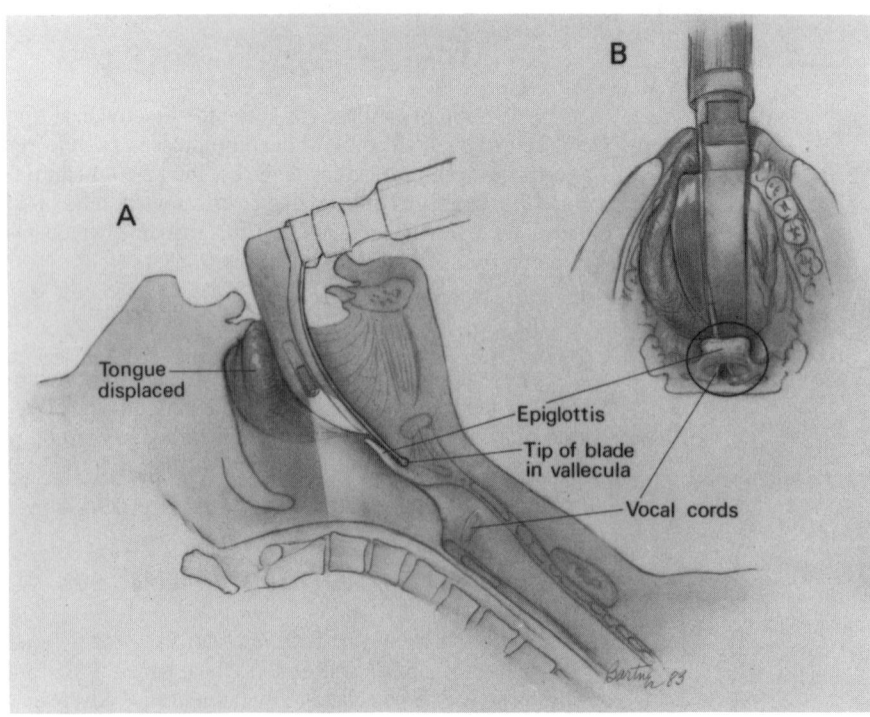

Figure 3 Sagittal view (A) and laryngoscopist's view (B) of the upper airway during proper placement of the curved laryngoscope blade (MacIntosh). The tongue is pushed aside by the lateral surface of the blade, and the tip of the blade is placed into the vallecula, giving a view of the vocal cords. (Republished with permission from Natanson C, Shelhamer J, Parrillo J. JAMA 1985; 253:1160–1165.)

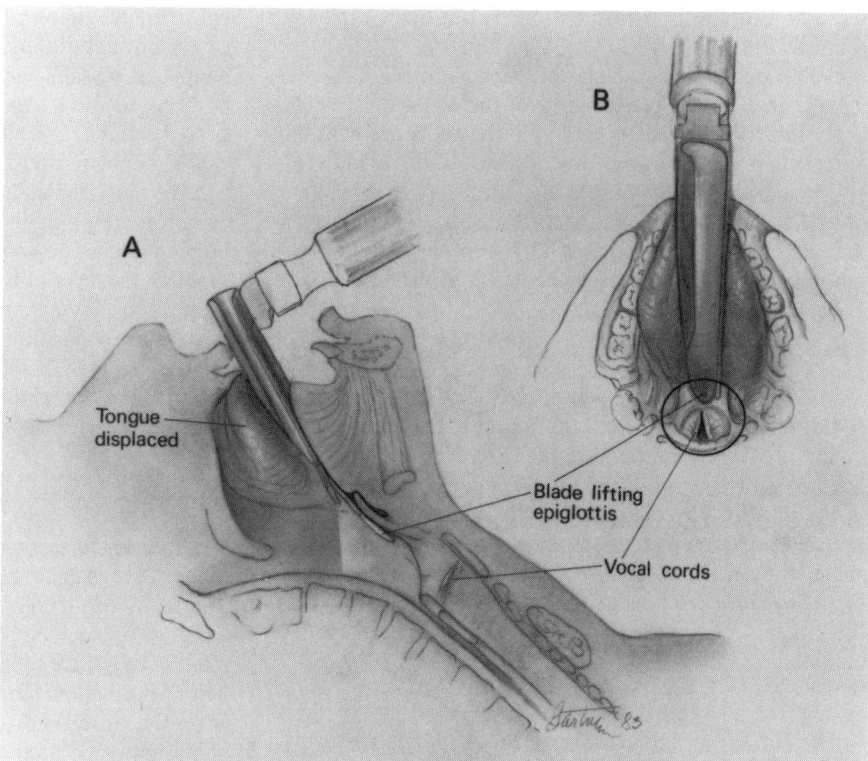

Figure 4 Sagittal view (A) and laryngoscopist's view (B) of the upper airway during proper placement of the straight laryngoscope blade. The tongue is pushed aside by the lateral surface of the blade, and the tip of the blade lifts the epiglottis, giving a view of the vocal cords. (Republished with permission from Natanson C, Shelhamer J, Parrillo J. JAMA 1985; 253:1160–1165.)

and disadvantages that can improve or diminish one's view of the airway. Many types and sizes of endotracheal tubes are also available.

Laryngoscope Handle

The laryngoscope handle generally contains the power source for the light of the laryngoscope blade. The blades connect to the handles via a hinge, which has an electrical contact for blade illumination.

Laryngoscope Blades

The blade is the part of the laryngoscope which, when inserted into the mouth, positions oral and pharyngeal structures so that the clinician has a direct view of the larynx. There are two types of laryngoscope blades: curved (see Fig. 3) and straight (see Fig. 4). Selecting the proper blade size is essential for optimal laryngoscopy. Blades are available in several sizes and are numbered (higher numbers represent larger blades). For children, consult a pediatric text for suggested blade sizes by age.

Curved Blades

The most commonly used curved blade is the MacIntosh blade, which novices frequently find easier to use. This blade has a large surface area, allowing easy manipulation of the tongue and creating more space in the oral cavity to enable the endotracheal tube to pass through the oropharynx into the trachea. For the average-sized adult,

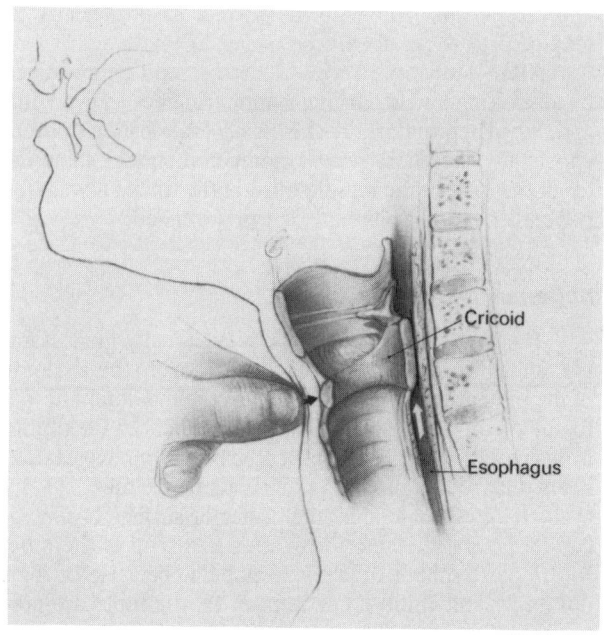

Figure 5 The Sellick maneuver. Pressure is applied directly against the anterior rim of the cricoid causing compression of the esophagus and preventing passive regurgitation. (Republished with permission from Natanson C, Shelhamer J, Parrillo J. JAMA 1985; 253:1160–1165.)

the Size 3 blade is used most often, but Size 4 may be required for adults with very long tongues.

The major disadvantage of the curved blade is that it may give only a partial view of the vocal cords. The tip of the curved blade is placed in the vallecula with the epiglottis posterior to the lower surface of the blade. The epiglottis may partially block the clinician's view so that only the arytenoids are seen (see Fig. 3B), and thus even though the vocal cords are not fully seen, the endotracheal tube is passed above the arytenoids into the trachea.

Straight Blades

Several straight blades (e.g., Miller, Flagg, and Wis-Forreger) are available, with only minor differences among them. If Miller blades are used, Size 2 or 3 is required for the average-sized adult. The advantage of these blades is that they lift the epiglottis directly out of sight (see Fig. 4B) and provide an excellent view of the vocal cords. Because of their narrower surface area, however, the use of straight blades requires greater technical skill to position the tongue out of view compared with the use of curved blades.

Endotracheal Tubes

Endotracheal tubes are inserted through the larynx into the trachea and are used to conduct gases to and from the trachea. Some clinically important features of these tubes are their diameter, length, material content, shape, and cuff.

Diameter

The appropriateness of an endotracheal tube is determined by the internal diameter of the tube. Internal diameters range from 2.5 to 10 mm by 0.5-mm increments. Some manufacturers also specify the external diameter using the French scale (external diameter in millimeters × 3.14). Tubes with the same internal diameter may have different external diameters, as the thickness of the tubing may vary. The external diameter is especially important for the child whose larynx and trachea cannot accommodate large tubes. Manufacturers generally specify the external diameter of tubes that have an internal diameter of 6 mm or less.

The internal diameter determines the resistance associated with the tube (smaller diameters produce greater resistance). This resistance may be important in some spontaneously breathing patients (especially those with high peak inspiratory flows), but this resistance is not as important in patients receiving mechanical ventilation (in which case the ventilator provides the additional work of breathing).

It is not always possible to determine the proper tube size before intubation. The average adult trachea easily accommodates an internal diameter of 7 to 8 mm (men, 8 to 9 mm; women, 7 to 8 mm). During difficult intubations, one may reattempt intubation with a smaller internal diameter tube (6 to 7 mm), which often passes more easily through the mouth and vocal cords. When reintubation can be safely accomplished, this smaller tube should be changed for a larger one if airway resistance or secretions becomes an important problem.

Except in unusual circumstances, small children receive uncuffed endotracheal tubes until they are 6 to 8 years of age or until they require a 5.5 to 6.0 mm tube. Formulae used to estimate tube size for children can be found in most pediatric texts. When one is intubating children, tubes having smaller and larger diameters than the initial tube used should be readily available. In children, the trachea is usually best fit with the tube that produces a gas leak (external to the tube) when 15 to 30 cm of water positive pressure is applied.

Length

Manufacturers produce endotracheal tubes that are longer than is anatomically necessary for most adults. To avoid endobronchial intubation (with too long a segment of tube) or accidental extubation (with too short a segment of tube), the tube length required should be estimated before intubation. Oral endotracheal tubes are measured from the distal end (cuff end) to the end extending out of the patient's mouth or nose. Generally, the length of the endotracheal tube at the front incisor teeth should approximate the distance from 3 to 4 cm above the bifurcation of the trachea. This length can be estimated from examination of the patient's chest and neck, since the angle of Louis is approximately at the level of the tracheal bifurcation. For average-sized adults, this distance is usually 18 to 24 cm. To obtain the correct nasotracheal tube length, 3 to 4 cm should be added to this length.

After intubation, proper length should be evaluated by ausculting and observing symmetric chest movement, and, when appropriate, by chest x-ray examination or bronchoscopy. The chest x-ray examination should show the tip of the tube in the middle third of the trachea when the patient's head is neither flexed or extended.

Materials and Shape

The ideal endotracheal tube is chemically inert, durable, and resistant to collapse; it conforms to the anatomy of the patient when in place and has the maximal internal diameter for a given external circumference. Flexibility is desirable in the endotracheal tube because mucosal trauma arises from compression of tissue by the tube, usually at the base of the tongue, the posterior surface of the vocal cords, and the anterior trachea at the tip of the tube. In the past, rubber tubes were popular because of their durability and ability to be reused. Plastic tubes are now preferred because they are less likely to produce laryngeal and tracheal trauma. Plastic endotracheal tubes can be kept in patients for 3 weeks or more. Preshaped plastic tubes (e.g., Lindholm and RAE tubes) are available that theoretically minimize pressure against the posterior wall of the larynx and the anterior wall of the trachea.

Cuffs

For adults and for children in whom it is specifically indicated, the cuff on an endotracheal tube inflates to create a seal with the trachea, thus producing a closed system for positive pressure ventilation. This seal also reduces but does not eliminate the risk of aspiration of oropharyngeal or gastric materials. In the past, low-volume, high-pressure cuffs were used on endotracheal tubes, but were found to cause extensive ischemic damage to the tracheal wall. Consequently, high-volume, low-pressure cuffs were developed to maintain an intraluminal pressure less than the capillary hydrostatic pressure (20 mm Hg) and thus limit ischemic damage to the trachea. When cuffs are inflated, they form a seal with a minimum force per unit area of tracheal mucosa. Cuff pressures should be monitored regularly and kept below 20 to 30 mm Hg. Foam cuffs have also been developed to provide a seal at low pressure.

PHARMACOLOGIC AGENTS

Because laryngoscopy and intubation are noxious stimuli, patients who are conscious require medication for these procedures. Sedative-hypnotics (which decrease the level of consciousness), analgesics (which decrease pain), muscle relaxants (which prevent movement), and anesthetics (which produce a combination of these effects) are commonly needed to make intubation tolerable for patients, to maximize patient cooperation, and to provide optimal intubating conditions. In many cases, these drugs are given in combination. When giving these medications, physicians should continually observe patients, as they can easily have complications (see below).

Narcotic Analgesics

Narcotics decrease the patient's perception of pain. In addition, these drugs are cough suppressants and decrease the discomfort caused by the patient's awareness of dyspnea. Narcotics create a sense of tranquility and euphoria, but do not reliably produce sleep.

In intensive care units, morphine and fentanyl are commonly used narcotics. The initial dose of morphine is 0.01 to 0.1 mg per kilogram administered as an intravenous bolus, which has effects lasting several hours. If an adequate effect is not obtained, subsequent doses of 0.01 to 0.1 mg per kilogram administered intravenously can be given after 3 to 5 minutes. The most common adverse side effects of morphine are profound respiratory depression and hypotension, which is partly produced by histamine release. Fentanyl, a synthetic narcotic, is extremely lipid-soluble and has a more rapid onset and a shorter duration of action than morphine. Unlike morphine, fentanyl does not cause significant histamine release and therefore produces fewer cardiovascular effects. Fentanyl, which is ten times more potent than morphine, is usually given in doses of 25 to 50 µg as an intravenous bolus. If adequate analgesia is not obtained, the same dose can be repeated after 1 to 2 minutes. Its short duration of action, faster onset, extremely potent analgesic properties, and decreased propensity to cause hypotension make fentanyl preferable for short procedures in critically ill patients.

A specific narcotic antagonist, naloxone, can be given to reverse unmanageable complications (e.g., complete airway obstruction in patients who cannot be intubated) that are attributed to narcotics. Because of the side effects of this drug, however (e.g., severe hypertension, pulmonary edema, reversal of analgesia), we do not recommend its routine use.

Sedative Hypnotics

Sedative hypnotics, such as thiopental sodium, diazepam, and midazolam, are central nervous system depressants that decrease the patient's level of consciousness and may cause amnesia. Hypnotics help reduce anxiety during procedures and potentiate some effects of narcotics, although they should not be given in place of analgesics. Unlike narcotics, hypnotics presently have no specific antagonist for clinical use.

Thiopental sodium is a short-acting barbiturate with effects that range from mild sedation to coma. Because this agent is not an analgesic, patients under its effects may respond to painful stimuli (e.g., movement, increased autonomic tone), even though they may not remember the pain after the procedure. The average intubating dose is 3 to 4 mg per kilogram administered as an intravenous bolus, but this dose must be markedly decreased for patients with limited cardiovascular reserve or reduced intravascular volume. Thiopental sodium has a rapid onset of action (30 to 50 seconds) from a single bolus injection of the drug. The duration of action is also short, with the effects abating within 10 to 15 minutes. The rapid onset and short duration of its effects make this agent useful for short procedures such as intubation. Furthermore, when patients with increased intracranial pressures and a stable cardiovascular system are given thiopental sodium, they do not have as great an increase in intracranial pressure associated with intubation.

Thiopental sodium should be used with caution in the critically ill patient, as it can markedly decrease blood pressure. For critically ill patients, small incremental doses (25 to 50 mg IV) may be given slowly (every 1 to 2 minutes) until the desired level of sedation is achieved. This agent may also cause respiratory depression and, if the drug extravasates from the intravenous line, extensive tissue necrosis.

Diazepam is a long-acting benzodiazepine sedative (with long-acting active metabolites) that can potentiate narcotic effects and cause amnesia. Diazepam has mild alpha-adrenergic blocking effects and thus may cause hypotension. It also contributes to respiratory depression, especially when given with narcotics. The diluent for diazepam (propylene glycol and ethanol) is irritating to veins and causes pain on injection. To sedate critically ill patients, diazepam is given in 0.5- to 1.0-mg intravenous boluses every 2 to 5 minutes (lower doses are given to elderly or severely compromised patients) until the desired effect is achieved.

Midazolam is a shorter-acting benzodiazepine than diazepam. Unlike diazepam, midazolam is not dissolved in propylene glycol and does not produce pain on injection. Like diazepam, midazolam may produce respiratory depression and hypotension. It is given in 0.25- to 1.0-mg intravenous boluses every 2 to 5 minutes (lower doses are given to elderly or severely compromised patients) until the desired effect is achieved.

Anesthetics

By blocking sensations, general and local anesthetics prevent movement in response to surgical stimuli. These drugs reversibly promote hypnosis (general anesthetics only), analgesia, muscle relaxation, and control of visceral reflex responses. In the critical care setting, the general anesthetic ketamine and the local anesthetics cocaine and lidocaine are particularly useful.

Ketamine is related to the hallucinogens (phencyclidine) and provides profound analgesia even in small doses. The intubating dose is 1 to 2 mg per kilogram IV (or 4 to 10 mg per kilogram IM). As with thiopental sodium, the onset of action is rapid (30 to 40 seconds) and the duration of action is short (10 to 15 minutes). Ketamine increases sympathetic tone, which tends to preserve blood pressure, making this drug particularly useful for hypovolemic, hypotensive patients. The sympathomimetic effects of ketamine typically predominate over its mild direct myocardial depressive effects. However, the hypertensive effects of ketamine make it relatively contraindicated in patients with hypertension, cerebral vascular disease, or disorders associated with increased intracranial pressure. Another disadvantage of ketamine is its dissociative effect, which has been reported to cause distressing hallucinations in some patients as they emerge from anesthesia. This side effect of ketamine may be especially undesirable for patients with a psychiatric history. Ketamine's rapid onset, short duration of action, profound analgesic properties, and preservation of blood pressure make it useful for critically ill patients undergoing short procedures such as tracheal intubation.

Cocaine is a local anesthetic that is useful for nasal intubations, as it provides topical anesthesia and promotes vasoconstriction and shrinkage of the nasal mucosa. Cocaine used for nasal intubations produces more patient comfort, allows the tube to pass through the nasal airway more easily, and reduces bleeding. In adults, the total topical dose should be less than 200 mg, as larger doses may be associated with seizures.

Lidocaine can be used either topically or subcutaneously. To obtain topical anesthesia in the oropharynx, a 4 to 10 percent concentration of lidocaine can be applied. In therapeutic doses, lidocaine may cause mild myocardial depression, but has few respiratory effects. The major toxicity of lidocaine is related to its systemic absorption, which may cause seizures. Seizures can occur in an average-sized adult when topical doses of more than 500 mg are used. Sedatives, such as diazepam or thiopental sodium, may markedly raise the seizure threshold (reducing the likelihood of seizures) of patients given local anesthetics.

Muscle Relaxants

Muscle relaxants reversibly paralyze skeletal musculature and prevent movement, thus facilitating laryngoscopy and intubation. The use of muscle relaxants to paralyze ventilatory effort can be extremely dangerous if the clinician lacks extensive experience and skill in intubation techniques, positive pressure mask ventilation, and overcoming airway obstruction. These drugs should be used with extreme caution in patients with a partially obstructed airway. We recommend that muscle relaxants be administered by only those physicians who have substantial experience in mask ventilation and intubation of the trachea in critically ill patients.

Succinylcholine Chloride

Succinylcholine chloride is a depolarizing neuromuscular relaxant that acts as an agonist on acetylcholine receptors at the neuromuscular junction and other tissues. Because this drug is not metabolized as rapidly as acetylcholine, end-plate depolarization lingers, causing inexcitability of the muscle membrane. Because succinylcholine chloride has a rapid onset and short duration of action (Table 1), it is an ideal drug for short procedures in the intensive care unit.

This agent also has numerous side effects that limit its general use in intensive care units. First, some patients receiving succinylcholine chloride may develop *dangerous hyperkalemia*. The drug normally increases the potassium level by 0.5 to 1.0 mEq per liter. Greater increases may occur in patients with burns, upper and lower neuron disease, trauma, muscle diseases, or closed head injury, and in those who have had prolonged bedrest. Patients are susceptible to these increases in potassium for as long as 9 months after sustaining the injury. Second, succinylcholine chloride produces *muscle fasciculations*, which occur before inexcitability, and *muscle pains*, which may be prevented with a small dose (a defasciculating dose) of a nondepolarizing relaxant (e.g., 3 mg of curare or 1 mg of pancuronium) given 3 minutes before succinylcholine administration. In some patients, however, this small dose of curare may cause significant weakness and respiratory compromise. Patients should therefore be observed continuously after being given a defasciculating dose of a nondepolarizing relaxant. Third, because of its lack of specificity for the neuromuscular junction, succinylcholine chloride may produce *ganglionic stimulation*. This effect occurs particularly after a second dose and is commonly manifested as tachycardia and hypertension in adults, and bradycardia in children and adults. Pretreatment with atropine may prevent this bradycardic response. Fourth, because succinylcholine chloride produces *increased intraocular pressure* from contraction of the extraocular muscles, this drug is generally not given to

Table 1 Clinical Characteristics of Neuromuscular-Blocking Drugs for Intubation

Drug	Intubating Dose (mg/kg)	Onset (min)	Termination of Effect	Recovery Time	Side Effects
Succinylcholine chloride	1.0–1.5	1.0–1.5	Rapid metabolism with recovery in 8–10 min	Recovery may be prolonged in patients with abnormal pseudocholinesterase	Hyperkalemia, bradycardia (particularly after the second dose), tachycardia, hypertension, increased intraocular pressure, triggers malignant hyperthermia
Pancuronium	0.1–0.15	2.0–5.0	70%–80% renal, 15%–20% biliary excretion and hepatic metabolism	Recover in 80–100 min	Tachycardia
Vecuronium	0.1–0.2	2.0–3.0	10%–20% renal, 80% biliary excretion and hepatic metabolism	Recovery in 25–30 min; recovery time is only moderately increased in renal failure	
Atracurium besylate	0.4–0.6	2.0–3.0	Ester hydrolysis; elimination is independent of renal function	Recovery in 25–30 min; recovery time is not increased in renal failure	Releases histamine and causes hypotension with large rapid bolus doses

patients with open injuries of the eye. Finally, in susceptible patients, this agent triggers *malignant hyperthermia* and should therefore be avoided in patients with a family history of this condition.

Nondepolarizing Relaxants: Pancuronium, Atracurium, and Vecuronium

These drugs, which are longer acting and have a slower onset than succinylcholine chloride (see Table 1) may be used when succinylcholine chloride is contraindicated. They are competitive for acetylcholine receptor sites at the neuromuscular junction and thereby decrease acetylcholine binding. The relaxant effect of these drugs spontaneously reverses as the drug diffuses away from the site of action and is excreted. However, this reversal may be accelerated by agents that inhibit acetylcholinesterase (an enzyme that metabolizes acetylcholine), thereby increasing the competition of acetylcholine with the relaxant for these binding sites.

PREPARATION FOR INTUBATION

Proper preparation of the patient and equipment minimizes complications during intubation. It is also important to review the intubation plan with all assistants (e.g., nurses and respiratory therapists).

Patient Evaluation

Each critically ill patient must be assessed so that the method of intubation that is most appropriate and least dangerous to the patient can be selected. During this evaluation, the following questions should be addressed: (1) "How much time is available for intubation?" (2) "Does the patient have a full stomach?" (3) "To what extent will intubation and positive pressure ventilation compromise cardiovascular status?" (4) "Will the patient be difficult to intubate?" and (5) "Are there special problems related to the patient's disease?"

"How Much Time is Available for Intubation?"

If the patient is responsive and in a stable cardiovascular state, a complete evaluation can be performed. If the patient's condition permits sufficient time, the clinician can fully prepare the patient, consider various techniques of intubation, and obtain informed consent. With cardiopulmonary arrest or indications of inadequate cerebral perfusion, however, the clinician may only have time for minimal preparation. In these cases, mask ventilation and the unconscious oral technique of intubation should be carried out as quickly as possible (this is discussed in greater detail later in this chapter).

"Does the Patient Have a Full Stomach?"

Patients with a full stomach are at risk for aspiration during intubation, and this condition can profoundly compromise airway management as well as ventilatory status. Adult elective surgical patients are considered to have an empty stomach after a 6- to 8-hour fast. However, patients with certain conditions such as obesity, pain, bowel obstruction or ileus, pregnancy, and diabetes are more likely to have high gastric volumes even after a prolonged fast. For patients with a full stomach, there are specific techniques for intubation (e.g., the rapid sequence, blind nasal, or awake oral approach) that minimize the risk of aspiration.

"To What Extent Will Intubation and Positive Pressure Ventilation Compromise Cardiovascular Status?"

Laryngoscopy, intubation, and positive pressure ventilation may produce several cardiovascular effects, such as (1) increased sympathetic tone in response to laryngoscopy; (2) vasovagal responses (hypotension and bradycardia) caused by tenth cranial nerve stimulation; (3) decreased sympathetic tone in response to medications; (4) increased or decreased arterial carbon dioxide partial pressure, possibly affecting vascular tone and blood pressure, caused by changes in minute ventilation; and (5) decreased venous return, causing decreased cardiac output from positive pressure ventilation. Topical local anesthetics given before nasal or oral intubation may blunt some of these cardiovascular responses and may reduce the need for hypotension-producing sedatives or narcotics.

"Will the Patient be Difficult to Intubate?"

To anticipate problems with laryngoscopy or intubation, one should examine the patient's airway. A history of difficult intubation (e.g., from a previous surgery) increases the likelihood of another difficult intubation. Particular congenital anomalies, such as hypoplasia or hyperplasia of the mandible, prominent maxillary incisors, maxillary hyperplasia, inadequate oral aperture (<4 cm), a short neck, and a relatively large tongue are associated with difficult intubation. If the distance between the thyroid cartilage and the chin is less than three fingerbreadths (with the head in the neutral position), then the patient may have insufficient space for the tongue during laryngoscopy, and intubation will probably be difficult. Patients should also have adequate mobility of the neck and cervical spine for proper head positioning, since inadequate mobility is associated with rheumatoid arthritis, ankylosing spondylitis, osteoarthritis, and cervical spine fractures. If the history and physical examination suggest a potentially difficult intubation, additional equipment (e.g., smaller endotracheal tubes, bronchoscope) and assistants (e.g., clinician skilled in cricothyroidotomy or tracheotomy) should be readily available.

"Are There Special Problems Related to the Patient's Disease?"

A patient's underlying illness may greatly affect the ease of intubation, the response to medications, and associated complications. Patients with coagulopathies (thrombocytopenia or factor deficiencies) are at risk for significant nasopharyngeal bleeding during nasal intubation. A patient with hyperkalemia or neuromuscular disease may be at greater risk for dangerous succinylcholine chloride–induced hyperkalemia. An inebriated or uncooperative patient is a poor candidate for blind nasal intubation. A patient with atherosclerotic coronary artery disease may be at high risk for myocardial ischemia during intubation if given inadequate anesthesia. Each patient's history must therefore be carefully reviewed along with the risks and complications of the drugs and techniques used.

Equipment Preparation

The following steps should be taken to prepare for the intubation:

1. An oxygen source with a mask and bag for manual ventilation should be made available.
2. An adjustable bed should be used so that the patient can be placed in the Trendelenburg position to minimize aspiration and treat hypotension.
3. The patient should receive a securely positioned intravenous line 18-gauge or larger for a normal saline or lactated Ringer's infusion given via a macro-drip. This line should be separate from lines used to administer medications. The administration rates of any vasoactive drugs or other medications should not be altered by this infusion. In addition, if the patient becomes hypotensive, this intravenous line can be used for rapid fluid administration.
4. We believe that, ideally, monitoring for intubation should consist of electrocardiography (for monitoring of continuous cardiac rhythm), a blood pressure cuff (for monitoring of blood pressure), and a pulse oximeter (for monitoring of continuous arterial oxygen saturations). In critically ill patients, an intra-arterial catheter, which provides precise continuous arterial blood pressure data, should be used, because intubation can result in cardiovascular instability that requires immediate intervention. Although not essential for all intubation procedures, an end-tidal carbon dioxide monitor may be important, as it can confirm correct endotracheal tube placement by measuring the carbon dioxide concentration in expired gas. If these monitors detect carbon dioxide in expired gas, then esophageal intubation is unlikely, as carbon dioxide is not normally a constituent of upper gastrointestinal gas or inspired air.
5. Suction equipment with a large-bore catheter should be available, as suction may be necessary to clear airway secretions. Without effective suction, secretions may obstruct the laryngoscopist's view, and oral or gastric contents may spill into the trachea.
6. A complete set of intubation equipment should be readily available. Appropriate equipment includes several sizes of endotracheal tubes (smaller than predicted), stylets, lubricant, bite blocks, oral and nasopharyngeal airways, a laryngoscope with operational light source, and a selection of blade sizes (straight and curved). All equipment should be checked in advance to make certain that they function properly, and the cuff of the en-

dotracheal tube should be tested for leaks and the volume required. These items should be available at the bedside before the intubation begins.
7. All potentially necessary drugs should be drawn up into a syringe and clearly labeled. Anesthetics, muscle relaxants, and drugs for emergency use should be immediately accessible for injection. If the patient is likely to require treatment of hypertension or hypotension, vasoactive drugs and fluids should also be available at the bedside.
8. Medical personnel who can perform CPR should be available. Cardioversion equipment, pacemakers, and venous access kits should also be readily available.
9. Ideally, two medical assistants should be available to help the laryngoscopist. One person can observe monitors and operate the controls that raise and lower the bed. The second assistant should stand beside the laryngoscopist to assist in manipulating the airway, perform the Sellick maneuver (see Fig. 5), provide needed equipment, and assist in suctioning. With two assistants, the laryngoscopist is able to concentrate on maintaining the airway and intubating the patient.

TECHNIQUE OF LARYNGOSCOPY

Direct laryngoscopy involves positioning the patient's head, inserting the laryngoscope, and positioning the tip of the epiglottis anteriorly.

Positioning the Head

To achieve the best possible view of the vocal cords, one should make the route from mouth to larynx a straight line (Fig. 6). This view is produced by flexion of the head at the neck and extension of the head at the atlanto-occipital joint, known as the "sniffing position." For adults, this position can be achieved by elevating the head on a small pillow. In young children, who have a relatively large occiput, a pillow placed under the shoulders can properly position the head.

Inserting the Laryngoscope

Right-handed and most left-handed operators hold the handle of the laryngoscope in the left hand. For unconscious patients, the right hand is used both to open the patient's mouth and to spread the lips. The blade is inserted between upper and lower teeth at the right side of the mouth. The blade is then advanced to the midline, along the right side of the tongue, until the epiglottis is seen.

Positioning the Epiglottis Anteriorly

The tip of the epiglottis hangs posteriorly in a supine patient, so that the view of the larynx is obstructed. The tip of the blade is used to move the epiglottis anteriorly. The curved blade's tip is placed in the vallecula with the epiglottis positioned posterior to the blade's lower surface (see Fig. 3). In most patients, this maneuver indirectly springs the epiglottis anteriorly by placing traction on the hyoepiglottic ligament. The straight blade's tip directly lifts the epiglottis out of sight and gives the laryngoscopist an excellent view of the vocal cords (see Fig. 4). By lifting the handle directly upward and forward (along its axis), taking care not to damage the teeth, the operator pushes the tongue toward the base of the mandible and obtains the best view of the larynx. If these maneuvers do not produce a good view of the vocal cords, an assistant can push downward on the larynx (cricoid pressure), which may bring the larynx into sight.

INTUBATION TECHNIQUES

There are many accepted techniques for intubation. Endotracheal tubes may be placed orally or nasally. The patient may be fully awake or receive some combination of analgesics, sedatives, and anesthetics (local or general). The patient may be spontaneously breathing or paralyzed. Five intubation techniques that may be useful in the intensive care unit are the blind nasal, the rapid (crash) sequence, the awake oral, the fiberoptic, and the unconscious oral approaches.

Blind Nasal Intubation

This technique is called "blind" nasal intubation because it is done without laryngoscopy. It is used for patients who are awake and breathing spontaneously. If the procedure cannot be accomplished quickly, an oral intubation (with laryngoscopy) may be performed instead.

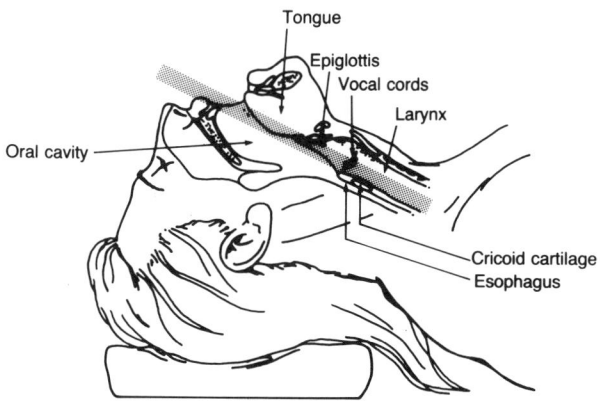

Figure 6 "Sniffing" position. In adults, the best alignment of the oral cavity, oral pharynx, and larynx usually occurs when the patient's head is raised (2 to 4 inches) on a small pillow and the atlanto-occipital joint is extended. In this figure, the epiglottis and tongue are shown as though they are positioned by the laryngoscope, out of sight of the larynx.

Procedure

Before intubation, the nasopharynx is topically anesthetized. Cocaine can be placed in the nasopharynx by soaking cotton swabs with a 1 to 10 percent solution. The cocaine-soaked cotton swabs are slowly advanced from the nares past the nasal turbinates to the posterior pharynx. The lubricated nasal endotracheal tube is then passed through the nose into the posterior pharynx. The tube is further advanced with each inspiration to and through the vocal cords. The clinician monitors progress through the airway by listening for air movement within the tube and watching water condense on the tube during expiration as the tube moves down the airway.

Advantages

Blind nasal intubation is useful because it allows the patient to continue breathing spontaneously and may be performed with the patient in any one of many positions. For example, the flexibility of this procedure is beneficial in patients with pulmonary edema who may need to sit upright during intubation. With good topical anesthesia, few drugs are necessary with this technique, thus the cardiopulmonary side effects of anesthetics, narcotics, and sedatives (hypotension, respiratory depression) are avoided and the patient's mental status is not altered. This procedure allows patients to remain alert and protect their airway. In patients with a full stomach, the risk of aspirating gastric contents is also decreased.

Disadvantages

This procedure may take longer than other techniques, and this is a disadvantage in patients requiring immediate intubation. The major risk of the blind nasal intubation is trauma to nasal mucosa and the oropharynx (especially in patients with coagulopathy). Extensive bleeding can cause further respiratory compromise and make direct visualization of the airway structures difficult. Sinusitis is a frequent complication of prolonged nasotracheal intubation. In addition, this procedure usually requires tubes with a smaller diameter than could be used for an oral intubation.

Rapid Sequence Induction

The rapid sequence approach or "crash intubation" is used to decrease the risk of tracheal aspiration of gastric contents. Thorough preparation for this procedure is extremely important. It must be cautioned that administering analgesics, sedatives, and anesthetics to a patient with a full stomach greatly increases the risk of aspiration. These drugs decrease the patient's level of consciousness and may blunt airway reflexes at a time when airway manipulation may cause regurgitation. In addition, these drugs themselves may induce vomiting.

Procedure

If time allows, the patient should be preoxygenated with 100 percent oxygen by mask for 5 to 6 minutes. Drugs are then given intravenously in rapid sequence. A muscle relaxant is required (succinylcholine chloride). An analgesic (morphine or fentanyl), sedative (valium or thiopental sodium), or anesthetic (ketamine) may also be given as dictated by the patient's condition (e.g., level of awareness, cardiovascular stability). Administering the muscle relaxant simultaneously with other drugs minimizes the time during which the patient is at risk for active regurgitation and aspiration before full paralysis takes place. After the drugs are administered, the bedside assistant should apply the Sellick maneuver (see Fig. 5) to prevent aspiration secondary to passive regurgitation. During this procedure, mask ventilation should be avoided because it may cause gastric distention and precipitate regurgitation. After the muscle relaxant takes effect, laryngoscopy and intubation (with a stylet in place in the endotracheal tube) are performed. The endotracheal tube cuff is inflated, the stylet removed, ventilation begun, and the Sellick maneuver released.

Advantages

The major advantages of rapid sequence intubation are (1) that the time during which the patient is at risk for aspiration of gastric contents is minimized; (2) that the procedure can be performed rapidly; and (3) that because the vocal cords can be seen directly, trauma to the airway is minimized.

Disadvantages

Some of the disadvantages of this technique include the possibility of cardiopulmonary compromise caused by the drugs or by unfavorable patient positioning (i.e., placing a patient in pulmonary edema supine and increasing venous return) and by the inherent risks of paralyzing any patient, especially a critically ill patient with limited cardiac and respiratory reserve. The procedure should be performed only by those physicians who can ventilate the patient by mask if initial intubation is unsuccessful.

Awake Oral Intubation

Procedure

Awake oral intubation in an alert patient requires some combination of topical anesthetics (cocaine, lidocaine), mild sedation (valium, thiopental sodium), an analgesic (morphine, fentanyl), and in selected cases, a nerve block (superior laryngeal). It takes considerable time and care to obtain adequate anesthesia of the oropharynx, and optimal cooperation from the patient is necessary. After drug administration, laryngoscopy, tube placement, and verification of the position are done. Often additional analgesics or sedatives are required after intubation.

Advantages

If there is any doubt about the ease with which intubation can be performed (especially when the patient has a full stomach) or with which a patent airway can be maintained, this procedure should be used since it allows the patient to remain awake and breath spontaneously. This technique is also useful for the laryngoscopist who is inexperienced with the use of potent anesthetics and muscle relaxants.

Disadvantages

The laryngoscope blade in the posterior pharynx is a strong stimulus. Without adequate topical anesthesia, the blade may precipitate gagging and vomiting, severe pain and hypertension, or myocardial ischemia. Care should be taken when using this procedure in patients with a full stomach because the overuse of sedatives and narcotics may blunt airway reflexes, depress mental status, and make the patient unable to protect the airway and avoid aspiration of stomach contents.

Unconscious Oral Intubation

Unconscious oral intubation is performed during cardiac or respiratory arrest. No drugs are required, and laryngoscopy with cricoid pressure, intubation, and ventilation should be undertaken as quickly as possible. The option of mask ventilation with cricoid pressure before intubation should be considered; however, the patient may vomit and aspirate during cardiopulmonary resuscitation.

Fiberoptic Laryngoscopy

Procedure

After the fiberoptic laryngoscope is used to locate the larynx and enters the trachea, a tracheal tube can be passed over the scope into the trachea. To replace an endotracheal tube, the clinician first places a new one over the scope. The tip of the scope is then positioned next to the endotracheal tube already in place in the trachea. The old tube is removed, and the new one is then advanced into the trachea, using the scope as a guide.

Advantages

A fiberoptic laryngoscope (or bronchoscope) can be used to facilitate difficult intubations. This technique can also be used for critically ill patients on ventilators so that they do not lose their airway during tube replacement.

Disadvantages

Successful use of a fiberoptic laryngoscope requires extensive experience. In patients with bleeding or excessive secretions, the clinician may have difficulty seeing airway structures. If the patient is not breathing spontaneously or has been paralyzed (causing collapse of oral structures), it may be difficult to locate the epiglottis and vocal cords.

CONSIDERATIONS AFTER INTUBATION

Verification of Tube Position

It is critical to ensure that the endotracheal tube is properly positioned after intubation. Rapid verification of proper tube placement may be difficult in obese patients. As no single sign is 100 percent accurate, several of the following clinical signs should be used to verify tube position:

1. If the laryngoscopist has seen the tube pass between the vocal cords, proper tube placement is likely.
2. End-tidal carbon dioxide monitors measure carbon dioxide expiration and therefore test for proper tube position.
3. After intubation, the apices of the chest should move with ventilation.
4. The apex of each axilla should be auscultated for bilateral breath sounds. The abdomen (stomach) should be examined for distention and auscultated for sounds. Distention over the abdomen may indicate improper tube placement.
5. Water condensation in the endotracheal tube with each exhalation suggests proper tube placement.
6. The position of the endotracheal tube can be ascertained by adding a few extra milliliters of air to the cuff and palpating the cuff at the level of the sternal notch. This position ensures placement of the tube below the vocal cords and above the carina. A chest x-ray examination should be obtained to document the distance from the tip of the endotracheal tube to the carina.
7. After intubation, a second look with a laryngoscope is one way of ascertaining proper placement.

Secure the Tube

A bite block should be placed between the patient's teeth to prevent the patient from biting down and occluding the lumen of oral tubes. The tube should be fixed securely to the patient (taping the tube to facial skin or using a nonadhesive tube fixation device) to prevent accidental extubation or advancement. Any traction on the tube should also be prevented.

SUGGESTED READING

Sellick BA. Cricoid pressure to control regurgitation of stomach contents during induction of anesthesia. Lancet 1961; 2:404–406.

Miller RD, et. Anesthesia. 2nd ed. New York: Churchill Livingstone, 1981.

Firestone LL, ed. Clinical anesthesia procedures of the Massachusetts General Hospital. Boston: Little Brown & Company, 1988.

Clements JA, Nimmo WS. Pharmacokinetics and analgesic effects of ketamine in man. Br J Anaesth 1981; 53:27.

Gravenstein JS, Paulus DA, ed. Monitoring practice in clinical anesthesia. 2nd ed. Philadelphia: JB Lippincott, 1987.

BRONCHOSCOPY IN THE INTENSIVE CARE UNIT

FREDERICK P. OGNIBENE, M.D.

Bronchoscopy is an important diagnostic and therapeutic procedure for the treatment of patients who are in an intensive care unit. It is a procedure in which both bronchoalveolar lavage and transbronchial biopsy yield important information for the diagnosis of pulmonary pathologic processes. It allows for the rapid diagnosis of neoplastic, infectious, and noninfectious inflammatory processes in the lung, and is an established, safe procedure that can be performed in either a spontaneously breathing patient or in a patient requiring mechanical ventilation. Bronchoscopes are available in a variety of sizes based on the external diameter of the bronchoscope. If a bronchoscope with a large suction channel and the ability to perform transbronchial biopsies is desired, then bronchoscopes with an external diameter of 4.9 to 6.0 mm are available. A smaller bronchoscope with a 3.6-mm external diameter has suction capabilities only and is ideal for use in small adults, children, and patients with small-diameter endotracheal tubes. Recent advances in the ability to monitor oxygen saturation noninvasively have added to the safety of this procedure.

INDICATIONS

Bronchoscopy has a significant role in the therapy of airway management. The major indications for bronchoscopy are listed in Table 1. Bronchoscopy may be used to facilitate difficult endotracheal intubations. In such a situation, an endotracheal tube may be passed over the bronchoscope to its proximal end, and the bronchoscope is then placed into the trachea under direct visualization. After the bronchoscope has entered the trachea, the endotracheal tube is gradually advanced through the vocal cords and secured into place above the carina. This is particularly effective when one is unable to visualize the appropriate upper airway landmarks by direct laryngoscopy. In addition, if one is uncertain of the placement of an endotracheal tube, a bronchoscope can be passed through an existing endotracheal tube in order to confirm the location of the tube in the appropriate position above the carina yet below the vocal cords. Using a flexible pediatric-size bronchoscope, this is an important technique, especially in infants and children in whom tube placement and tube stability are among the most difficult issues of airway management.

Atelectasis, which is typically caused by local retention of pulmonary secretions, is common in patients receiving mechanical ventilation, in those who are weak or debilitated, and in certain postoperative patients such as those who have undergone thoracoabdominal surgical procedures. Atelectasis can result in abnormalities of pulmonary gas exchange leading to hypoxemia, and it can also be a focus for pneumonia. Conventional nasotracheal suctioning or blind endotracheal suctioning may not be effective in clearing secretions. As a consequence, bronchoscopy allows for the removal of secretions and, it is hoped, for the subsequent improvement in both roentgenographic findings and improvement in pulmonary gas exchange. The left lower lobe and the left mainstem bronchus are the most common sites of atelectasis, and retained secretions, respectively. If more significant secretion retention occurs, actual lobar collapse may result. Although bronchoscopy has not been determined to be advantageous over vigorous pulmonary toilet and blind suctioning in the treatment of atelectasis, in certain situations there probably is a role for bronchoscopy and the removal of retained secretions. If there is atelectasis with air bronchograms, which suggests that central airway plugging is probably not the problem, then bronchoscopy is not likely to be helpful. However, if there is atelectasis without visible air bronchograms, which suggests that mucous plugging of the airways is likely, then bronchoscopy with aggressive suctioning is likely to improve atelectasis.

Bronchoscopy is also effective in the removal of foreign bodies that have been aspirated. In some situations, once the object has been localized by fiberoptic bronchoscopy, a patient may have to undergo rigid bronchoscopy in the operating room in order to remove the foreign body effectively. Fiberoptic bronchoscopy has also been used to identify a focus of hemorrhage in patients with hemoptysis. If there is active bleeding, placement of the bronchoscope in a wedged position into the area of hemorrhage can often lead to effective tamponade at the site of bleeding. In addition, if bleeding is no longer an active process, the bronchoscope can be used to remove retained clot leading to secondary improvement in pulmonary function.

Bronchoscopy also has an important diagnostic role in the intensive care unit. First, because of direct visualization, it allows the identification of endobronchial or other structural lesions that may be the cause of either retained secretions or hemorrhage. Bronchoscopy can also local-

Table 1 Indications for Bronchoscopy in the Critical Care Setting

Therapeutic
  Difficult endotracheal intubation
  To confirm endotracheal tube position
  Atelectasis/acute lobar collapse
  Aspiration (foreign body or gastric contents)
  Hemoptysis

Diagnostic
  Atelectasis
  Hemoptysis
  Neoplasia
    Suggestive x-ray
    Abnormal sputum cytology
  Diffuse interstitial lung disease
  Evaluation of unresolved pneumonia

ize and confirm a neoplastic process that may have been suspected on the basis of either an abnormal chest roentgenogram or an abnormal sputum cytology. Lesions that are identified endobronchially may be brushed for cytology or biopsied via a bronchoscopic approach.

Bronchoscopy with bronchoalveolar lavage and transbronchial biopsy is also useful in the early evaluation of pulmonary interstitial disease. The list of differential diagnoses leading to a diagnosis of diffuse pulmonary infiltrates is long, especially for immunocompromised patients. However, bronchoscopy can be extremely useful in the diagnosis of both neoplastic and inflammatory processes in critically ill patients. When patients with diffuse pulmonary infiltrates become critically ill, requiring intensive care and/or intensive monitoring, they are frequently quite ill medically and have concomitant multiorgan system failure. As a consequence, the effective and rapid diagnosis of the pulmonary dysfunction is essential to their receiving optimal care. Bronchoscopy is a relatively safe and rapid initial procedure to undertake to determine the etiology of the diffuse pulmonary infiltrates. If there is no medical or technical contraindication to the procedure, bronchoscopy should be the initial diagnostic pulmonary procedure in these patients, since the morbidity of bronchoscopy is much less than that of an open lung biopsy. After a diagnosis has been established and appropriate therapy initiated, however, there may be critically ill patients who do not show an appropriate response and who have either unresolved pneumonia or a complicating process. For these patients, bronchoscopy also provides useful diagnostic information by allowing one to obtain specimens directly in order to determine whether the persistence of the pulmonary dysfunction is caused by the initial process or whether a superimposed infectious process has occurred that is not being treated effectively by the initial therapy.

APPROACH

All critically ill patients and most moderately ill patients who may benefit from intensive care unit monitoring should undergo bronchoscopy in an intensive care unit. All patients should be electrocardiographically monitored continuously, and they should either have an intra-arterial catheter placed for continuous blood pressure monitoring as well as for frequent assessment of arterial blood gases, or they should be monitored with a cutaneous pulse oximeter that measures oxygen saturation. Any decrease in saturation, indicating hypoxemia, should be noted and treated aggressively. Frequent monitoring of blood pressure is also mandatory. In patients requiring mechanical ventilation, the existing endotracheal tube (if adequate in diameter size) is used for the examination of the tracheobronchial tree. If they have adequate ventilatory reserve, nonintubated patients may have a bronchoscopy performed either via a transnasal or a transoral approach. If a patient is exhibiting hypoxemia and/or hemodynamic instability, however, an oral endotracheal tube should be electively placed before the procedure. This is especially true if transbronchial biopsies are to be performed in an already hypoxemic patient. Placement of an endotracheal tube allows for optimal airway protection and also provides for the safe delivery of an adequate tidal volume in order to optimize ventilation and oxygenation. The diameter of the endotracheal tube is important and can have physiologic consequences; an appropriate diameter is necessary to maintain effective ventilation after the bronchoscope has been placed in the tube. The appropriate diameter can be determined based on the principle of the residual cross-sectional area of the endotracheal tube. The residual cross-sectional area is that area that remains after the bronchoscope is placed in the endotracheal tube, and it is the area available to assure ventilation. For example, an endotracheal tube having a 7.5-mm internal diameter with a 6-mm bronchoscope in place has a resultant cross-sectional area that is equivalent to an endotracheal tube size of 4 to 4.5 mm. That resultant cross-sectional area is probably not adequate for effective ventilation in an adult, and high positive airway pressures may be generated that could result in barotrauma leading to either pneumothorax or pneumomediastinum. In patients already receiving ventilation, it may be necessary to change the existing endotracheal tube to one of a larger size before bronchoscopy in order to avoid problems secondary to a low cross-sectional area. Although pediatric-sized bronchoscopes have a smaller external diameter (3.6 mm) and therefore can be placed in small endotracheal tubes, they are not as effective in suctioning retained secretions and do not have a biopsy channel; for this reason, transbronchial biopsies cannot be performed. As a general rule, if one has to perform a bronchoscopy through an endotracheal tube, it is desirable to use the largest endotracheal tube possible to allow for the most effective ventilation during the procedure and to provide the most effective clearance of secretions if necessary. Provided that they do not have excessive hypoxemia, patients who are undergoing only bronchoalveolar lavage may undergo bronchoscopy via either the transnasal or transoral approach.

Before one undertakes the procedure, it is essential that the patient is provided with adequate analgesia and anesthesia. The topical anesthetic agents usually used are 1 percent lidocaine and 4 percent liquid cocaine. They provide effective anesthesia for the oropharynx and nasopharynx. The topical cocaine is typically applied to the nares with a nasal applicator, and the lidocaine is aerosolized via a nebulizer into the posterior oropharynx such that effective topical anesthesia is achieved. In addition, one may elect to use systemic medications for the procedure. Typically these medications include benzodiazepines and narcotics. Diazepam (5 to 10 mg) used in conjunction with fentanyl (50 to 150 μg) is an example of a benzodiazepine and narcotic combination.

If I am performing the procedure via an endotracheal tube, then before the procedure, I place a swivel adaptor on the proximal end of the endotracheal tube to allow entry of the bronchoscope into the endotracheal tube without the loss of a significant tidal volume from the proximal end of the endotracheal tube. One hundred percent oxygen is delivered to the patient before and during the bronchoscopy in order to maintain an acceptable level of oxygen. Tidal volumes may be delivered either mechanically through a ventilator or they may be achieved through compression of a Jackson-Reese manual resuscitator during the procedure. It is important to note that if one suctions through a bronchoscope, a deficit of 200 to 300 ml of the inhaled tidal volume may result. As a consequence, it is important to monitor a patient for effective ventilation as well as for oxygenization during the procedure. If a patient is not intubated and breathing spontaneously, then oxygen in a concentration of 50 to 100 percent is delivered via an aerosol mask during the procedure. It is important to maintain this flow of oxygen since even relatively healthy patients may experience transient hypoxemia during and after a bronchoscopic procedure. If a patient is undergoing bronchoscopy without an endotracheal tube in place, endotracheal tubes and laryngoscopes should be readily accessible so that emergent laryngoscopy and oral intubation may be performed if there are problems with hypoxemia, ventilatory failure, or significant hemorrhage during the procedure.

Once the airway is secure and proper ventilation is guaranteed, the bronchoscope is passed into the tracheobronchial tree. The initial part of the procedure is the anatomic identification of major landmarks (carina and right and left mainstem bronchi) and the performance of a thorough bilateral anatomic examination of the tracheobronchial tree. It is important to establish the correct right-left orientation and to identify endobronchial lesions or obstructions, such as mucous plugging or endobronchial tumors that may be the cause of atelectasis or lobar collapse. If there is a specific lobar abnormality noted on the chest roentgenogram, the procedure should be directed primarily toward that affected lobe. Any obstructing endobronchial lesions should be identified, brushed, and biopsied if clinically feasible. If retained secretions are present, sterile 0.9 percent sodium chloride may be instilled to mobilize these secretions and clear the airway. If there is evidence of a lobar pneumonia, the specimens obtained should be sent to microbiology for appropriate stains and cultures.

In a patient with diffuse pulmonary infiltrates, especially a patient who is immunocompromised, the differential diagnosis of the infiltrates is extensive. It is important to make an early and reliable diagnosis before pulmonary function progressively deteriorates. After the anatomic examination, bronchoalveolar lavage of one or more lobar subsegments should be performed. With this technique, 35-ml aliquots of 0.9 percent sodium chloride are instilled via the biopsy channel of the bronchoscope while it is in a wedged position and are then aspirated into a sterile sputum trap. Aspiration of at least 50 percent of the instilled sodium chloride is considered an adequate yield for bronchoalveolar lavage. Up to 300 ml of 0.9 percent sodium chloride may be safely instilled in an adult. The lavage specimens should be microbiologically and cytologically evaluated, using special stains and cultures. In immunosuppressed patients, lavage has proven to be an effective technique for diagnosing pneumonia secondary to routine bacterial or fungal pathogens, *Pneumocystis carinii*, cytomegalovirus, and various species of mycobacteria. In addition, malignant processes, chemotherapeutic changes, or pulmonary parenchymal hemorrhage can likewise be diagnosed by means of lavage. Because lavage does not involve obtaining tissue, it can be performed safely in patients with severe thrombocytopenia or a coagulopathy. It is also a procedure that can be performed quickly with minimal risk of pneumothorax and can therefore be performed in patients who are receiving mechanical ventilation and who may also be receiving a high fractional percentage of inspired oxygen or positive end-expiratory pressure (PEEP).

In patients with diffuse pulmonary infiltrates who do not have medical contraindications, transbronchial biopsies should also be performed to obtain pulmonary tissue. This material could provide additional diagnostic information. Biopsies are most safely performed under fluoroscopy, which helps guide placement of the biopsy forceps and may limit the risk of pneumothorax. Pulmonary tissue obtained by transbronchial biopsies should be processed histopathologically to assess alveolar and interstitial architecture. In addition, these histopathologic sections are used to assess the infectious etiology of the diffuse infiltrates. Multiple stains are required because of the broad range of infectious and noninfectious etiologies of diffuse pulmonary infiltrates (Table 2). Bronchoalveolar lavage and transbronchial biopsy are additive in the diagnostic yield in these patients.

Repeat bronchoscopic procedures are sometimes warranted in critically ill patients. In patients with copious secretions, they are often necessary in order to clear the airways of retained secretions that persist despite blind suctioning. In addition, a repeat bronchoscopy may be needed in order to perform an adequate anatomic examination in a patient with hemoptysis in whom blood or bloody secretions may obscure visualization during the initial bronchoscopic examination. Another important reason for repeating the examination is to obtain lavage and/or biopsy samples to assess results of antimicrobial therapy in documented instances of infectious pneumonia or to evalu-

Table 2 Histopathologic Stains Useful in the Diagnosis of Diffuse Pulmonary Infiltrates Caused by Microorganisms

Staining Technique	Organisms
Hematoxylin and eosin	Viruses (i.e., cytomegalovirus inclusion bodies); may reveal alveolar exudate with *P. carinii*
Toluidine blue	*P. carinii*
Gomori methenamine silver	*P. carinii*, fungi
Fite	Mycobacteria
Giemsa or Brown-Brenn	Bacteria
Periodic-acid-Schiff	Encapsulated fungi

ate patients with infectious, neoplastic, or inflammatory pulmonary disease who develop a worsening of pulmonary function despite directed therapy. Because this deterioration may be caused by a secondary nosocomial process, most commonly an infection, a repeat bronchoscopic examination is indicated. In an effort to improve the diagnostic interpretation and yield from bronchoscopy in patients who may have a nosocomial pneumonia, the telescoping microbiology brush is a useful tool. It allows one to obtain a deep, protected specimen that has not been contaminated by passage through the upper airway or endotracheal tube, which may frequently be colonized by bacteria or *Candida*. In addition, when lavage is cultured and data are expressed in colony-forming units of bacteria there is a significant association between greater than 10^5 colony-forming units per milliliter and clinically active bacterial pneumonia. This is another way of distinguishing a true nosocomial pneumonia from bacterial colonization.

COMPLICATIONS AND CONTRAINDICATIONS

The complications of bronchoscopy may be related either to the medications given or to the procedure itself (Table 3). In intubated patients, the airway is protected by the endotracheal tube; however, sedative and analgesic agents may lead to respiratory depression and the need for mechanical or supplemental ventilation. Patients who are receiving mechanical ventilation may have the desired respiratory rate and tidal volume, but those who are not receiving ventilation may need assisted ventilation (e.g., a Jackson-Reese manual resuscitator) if they have respiratory depression secondary to the use of medications. Another potential side effect of sedative and analgesic agents is hypotension. Hypotension may be caused by decreased left ventricular preload secondary to the venous pooling effect of some narcotic agents as well as to diminution of intrinsic catecholamine drive. Hypotension caused by the use of narcotics may be reversed with the administration of naloxone; vigorous fluid replacement may also be necessary to restore a normal blood pressure. Hyperexcitement and, more seriously, seizures may be side effects of the topical anesthetic agents lidocaine and cocaine. The blood concentration after topical anesthesia may be as high as approximately 30 to 50 percent of that obtained after intravenous administration of the drugs. Only the minimal amount of the drug necessary to achieve topical anesthesia should be administered; a total of approximately 300 mg lidocaine is a generally safe maximal dose in a full-sized adult.

Complications of the bronchoscopic examination of the airway are rare. Transient vasovagal responses have been reported. Although laryngospasm and bronchospasm caused by the bronchoscope can be severe, they are usually seen in patients with underlying obstructive or bronchospastic pulmonary disease. Bronchodilators or atropine may be required to prevent or reverse bronchospasm. Transient hypoxemia occurs during bronchoscopy, but significant oxygen desaturation is prevented by the delivery of supplemental oxygen. Because ventricular and atrial arrhythmias secondary to the hypoxemia may occur, it is important to monitor heart rate and rhythm during the procedure as well as to assess arterial blood gases frequently.

Diagnostic bronchoscopic procedures can also produce complications. Bronchoalveolar lavage may be as-

Table 3 Complications of and Contraindications to Bronchoscopy in the Critical Care Setting

Complications		Contraindications	
Cause	Complication	To Routine Bronchoscopy	To Transbronchial Biopsy
Medications	Respiratory depression Hypotension Hyperexcitement or seizures	Asthma Unstable angina or recent myocardial infarction Poor cooperation Uncorrectable hypoxemia or hypercapnia	Bleeding diastheses (i.e., thrombocytopenia or coagulopathy) Uremia Pulmonary hypertension Ventilation with high PEEP
Routine bronchoscopy	Vasovagal response Laryngospasm Bronchospasm Hypoxemia Cardiac arrhythmias		
Bronchoalveolar lavage	Worsening infiltrate Transient hypoxemia Transient fever		
Transbronchial biopsy	Pneumothorax Hemorrhage Pneumonia		

sociated with transient hypoxemia, fever, or worsening of the pulmonary infiltrate at the site of the lavage. Pneumonia may also occur, although rarely, as a consequence of a bronchoalveolar lavage or bronchial brushing, especially when there is an underlying endobronchial or partially obstructing lesion.

Among the bronchoscopic procedures, transbronchial biopsies have the highest potential for morbidity and, in rare instances, mortality. Pneumothorax occurs in approximately 5 percent of all patients who undergo transbronchial biopsy. About half of these cases resolve spontaneously, whereas the other half require a tube thoracostomy in order to reinflate the collapsed lung. In addition, hemorrhage may also complicate transbronchial biopsy. Significant hemorrhage (more than 50 to 100 ml of blood) is reported in as many as 3 percent of patients. Serious or life-threatening hemorrhage is rare, however, unless there is an underlying reason for the bleeding, such as thrombocytopenia, coagulopathy, or uremia. Because the site of the bleeding is distal to the tip of the bronchoscope, the bronchoscope may be wedged into the subsegmental bronchus that is the source of the bleeding in order to provide tamponade to the site, to control bleeding, and to protect the rest of the tracheobronchial tree. It is important always to maintain visualization with the bronchoscope and to control the bleeding if hemorrhage has occurred.

There are few contraindications to routine bronchoscopy, anatomic examination, and bronchoalveolar lavage. Asthma is a contraindication to bronchoscopy because of the high risk of bronchoscope-induced bronchospasm. Patients with unstable angina or those who have had a recent myocardial infarction should also undergo bronchoscopy only if it is essential. Close attention to cardiac rhythm and to the level of oxygen saturation may avoid precipitation of a dysrhythmia or angina in these patients.

Transbronchial biopsies should not be performed in patients who have a risk of bleeding. A minimum platelet count of 50,000 with normal prothrombin and partial thromboplastin times usually guarantees hemostasis. Uremia or medications with antiplatelet properties cause platelet dysfunction and, consequently, bleeding, and therefore these are additional contraindications to transbronchial biopsy. Patients with pulmonary hypertension may bleed more after transbronchial biopsy, theoretically because of increased perfusion in the pulmonary capillary circulation. The risk of pneumothorax is also heightened in patients undergoing positive-pressure mechanical ventilation and in patients receiving high levels of PEEP (i.e., >10 cm H_2O). Because of these added risk factors, transbronchial biopsies should be performed with caution in patients receiving mechanical ventilation. In a patient requiring mechanical ventilation, one approach is to perform biopsies during pharmacologically-induced apnea. During the biopsy, the apneic patient is not given mechanical breaths for a few seconds, thus allowing for a safer biopsy procedure.

SUGGESTED READING

Barrett CR. Flexible fiberoptic bronchoscopy in the critically ill patient: methodology and indications. Chest 1978; 73(suppl):746–749.
Crystal RG, Reynolds HY, Kalica AR. Bronchoalveolar lavage: the report of an international conference. Chest 1986; 90:122–131.
Dietrich KA, Strauss RH, Cabalka AK, et al. Use of flexible fiberoptic endoscopy for determination of endotracheal tube position in the pediatric patient. Crit Care Med 1988; 16:884–887.
Niederman MS, Craven DE, Fein AM, Schultz DE. Pneumonia in the critically ill hospitalized patient. Chest 1990; 97:170–181.
Papin JA, Grum CM, Weg JG. Transbronchial biopsy during mechanical ventilation. Chest 1986; 89:168–170.
Shelley MP, Wilson P, Norman J. Sedation for fiberoptic bronchoscopy. Thorax 1989; 44:769–776. Editorial.
Thorpe JE, Baughman RP, Frame PT, et al. Bronchoalveolar lavage for diagnosing acute bacterial pneumonia. J Infect Dis 1987; 155:855–861.

ARTERIAL BLOOD GASES

FREDERICK P. OGNIBENE, M.D.

The analysis of arterial blood samples provides information regarding acid-base status, the degree of oxygenation, and the adequacy of ventilation. Because arterial blood samples are safely and easily obtained in an intensive care unit, they are one of the most common laboratory parameters used in the clinical evaluation of a patient. Arterial blood gas data indicate how well the patient's pulmonary and renal systems are functioning and provide information regarding trends in metabolic and pulmonary parameters in response to therapeutic interventions. Arterial blood gases also provide much more reliable information regarding a patient's ventilatory function than that which can be provided simply by a clinical examination.

This chapter focuses on the information provided by an arterial blood gas, discusses an approach to assessing responses to therapy, and presents insights into new technologies which provide noninvasive ways of measuring some of the parameters provided by a standard arterial blood gas.

ACID PRODUCTION AND BUFFER SYSTEMS

Blood pH is determined by processes that alter the concentration of hydrogen ions as well as by the ability of buffer systems to maintain the pH based on a response to changes in hydrogen ion concentrations. Buffers include naturally occurring components of blood such as plasma proteins, hemoglobin, and the bicarbonate ion. The carbonic anhydrase system freely allows for a balance between carbonic acid and bicarbonate. In addition to buffers, adequate pulmonary function and renal function are essential to the handling of not only increments in acid production but also the buffering systems used to offset these increments.

As long as renal function and pulmonary function are adequate in the presence of an intact circulation, the bicarbonate buffering system can generally correct for moderate increments in hydrogen ion concentration simply by producing more carbon dioxide and consequently eliminating that gas. Intrinsic buffer systems reduce but do not eliminate the hazards of an acute acidosis or alkalosis.

Most fats and carbohydrates are metabolized to water and carbon dioxide. Since carbon dioxide is generally a freely diffusible gas, the carbon dioxide tension is set by the degree of alveolar ventilation. Hyperventilation can rapidly decrease carbon dioxide tension, and hypoventilation consequently leads to an increase in arterial carbon dioxide tension. In most situations, a steady state allows for the excretion of hydrogen ions and the retention of bicarbonate, which leads to a readjustment in pH when carbon dioxide tension is altered. However, acidosis and alkalosis are the end result of pathophysiologic processes that lead to abnormalities in normal acid-base relationships. For example, if there is a fixed acid load that cannot be adequately excreted by the kidney or if there is an inordinate amount of acid generated and presented to the kidney, then there must be adequate pulmonary compensation to handle carbon dioxide generation and elimination and thereby readjust the pH. It is important to remember that sulphur-containing amino acids, phospholipids, and other endogenous acids cannot be metabolized to carbon dioxide and water using the carbonic anhydrase buffer system. As a consequence, these acids must be excreted by the kidney.

Three principal renal tubular mechanisms lead to renal acid excretion. The role of the kidney is to secrete acid, to reabsorb filtered bicarbonate, and to excrete phosphate, chloride, and ammonia in association with hydrogen ions. Although this regulation by the kidney can take as long as 24 hours to occur, intact renal function is essential to maintaining acid-base homeostasis. Although renal compensatory responses to respiratory disorders may take considerable time, the respiratory response to acid-base derangements occurs rapidly.

METABOLIC ACID-BASE DERANGEMENTS

Metabolic acidoses can be classified into two physiologic subsets based on the pattern of serum electrolytes. This pattern involves the use of unmeasured anion determination or "anion gap." Although the principle of electroneutrality is physiologically obligate, the concept of "anion gap" provides a simple clinical approach to the assessment of a metabolic acidosis. One can calculate unmeasured anions using the following formula:

$$\text{anion gap} = Na^+ - [HCO_3^- + Cl^-]$$

In "normal" situations, the anion gap is typically less than 12 mEq per liter. A metabolic acidosis can occur with either a normal anion gap or an increased anion gap. A normal anion gap is typically seen when there is an elevated serum chloride level. Using these categories, one often can easily differentiate the etiologies of metabolic acidosis. Table 1 stratifies some of the etiology of the metabolic acidosis based on the determination of the anion gap. Once a diagnosis is established, therapy is directed specifically against that underlying etiology. It is important to know that therapy with sodium bicarbonate should be used cautiously, utilizing the arterial blood gas as a guide to therapy. There are data emerging that indicate that overly aggressive therapy with bicarbonate can lead to more significant physiologic derangements. These include worsening of alkalemia, negative inotropy, hyperosmolality, sodium overload, and paradoxical acidosis of the cerebrospinal fluid. When indicated, one can administer sodium bicarbonate based on the determination of the bicarbonate deficit. However, the calculated bicarbonate deficit should not be totally repleted all at once; rather one-half of the measured deficit should be administered, and this should be followed by a subsequent check of the arterial blood gas to look for a pH response. The clinical indications for therapeutic intervention with sodium bicarbonate are (1) evidence that acidosis is leading to dangerous electrophysiologic abnormalities, (2) electrolyte imbalance, or (3) altered response to exogenous drugs such as inotropic agents.

A metabolic alkalosis is present whenever there is an elevation in the serum bicarbonate level that is inappropriate for the arterial pH. A metabolic alkalosis may occur secondary to the loss of hydrogen ions from the body, excessive gain of bicarbonate, or a loss of chloride ions that is disproportionate to the loss of bicarbonate. Based on these anion depletions, metabolic alkalosis can be generally classified as either a chloride-responsive alkalosis or a chloride-resistant alkalosis (Table 2). Chloride-resistant

Table 1 Differential Diagnosis of Metabolic Acidosis Based on the Anion Gap

Increased unmeasured anion
  Azotemia
  Diabetic ketoacidosis
  Ethylene glycol intoxication
  Lactic acidosis
  Methanol intoxication
  Salicylate intoxication

No increase in unmeasured anions (hyperchloremic)
  Ammonium chloride ingestion
  Carbonic anhydrase inhibitors (bicarbonaturia)
  Diarrhea
  Pyelonephritis (chronic diminished tubular secretion of hydrogen ion)
  Renal tubular acidosis
  Ureterosigmoidostomy

Table 2 Differential Diagnosis of Metabolic Alkalosis Based on Chloride Responsiveness

Chloride-Responsive Alkalosis
  Vomiting
  Diuretic therapy (except potassium sparing)
  Nasogastric suctioning
  Posthypercapnic state
  Villous adenoma
  Chloridorrhea (diarrhea rich in chloride, typically congenital)

Chloride-Resistant Alkalosis
  Corticosteroid therapy
  Cushing's disease
  Ectopic adrenocorticotropic hormone production
  Primary hyperaldosteronism
  Severe potassium depletion

alkaloses typically occur in settings of mineralocorticoid excess or severe potassium ion depletion.

A metabolic alkalosis can cause symptoms in both the central nervous system and the cardiovascular system. Lethargy, confusion, and agitation may all be seen in the setting of metabolic alkalosis. The major cardiovascular side effect is arrhythmia, which may be either atrial or ventricular in origin.

A chloride-responsive alkalosis can be treated with replacement of chloride ion, in the form of either sodium chloride or potassium chloride. Potassium chloride is somewhat preferable because it also allows for repletion of the deficit in potassium, which may be substantial. If there are situations in which more aggressive correction of the metabolic alkalosis is needed, the use of hydrochloric acid (HCl) can be undertaken. HCl is delivered in a dilute form, typically 0.1N HCl, and is administered via a central venous line.

RESPIRATORY ACID-BASE DERANGEMENTS

In a primary respiratory acidosis, the arterial carbon dioxide pressure ($PaCO_2$) is elevated because of ventilatory dysfunction. As already mentioned, compensatory changes in the level of bicarbonate occur to help minimize the effects of the elevation in $PaCO_2$ on hydrogen ion concentration. When a primary respiratory acidosis is present, it is important to determine the duration of the acidosis. During an acute respiratory acidosis, there is not enough time for renal mechanisms to correct the pH. As a consequence, when the level of arterial carbon dioxide increases acutely, the fall in pH is dramatic. In this setting, the measured bicarbonate level is not greatly changed relative to the normal state. In the acute setting, there is an approximate increase of only 1 mEq per liter in bicarbonate concentration for every 10 mm Hg increase in the $PaCO_2$. This response to alveolar hypoventilation is very predictable, and if a variability in the expected level of measured bicarbonate exists, then one has to postulate that there is a mixed acid-base disturbance (i.e., a superimposed metabolic component).

In the setting of a persistent respiratory acidosis, the kidneys readjust the serum bicarbonate level by limiting its excretion in an attempt to bring the pH back toward normal. As a consequence, the pH is protected. If there is a steady state, a chronic respiratory acidosis occurs. In this setting, the pH trends toward normal because of the increment seen in the serum bicarbonate. It takes 2 to 4 days to maximize the renal compensation for a respiratory acidosis.

In the setting of a chronic respiratory acidosis, although the pH trends toward normal, it never does achieve that normal value. If a pH is determined to be greater than 7.4, there must be a superimposed process in addition to the renal compensation for the respiratory acidosis. One must therefore again consider a mixed acid-base disturbance. The acute causes of respiratory acidosis are those diseases that lead to hypercapnic respiratory failure, and consequently therapy is aimed toward treatment of the underlying ventilatory failure.

In a primary respiratory alkalosis, the $PaCO_2$ decreases with a compensatory decrease in serum bicarbonate. Typically, for a 10 mm Hg decrease in the $PaCO_2$ in the setting of hyperventilation, there is an accompanying decrement in bicarbonate of 2 mEq per liter. A primary respiratory alkalosis can occur in the setting of either a normal or elevated alveolar-arterial oxygen gradient. Table 3 lists some common causes of respiratory alkalosis and categorizes them as those with normal alveolar-arterial gradients and those with elevated alveolar-arterial gradients. The general approach to treating a respiratory alkalosis is to treat the underlying condition.

ARTERIAL OXYGENATION

In addition to the acid-base parameters provided by an arterial blood gas, parameters of gas exchange, (i.e., arterial oxygen and arterial carbon dioxide tensions) are also measured. Respiratory failure is defined as a severe abnormality in either (or both) of these measurements of

Table 3 Differential Diagnosis of Respiratory Alkalosis Based on the Alveolar-Arterial Gradient

Normal gradient
  Altitude elevations
  Severe anemia
  Central nervous system dysfunction
  Hyperventilation (mechanical or psychogenic)
  Pregnancy
  Salicylate intoxication

Elevated gradient
  Asthma
  Hepatic failure
  Interstitial pulmonary diseases
  Pneumonia
  Pulmonary edema
  Pulmonary embolism
  Sepsis

gas exchange. To help interpret a decrease in the arterial oxygen pressure (PaO_2), one can utilize a number of indices in addition to the arterial blood gas itself. These include the alveolar-arterial oxygen gradient and the ratio of arterial oxygen tension to fractional inspired oxygen (FIO_2)(PaO_2/FIO_2). The latter is much more helpful in situations of significant intrapulmonary shunting in which further increments of FIO_2 lead to further increases in the alveolar-arterial gradient.

Hypoxemia can be attributed to any of five basic conditions: (1) delivery of a low partial pressure of oxygen, (2) alveolar hypoventilation, (3) ventilation-perfusion mismatching, (4) right-to-left shunting, and (5) diffusion impairments. Hypoventilation, ventilation-perfusion mismatching, and right-to-left shunting are the most important causes of hypoxemia.

Three major situations can lead to an elevation in $PaCO$(hypercapnia). These include breathing a gas rich in carbon dioxide, alveolar hypoventilation, and very severe ventilation-perfusion mismatching.

The purpose of monitoring arterial oxygenation is to ensure adequate tissue oxygenation. The most critical factors in maintaining tissue oxygenation are optimal cardiac output, adequate tissue perfusion, and adequate arterial oxygenation (which can be enhanced significantly by the maintenance of hemoglobin concentration). The determination of mixed venous oxygen tension from pulmonary arterial blood can be of additional benefit in the assessment of a patient's cardiovascular status. In the setting of progressive cardiovascular dysfunction, the mixed venous oxygen tension decreases. Frequently, deterioration in cardiovascular function may be manifested by an initial decrement in the mixed venous oxygen tension before any change in the arterial oxygen content occurs.

Oxygen therapy is essential for the treatment of hypoxemia and can also aid in determining the etiology of the disorder. In situations of ventilation-perfusion mismatching, the PaO_2 typically shows a dramatic response to oxygen therapy, whereas the patient with right-to-left shunting shows either much less response or no response at all. The differentiation of ventilation-perfusion mismatching from right-to-left shunting as the cause of hypoxemia is crucial to the treatment of this disorder.

ACID-BASE BALANCE DURING CARDIOPULMONARY RESUSCITATION

During cardiopulmonary resuscitation, cardiac output is low, and there is a consequent decrease in tissue oxygen delivery. Because of the subsequent anaerobic metabolism, lactic acid production occurs, leading to the generation of hydrogen ions. It is important to note that during this anaerobic metabolism, the carbon dioxide concentration increases much more rapidly intracellularly than in blood. This intracellular carbon dioxide diffuses freely from the cells into capillary blood and returns to the heart and lungs in venous blood. During cardiopulmonary resuscitation, a mixed venous blood gas typically reveals acidemia with hypercarbia. However, with hyperventilation during resuscitation, arterial blood is typically less acidotic than venous blood. In well-performed cardiopulmonary resuscitation, arterial blood pH is typically normal or even mildly alkalotic, although the venous blood remains acidotic. Arterial acidosis during cardiopulmonary resuscitation is usually caused by ineffective or inadequate ventilation. Therefore the best therapy is to optimize manual chest compression techniques as well as to hyperventilate the patient.

In the past, liberal administration of sodium bicarbonate was recommended during cardiopulmonary resuscitation. Sodium bicarbonate administration can generate a large amount of carbon dioxide, however, which diffuses into the cells more readily than bicarbonate itself, leading to a further increment in intracellular partial pressure of carbon dioxide (PCO_2). This leads to a further decrement of intracellular pH and subsequent deterioration in cellular function. This elevation of intracellular PCO_2 can have adverse effects on both the central nervous system and cardiovascular system. Intracellular acidosis in myocardial muscle cells leads to decrements in cardiac contractility, cardiac output, and blood pressure. As already noted, bicarbonate administration can also lead to significant hyperosmolality, alkalemia, and sodium overload. Bicarbonate therapy is therefore not recommended as initial therapy in the routine management of a cardiac arrest. This is also true for unwitnessed cardiac arrests.

Bicarbonate should be used only after defibrillation, cardiac compression, ventilatory support, and other pharmacologic interventions have been administered. If it is to be used, an initial dose of 1 mEq per kilogram is recommended. Subsequent doses should be no more than one-half of the original dose. During the postresuscitation management of the patient, further bicarbonate therapy should be based solely on arterial blood gas determinations. Alternative buffer agents such as tris (hydroxymethyl) aminomethane (THAM) can effectively correct metabolic acidosis in an animal model of cardiopulmonary resuscitation. However, its value in human resuscitation has not been documented. In addition, dichloroacetate (DCA) has been shown to decrease serum lactate concentrations by stimulating the pyruvate dehydrogenase pathway. However, its value during cardiopulmonary resuscitation has also not been determined.

ARTERIAL BLOOD GAS MEASUREMENTS/MONITORING

Important in the assessment of arterial blood gases is the maintenance of excellent quality control. The quality of results depends on both the sophistication of the machine being used and on the operator. Blood gas equipment should therefore be frequently checked against control values such that a good quality control program exists and accuracy of the machinery is guaranteed. This usually requires a staff of fully trained technicians who are also aware of the importance of quality control. Blood gas machines run by untrained personnel clearly are prone to many errors and are not recommended in clinical situations.

There is no question that body temperature has an effect on blood gas tension. Blood gas determinations based on a body temperature of 37°C are not reflective of in vivo blood gas tensions when there is an abnormal body temperature. Hence, correction of arterial blood gases based on body temperature is important, especially when there are temperature extremes such as those of hypothermia or hyperthermia. If a patient's body temperature is outside of the normal range, then the values of PaO_2 and $PaCO_2$ should be corrected. The oxygen content and bicarbonate level in base excess calculations are typically independent of temperature variation.

NONINVASIVE TECHNIQUES

Numerous technical advances have occurred that provide noninvasive and continuous means by which to monitor both $PaCO_2$ and PaO_2. The most significant techniques involve oximetry, capnography, and transcutaneous gas electrodes. Pulse oximetry provides a readily accessible tool for the noninvasive measurement of the oxyhemoglobin saturation. A pulse oximeter is a dual-wavelength spectrophotometer with plethysmographic capabilities. The oximetry technique has added another dimension to our ability to monitor oxygen saturation noninvasively. This has led to increased safety and less patient risk in settings such as operating rooms and intensive care units (especially pediatric environments). It is important to remember, however, that pulse oximeters should be used primarily for detecting trends in arterial oxygenation and saturation and should not substitute for arterial blood gas determinations.

Pulmonary artery oximetry allows for continuous determination of the mixed venous oxygen saturation. The mixed venous oxygen saturation is dependent on the relationship between oxygen delivery and oxygen consumption. The ability to monitor mixed venous oxygen saturation continuously allows one to detect subtle changes in cardiovascular function before overt cardiovascular collapse or arterial desaturation occurs. For maximum effectiveness, it is important to monitor mixed venous and arterial saturations continuously.

Capnography allows for noninvasive measurement of the end-tidal carbon dioxide (CO_2) tension, which is typically several torr less than the $PaCO_2$. End-tidal CO_2 varies with increasing physiologic dead space, which increases the gradient between arterial and end-tidal CO_2. In this clinical situation, capnographic measurements may be limited. End-tidal CO_2 monitoring is most effectively used noninvasively to reflect $PaCO_2$ if dead space is constant, and it can also be used to follow trends in dead space ventilation. It is particularly useful in patients requiring therapeutic hyperventilation (e.g., elevations in intracranial pressure) and for noninvasive apnea monitoring.

A final noninvasive mode of measuring and tracking both arterial oxygen and arterial CO_2 content is the use of transcutaneous gas electrodes. Transcutaneous monitoring is a continuous way to trend both PaO_2 and $PaCO_2$; transcutaneous monitors typically overestimate the true $PaCO_2$. Because transcutaneous measurements require a heating element in the electrode, burns to skin have occurred. Burns can be limited by keeping electrode temperatures at less than 44°C and by changing the site of the electrode every 4 hours. Unlike capnographic measurement of end-tidal CO_2, which requires an endotracheal tube attachment, transcutaneous CO_2 monitors can be used in nonintubated patients.

SUGGESTED READING

Bersin RM, Chatterjee K, Arieff AI. Metabolic and hemodynamic consequences of sodium bicarbonate administration in patients with heart disease. Am J Med 1989; 87:7–14.
Madias NE, Wolf CJ, Cohen JJ. Regulation of acid-base equilibrium in chronic hypercapnia. Kidney Int 1985; 27:538–543.
Narins RG, Emmett M. Simple and mixed acid-base disorders: a practical approach. Medicine 1980; 59:161–187.
Shapiro BA, Cane RD. Blood gas monitoring: yesterday, today, and tomorrow. Crit Care Med 1989; 17:573–581.
Weil MH, Rackow EC, Trevino R, et al. Difference in acid-base state between venous and arterial blood during cardio-pulmonary resuscitation. N Engl J Med 1986; 315:153–156.

MECHANICAL VENTILATION

ROBERT A. BALK, M.D.

Critically ill patients frequently require the use of mechanical ventilatory support. During the first half of this century, ventilatory support was difficult to provide and typically involved the use of negative pressure ventilators. During the polio epidemic of the late 1940s and early 1950s, the concept of respiratory support using positive pressure ventilators was put into widespread use. This technique helped solidify the concept of the centralized intensive care units we know today.

During the past two decades there have been a tremendous number of advances and innovations in the design and use of mechanical ventilators. The use of microprocessor technology and a better understanding of the physiology of mechanical ventilation have to a great extent been responsible for this major progress in ventilatory support.

Despite these advances, however, several controversial issues remain regarding the use and proper application of these technologic and scientific advances. This chapter serves as an introduction to the use of mechanical ventilatory support. With the large number of recent developments in this field, it would be impossible to discuss them in depth in this brief chapter. The interested reader is referred to the various suggested readings cited at the end of this chapter for a more in-depth discussion of the specifics of mechanical ventilatory support.

TYPES OF VENTILATORS

The first mechanical ventilators that were developed created a negative pressure relative to the atmospheric pressure around the patient and/or the patient's chest. The iron lung is the typical example of the negative pressure ventilator. Unfortunately, these ventilators limited the access of the health care professional to the patient and were very cumbersome.

The major type of mechanical ventilator used today is the positive-pressure ventilator. This ventilator supplies the patient with conditioned gas under positive pressure. An artificial airway is required to facilitate the delivery of the pressurized conditioned gas mixture to the tracheobronchial tree. The typical intubation routes employed for this purpose include an oral endotracheal tube, nasotracheal tube, or a tracheostomy tube. A variety of positive-pressure ventilators are used today. They are defined by the parameter that terminates the normal inspiratory cycle. The four types of positive-pressure ventilators commonly used include pressure-cycled, volume-cycled, time-cycled, and flow-cycled ventilators. The volume-cycled and time-cycled ventilators are the most popular of the positive-pressure ventilators. The reasons for this popularity may include the ease of use and the ability to deliver a constant tidal volume (V_T) despite changes in the patient's compliance or airways resistance.

The traditional concept of mechanical ventilatory support revolves around the delivery of a sufficiently large tidal volume of air (usually greatly exceeding a patient's spontaneous resting V_T) delivered a set number of times per minutes. The high-frequency ventilators are designed to delivery a V_T of conditioned gas that is much smaller than the dead space volume at rates from 60 to 6,000 breaths per minute (1 to 100 Hz). High-frequency ventilation is accomplished using high-frequency positive-pressure ventilation, high-frequency jet ventilation, or high-frequency oscillation. Since a V_T smaller than the dead space volume is used in all of the methods of high-frequency ventilation, the traditional concept of convective gas exchange does not adequately explain the ability to achieve adequate oxygenation, ventilation, and acid-base balance. The concept of augmented diffusion of gases through a variety of mechanisms has been used to explain the method of gas exchange with high-frequency ventilation.

INDICATIONS

There are a variety of indications for the use of mechanical ventilation in the critically ill patient; these include (1) respiratory failure, (2) ventilatory failure, and (3) support of the respiratory system to decrease the work of breathing and allow better oxygen delivery to the other organ systems during systemic illness. The most common indications are for the treatment of patients with acute respiratory or ventilatory failure. As discussed in the chapters in this text dealing specifically with these conditions, not all of these patients require the use of assisted ventilation, but a significant percentage do. At times it is also prudent to intubate and mechanically ventilate patients with nonpulmonary conditions (e.g., sepsis, cardiac dysfunction) in an attempt to decrease the work of breathing and allow a greater percentage of the cardiac output to be supplied to the heart, brain, and kidneys. While this practice is still controversial, in theory it is a rational approach and one that coincides with my own biases.

INITIATION OF MECHANICAL VENTILATION

Mechanical ventilatory support has two major goals. The first is to maintain an alveolar ventilation appropriate for the patient's metabolic needs. The way to ensure that this is accomplished is to achieve a normal pH rather than a predetermined partial pressure of carbon dioxide in arterial blood ($PaCO_2$). The second goal of mechanical ventilation is to correct the hypoxemia and improve the tissue oxygen delivery.

The initiation of mechanical ventilatory support can be a time of patient instability. This may relate to the circumstances that necessitated the intubation and the institution of ventilatory support or the uncertainty of the initial ventilator parameters. Because of these concerns, my bias is using 100 percent oxygen as the fraction of inspired oxygen in the conditioned gas (FIO_2). Proper oxygenation of the patient's blood is usually assured by this maneuver. It also allows for the calculation of shunt fraction or venous admixture if that is desired. The short period of high oxygen tensions does no harm and provides the clinician with some peace of mind. Once the initial arterial blood gases are available, the FIO_2 can be tailored to more appropriately fit the individual patient's needs.

The initial rate should be set so as to achieve a minute ventilation ($\dot{V}E$) that will maintain a normal acid-base status. This rate is typically between 8 and 16 breaths per minute; however, it is important that the true goal be the attainment of the proper pH for the patient's metabolic needs. Patients who normally retain carbon dioxide should not receive ventilation to a $PaCO_2$ that is within the normal range, as doing so produces an alkalosis that may predispose the patient to cardiac arrhythmias and seizures and may eventually lead to weaning difficulties. Similarly, a patient who has a metabolic acidosis normally compensates with a respiratory alkalosis. If the pH is not used as a guideline and this patient instead receives ventilation to a normal $PaCO_2$, the end result will be an uncompensated metabolic acidosis. This initial rate recommendation is purely a guideline for the usual patient. Again, once the results of the initial arterial blood gas are available, the ventilator settings can be tailored to meet the individual patient's specific needs.

The initial V_T should be 10 to 12 ml per kilogram of body weight. A V_T greater than 15 ml per kilogram should be avoided since it is associated with an increased risk of pulmonary barotrauma. When a V_T greater than 8 ml per kilogram is used, it is not necessary to incorporate sighs into the ventilator management. Sighs were initially used to prevent the development of atelectasis. When used, a typical sigh volume is one and a half to two times the V_T, and the frequency is one to three sighs every 15 minutes or every 100 breaths, depending on the type of ventilator used.

The flow rate of the inspired gas and the inspiration/expiration (I/E) time should also be adjusted to achieve adequate airway pressures and ventilation. Flow rates that are too high may result in peak inflation pressures that are too high, and this may be an important determinant for the production of pulmonary barotrauma. Flow rates that are too low may increase the duration of inspiratory time at the expense of expiratory time and may not allow adequate time for expiration to occur. Under normal circumstances, expiratory time should be about twice as long as inspiratory time. If expiration has not been completed before the next inspiration takes place, the breaths may stack up on each other and produce elevations in the end-expiratory pressure. This phenomenon is termed auto PEEP, intrinsic PEEP, or occult PEEP. Auto PEEP typically occurs in patients with increased lung compliance (Cl) or increased airways resistance (Raw), when the time constant of the lung/airway (T.C. = Cl × Raw) is exceeded. When carefully evaluated, more than half of the patients receiving mechanical ventilatory support may exhibit auto PEEP.

MODES OF VENTILATION

One of the areas of controversy concerns the proper mode of ventilation to use in an individual patient. Several different modes of ventilation are currently available (Table 1), and a number of these modes can even be used in conjunction with one another, such as intermittent mandatory ventilation (IMV) with pressure support. In this chapter, the discussion of ventilator modes is limited to assist/control, synchronized intermittent mandatory ventilation (SIMV), and pressure support. The choice of a ventilator mode often reflects the clinician's biases and past experiences. Unfortunately, there is a paucity of well-controlled studies that actually compare the different modes in similar clinical situations and patients. It is therefore easy to understand the controversy surrounding the use of a given mode of ventilation in a certain clinical situation.

Table 1 Modes of Mechanical Ventilation*

Controlled ventilation
Assist/control
Intermittent mandatory ventilation
Synchronized intermittent mandatory ventilation
Continuous positive-pressure ventilation
Pressure support
Pressure-release ventilation
Mandatory minute ventilation
Continuous flow-by
Inverse ratio ventilation

*Some modes may be used in conjunction with one another (e.g., IMV with pressure support).

The assist/control mode delivers a preset V_T at a preset rate to the patient. Additionally, each time the patient generates a negative inspiratory pressure (usually -2 to -4 cm water), the ventilator delivers the preset V_T. This mode allows for controlling the patient's V_E when it is coupled with pharmacologic control (sedatives with/without paralyzing agents). My bias is usually to use this mode during the initiation of mechanical ventilatory support, especially if the patient has been sedated or is unstable hemodynamically. The assist/control mode is associated with less work of breathing compared with the IMV or SIMV modes. This permits the patient more rest, and less demand is placed on the cardiovascular system to deliver cardiac output to the muscles of respiration. Theoretically, this allows a greater percentage of the cardiac output to be available to the heart, brain, liver, and kidneys.

IMV delivers a preset V_T at a preset rate each minute, but the patient may take additional conditioned gas at his own rate and at his own V_T between the machine-delivered breaths. When SIMV is used, the machine tries to synchronize a machine-delivered breath with one of the patient's own inspiratory efforts. This is meant to be more comfortable for the patient and avoids the possibility of the machine breath being delivered immediately after the patient has taken a full inspiration. IMV was originally developed as a means of weaning the patient from mechanical ventilatory support, but has currently become popular as a mode of ventilatory support. Proponents of IMV argue that it is more comfortable for the patient and requires less use of sedatives. Since positive-pressure breaths are given only during the machine breath cycles, there is less potential cardiac depression from decreased venous return that may occur from the increase in intrathoracic pressure. The claims that IMV achieves better blood gases or decreases the time of mechanical ventilatory support have not been proven in well-controlled studies.

The realization that there was a significant work load placed on the patient in overcoming the resistance of the endotracheal tubing and the opening and closing of the various valves that regulate airflow from the ventilator led to the development of pressure-support ventilation. A selected amount of pressure can be applied to the conditioned gas that the patient can access during spontaneous breaths. This pressurized gas source helps offset the increased work load imposed by the physical impediments previously described. The patient is given the responsibility of setting his own V_T; however, increasing the amount of pressure support can help support patients who otherwise could not achieve the desired V_T. Again, we are hampered by a lack of well-controlled studies to support the use of pressure-support ventilation in a given clinical situation. It does appear that pressure-support ventilation is more comfortable for certain patients and is associated with the least work of breathing. Even patients receiving assist/control ventilation who are generating large negative inspiratory pressures before the ventilator can be triggered to deliver a V_T sufficient to turn off their inspiratory effort may be generating 25 to 50 percent of the work of breathing that would be produced during spontaneous respiration.

MAINTENANCE OF MECHANICAL VENTILATION

As stated, the goal of mechanical ventilation is to achieve adequate ventilation, oxygenation, and acid-base status. To help determine the adequacy of the mechanical ventilatory support, arterial blood gases (ABG) should be obtained periodically and adjustments should be made in accordance with the results. After a change is made, one usually waits 20 minutes before checking the ABG. This allows the various gases time to equilibrate in the majority of the alveoli in patients with ventilation/perfusion abnormalities. In those patients who are being treated with positive end-expiratory pressure (PEEP), the full benefit may not be achieved for several hours while the recruitment process occurs.

The adequacy of the ventilation and acid-base status are directly related to the alveolar ventilation which is being delivered to the patient. The alveolar ventilation ($\dot{V}_A$) is the net of the $\dot{V}_E$ minus the dead space ventilation (V_D). The $\dot{V}_E$ is the product of the tidal volume (V_T) and the respiratory rate. The $\dot{V}_E$ is proportional to the $\dot{V}_A$, and both are inversely proportional to the $PaCO_2$. These relationships can be utilized to help direct needed changes in the ventilator settings to obtain the desired ABGs through the use of the following equation:

$$\text{desired respiratory rate} = \text{initial rate} \times \frac{\text{initial } PaCO_2}{\text{desired } PaCO_2}$$

With large amounts of V_D, this approximation may not be as useful unless one takes into account the actual $\dot{V}_E$ needed to produce the desired change in $PaCO_2$. The amount of V_D can be calculated using the Enghoff modification of the Bohr equation:

$$\frac{V_D}{V_T} = \frac{PaCO_2 - P\bar{E}CO_2}{PaCO_2}$$

where $P\bar{E}CO_2$ is the partial pressure of carbon dioxide in mixed expired air. Some patients manifest an inappropriate respiratory alkalosis and overshoot the normal compensatory mechanisms, producing an alkalotic pH. This situation can potentiate cardiac arrhythmias and seizures, and if it persists, can also lead to difficulty weaning the patient from the mechanical ventilatory support when this becomes necessary. To correct this situation, you can sedate the patient to control the respiratory drive, add dead space to the ventilator tubing, or switch to an IMV, SIMV, or mandatory minute ventilation (MMV) mode of ventilation. There are instances when simply switching modes will not correct the problem, and the addition of extra dead space to the ventilator tubing can cause difficulties if the patient's breathing pattern changes in the future.

The patient's oxygenation status is assessed by the partial pressure of oxygen in arterial blood (PaO_2). Since the main objective of oxygenation is primarily the delivery of oxygen to the tissues, the goal is to obtain a PaO_2 that reflects a hemoglobin saturation of 90 percent. Tissue oxygen delivery is defined as the product of the cardiac output and the oxygen content of arterial blood ($DO_2 = Q_T \times CaO_2$). The CaO_2 is comprised of the oxygen bound to hemoglobin and the oxygen dissolved in blood ($CaO_2 = Hgb \times 1.34 \times SaO_2 + 0.003 \times PaO_2$). As can be seen from this equation, very little oxygen is dissolved in blood. The majority is carried bound to hemoglobin. It therefore becomes important to achieve adequate oxyhemoglobin saturation without the potential risk of oxygen toxicity from using too high an FIO_2. Little is known of the risks and consequences of a high FIO_2 in an injured lung, but in a normal healthy lung there appears to be some risk of oxygen toxicity associated with the prolonged use of an FIO_2 of greater than 50 percent. By using the least FIO_2 necessary to ensure adequate oxygen delivery to the tissues, one limits the possibility of oxygen toxicity.

A common method of determining the degree of oxygenation impairment is the calculation of the alveolar-arterial oxygen gradient [$D(A-a)O_2$] (Table 2). Unfortunately, this value is not FIO_2 independent and the gradient will be seen to widen as the FIO_2 is increased. The use of arterial/alveolar (a/A) ratio (PaO_2/PAO_2) is independent of the FIO_2. The normal value of the a/A is greater than or equal to 0.75. This value can be used to assess changes in oxygenation status as well as to assist with the tailoring of the FIO_2. Another method for evaluating the oxygenation abnormality is to calculate the shunt fraction or amount of venous admixture of the arterial blood (see Table 2).

POSITIVE END-EXPIRATORY PRESSURE

Patients with diffuse lung disease that requires a high FIO_2 may benefit from the addition of PEEP to their ventilatory support. The application of various levels of positive pressure at the end of expiration helps maintain the patency of the airways and alveoli. The radial traction

Table 2 Common Formulae Used to Monitor Mechanical Ventilation

$\dot{V}E = V_T \times Rate$

$\dot{V}E = \dot{V}_A + \dot{V}_D$

$\text{desired rate} = \text{initial rate} \times \dfrac{\text{initial PaCO}_2}{\text{desired PaCO}_2}$

$\dfrac{\dot{V}_D}{V_T} = \dfrac{PaCO_2 - P_ECO_2}{PaCO_2}$

$D(A\text{-}a)O_2 = P_AO_2 - PaO_2$

$P_AO_2 = P_IO_2 - \dfrac{PaCO_2}{R}$

$P_IO_2 = (P_B - P_{H_2O}) \times F_IO_2$

$P_AO_2 = P_IO_2 - PaCO_2 \left[F_IO_2 + \dfrac{1 - F_IO_2}{R} \right]$

The normal value of the $D(A\text{-}a)O_2 < \dfrac{age + 12}{4}$

$\dfrac{PaO_2}{P_AO_2} > 0.75$

$\dfrac{PaO_2i}{P_AO_2i} = \dfrac{PaO_2f}{P_AO_2f}$

$CaO_2 = SaO_2 \times Hgb \times 1.34 + PaO_2 \times 0.003$

$\dfrac{\dot{Q}s}{\dot{Q}_T} = \dfrac{C_IO_2 - CaO_2}{C_IO_2 - C\bar{v}O_2}$

---

forces from the PEEP distended and overly distended alveoli pull open collapsed and partially collapsed alveoli in a process called recruitment. The full recruitment effect from a certain level of PEEP is not manifested instantaneously, but requires several hours until the maximal effect is realized.

The major use of PEEP is in the support of the patient with diffuse parenchymal lung disease, such as noncardiogenic pulmonary edema. It is important to use PEEP in the setting of diffuse disease since it will otherwise be preferentially directed toward the relatively compliant normal lung tissue rather than toward the stiffer, noncompliant diseased lung. The end result is the misappropriation of ventilation and perfusion with the normal compliant alveoli receiving the majority of the ventilation with little perfusion, and with the diseased alveoli receiving the majority of the perfusion with little ventilation. This ventilation/perfusion imbalance can actually result in a worsening of oxygenation and ventilation.

The potential benefits of the addition of PEEP include an increase in functional residual capacity, an increase in pulmonary compliance, decreased dead space ventilation, decreased shunt fraction, and the ability to maintain adequate oxygenation using a less toxic F_IO_2. There is speculation that PEEP may help conserve alveolar sur-

factant and improve its function. PEEP also has several proponents asserting that it has a beneficial as a form of prophylaxis for the development of the adult respiratory distress syndrome (ARDS); however, a well-controlled clinical study has not substantiated these claims.

Unfortunately, the use of PEEP is also associated with several potential adverse effects. As previously mentioned, PEEP may actually worsen oxygenation and ventilation when used inappropriately. The positive pressure of the intrathoracic region can impair venous return and decrease the filling pressure (preload) of the right ventricle. This can result in a decrease in the cardiac output. Cardiac output is the other major component of tissue oxygen delivery, and its decrease can negate any benefit of improved oxygenation. PEEP can also increase the right ventricular afterload, shift the interventricular septum to the left altering the compliance characteristics of both ventricles, decrease myocardial blood flow, and decrease left ventricular afterload. The use of PEEP can potentiate cerebral edema by decreasing venous drainage from the head. PEEP is also associated with an increased incidence of pulmonary barotrauma.

PEEP is still one of the primary supportive measures employed in patients with ARDS. Unfortunately, there is no consensus on the amount of PEEP to apply and the proper parameter by which to judge its therapeutic effect. Some advocate giving enough PEEP to produce an arterial oxygen percent saturation (SaO_2) greater than 90 percent on 50 percent F_IO_2. Others would titrate the PEEP to reduce the shunt fraction to less than 15 percent or to provide maximal improvement in lung compliance. My own bias is to use PEEP to obtain adequate tissue oxygen delivery using less toxic F_IO_2, preferably an F_IO_2 of 50 percent or less.

MONITORING

It is impossible to overemphasize the importance of properly trained personnel caring for patients who require mechanical ventilatory support. Adverse occurrences are fairly frequent and can have disastrous consequences. Mechanically ventilated patients may have hemodynamic instability or may be treated with sedatives and even paralyzing agents. These patients should be cared for in an intensive care unit or special care unit where they can be observed by specially trained personnel and monitored as needed.

Included in the proper monitoring of mechanically ventilated patients is the physical examination of the patient and evaluation of the clinical data. It is advisable to monitor the electrocardiogram in these patients. My bias is to obtain a daily chest x-ray film, especially if the patient has an endotracheal tube in place. It is important to know the location of the various tubes and vascular catheters that are inserted in these acutely ill patients. It is also of importance to be able to detect changes—either improvement or worsening of old processes—as well as new, unsuspected abnormalities.

As previously stated, the ABG is the mainstay of monitoring the adequacy of the oxygenation, ventilation, and acid-base status of these patients. No other test yields as much information. Unfortunately, ABGs are invasive, are associated with potential morbidity, are often expensive, and are associated with some delay in the reporting of results. Attempts are currently underway to monitor continuous ABG data using intra-arterial electrodes. The oxygenation status of the patient can be assessed using noninvasive monitors such as pulse oximeters and transcutaneous, conjunctival, and tissue oxygen tension monitors. The pulse oximeters have been well accepted in clinical medicine. They are easy to use, reliable, portable, noninvasive, and cost-effective monitors. They continuously display the oxygen saturation and, in the majority of circumstances, have good correlation with the SaO_2 as measured by co-oximetry.

The noninvasive assessment of carbon dioxide (CO_2) has not been as successful as the evaluation of the oxygenation status. The mixed expired CO_2, end-tidal CO_2, and the transcutaneous CO_2 tension can all be monitored. The end-tidal CO_2 ($P_{ET}CO_2$) has been the most widely used noninvasive method in adult medicine and does seem to correlate fairly well in the normal patient, as in its use as an operating or recovery room monitor. However, in critically ill patients with ventilation and/or perfusion abnormalities there is frequently poor correlation between the $P_{ET}CO_2$ and the $PaCO_2$.

It is also useful to monitor the physiologic changes that occur during the use of mechanical ventilatory support (Table 3). These include the ventilator parameters, compliance curves, airway resistance, and changes in oxygenation, ventilation, dead space ventilation, and shunt fraction. The detection of occult PEEP is useful to avoid its potential detrimental effects on hemodynamic function and lung volume. The monitoring of weaning parameters can also give information concerning changes in pulmonary function.

COMPLICATIONS

Mechanical ventilatory support is typically instituted in critically ill patients who are at risk for a variety of potential complications. Some of the more common complications and adverse events occurring in patients receiving supported ventilation are listed in Table 4. Attention should be directed to the prevention, identification, and treatment of these adverse sequelae as early as possible. Although this chapter does not specifically address each of these situations, there are several thorough reviews and studies that can be consulted for more detailed information.

It is my practice to treat all mechanically ventilated patients with "mini-dose" heparin for deep venous thrombosis and pulmonary embolism prophylaxis unless there is a contraindication to heparin use or the patient requires full-scale anticoagulation for some specific entity. I am also an advocate of stress ulcer prophylaxis with either

Table 3 Physiologic Monitors of Mechanical Ventilation

Ventilator parameters
   V_T
   Rate
   FiO_2
   I/E
   Peak and plateau pressure
Compliance
   Dynamic characteristic
   Static (plateau)
Airway Resistance
Occult PEEP
ABG
D(A-a) O_2
PaO_2/PAO_2
V_D/V_T
$\dot{Q}_S/\dot{Q}_T$
Weaning parameters

Table 4 Complications Associated With Mechanical Ventilation

Pulmonary complications
   Pulmonary emboli and deep venous thrombosis
   Pulmonary barotrauma
   Complications of endotracheal tube and tracheostomy tubes
   Complications associated with invasive monitoring
   Complications associated with ventilator malfunction or human error

Cardiovascular complications
   Decreased cardiac output
   Hypotension
   Arrhythmias

Gastrointestinal complications
   Stress ulceration and gastrointestinal bleeding
   Gastric distention
   Ileus
   Pneumoperitoneum

Renal complications
   Renal failure
   Fluid retention
   Hyponatremia

Infectious complications
   Nosocomial pneumonia
   Sepsis

Hematologic complications
   Anemia
   Thrombocytopenia
   Disseminated intravascular coagulation

Nutritional complications
Endocrine abnormalities
Hepatic abnormalities
Neurologic abnormalities
   Intensive care unit psychosis
   Altered mentation
   Critical illness polyneuropathy

H₂ receptor antagonists or cytoprotective agents as opposed to antacid therapy. The use of continuous enteral nutrition to prevent stress ulceration has been suggested, but it needs to be confirmed by further study. This approach may be preferential, since the provision of adequate and appropriate nutritional support is important for the preservation of respiratory muscle function. If this aspect is ignored, difficulty with weaning may be encountered.

In patients treated with mechanical ventilation, the incidence of pulmonary barotrauma is estimated to be 5 to 15 percent. The production of barotrauma is probably related to high inflation pressures with the subsequent rupture of small alveoli. The incidence is highest when volume-cycled ventilators are used with high inflation volumes ($V_T > 15$ ml per kilogram) and in patients with necrotic pulmonary infections or after acid aspiration.

Because of the various technologic advances over the past few decades and the improvement in our abilities to provide adequate patient support, two of the major causes for death in critically ill patients are now multiple systems organ failure (MSOF) and nosocomial infection. Patients requiring ventilatory support fall into the high-risk group for both of these disorders. It becomes an important part of the care plan to ensure that organ system function is preserved, and maintaining an adequate cardiac output and proper tissue oxygen delivery become paramount goals to ensure that MSOF does not develop. Careful attention to sterile technique and proper infection control measures help prevent nosocomial infections.

Once the patient's condition has stabilized and the process that necessitated the use of ventilatory support has improved sufficiently to allow the patient to support his own spontaneous respirations, the patient should be weaned from the mechanical ventilator. A variety of weaning strategies are available, and there are an equal number of controversies concerning the weaning process. Fortunately, the great majority of patients are weaned with little difficulty regardless of the weaning strategy used. The process of weaning from mechanical ventilatory support is addressed in greater detail in a subsequent chapter of this text.

SUGGESTED READING

Groeger JS, Levinson MR, Carlon GC. Assist control versus synchronized intermittent mandatory ventilation during acute respiratory failure. Crit Care Med 1989; 17:607–612.
MacIntyre NR. New forms of mechanical ventilation in the adult. Clin Chest Med 1988; 9:47–54.
Pingleton SK. Complications of acute respiratory failure. Am Rev Respir Dis 1988; 137:1463–1493.
Plummer AL, Gracey DR. Consensus conference on artificial airways in patients receiving mechanical ventilation. Chest 1989; 96:136–138.
Powner DJ. Pulmonary barotrauma in the intensive care unit. J Intens Care Med 1988; 3:224–232.
Schuster DP. A physiologic approach to initiating, maintaining, and withdrawing mechanical ventilatory support during acute respiratory failure. Am J Med 1990; 88:268–278.

BEDSIDE EVALUATION OF RESPIRATORY FUNCTION

DANIEL P. SCHUSTER

The major goal of any bedside evaluation of respiratory function is to evaluate the ability and efficiency of the lungs to achieve acceptable oxygen absorption and carbon dioxide elimination. In addition, inextricably linked to this gas exchange function of the lung is the ability of the entire respiratory system (including components of the central and peripheral nervous system, diaphragm, and other respiratory muscles, chest wall, and lung parenchyma) to serve as a ventilatory pump, providing the necessary energy and work to move air in and out of the chest for the purpose of gas exchange.

Ultimately, the onset of respiratory failure is marked by the failure to meet the normal homeostatic goals of gas exchange—that is, a failure either to fully oxygenate the circulating mass of hemoglobin or to eliminate enough carbon dioxide to maintain normal acid-base balance. The goal of monitoring respiratory function is to diagnose impending failure in a timely fashion and to evaluate responses to treatment so that they may be properly adjusted.

NEW TECHNOLOGIES

In addition to the traditional methods of evaluating respiratory function (e.g., physical examination, arterial blood gases), several new technologies have recently been introduced which have already had a significant impact on standard practice. Three important examples include pulse oximetry, carbon dioxide (CO_2) capnography, and respiratory inductance plethysmography.

The most dramatic example is pulse oximetry. In general, oximetry refers to those techniques used to estimate the fractional oxygen saturation of hemoglobin. These techniques are based on the fact that maximum light absorption by the different hemoglobin species (e.g., reduced hemoglobin, oxygen-saturated hemoglobin, methemoglobin) as well as by various tissues occurs at different wavelengths of light. Unlike conventional oximetry, however, pulse oximetry does not require a separate wavelength of light for each type of hemoglobin or tissue. Instead, only two wavelengths of light are needed, given the additional assumption that any pulsatile change in light absorption is specifically caused by the effects of arterialized blood. Oxyhemoglobin saturation is actually calculated from the ratio of pulse-added light absorbance at each of the two wavelengths of light. This ratio is then converted into an estimate of saturation using an empirically derived nomogram. (The calculation also assumes, sometimes incorrectly, that the only hemoglobin species present are reduced and oxyhemoglobin.) This innovation eliminates any need to "arterialize" the portion of skin being examined to eliminate effects of venous blood, and it also eliminates any need for bedside calibration, since there is little interindividual variation in the light-absorbing effects of blood per se.

The accuracy of pulse oximetry is approximately ± 3 to 5 percent at true saturations greater than 70 percent (recall that a hemoglobin saturation of 70 percent corresponds to an arterial oxygen pressure (PaO_2) of about 38 mm Hg at a normal pH and temperature). Its accuracy clearly falls off in the presence of significant amounts of carboxy- or methemoglobin. Jaundice apparently has little effect. Because the technique depends on pulse detection, low cardiac output states—especially with peripheral vasoconstriction—can be associated with inaccurate readings or even the inability to produce a reading at all. In general, if an accurate heart rate is recorded by the device, the arterial saturation calculation is also likely to be correct.

A second important technique, not actually very new but still underutilized, is that of CO_2 capnography. In general, this technique is most easily and accurately accomplished in the intubated patient. The actual measurement of end-tidal CO_2 concentration can be made with mass spectrometry or more cheaply with infrared methods. In normal individuals, the end-tidal CO_2 correlates closely with the mean alveolar CO_2 and the arterial-alveolar CO_2 gradient is less than 5 mm Hg. This gradient increases in patients with ventilation-perfusion mismatching, increased physiologic dead space, or changes in hemodynamics. As long as these confounding factors are stable, however, a rising end-tidal CO_2 can be assumed to indicate progressive alveolar hypoventilation and a rising arterial CO_2 partial pressure (PcO_2). Indeed, since the end-tidal CO_2 value is always less than that of the arterial CO_2, a high value for the end-tidal CO_2 virtually always indicates hypercapnea. Thus, although the *initial* end-tidal CO_2 in a recently intubated patient may be difficult to interpret, an *increasing* end-tidal CO_2 in an otherwise stable patient (e.g., during a trial of weaning from mechanical ventilation) usually indicates progressive hypercapnia, which can then be verified by direct arterial blood gas analysis.

The infrared probes used to measure exhaled CO_2 can either be placed in the mainstream of the exhaled gas or can be sidestream analyzers. (Although it is possible to also sample pharyngeal gas in nonintubated patients, this is still used most commonly in patients requiring mechanical ventilatory support.) Unfortunately, the sidestream analyzers often malfunction because of aspirated secretions. The mainstream analyzers, on the other hand, are heavier and add additional dead space to the system tubing.

It is important to keep several points in mind when interpreting capnographic measurements. Because considerable breath-to-breath variability is common, an end-tidal CO_2 value averaged over a reasonable period of time (several minutes) is usually more valid than a single breath value. The entire capnographic tracing should also be inspected. If the tracing fails to reach a plateau, as is common during rapid, shallow breathing or with significant obstructive airway disease, the arterial end-tidal CO_2 gradient widens, even without a significant change in underlying lung disease. Again, as is so common in all types of monitoring, a trend analysis is more valuable than a single isolated value.

Finally, many new monitoring units include modules for continuous measurement of respiratory rate by changes in chest wall impedance. Since the first evidence of impending respiratory failure is often an increase in the respiratory rate, such monitoring offers an easy, objective, continuous, and relatively cheap means of monitoring. A more elegant approach is that of respiratory inductance plethysmography, in which wire coils are strapped around the chest and abdomen. Changes in cross-sectional area cause the electrical impedance to change, and this can be used to calculate the respiratory rate, tidal volume, and the interaction of chest wall and abdomen. Thus it is possible to evaluate the onset of respiratory alternans and paradoxical breathing with this technique. Since these signs sometimes precede hypercapnea, monitoring for their occurrence may be valuable when difficult patients with chronic lung disease are weaned from mechanical ventilatory support.

MONITORING FOR IMPENDING RESPIRATORY FAILURE

A wide variety of techniques are now available for evaluating respiratory function at the bedside (Table 1). In the routine clinical setting, however, many are difficult to apply or interpret. In the nonintubated patient at risk for acute respiratory failure, this evaluation still begins with insightful observations by the physician and nurse.

Physical signs of hypoxemia (e.g., cyanosis, tachycardia, mental status changes) and of hypercapnia (e.g., central nervous system depression, headache) are well known to be poorly sensitive and nonspecific. Still, when present and especially when linked to appropriate historical information, arterial blood gases must be measured to verify the presence and severity of the gas exchange defect.

The diagnosis of acute respiratory failure still depends on arterial blood gas documentation of hypoxemia or hypercapnia. Although a PaO_2 less than 40 to 50 mm Hg despite supplemental oxygen is almost always an absolute indication for endotracheal intubation, hypercapnia requires more clinical judgment. Even though hypercapnia

Table 1 Techniques for Bedside Evaluation of Respiratory Function

Usefulness of Technique	Gas Exchange			Work Load			Capacity		
	Endpoint Variables	Efficiency	Metabolic Activity	External Load/Performance	Strength	Breathing Patterns	Ventilatory Drive	Reserve	
Routinely useful	Arterial blood gases Pulse oximetry Capnography	P_aO_2/F_iO_2 P_aO_2/P_AO_2		Minute ventilation (V_E) Airway pressures Peak Intrinsic PEEP	Vital capacity MIP	Rate Tidal volume	$\dot{V}_E$ Rate	Signs of stress (paradox, alternans, tachypnea) Acces. mm use	
Occasionally useful	Mixed venous oximetry	$P(A\text{-}a)O_2$ $\dot{Q}_S/\dot{Q}_T$ V_D/V_T	Oxygen consumption CO_2 production	Compliance					
Usefulness uncertain	Transcutaneous PO_2 Transconjunctival PO_2 Transcutaneous P_{CO_2}		Diaphragm electromyogram (EMG)	Work-of-breathing Pressure-time product Transdiaphragmatic pressure (Pdi) Esophageal manometry Airway resistance Inflation impedance	Pdi_{MAX}	T_i/T_{TOT}	T_i/T_{TOT} EMG $P_{0.1}$	EMG Tension-time index	

Acces. mm = accessory muscles of respiration; EMG = electromyography; MIP = maximum inspiratory pressure; $\dot{Q}_S/\dot{Q}_T$ = intrapulmonary shunt fraction; T_i/T_{TOT} = inspiratory time fraction of total respiratory cycle; $P_{0.1}$ = inspiratory airway pressure generated after 0.1 second.
Adapted from Marini JJ. Monitoring during mechanical ventilation. Clin Chest Med 1988; 9:73–100.

leads to respiratory acidosis and mental status changes, these alone are rarely life threatening. Nor does acidemia by itself necessarily imply acute failure, since some acidemia is also common with severe *chronic* hypercapnia, because few patients are able to retain sufficient bicarbonate to normalize arterial pH if the arterial CO_2 pressure ($PaCO_2$) is greater than 60 to 70 mm Hg, in the absence of a forced diuresis, gastric suctioning, or vomiting.

Progressive hypercapnia (and acidosis), however, are important harbingers of impending central nervous system depression, additional alveolar hypoventilation, apnea, and finally, hypoxemia. Hypercapnia with acidemia is a signal that the patient is unable to excrete CO_2 effectively, whatever the reason. Further deterioration is likely to occur rapidly and is important because little additional ventilatory reserve is present. By contrast, hypercapnia alone, *without* acidemia or central nervous system depression, is rarely sufficient reason to initiate mechanical ventilatory support.

Hypoxemia in the hypercapnic but spontaneously breathing patient presents a special problem. Worsening hypercapnia and CO_2-narcosis after oxygen administration to hypoxemic, hypercapnic patients with chronic obstructive pulmonary disease (COPD) is a well-known sequence. Although hypoxic ventilatory drive may be inhibited by administration of oxygen, worsening ventilation-perfusion matching resulting from the release of hypoxic vasoconstriction may actually be a more common cause for the increase in CO_2 retention. In some cases, the association is undoubtedly temporal and not causal, as respiratory muscle fatigue develops despite initial therapy. Acidosis (pH < 7.30) and hypoxemia on admission are more important as risk factors for eventual mechanical ventilatory support than the $PaCO_2$ per se. Regardless of the mechanism, however, relatively few patients with hypercapnia actually develop CO_2 narcosis if hypoxemia is relieved with *controlled* oxygen therapy (e.g., 2 to 4 L per minute of nasal oxygen, Venti-masks, or controlled oxygen via high-humidity systems).

Finger pulse oximetry, with continuously monitored arterial oxygen saturation, allows the fraction of inspired oxygen (FIO_2) to be titrated with additional safety. Supplemental oxygen can be quickly titrated to achieve an arterial saturation of more than 85 to 90 percent ($PaO_2 > 55$ mm Hg). If this degree of saturation cannot be achieved without worsening hypercapnea *and* respiratory acidosis (as documented by arterial blood gases), then tracheal intubation and mechanical ventilatory support must be initiated.

Mechanical ventilatory assistance should also be initiated if the work required for the maintenance of adequate gas exchange is greater than that which can be sustained indefinitely, even if gas exchange is still satisfactory. Unfortunately, it is difficult to quantify with accuracy an "excessive" work-of-breathing. Clinical clues include tachycardia, diaphoresis, accessory respiratory muscle use, a widened paradoxical pulse, a distressed facial expression, and a respiratory rate of more than 30 to 35 breaths per minute. When a combination of these signs are present, intubation and mechanical ventilatory assistance are usually required, unless the underlying cause (e.g., bronchospasm or, occasionally, heart failure) can be rapidly reversed.

MONITORING DURING MECHANICAL VENTILATION

Ensuring adequate gas exchange is, of course, the first priority during mechanical ventilation. Traditionally, this has been accomplished with intermittent arterial blood gas analyses. More recently, as described above, it has become possible to monitor gas exchange continuously, using a combination of pulse oximetry and CO_2 capnography, within the limits of each technology. It is likely that as each of these technologies becomes incorporated into monitoring equipment, they will become part of routine and standard practice. Although the monitoring of trends and changes with these technologies is unquestionably valuable, significantly reducing the number of needed arterial blood gas analyses, it is still necessary to measure periodically the partial pressure of oxygen (PO_2) and PCO_2 directly.

The arterial PO_2 and PCO_2 are *endpoints* for gas exchange. However, to evaluate and interpret changes in these partial pressures or to evaluate the *efficiency* of gas exchange, additional information is required. The alveolar-arterial PO_2 gradient (or difference) is often used for this purpose; the arterial-alveolar PO_2 *ratio* (a/A ratio) is actually a better measure, since it is less sensitive to changes in FIO_2. Calculation of the intrapulmonary venous admixture or shunt is another means of quantifying the efficiency of oxygenation. However, this measurement requires data obtained from invasive hemodynamic monitoring. Although frequently such data are available, it is not clear that a venous admixture calculation is necessary for appropriate management of the patient with acute respiratory failure, since clinical algorithms based on this measurement have never been shown to be uniquely useful. In a similar manner, the efficiency of CO_2 excretion can be quantified by the calculation of the physiologic dead space to tidal volume ratio (V_D/V_T). This requires the collection of an accurate mixed exhaled PCO_2 over time, still a cumbersome process. Furthermore, the *clinical* utility of this measurement has also never been established.

The measurement of airway pressure is especially important during mechanical ventilation. High peak airway pressures (>45 cm H_2O) are a significant risk factor for barotrauma during mechanical ventilation. Barotrauma is apparently less common with peak airway pressures of less than 40 to 45 cm H_2O. Other factors, such as the underlying disease, may be equally important, but are not as easy to quantify.

The *peak* airway pressure is determined by both respiratory system compliance and airways resistance, which in turn determine the so-called "dynamic characteristic" (simply the V_T divided by the peak airway pressure). The normal dynamic characteristic is at least 50 ml per centimeter of H_2O, and is reduced by at least half in cases of severe lung disease, such as the adult respiratory distress syndrome. Therefore, a "normal" tidal volume (i.e., used during spontaneous breathing) of 5 to 7 ml per kilogram should generate about 7 to 10 cm H_2O pressure during mechanical ventilation.

Theoretically, when airways resistance alone elevates the peak airway pressure, the lung parenchyma distal to the resistance is relatively protected by the pressure drop across the resistance. To determine the contribution of airway resistance to the peak airway pressure, exhalation can be momentarily stopped immediately after the V_T is delivered ("plateau pressure"). For proper interpretation, a regular respiratory pattern at a relatively slow rate is required in a reasonably relaxed cooperative patient. Unfortunately, this combination is often not present. Furthermore, any interpretation of these static and dynamic contributions to the peak airway pressure is complicated by regional variations in lung compliance and airways resistance. Thus the peak airway pressure is still the most easily obtained, clinically valid, and interpretable airway pressure variable, and the tidal volume should be adjusted to keep the peak airway pressure, if possible, below about 45 cm H_2O.

While peak airway pressure is related to the development of barotrauma, arterial hypotension is related to the *mean* airway pressure via a decrease in either venous return or right ventricular function. Mean airway pressure is the time-integral of airway pressure. It *increases* with decreased respiratory system compliance, increased airways resistance of V_T, rapid breathing rates, the use of machine positive end-expiratory pressure (PEEP), and inspiratory flow rates or patterns that contribute to "intrinsic" PEEP.

Respiratory rate and PEEP (both intrinsic and extrinsic) have perhaps the greatest effect of mean airway pressure. Breathing frequency, together with V_T and inspiratory flow rate, determine the inspiratory/expiratory time (I/E) ratio, which has an important but often unappreciated effect on the development of so-called "auto" or "intrinsic" PEEP. With intrinsic PEEP, distal airway pressures are positive at end exhalation (sometimes >15 cm H_2O), even though the machine's proximal airway pressure manometer indicates zero pressure. Intrinsic PEEP probably represents very low flow through obstructed airways, related to the well-known problem of "air-trapping," and is compounded by ventilation through narrow endotracheal tubes. Significant airway obstruction, rapid respiratory rates, slow inspiratory flow rates, and relatively equal I/E ratios all tend to produce intrinsic PEEP. The largest V_T possible without excessive peak airway pressures, the slowest respiratory rate consistent with effective CO_2 elimination, and inspiratory flow rates fast enough to decrease the I/E ratio all minimize the development of intrinsic PEEP, as all allow a longer expiratory time. To measure intrinsic PEEP, the expiratory port of the ventilator must be occluded just before the next inhalation and often the patient must be sedated or paralyzed. Instead, it is often more practical simply to recognize the situations that promote the development of intrinsic PEEP.

MONITORING DURING WEANING

Various weaning parameters have been used to judge progress and to predict the potential for eventual success in weaning patients from mechanical ventilatory support. Those most commonly employed are respiratory rate, minute ventilation during spontaneous breathing, vital capacity, and maximum inspiratory force. However, when applied to patients, in actual practice these parameters are unfortunately both nonspecific and insensitive as predictors of weaning success. In some cases, part of the problem is the difficulty in making these measurements with accuracy. Patient cooperation is particularly difficult to ensure. Techniques to improve accuracy despite a lack of patient cooperation have been published, but they still do not replace the effort generated by a cooperative patient. Still, some useful information can be gathered by measuring these variables. A spontaneous, mechanically unassisted minute ventilation of less than 10 L per minute with a respiratory rate of less than 25 to 30 breaths per minute implies that a relatively low level of respiratory work is needed to maintain adequate gas exchange. A vital capacity of greater than 10 ml per kilogram and a maximum inspiratory pressure more negative than $^-25$ cm H_2O may be useful as indices of respiratory muscle strength, but may also predict the potential for effective coughing (often critical to successful extubation). Patients who consistently achieve these goals during periods of unassisted ventilation have a high likelihood of remaining extubated. Failure to meet these goals has less predictive value because of the issue of patient cooperation.

SUGGESTED READING

Grum CM, Chauncey JB. Conventional mechanical ventilation. Clin Chest Med 1988; 9:37–46.
Grum CM, Morgenroth ML. Initiating mechanical ventilation. J Intens Care Med 1988; 3:6–20.
Marini JJ. Monitoring during mechanical ventilation. Clin Chest Med 1988; 9:73–100.
McGough EK, Boysen PG. Benefits and limitations of pulse oximetry in the ICU. J Crit Illness 1989; 4:23–31.
Morgenroth ML, Grum CM. Weaning from mechanical ventilation. J Intens Care Med 1988; 3:109–120.
Schuster DP. A physiologic approach to initiating, maintaining, and withdrawing mechanical ventilatory support during acute respiratory failure. Am J Med 1990; 88:268–278.

ECHOCARDIOGRAPHY

PHILIP R. LIEBSON, M.D.

SCOPE AND TECHNIQUE

Echocardiography is a versatile, comprehensive, noninvasive diagnostic tool for determining the structure and function of the pericardium and cardiac chambers and valves, and evaluating the proximal aorta, pulmonary artery, and inferior vena cava. Echocardiographic instrumentation has progressed to the extent that a portable machine can combine the techniques of M-mode and two-dimensional (2-D) echocardiography with pulse wave (PW), continuous wave (CW), and realtime color Doppler capabilities, using either a transthoracic or transesophageal approach. Although there are standard echocardiographic views, the tomographic planes which may be evaluated by echocardiography are infinite. Unlike radionuclide angiography, cineangiography, and chest radiography, which superimpose three-dimensional cardiac data into one plane, the tomographic visualization of echocardiography allows analysis of specific portions of cardiac structures, sometimes in minute detail.

Echocardiography is accomplished with a transducer which is placed either directly onto the surface of the body or at the tip of a transesophageal catheter. Two applications of ultrasonographic reflection are evaluated. M-mode and 2-D techniques apply short pulses of ultrasonographic energy generated by the transducer, traveling into the body and reflecting back to the transducer from acoustic interfaces. An electronic image is generated that provides either an ice pick image through the depth of a cardiac structure (M-mode) or a sector scan (2-D). Alternatively, by analyzing the change in ultrasonographic frequency when ultrasonographic waves bounce off moving red blood cells and return to the transducer (Doppler effect), one can assess the velocity direction of blood flow. PW Doppler allows range resolution but is limited in the assessment of peak velocities of flow in a given location. CW Doppler allows analysis of peak velocity but is spatially ambiguous. These techniques therefore complement each other in blood flow analysis.

M-mode is useful for determining changes in motion within brief periods, since approximately 1,000 impulses are analyzed per second. It can demonstrate fine motion of the mitral valve and ventricular walls, which may be used for timing of events. 2-D scans are actually M-mode studies swept rapidly through a sector, providing a frame or sector scan with each sweep. Each frame takes approximately 30 to 60 msec to complete, so that for any specific location, far fewer samples are taken per second than for an isolated M-mode study. An M-mode or 2-D image is enhanced when the beam is perpendicular to an acoustic interface. This allows the beam to reflect directly back to the transducer. A Doppler velocity is maximal when the beam passes parallel to the motion of blood flow. The standard views for M-mode and 2-D echocardiography are therefore not necessarily the best views for assessing maximal blood flow. The comprehensive images of real-time color Doppler now save considerable time in providing information about the best location for placing the PW and CW Doppler beams for more definitive analysis of blood flow patterns. PW Doppler is useful for demonstrating the spatial velocity profiles of normal valves and mapping regurgitant lesions. CW evaluates high velocity in stenosis and regurgitation. A small stand-alone CW transducer (nonimaging) can be used in the suprasternal notch for evaluating aortic flow, and has an excellent signal-noise ratio.

M-mode studies are obtained from the real-time 2-D sector scan on the machine, using a cursor on the video 2-D image to position the M-mode study. Similarly, a cursor from the 2-D video image can be used to direct the CW or PW Doppler beam. A spatial map of blood flow is accomplished using a real-time color Doppler scan superimposed on the 2-D image.

The ultrasonographic beam moves best through muscle and tends to be markedly absorbed as it moves through bone or scattered as it moves through air. The optimal view for evaluation is therefore through muscle rather than through bone or cartilage. Consequently, thoracic echocardiographic windows are limited. Standard views for echocardiographic study that allow windows include the left parasternal interspaces, usually the third or fourth, the left side of the chest slightly inferior to the apex beat, the epigastric area just below the xiphoid process, and the suprasternal notch area. Occasionally other views are used. For example, with a large pleural effusion, right parasternal views and left posterior chest views can sometimes be used to visualize the heart.

Transesophageal echocardiography (TEE) uses a transducer fixed to the tip of a modified flexible gastroscope without fiberoptics. The transducer is located either in the high gastric area or lower esophagus, allowing superb visualization of the descending thoracic aorta in the left side of the heart. Because the transducer is so close to the surfaces that are to be visualized, higher-frequency transducers can be used to allow better resolution than that provided by transthoracic echocardiography. TEE is particularly useful if the geometry of the chest prevents adequate transthoracic visualization. This might occur in patients with pulmonary emphysema or chest cage abnormalities, with the use of chest dressings, or even during procedures undertaken simultaneously (on the chest) such as external cardiac massage. TEE appears to be especially helpful in the assessment of mitral and aortic prosthetic valve function. For example, although heavy echoes from a prosthetic mitral valve obscure Doppler flow patterns in the transthoracic position, the recent developments of biplane (longitudinal and transverse) transducers and CW probe capabilities in TEE promise to increase considerably the range and resolution of this approach.

When an echocardiogram is being ordered in a critical care unit, it is important that the echocardiographer or technician understand the precise reason for the study.

Because a multiplicity of tomographic views and flow patterns can be obtained, the echocardiographic evaluation must be directed at a specific question. This allows the most efficient examination, especially under circumstances in which rapid diagnosis is needed. The use of mechanical ventilators, especially with positive end-expiratory pressure, decreases the transthoracic echo window considerably.

It is helpful to have a portable machine stored in the critical care area for easy access, but if this is not possible, every effort should be made to have an instrument stored in area within 15 minutes' distance of the patient's bed. Echocardiography can be performed at the bedside. In anticipation of such a study, it is helpful to clear the area on the left side of the bed, since the most efficient examination is made with the machine and technician on the patient's left, with the patient in the left lateral cubitus position. An echocardiographic examination may take as long as 1 hour, depending on the specific reason for the evaluation and the ease with which the cardiac structures are visualized. In anticipation of the study, it is also helpful to move any leads from the left parasternal or apical areas of the chest and to free up redundant dressings in the parasternal area. The echocardiographic evaluation is recorded on either a videotape or a strip chart recorder. The latter is useful for the evaluation of the M-mode study and calculation of some of the Doppler flow determinations. With the increasing use of on-line calculations during examination, it is less likely that strip chart recordings will be needed in the future.

Echocardiography can be used for (1) emergent or urgent critical situations; (2) obtaining definitive diagnostic information; and (3) obtaining prognostic information (Table 1). Emergency echocardiography in a critical care unit is useful for the diagnosis of the following problems: (1) acute hypotension, (2) chest pain, (3) acute dyspnea or heart failure, (4) syncope, (5) new neurologic deficiencies, (6) new auscultatory findings, and (7) acute clinical deterioration. Echocardiography provides specific information with regard to (1) ventricular dysfunction, (2) cardiac tamponade or pericardial constriction, (3) complication of myocardial infarction, (4) acute valvular dysfunction, (5) prosthetic valve dysfunction, (6) vegetation or myocardial abscess, (7) thoracic aortic dissection, (8) source of embolus, (9) myocardial contusion or laceration, and (10) intracardiac tumors.

EMERGENCIES AND URGENCIES

Pericardial Tamponade and Constriction

Echocardiographic evaluation is highly sensitive and specific for the presence and severity of a pericardial effusion (Fig. 1). In addition, the finding of sudden inward diastolic motion of the anterior wall of the right ventricle in early diastole or of the right atrium in late diastole suggests the presence of pericardial tamponade (Fig. 2). With increasing severity of tamponade, the inward diastolic mo-

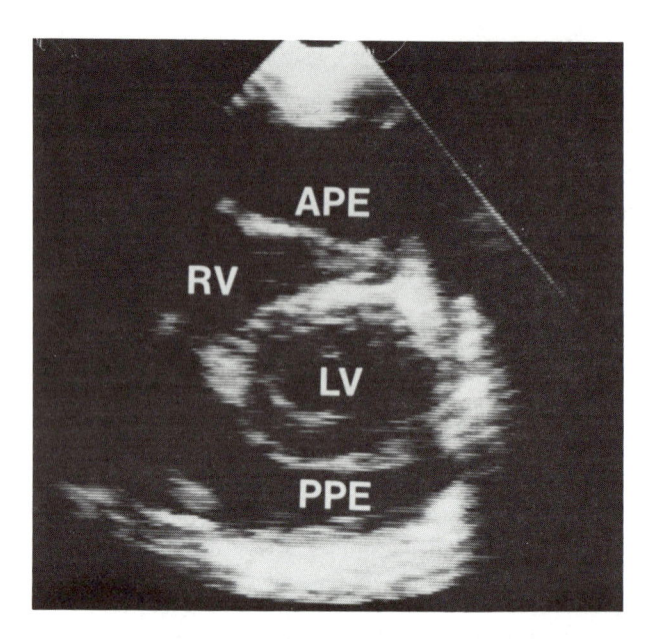

Figure 1 Two-dimensional study of large pericardial effusion. APE = anterior pericardial effusion; LV = cross-section view of left ventricle; PPE = posterior pericardial effusion; RV = right ventricle. Republished with permission from Liebson PR. What echocardiography can tell you about dyspnea. J Respir Dis 1986; 7:35–45.

tion may be seen first in the right atrial wall, then in the right ventricular inflow tract wall, and then in the right ventricular outflow tract wall. Doppler study aids in the diagnosis by demonstrating an exaggerated inspiratory increase in tricuspid and pulmonary flow velocities and an

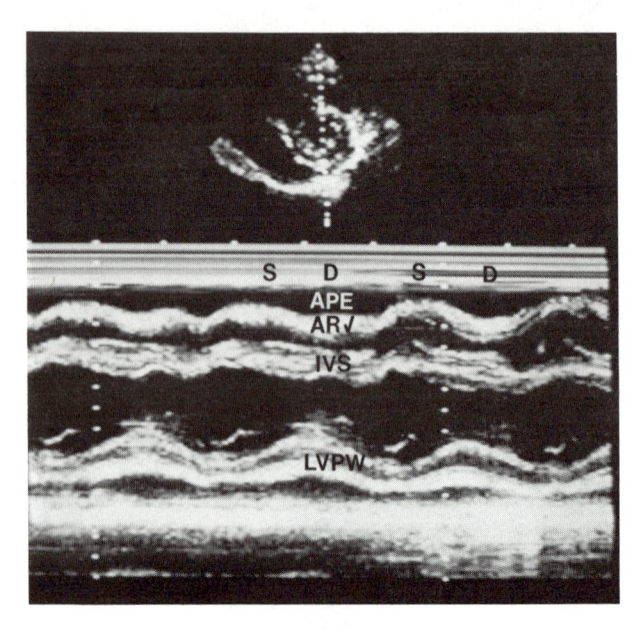

Figure 2 M-mode study of moderate pericardial effusion with tamponade. Note downward (posterior) movement of anterior right ventricular wall in diastole. APE = anterior pericardial effusion; ARV = anterior right ventricular, D = diastole; IVS = intraventricular septum; LVPW = left ventricular posterior wall; S = systole.

Table 1 Echocardiography in the Critical Care Setting

	Emergencies		Definitive Serial Evaluation		Obtaining Prognostic Information	
Clinical Setting	Capabilities		Clinical Setting	Capabilities	Clinical Setting	Capabilities
Enlarged heart shadow and hypotension	Determines presence and degree of pericardial effusion, evidence for tamponade, pericardial vs. pleural effusion		Vegetations	Detects changes in size, evidence of valve regurgitation or prosthetic valve dehiscence	Acute myocardial infarction	Evaluation of ejection fraction vs. aneurysm, clot, infarct at a distance, infarct expansion
Shock	Differential diagnosis of cardiogenic vs. septic shock, assesses LV structure and function, evaluates valvular occluding lesions		Acute myocardial infarction	Detects changes in systolic or diastolic LV performance, effects of vasoactive therapy, prognosis	Mitral valve prolapse	Evidence for flail leaflet or severe mitral regurgitation, redundancy of valve
Acute pulmonary edema	Determines cardiac causes (e.g., acute aortic and mitral regurgitation, acute ventricular septal defect, acute myocardial infarction, differentiation of dilated vs. restrictive cardiomyopathy)		Cardiomyopathy	Differentiates among hypertrophic, restrictive, dilated cardiomyopathies and allows selection of appropriate therapy	Cardiomyopathy	Prognosis primarily from LV size and systolic performance
Thoracic aortic dissection	TEE may increase sensitivity of diagnosis to more than 90%. Determines location of flaps, flow in both lumens		Valvular heart disease	Determines severity of stenosis and regurgitation before definitive catheterization	Chronic aortic or mitral regurgitation	Need for surgery based upon end systolic LV dimension and degree of regurgitation
Pulmonary flow/embolus	Provides evidence of RA and RV dilatation, possible IVC, RA, or RV sources of embolus, assessment of peak PA pressure by analysis of tricuspid regurgitant Doppler velocity		Pulmonary hypertension	Serial evaluation of peak PA pressures if tricuspid regurgitation is present		
Valve dysfunction	Provides evidence of vegetations, abscess, ring dehiscence, valvular stenosis, or regurgitation, including prosthetic valves. Differentiates acute from chronic regurgitation		Pericardial effusion	Development and resolution		

Table continues on the following page

Table 1 (*Continued*)

Emergencies		Definitive Serial Evaluation		Obtaining Prognostic Information	
Clinical Setting	Capabilities	Clinical Setting	Capabilities	Clinical Setting	Capabilities
Edema and ascites	Determines right heart causes, including TV and PV lesions, RA dysfunction, clots or masses in RA or IVC; provides evidence of constrictive pericarditis or restrictive cardiomyopathy	Aortic dissection	(TEE) detects changes and recurrence		
Acute myocardial infarction	Evaluates LV function, complications including papillary muscle rupture, IV septal rupture, pseudoaneurysm, aneurysm, clot, right ventricular infarction, infarct expansion, segmental wall motion abnormalities				
Chest trauma	Determines valve dysfunction, myocardial contusions or lacerations, hemopericardium				
Rhythm disturbances	Determines LV function, LA and RA size, presence of clots, location of pacemaker catheter tip, presence of aortic ring calcification, MV prolapse				

IV = interventricular; IVC = inferior vena cava; LA = left atrium; LV = left ventricle; PA = pulmonary artery; PV = pulmonic valve; RA = right atrium; RV = right ventricle; TV = tricuspid valve.

exaggerated decrease in mitral and aortic flow velocities, usually with a difference of more than 40 percent in each case. Echocardiography can also be used for determining the location of the pericardiocentesis needle, and finally, for the serial evaluation of changes in pericardial fluid.

Echocardiography has a role in the diagnosis of constrictive pericarditis as well. Suggestive findings consist of increased pericardial echo density, abrupt early diastolic anterior motion of the interventricular septum, and abrupt posterior motion of the left ventricle posterior wall on M-mode study. Changes in rapid early diastolic left ventricle Doppler flow patterns and abrupt cessation of flow in early to mid-diastole are also suggestive. Echocardiography can be used to detect pericardial tumors, organized intrapericardial clots, and fibrous adhesions, which likewise indicate constrictive pericarditis, Right-sided intracardiac tumors can mimic clinical findings of tamponade or constriction, and can be diagnosed readily by 2-D echocardiography. Computed tomography (CT) is much more sensitive in the diagnosis of thickened pericardium per se.

Hypotension

In both septic and cardiogenic shock, left ventricular function may diminish and this can be determined by 2-D and M-mode evaluation of systolic performance. Standard views, such as the parasternal long and short axis views and the apical four-chamber view, allow analysis of segments of the left ventricle so that a semiquantitative reference score of left ventricular dysfunction can be obtained. Myocardial infarction characteristically produces thinning of the involved segment of the ventricular wall during systole, rather than normal thickening. Global left ventricular systolic performance can be evaluated by 2-D views using standard geometric formulae, especially when helped by computerized off-line analysis capabilities. Even without such an analysis, ejection fraction can be estimated using standard 2-D views, with the ejection fraction subdivided for practical purposes into (1) greater than 50 percent, (2) 30 to 50 percent, and (3) less than 30 percent (Fig. 3). This information is helpful in the diagnosis and prescription of appropriate drug therapy. Both cardiogenic and septic shock are associated with the dilatation of the ventricles and reduced ejection fraction. Septic shock is more likely to demonstrate eventual return of ventricular size and functions to normal. Hypovolemic shock is associated with small hyperdynamic ventricles.

Hypotension can also be caused by complications of acute myocardial infarction such as acute septal perforation, papillary muscle rupture, ventricular free wall rupture, and right ventricular infarction. Acute septal perforation can be diagnosed best by color Doppler. In such a case a transesophageal approach is sometimes helpful. This technique can be used in conjunction with demonstration of a step-up in pulmonary artery oxygen saturation using a Swan-Ganz (flow-directed) pulmonary catheter. Papillary muscle rupture associated with a flail mitral leaflet and mitral regurgitation can easily be demonstrated by 2-D and Doppler imaging. A ventricular pseudoaneurysm may occur after rupture of the left ventricular free wall, with blood collecting in a loculated area of pericardium (Figs. 4 and 5). Finally, right ventricular infarction can be demonstrated by a dilated poorly contracting right ventricle.

Other causes of hypotension determined by echocardiography include a clot or tumor impinging on a valve orifice, especially a large vegetation or an atrial myxoma (Fig. 6). A malfunctioning prosthetic valve is another cause of hypotension or transient syncope.

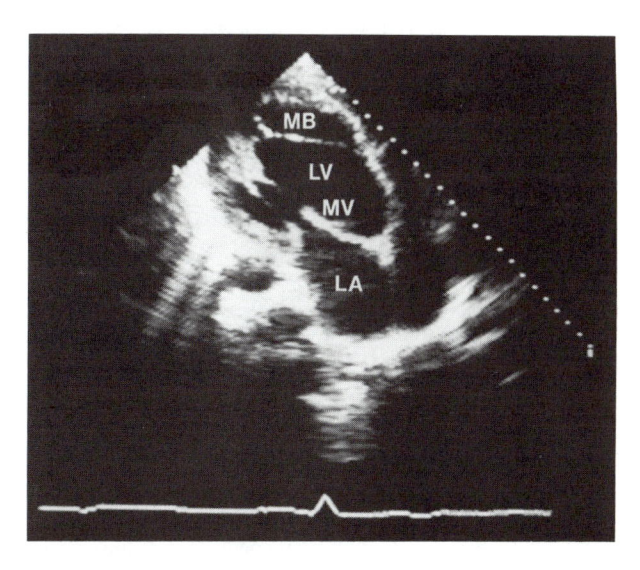

Figure 3 Dilated cardiomyopathy. The left ventricular ejection fraction was less than 20 percent. MB = muscle band; LA = left atrium; LV = left ventricle; MV = mitral valve.

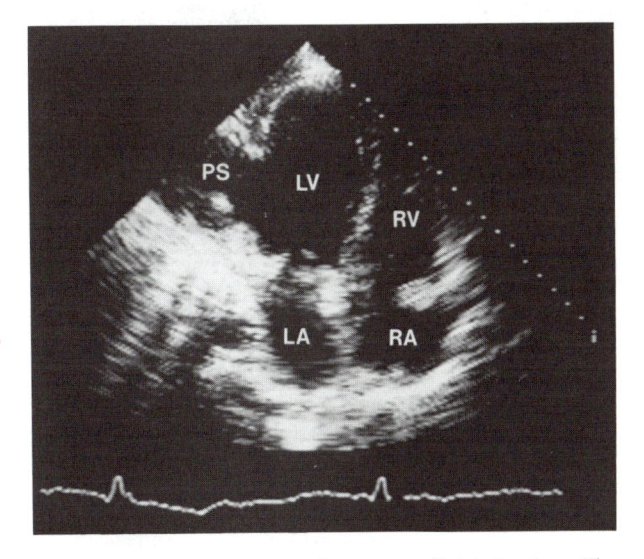

Figure 4 Pseudoaneurysm after myocardial infarction. The pericardial sac contains blood from rupture of the left ventricular free wall. LV = left ventricle; PS = pseudoaneurysm; LA = left atrium; RA = right atrium; RV = right ventricle.

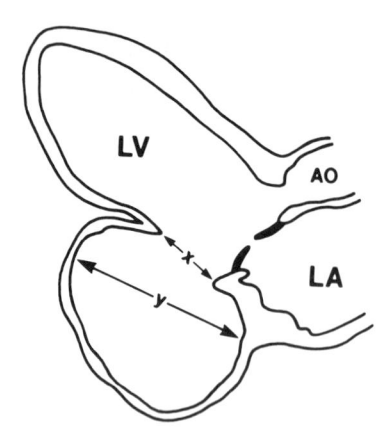

Figure 5 Pseudoaneurysm. y = small neck of pseudoaneurysm (x); AO = aorta; LA = left atrium; LV = left ventricle. Republished with permission from Knowlton AA, et al. Ventricular pseudoaneurysm: a rare but ominous condition. Cardiovasc Rev Rep 1985; 6:511–518.

Congestive Heart Failure and Acute Pulmonary Edema

In acute pulmonary edema, the echocardiogram can be used to differentiate cardiac causes from noncardiac causes. The Doppler evaluates the presence and degree of aortic regurgitation, mitral regurgitation, or ventricular septal defect, which may underlie acute congestive heart failure. TEE is useful in the diagnosis of ventricular septal defect caused by rupture of the septum in acute myocardial infarction, a condition for which early surgery may be needed. Flail valve leaflets causing acute regurgitation can be easily diagnosed by TEE. Color Doppler assessment of acute aortic regurgitation is more sensitively evaluated by TEE than by transthoracic assessment. Findings of valve incompetence or left-to-right shunt may accompany myocardial infarction, infective endocarditis, myxomatous degeneration of heart valves, or aortic valve disruption from acute dissection of the proximal aorta. 2-D echocardiography is especially helpful in differentiating restrictive cardiomyopathy from dilated cardiomyopathy, both of which can produce congestive heart failure. Restrictive cardiomyopathy is associated with a small left ventricle chamber, usually with normal or thickened walls and dilated cardiomyopathy with dilated, globally hypokinetic ventricles. The differential diagnosis is important because of differences in therapeutic approach.

Aortic Dissection

Although aortic dissection (Fig. 7) is definitively diagnosed by aortography or CT, sensitivity for evaluation has been considerably increased by echocardiography with the advent of TEE. Using a combined thoracic and esophageal approach, one can evaluate the entire thoracic aorta, especially if biplane TEE is available. Color Doppler visualization has been used to demonstrate the location of the tear by means of color flow patterns. In one study of thoracic aortic dissection, TEE was compared with CT and aortography for sensitivity and specificity of diagnoses. TEE had a sensitivity of 99 percent and a specificity of 98 percent, compared with the sensitivity and specificity of 83 percent and 100 percent, respectively, for CT, and of 88 percent and 94 percent, respectively, for aortography. TEE is especially helpful in the serial evaluation of dissection, particularly when surgery is not contemplated, as in the case of isolated descending thoracic aorta dissection.

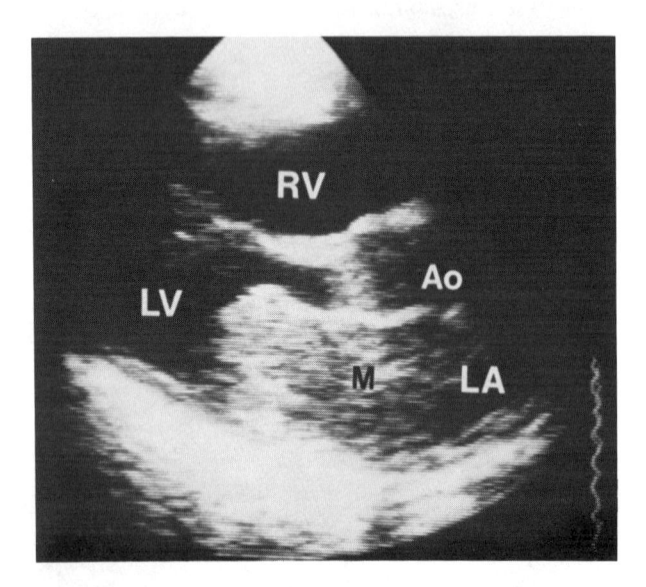

Figure 6 Left atrial myxoma (M) causing hypertension. Ao = aorta; LA = left atrium; LV = left ventricle; RV = right ventricle. Republished with permission from Liebson PR. What echocardiography can tell you about dyspnea. J Respir Dis 1986; 7:35–45.

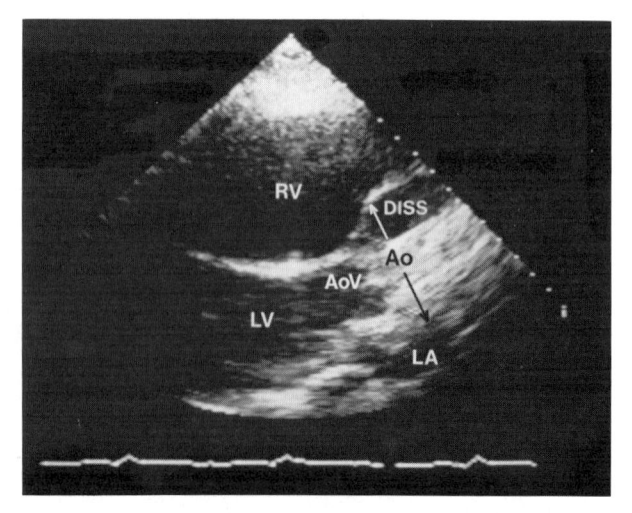

Figure 7 Anterior dissection of aortic root. Modified parasternal long axis view. Ao = aorta; AoV = aortic valve; DISS = dissection; LA = left atrium; RV = right ventricle.

Prosthetic Valve Dysfunction

Each class of prosthetic valves has a characteristic Doppler velocity that is normally greater than the velocity through a native valve (Table 2). In the assessment of prosthetic valve dysfunction, it is helpful to obtain a baseline echocardiogram soon after valve surgery for comparison. However, this is rarely available. Some degree of regurgitation is normally noted with both mitral and aortic valve prostheses. Dysfunction is suggested by rocking of the prosthetic valve ring on 2-D study and Doppler evidence for excessive regurgitation or a markedly increased CW Doppler velocity suggesting stenosis. A comprehensive echocardiographic examination provides the surgeon with both anatomic and prognostic information. The finding of abscesses and large vegetations on the prosthetic valve would more likely indicate the need for surgery. Left ventricular ejection fractions of less than 30 percent determined by echocardiography would suggest an increased risk perioperatively.

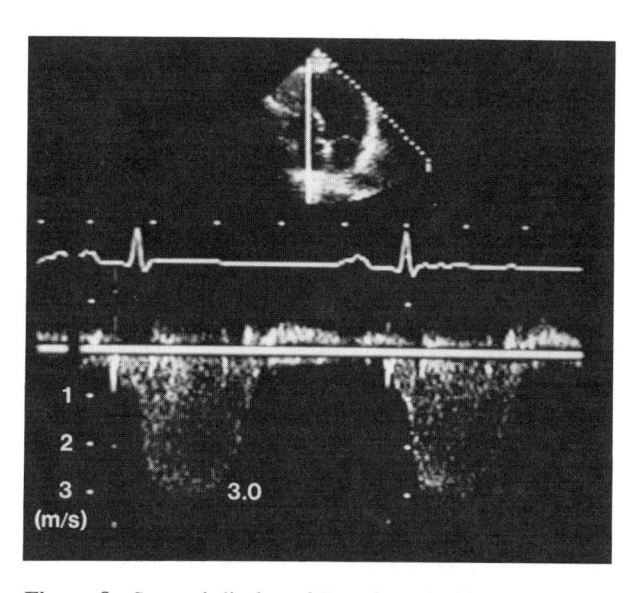

Figure 8 Spectral display of Doppler velocities (meters per second). Tricuspid regurgitation. Estimated peak pulmonary artery pressure = 4 (3.0)^2 + right atrial mean pressure estimate (see text).

Pulmonary Hemodynamics

When tricuspid regurgitation is present, the evaluation of peak Doppler velocity allows estimation of peak pulmonary artery pressure (Fig. 8). A peak transvalvular gradient (G) can be accurately diagnosed using a modification of the Bernoulli equation, $G = 4V^2$, where V = peak Doppler velocity. Because as many as 80 percent of normal subjects have Doppler evidence of tricuspid regurgitation, evaluation of tricuspid flow should provide a high yield. The estimated pulmonary artery peak pressure is equal to the calculated gradient plus the mean right atrial pressure. Right atrial pressure can be estimated by 2-D evaluation of the inferior vena cava (Fig. 9). If the inferior vena cava collapses during inspiration, the right atrial mean pressure is estimated to be 5 mm Hg; if it collapses partially, the right atrial estimated mean pressure is 10 mm Hg; and if it does not collapse during inspiration, the right atrial estimated mean pressure is 15 mm Hg. For example, if one finds a peak tricuspid regurgitant velocity of 4 m per second and a noncollapsing inferior vena cava, the estimated systolic transtricuspid gradient is 64 mm Hg. Right atrial mean pressure is estimated to be 15 mm Hg. The calculated systolic pulmonary pressure is 81 mm Hg. These estimates correlate closely with more direct evaluation of peak pulmonary arterial pressures.

Table 2 Normal Doppler Echocardiographic Values for Valve Prostheses

Prostheses	Valve	Mean Velocity (M/Sec)	Mean Gradient (mm Hg)	Mean Pressure Half-time (msec)	Mild Regurgitation
Mechanical					
Björk-Shiley	Mitral	1.6±0.3	2–5	65–150	11%–38%
(pivoting disk)	Aortic	2.6±0.5	14±6		17%–62%
Starr-Edwards (ball)	Mitral	1.8±0.4	5±2	65	30%–33%
	Aortic	1.8±3.2	25±4		33%–75%
St. Jude (bileaflet)	Mitral	1.6±0.3	5.5±2.0	70	20%–32%
	Aortic	2.5±0.5	26±12		30%–38%
Tissue					
Carpentier-Edwards	Mitral	1.6±0.2	4–12	90±20	
	Aortic	2.5±0.5	15±5		26%
Hancock	Mitral		7.5±2.0	110–130	4%
	Aortic		11±2		22%
Ionescu-Shiley	Aortic	2.6±0.5	16±5		12%
Porcine	Mitral	1.9±0.3	7±1	136±18	0%–19%(30%)
(average)	Aortic	2.6±0.6	17±10		9%–44%(26%)

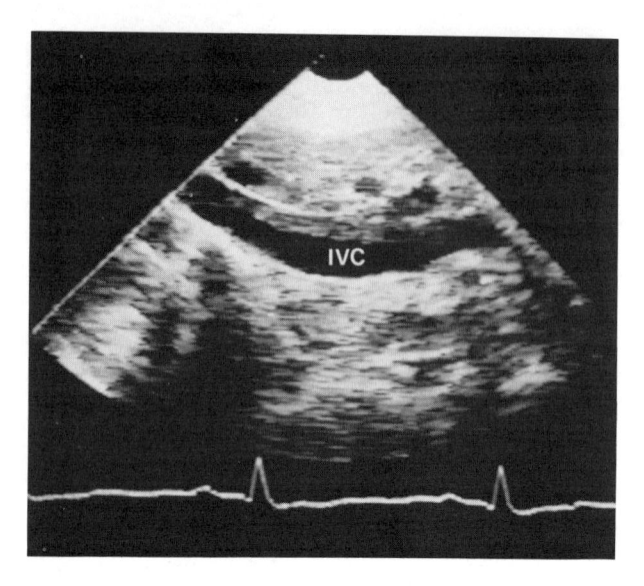

Figure 9 Right atrial mean pressure can be estimated by degree of inferior vena cava (IVC) contraction during inspiration.

Clots and Tumors

Although the yield for cardiac causes of peripheral emboli is usually low, the presence of severe mitral valve prolapse—especially with mitral regurgitation—or of clots in the left atrium or left ventricle may suggest a cardiac cause (Fig. 10). TEE is helpful in diagnosing left atrial clots which are frequently obscured in the transthoracic evaluation if they are present in the atrial appendage. In a patient without previous cardiac findings or chronic lung disease, suspicion of pulmonary embolus should be increased by the finding of dilated right atrium and right ventricle. Sometimes the pulmonary embolus originates from a clot in the right atrium or a hypernephroma or other tumor extending through the inferior vena cava into the right atrium.

Marked Peripheral Edema or Ascites

Two-dimensional echocardiography will indicate or exclude a cardiac cause. Specific diagnostic features suggestive of a cardiac cause include dilated inferior vena cava, right atrium, or right ventricle. The Doppler study is useful for diagnosing contributing causes such as tricuspid or pulmonic stenosis or regurgitation. Constrictive pericarditis is also a possible cause, although a markedly dilated right atrium or ventricle usually excludes this diagnosis.

Traumatic Heart Disease

Echocardiography is useful for determining the presence or absence of pericardial effusion, tamponade, and tears in the myocardial great vessels, septum, and valves. Myocardial contusions can sometimes be diagnosed by increased echogenicity and by regional contraction abnormalities in the involved myocardium.

Arrhythmias

Echocardiography can be helpful in evaluating some of the underlying causes and hemodynamics of dysrhythmias, and even in making diagnoses. M-mode assessment of the left atrial wall can be used for assessing atrial contraction, and if the echocardiogram shows rapid, regular ventricular activity with small, frequent atrial waves, the diagnosis of atrial flutter is suggested. The atrial dimension can be used to determine the likelihood of successful conversion of atrial fibrillation to normal sinus rhythm with the use of electric countershock. Occasionally, dislocation of a pacemaker wire tip from the right ventricle apex into the pericardium or even through the interventricular septum into the left ventricle can be diagnosed. The prognostic implication of complex ventricular arrhythmias can be assessed by 2-D evaluation of LV function. In a patient with infective endocarditis, the presence of a ring abscess can explain the development of atrioventricular block. Heart block can also be correlated with echocardiographic evidence of calcification near the aortic valve ring. The development of complex arrhythmias in children, adolescents, and young adults can be associated with mitral valve prolapse or hypertrophic obstructive cardiomyopathy, both of which are readily diagnosed by echocardiography.

DEFINITIVE OR SERIAL EVALUATION

In a critical care unit, determination of left ventricular structure and function is important in serial evaluation. The following characteristics of the left ventricle obtained by M-mode or 2-D echocardiography are useful

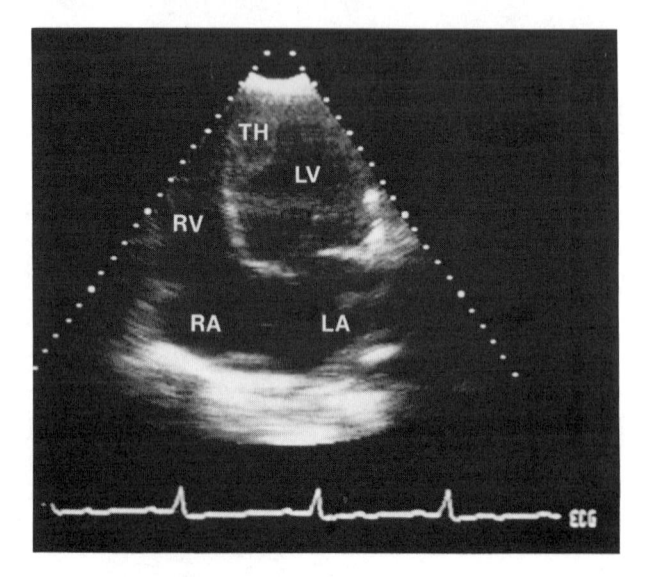

Figure 10 Thrombus in apex of left ventricle after myocardial infarction. LA = left atrium; LV = left ventricle; RA = right atrium; RV = right ventricle; TH = thrombus.

in this setting: (1) wall mass; (2) chest geometry, including the presence of concentric hypertrophy, disproportionate septal hypertrophy, dynamic (hypertrophic) subaortic stenosis, and eccentric hypertrophy; (3) global systolic function such as ejection fraction, end-diastolic volume, end-systolic volume, stroke volume, ejection fraction, left ventricular end-systolic stress, fractional shortening, and velocity of fiber shortening; and (4) segmental contraction characteristics. This information provides constructs of left ventricular contractile state, preload, and afterload. Peripheral vascular resistance can be estimated from echocardiography by calculation of the cardiac output (estimated stroke volume heart rate) and the mean arterial pressure. Changes in peak pulmonary artery pressure can be determined serially from the Doppler study of tricuspid regurgitation, as described previously.

Left ventricular diastolic performance can be assessed by evaluation of diastolic Doppler inflow with Doppler interrogation just distal to the mitral valve. The Doppler inflow velocity spectrum includes a large early peak velocity (E) from early ventricular filling and a smaller late peak velocity (A) from atrial contraction (Fig. 11). Normally, the E/A ratio is greater than 1 but tends to decrease with age. Severe congestive heart failure is associated with an increase of the E/A ratio. Decreased relaxation of the left ventricle in early diastole or decreased compliance to the left ventricle in late diastole are both associated with a decrease in the E/A ratio. Changes in diastolic performance can be serially evaluated in virtually all patients.

The effects of various interventions on left ventricular performance can be assessed. These include changes in left ventricular end-diastolic and end-systolic dimension, changes in contraction characteristics, and changes in the E/A ratio of diastolic inflow. The geometry of the left ventricle is especially important when one is considering diuretics and vasodilators for the treatment of congestive heart failure. If the left ventricle has a very small chamber size, as might occur with hypertrophic cardiomyopathy, restrictive cardiomyopathy, or congestive failure with severe concentric hypertrophy, especially in elderly patients, it is possible that administration of diuretics may cause the stroke volume to decrease considerably. Hypotension may ensue because of the abrupt decrease in preload caused by diuresis or by decreased impedance to outflow produced by vasodilators.

The cardiac valves can be comprehensively assessed using bedside echocardiography. Findings include assessment of valve structure, valvular thickness, presence of vegetations, and systolic and diastolic flow characteristics. The Bernoulli formula for estimated gradient ($G = 4V^2$) can be used for the determination of peak and mean velocities. Figure 12 demonstrates characteristic spectral velocity patterns through an aortic valve in systole and mitral valve in diastole in mitral and aortic stenoses. Both the peak and mean gradients can be estimated using the formula. The mean gradient can be estimated by summing the estimated gradient at short intervals and dividing the number of sample points. Excellent estimation of the mitral valve area in mitral stenosis can be obtained through the use of a pressure half-time formula based on the rate of velocity decrease from early diastolic peak velocity in the spectral profile of diastolic mitral flow (Fig. 13A) (Table 3). The aortic valve area in aortic stenosis has been estimated by a continuity equation in which the aortic valve area is based on calculations of the cross-sectional area of the left ventricular outflow tract (2-D), the average velocity of flow through the aortic valve, and the average velocity of flow at a point below the aortic valve in the outflow tract (Fig. 13B and C) (see Table 3).

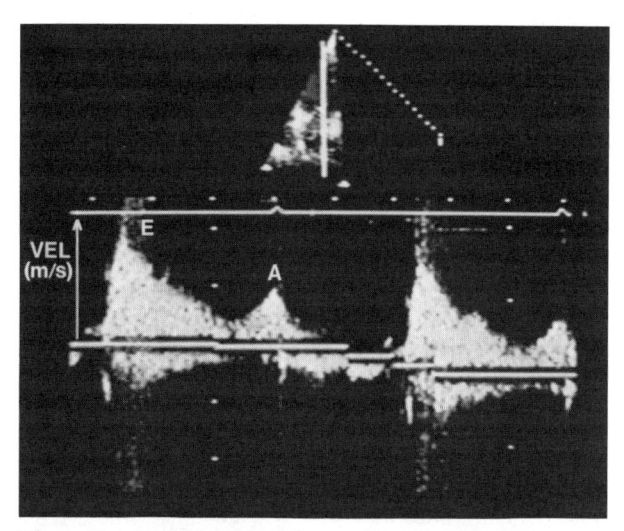

Figure 11 Spectral display of normal Doppler velocity pattern. Mitral inflow into left ventricle. Peak E/A ratio may be reversed or decreased with left ventricular diastolic compliance abnormalities. A = peak of emptying after atrial contraction; E = peak of early emptying; M/S = meters per second; VEL = velocities.

This approach can also be used for estimating stroke volumes through various valve orifices. Thus, it is possible to estimate stroke volume through the mitral, aortic, tricuspid, and pulmonic valves. This in turn would be useful for evaluating the degree of regurgitant flow or shunt flow.

Color Doppler provides a semiquantitative approach to determining the degree of regurgitant flow. It has been of less use in the quantification of intracardiac shunts. Injection of intravenous saline after agitation of the solution in the syringe, producing echogenic microbubbles, can also be useful for assessing right-to-left shunts at the atrial or ventricular level but is highly insensitive for left-to-right shunting.

It is frequently possible to diagnose large pleural effusions using 2-D echocardiography. This is important if a differential diagnosis of pericardial effusion is entertained, as illustrated in Figures 1 and 2.

OBTAINING PROGNOSTIC INFORMATION

The evaluation of left ventricular structure and function provides strong prognostic information. Evidence for

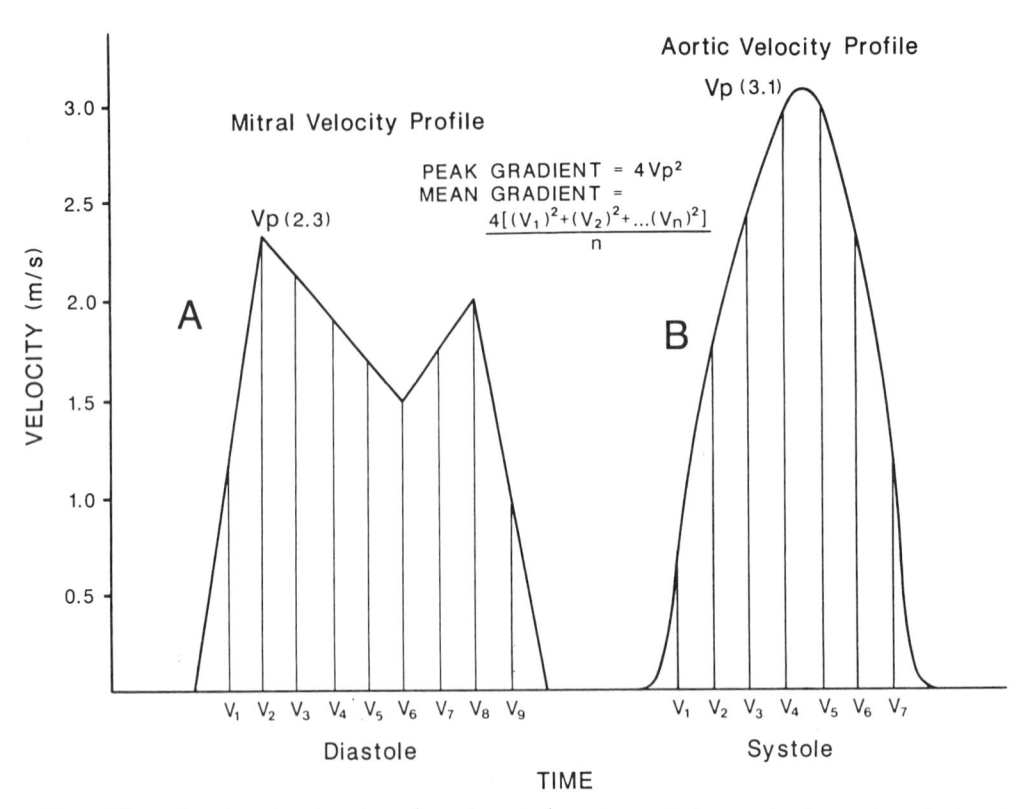

Figure 12 Estimation of peak and mean gradients by Doppler analysis. *A*, Mitral stenosis. Mitral peak velocity = 2.3 m per second. Estimated peak gradient is determined by application of the modified Bernoulli equation, as shown. The mean gradient is determined by the same equation using incremental determinants of velocities throughout diastole (V_1, V_2, ... V_n) and dividing by the number (n) of determinants. *B*, aortic stenosis. Aortic peak velocity = 3.1 m per second. The same principle applies for determining transaortic peak and mean velocities as with transmitral flow.

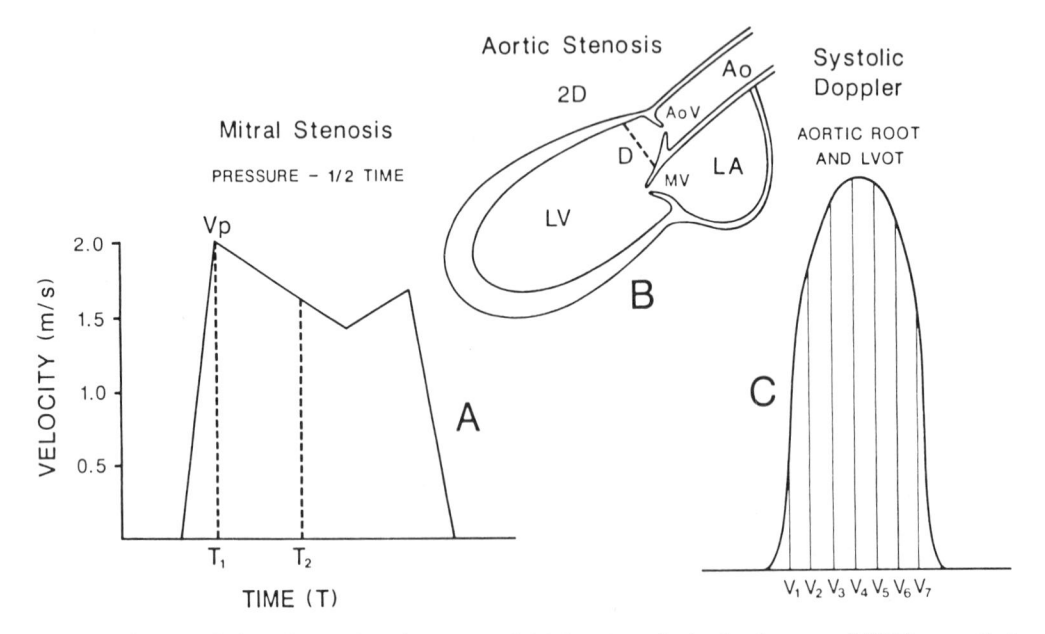

Figure 13 Calculation of stenotic valve areas. *A*, Estimation of mitral valve area (MVA) vs. mitral stenosis. Pressure half-time (T_1–T_2) is determined by time of peak velocity (T_1) to time on spectral velocity display when velocity = $V_p/\sqrt{2}$ MVA = 220/T_1–T_2 (msec). *B*, For determination of aortic valve area (AVA), the continuity equation is used. This requires determination of cross-sectional area of the left ventricular outflow tract (LVOT) by 2D (B), and mean flow velocity integrals of the aortic and left ventricular outflow tract Doppler profiles (*C*). (See also Table 3).

Table 3 Useful Quantitative Information from Doppler Evaluation

1.	Valve gradient (G)	$G = 4V^2$
2.	Mitral valve area (MVA) (mitral stenosis)	$MVA = \dfrac{220}{\text{Pressure } 1/2 \text{ time}}$
3.	Aortic valve area (AVA)	$AVA = \dfrac{\pi (D/2)^2 \, L_{VOT} \times {}^{FVI}L_{VOT}}{FVI_{Ao}}$
4.	Stroke volume through a valve (SV)	$SV = \pi (D/2)^2 \times FVI$
5.	Peak pulmonary pressure (PAP)	$PAP = 4V^2{}_{TR} \times RA \text{ mean pressure}$

$(D/2)^2$ = cross-sectional area of lumen; FVI = Doppler flow velocity integral profile; FVI_{Ao} = flow-velocity integral; $4V^2{}_{TR}$ = tricuspid regurgitant peak velocity; LVOT = left ventricular outflow tract; RA = right atrium.

---

increased left ventricular wall mass or left ventricular hypertrophy is associated with up to a tenfold increase in adverse cardiac outcome events over a period of years. The best use of echocardiography for short-term prognostic information is in the setting of acute myocardial infarction. It can be argued that echocardiography should be a mandatory examination in all patients suspected of having myocardial infarction. The examination allows baseline evaluation of left ventricular structure and function and determination of infarct expansion, which begins early in the infarct period and may lead to ventricular aneurysm. Echocardiography is also useful in the diagnosis of acute left ventricular clot formation, especially with anterior wall infarcts; for this condition, administration of anticoagulants appears to improve prognosis over the next 6 months. The diagnosis of aortic valve insufficiency by Doppler is especially important if intra-aortic balloon counterpulsation is being considered. Patients with global left ventricular systolic dysfunction are at high risk for immediate and long-term mortality.

SUGGESTED READING

Currie PJ. Transesophageal echocardiography: new window on the heart. Circulation 1989; 80:215–217.

King SW, Pandian NG, Gardin JM. Doppler echocardiographic findings in pericardial tamponade and constriction. Echocardiography 1988; 5:361–372.

Heldman D, Gardin JM. Evaluation of prosthetic valves by Doppler echocardiography. Echocardiography 1989; 6:63–77.

Kotler MN, Goldman AP, Parameswaran R, Parry WR. Acute consequences and chronic complications of acute myocardial infarction. Echocardiography 1989; 4:295–316.

Pandian NG, Weintraub A, Kusay BS, et al. Emergency echocardiography. Echocardiography 1989; 6:45–61.

NUCLEAR SCANNING

MARGARET M. PARKER, M.D.

Evaluation of cardiac function or myocardial perfusion is often important in the diagnosis and management of the critically ill patient. The availability of the portable gamma camera has made possible the bedside evaluation of cardiac function in even the most critically ill patient.

Radionuclide ventriculography (RNV) is accomplished by labeling the patient's red blood cells with technetium 99m or by using technetium-labeled human serum albumin. The collection of gamma counts is gated to the patient's electrocardiogram, and a time-activity curve of the counts emitted in each part of the cardiac cycle is generated. This curve is used to calculate the ejection fraction, the proportion of blood in the ventricle ejected with each heart beat. The individual images from each part of the cardiac cycle can be displayed in an endless-loop format to produce a cineangiogram, and different views of the heart can be obtained and analyzed for regional wall-motion abnormalities. In order to obtain a technically adequate study, the heart rhythm must be regular and stable. Frequent ventricular or atrial premature beats or atrial fibrillation, for example, will preclude a reliable study. In addition, the patient must be able to lie still for the period of time necessary to collect the study, usually 15 to 20 minutes. An adequate RNV can provide valuable information regarding right and left ventricular function in a critically ill patient.

RNV may be useful in a variety of clinical situations. Table 1 compares the usefulness of RNV with that of echocardiography in the critically ill patient. For the patient with cardiogenic shock, RNV provides an assessment

Table 1 Radionuclide Ventriculography Versus Echocardiography in the Critically Ill Patient

Clinical Setting	Radionuclide Ventriculography	Echocardiography
Cardiogenic shock	Assesses and quantifies global ventricular function Identifies regional wall motion abnormalities Detects ventricular aneurysm Evaluates right ventricular function	Qualitatively assesses global left ventricular function Identifies regional wall motion abnormalities Detects ventricular aneurysm Evaluates right ventricular function
Septic shock	Evaluates degree of depression of biventricular function Determines on follow-up study whether ventricular function has returned to normal	Evaluates degree of depression of biventricular function Determines on follow-up study whether ventricular function has returned to normal
Extracardiac obstructive shock	Usually normal	Identifies presence and amount of pericardial fluid or pericardial thickening
Hypovolemic shock	Usually normal	Usually normal
Congestive heart failure	Assesses global ventricular function and regional wall motion abnormalities	Assesses global ventricular function and regional wall motion abnormalities Evaluates wall thickness, septal hypertrophy, and valve structure

of global ventricular function and the presence of regional wall-motion abnormalities. A ventricular aneurysm appears as a dyskinetic segment of the ventricle. The right ventricle is dilated and hypokinetic in the patient who has suffered a right ventricular infarction.

Septic shock produces a reversible depression of right and left ventricular ejection fraction. RNV is useful in assessing the degree of ventricular depression and in follow-up evaluation to determine whether myocardial function has returned to normal, as usually occurs within 7 to 10 days in survivors of septic shock.

In patients with extracardiac obstructive shock (e.g., pericardial tamponade) and hypovolemic shock, ventricular function is usually normal. RNV does not have specific usefulness in these settings.

In patients with severe congestive heart failure, RNV is useful in distinguishing between ischemic cardiomyopathy, in which regional wall-motion abnormalities are usually seen, and idiopathic dilated cardiomyopathy, in which hypokinesis is generally global and biventricular. RNV cannot be used to evaluate wall thickness or valve structure, as can echocardiography.

Using the ejection fraction obtained from RVN with simultaneous hemodynamic measurements from a thermodilution pulmonary artery catheter, one can calculate several cardiovascular parameters that add to the understanding of the patient's cardiac physiology. As shown in Table 2, the stroke volume (the volume of blood ejected from the heart with each beat) can be calculated from the thermodilution-determined cardiac output. The end-diastolic volume can be calculated by dividing the stroke volume by the ejection fraction. The end-diastolic volume is a better measure of ventricular preload than the pulmonary artery wedge pressure, which is usually used as a measure of left ventricular preload.

Myocardial perfusion can be evaluated using thallium-201, a potassium analogue. In a critically ill patient, a perfusion defect on thallium scan may result from an acute myocardial infarction, unstable angina, coronary artery spasm, or a remote infarction. A single study cannot distinguish between these possibilities. Exercise thallium scanning with a follow-up reperfusion study may be useful in determining a patient's coronary perfusion status but is not practical in the critically ill patient. The effects of pharmacologic interventions on coronary perfusion may be potentially evaluated by a thallium study, but this technique has not yet been widely used for this purpose. Currently thallium scanning is of little, if any, usefulness in the intensive care unit, although a normal thallium perfusion scan within 24 hours of chest pain may be useful in ruling out a myocardial infarction.

Technetium 99m pyrophosphate is useful in detecting areas of myocardial infarction, as it accumulates in areas of calcium deposition. Usually acute myocardial in-

Table 2 Cardiovascular Parameters Calculated From Simultaneous Radionuclide Ventriculography and Catheter-Derived Hemodynamics

Stroke Volume = $\dfrac{\text{Cardiac Output}}{\text{Heart Rate}}$

Stroke Volume = End-Diastolic Volume − End-Systolic Volume

Ejection Fraction = $\dfrac{\text{End-Diastolic − End-Systolic Volume}}{\text{End-Diastolic Volume}}$

End-Diastolic Volume = $\dfrac{\text{Stroke Volume (from thermodilution cardiac output)}}{\text{Ejection Fraction (from RNV)}}$

farction can be diagnosed without infarct scanning, but technetium 99m pyrophosphate may be a diagnostic aid in the patient with equivocal enzyme or electrocardiographic findings, as in the patient who presents more than 24 hours after the onset of chest pain or in the patient with a left bundle branch block. Technetium 99m may also be useful in diagnosing right ventricular infarction, or in evaluating patients after coronary bypass surgery.

In many circumstances, nuclear scanning techniques may be helpful in the diagnosis and management of the critically ill patient. The techniques, however, require expensive equipment and technical support from the nuclear medicine department. While these techniques are clearly useful, they may not be practical for widespread use. If scanning is not available in the intensive care unit, other noninvasive techniques such as echocardiography may provide the necessary information and are generally more readily available.

SUGGESTED READING

Bulkley BH, Hutchins GM, Bailey I, et al. Thallium-201 imaging and gated cardiac blood pool scans in patients with ischemic and idiopathic congestive cardiomyopathy. Circulation 1977; 55:753–760.

Holman BL, Chisholm RJ, Braunwald E. The prognostic implications of acute myocardial infarct scintigraphy with technetium 99m pyrophosphate. Circulation 1978; 57:320–326.

Parker MM, Cunnion RE, Parrillo JE. Echocardiography and nuclear cardiac imaging in the critical care unit. J Am Med Assoc 1985; 254:2935–2939.

BEDSIDE HEMODYNAMIC MONITORING

WARREN R. SUMMER, M.D.
BENNETT P. deBOISBLANC, M.D.

The pulmonary artery catheter (PAC) was introduced for bedside hemodynamic monitoring during the 1970s and was immediately embraced as a valuable adjunct to patient management, with its usage tripling over the next decade. Over the past several years, the PAC has come under attack because of its expense and because of the lack of information on its cost effectiveness and risk/benefit ratio. In more than 3,000 acute myocardial infarction patients, evidence of increased acute mortality and prolonged duration of hospitalization has been associated with catheter insertion without any long-term benefit in survival. Similar data are being observed in general medical intensive care units, as well. Although these reports are retrospective in nature or lack concurrent randomized controls, they cannot be dismissed because there are no studies of hemodynamic monitoring demonstrating improved outcome. Significant consideration should therefore be given to the indication for PAC insertion and how long that information needs to be accrued during patient care.

Right atrial pressure (or central venous pressure) reflects systemic blood volume, venous tone, right ventricular performance, and pulmonary vascular resistance. It may remain normal during left ventricular failure, pulmonary congestion, and pulmonary hypertension. Left atrial pressure reflects central blood volume, pulmonary vascular compliance, left ventricular filling, and left ventricular performance. The right atria, pulmonary capillary wedge, and left atrial pressures move in the same direction except in primary pulmonary disease and right ventricular infarction, where they tend to diverge. Correlations between right atrial and left atrial pressure are good in normal individuals and in individuals with global cardiac dysfunction, but are not predictable in individuals with isolated left or right ventricular disease.

The PAC measures right-sided and left-sided cardiac pressures, pulmonary artery pressure, and cardiac output and allows for calculation of numerous derived hemodynamic variables. The PAC can aid the physician in better understanding the diagnosis of a particular patient, better defining the hemodynamic events occurring at a particular time in the progression of a disease, and in better monitoring of vasoactive drug and fluid management in selected individuals (Table 1).

INDICATIONS FOR PULMONARY ARTERY CATHETER USAGE

Diagnostic

Standard diagnostic indications for a PAC include unresolved questions of cardiogenic shock, papillary muscle rupture or dysfunction, right ventricular infarction, and

Table 1 Hemodynamic Variables in Common Cardiopulmonary Disorders

Disorder	RA	PA	PCW	PAD-PCW	Liters/min/m²	Comments
Normal range	0–5 mm Hg	9–18 mm Hg	5–12 mm Hg	1–2 mm Hg	2.8–4.2	
Septic shock	N, ↑	↑	N, ↑↓	↑	↑↑	High PAOP seen with volume overload or LV dysfunction.
Hypovolemic shock	↓	↓	↓	N	↓↓	Usually prompt improvement to infused volume unless actively bleeding
Cardiogenic shock	↑, N	↑	↑↑	N, ↓	↓↓	Extensive infarction; severe myocardiopathy
Cardiogenic pulmonary edema	↑, N	↑	↑↑↑	↓	↓	May not be volume overload in acute MI
Cardiac tamponade	↑↑	↑↑	↑↑	↓	↓↓	Equilization of left- and right-sided pressure. "Dip" and "plateau" in RV trace
Right ventricular infarct	↑↑	N	N	N	↓, N	Often responds to fluid challenge, RA > LA pressure
Adult respiratory distress syndrome	N, ↑	↑↑	N	↑↑	↑↑	Hyperdynamic state. PA mildly to moderately elevated. Early, persistent, and severe elevations associated with poor prognosis
COPD	N, ↑	↑	N	↑↑	N, ↓	PA usually < rp mm Hg; requires chronic hypoxia and responds to improved PaO_2. PCW elevated with underlying LV disease or due to ventricular interdependence. CO with dehydration, ASHD myopathy
Pulmonary embolism	↑↑	↑↑	N, ↓	↑↑↑	↓	Need to occlude more than 75% of pulmonary bed. Usually have additional underlying disease for significant elevation > 40 mm Hg. PCW normal, usually elevated with interdependence

LV = left ventricle; MI = myocardial infarction; PA = pulmonary artery mean pressure; PAD-PCW = pulmonary artery diastolic to pulmonary capillary wedge pressure gradient as reflection of pulmonary arterial resistance; PaO_2 = arterial oxygen pressure; PCW = pulmonary capillary wedge pressure or balloon occlusion pressure; RA = right atrium; RV = right ventricle.

cardiac tamponade. Knowing whether or not left atrial filling pressures are elevated can help in differentiating cardiogenic from noncardiogenic pulmonary edema and can aid in understanding the mechanisms of cardiopulmonary failure in patients with combined heart and lung disease. Detecting whether a patient is either hypovolemic or hypervolemic is aided by measurements of right and left atrial filling pressures. Patients with septic shock have a characteristic hemodynamic pattern of relatively normal filling pressures with a marked increase in cardiac output and a reduction in systemic vascular resistance (often with some increase in pulmonary vascular resistance). Recognition of this hyperdynamic state is occasionally helpful in establishing a diagnosis of the "sepsis syndrome." Measurements of intracardiac oxygen saturations are of value in diagnosing ventricular septal rupture after acute myocardial infarction. Finally, information derived from the PAC has been shown to have prognostic value, with an elevated pulmonary arterial resistance indicating a poorer prognosis in most critically ill patients.

Justification for using a PAC as an aid to diagnosis has been cited by physicians whose clinical assessment of hemodynamic parameters infrequently concurs with direct hemodynamic measurements. This discrepancy between the physicians' clinical impressions and actual measurements occurs at various levels of filling pressure and cardiac output and implies that clinical parameters do not correlate with hemodynamic events. More recently, Connors et al have reassessed the physician's ability to diagnose hemodynamic parameters. Using discriminate analysis, they have demonstrated that appropriate noninvasive historical, physical, and laboratory information can accurately assess initial hemodynamic status in all types of critically ill patients. In other words, it is often the physician's suboptimal processing of information that is faulty, not the availability of noninvasive diagnostic clinical information per se.

Monitoring

The other major indication for a PAC is optimization of therapy or early detection of hemodynamic change. Such information has been accrued most often in patients with cardiogenic shock, extensive myocardial infarction with or without hypertension, intra-aortic balloon counterpulsation, cardiac or major vascular surgery, congestive heart failure, adult respiratory distress syndrome, septic shock, burns, multi-organ system disease, and corpulmonale with acute respiratory failure. There is no argument that theoretically, changes in hemodynamic parameters, such as filling pressure, cardiac output, and systemic vascular resistance, can be better titrated and more easily detected with repeated hemodynamic measurements. However, no study has documented improved mortality by the use of invasive hemodynamic monitoring.

Finally, the PAC can be used to determine oxygen delivery, oxygen consumption, and resting energy expenditure (REE) as a means of assessing energy requirements and nutritional needs.

CHOICE OF CATHETER AND MODE OF INSERTION

Currently there are six commercially available PACs. Studies examining the different catheters find them relatively similar with regard to ease of insertion, reliability of thermodilution measurements, rate of infusion of fluids, luminal clotting, and maintenance of balloon integrity. All of the catheters have frequency responses that make determinations of systolic and diastolic pressures inaccurate at heart rates of more than 120 beats per minute. Several studies suggest that fiberoptic flow-directed catheters require longer insertion times, have more technical problems in obtaining wedge pressures, and are more expensive.

Several insertion sites have been used for the placement of catheters. The two most popular are the internal jugular vein and the subclavian vein. One prospective study reports no advantage for either route in terms of ease or time of insertion and initial and long-term complication rates. Higher success rates are, however, claimed for the jugular approach. Arterial puncture and pneumothorax, two major complications, occur less with the internal jugular approach, and this insertion site is therefore favored for patients with ventilatory insufficiency or bleeding diathesis. There are several insertion techniques used for internal jugular vein cannulation that can be easily learned. The internal jugular vein appears to be largest 1.5 cm inferior to the cricoid cartilage, with the patient's head rotated approximately 30 degrees to the contralateral side and the body placed 15 degrees in the Trendelenburg position. We often use a 22-gauge exploring needle to find the internal jugular vein and then insert the larger introducer needle while maintaining the exploring needle in the vessel as a directional guide. This technique lessens the vascular and neural trauma associated with large needle exploration.

Once vascular access has been obtained from the internal jugular vein or the subclavian vein, the PAC usually enters the right atrium after being advanced 15 to 20 cm. After it has entered the right ventricle, it usually takes less than 15 cm to reach the pulmonary artery. Several studies have demonstrated that it takes approximately 10 minutes for vascular cannulation to be achieved plus 10 minutes for positioning within the pulmonary artery. In most studies, 95 percent of attempts are ultimately successful, with less than half of the cases requiring repeated passes.

CENTRAL PRESSURE MEASUREMENTS

The PAC is most often used to measure central filling pressures: right atrial (RA), pulmonary artery (PA) and balloon occlusion pressures (PAOP). For this to be accomplished, the transducer must first be zeroed to air at midchest and calibrated. Inflation of the catheter balloon in the main pulmonary artery allows blood flow to propel the tip of the catheter into a lobar vessel which then becomes occluded. Once the vessel is occluded, the downstream blood in that vessel becomes an exploring manometer across the pulmonary capillary bed to some pulmonary venous site where blood flow from *nonoccluded* vascular beds enter. The pressure from this venous blood flow is transmitted back across the pulmonary bed through the exploring manometer to the catheter tip and transducer. It is important that the balloon-occluded vessel be relatively proximal in a lobar pulmonary artery so that the sensed venous blood flow is near the left atrium. Studies comparing proximal (central) PAOP versus distal (peripheral) PAOP have demonstrated more accurate estimations of left atrial pressure with proximal vessel occlusion. This is most important in conditions in which pulmonary venous resistance is high, producing a pressure drop across the venous bed to the left atria. Proximal placement of a PAC also reduces the chance of prolonged vascular occlusion, with resultant pulmonary infarction or balloon inflation in a small vessel causing arterial rupture and hemorrhage. In the absence of tachycardia and increased pulmonary arterial resistance, pulmonary arterial diastolic pressure (PADP) and left atrial pressure (LAP) are usually within 1 to 2 mm Hg. Under these circumstances, the PADP measurement can be used as an excellent approximation of the PAOP and LAP, obviating frequent balloon inflations, potential balloon rupture, distal catheter movement, and attendant complications. The PAOP should not be greater than the PADP. When the PAOP is 6 mm Hg greater than the PADP, it is always artifactual and minor repositioning or balloon reinflation corrects the discrepancies.

It must be remembered that the development of pulmonary edema depends on the pulmonary capillary pressure (PCP), which, weighted heavily toward left atrial pressure, it also influenced by the mean pulmonary artery pressure and is closely represented by the following formula:

$$PCP = LAP + 0.4 \, (P\overline{A}m - LAP)$$

In the presence of a significant downstream resistance distal to the fluid exchanging vessels, the measured balloon occlusion pressure may be significantly less than that of the true upstream capillary microvascular pressure. Several ways of conveniently estimating pulmonary capillary pressure have been suggested and may become clinically popular in the future.

LIMITATIONS

Measurements should be taken directly from the oscilloscope or written tracing at the end expiration during spontaneous or assisted respiration. End-expiratory pressures may be measured in spontaneously breathing tachypneic patients by having the patient sip fluid from a straw for 5 to 10 seconds. Artificially ventilated patients not requiring sedation may have oscilloscope pressure swings markedly attenuated by briefly overdriving the patient's ventilatory rate with the respirator. Patients should never be removed from ventilators, sedated, or paralyzed to record hemodynamic pressures.

While central pressure measurements have a narrow standard error in a laboratory setting, several problems with both accuracy and precision of pulmonary artery measurements are common in clinical settings.

Transducer Limitation

All transducers should be zeroed at midchest and calibrated electronically at least twice daily. Transducers should also be mechanically calibrated to standard pressure equivalents during each nursing shift. This is accomplished by opening the stop cock connected to the PAC to air and by elevating this open stop cock to a predetermined height above the midchest. The observed pressure should correlate with the electrical calibrations (27.2 cm = 20 mm Hg). It is also important that the transducers and amplifiers have appropriate frequency responses to prevent underdamping or overdamping. Increasing the paper speed of the recorder to 50 mm per second and quickly squeezing and releasing the infraflow flush produces a characteristic wave pattern from which frequency responses can be determined. Damping of a pressure tracing can occur from air bubbles, blood clots, loose fittings, catheter kinks, or a catheter tip malpositioned against the arterial wall. These complications make interpretation of hemodynamics inaccurate.

Physiologic Lung Limitation

Because PAOP measures pulmonary venous and/or left atrial events through an extended column of static fluid, a major limitation to accurate estimation of LAP occurs when the PAC is in a West lung zone 1 or 2 condition. Under these circumstances, alveolar pressure is either greater than pulmonary artery pressure or greater than pulmonary venous pressure and therefore occludes the column of fluid, preventing sensing of downstream pressure (Table 1). In zone 3 conditions, pulmonary venous pressure is greater than alveolar pressure, even when high levels of positive end-expiratory pressure (PEEP) are used (Table 2). It has been well documented that directly measured left ventricular end-diastolic pressure or LAP often does not correlate with PAOP measured in zone 2 areas when PEEP is over 10 cm of water. In this situation, measured PAOP exceeds true LAP. Changes in right atrial pressure (RAP) during PEEP do not correlate with changes in LAP, although both tend to change in the same direction. Both also increase in response to volume infusion. Interestingly, at high levels of PEEP, the RAP often correlates better with left ventricular end-diastolic pressure than does the PAOP, probably because of ventricular interdependence. To ensure that the catheter tip is not in a West zone 1 or 2 condition, a supine lateral chest x-ray examination can be done. If the PAC is below the left atrium, it is most likely in a zone 3 condition. In such radiographs, however, the PAC tip is often difficult to visualize. Seventy to eighty percent of PACs spontaneously float into the right lower lobe and can be seen on a routine A-P chest radiograph near the right hilum, indicating appropriate positioning during balloon inflation. Whenever there is a question that the PAC might reside in a zone 1 or 2 condition, we turn the patient into the lateral decubitus position on the side of the catheter tip to ensure that it is below the left atria, and we correlate the results with supine measurements.

Pulmonary Venous Limitation

Another major limitation of PAC balloon occlusion measurements is related to problems with pulmonary venous resistance or perivascular fluid pressures. Venous occlusion with thrombi is often present at autopsy and can frequently be demonstrated by wedge pulmonary angiograms in patients with adult respiratory distress syndrome. In addition, venous constriction has been observed in sepsis. Pulmonary edema with adult respiratory distress syndrome may increase interstitial pressure and result in increased pulmonary venous resistance. The more proximal the balloon occlusion of the pulmonary artery, the closer the measured pressure will be to true LAP, regard-

Table 2 Verification That Pulmonary Artery Occlusion Pressure is Equal to Pulmonary Venous Pressure (Zone 3 Condition)

	Positive Verification	*Negative Verification*
Pulmonary artery diastolic pressure	Decreases with occlusion	Unchanged or rises PAD = wedge
Wedge pressure contour	Atrial carotid and ventricular waves	Smooth
Withdraw blood freely	Yes	No return
Arterialization of blood from wedge	Yes	No
Variation of wedge pressure with respirator	< ½ airway change	> ½ airway change
PEEP transmission to wedge	< ½ PEEP change	> ½ PEEP change
Fluid challenge	Elevation in wedge	No change in wedge
Catheter tip position	Below left atria	Above left atria or undetermined

less of the venous resistance, unless there is actual critical closure within the pulmonary veins. Venous closure can occur after upstream balloon occlusion in the presence of high venous tone or high interstitial perivascular pressures that exceed LAP. Venous closure may mimic wedge pressure but may be recognized by a very rapid plateauing and marked damping of left atrial wave forms after balloon occlusion.

Pleural Pressure Limitation

One of the greatest "leaps of faith" in using pulmonary artery occlusion pressure is assuming a known or fixed relationship between estimated left ventricular end-diastolic pressure and left ventricular end-diastolic volume (LVEDP). In critically ill patients with or without ventilatory support, the predominant cause of the discrepancy is a change in pleural pressure. Transmural pressure (intracavitary pressure minus pleural pressure) is the actual distending pressure of a cardiac chamber and therefore more closely correlates with end-diastolic volume. It is generally agreed that end-expiratory pleural pressure represents the pleural pressure closest to zero, and it is at this time in the respiratory cycle that PAOP is most likely to reflect true left atrial transmural pressure.

Most pressure monitors have digital displays. Digital displays survey time intervals of pressure (usually 3 seconds or more), and provide time-based averages that prevent accurate consideration of the influence of the respiratory cycle. Thus the electronically averaged pressure can differ substantially from the actual left atrial transmural pressure. This discrepancy can be obviated by measuring intravascular pressure relative to the esophageal pressure (easily obtained but rarely performed) or attenuated by directly reading real-time pressure measurements from the tracing at end expiration. Some monitors are fitted with grid lines or have moveable lines to facilitate estimation of this pressure during respiratory fluctuation. Alternatively, drawing a line on a piece of tape allows accurate measurement of end-expiratory intravascular pressures directly from the oscilloscope. Removing a patient from mechanical ventilation to read vascular pressures obviates ventilator and PEEP interference but not necessarily variations from spontaneous respiration. It does not make sense to remove a patient from the ventilator, since severe hypoxemia may develop within 20 seconds. Furthermore, because of changes in venous return and pleural pressure, all hemodynamic parameters acutely change when ventilatory support is removed. Although muscle paralysis can remove spontaneous pleural pressure swings, it also produces a new hemodynamic state and is of little value in understanding ongoing hemodynamic events unless the patient requires prolonged neuromuscular blockade for other reasons.

Cardiac Limitation

The LAP usually reflects LVEDP, but with substantial mitral stenosis, mitral regurgitation, or aortic insufficiency, there may be a gradient between the mean LAP and true LVEDP. With prominent left atrial systole, the mean LAP may exceed the true LVEDP pressure. Measurements of ventricular pressure are merely estimates of ventricular volume and depend greatly on ventricular compliance. The normal left ventricular compliance is curvilinear, with compliance decreasing as volume increases. In critically ill patients, several factors can change ventricular compliance, including left ventricular wall mass, fiber stiffness, heart rate (especially in the elderly), body temperature, osmolarity, blood pressure, and right ventricular volume. Ventricular interdependence, the effect of right ventricular volume on left ventricular compliance, appears to be a major cause of the discrepancy between measured LAP and left ventricular volumes. Cardiac tamponade also substantially reduces ventricular compliance, resulting in very high intravascular pressures recorded at a time when ventricular stretch is minimal. Thus in a variety of circumstances, a shift in the ventricular compliance produces changes in pressure that poorly reflect changes in volume. Given the preceding complexities, it is not surprising that the correlation between end-diastolic ventricular volume determined from gaited heart pool scans and PAOP obtained by a PAC is not linear, and that occasionally there is no direct correlation whatsoever.

CARDIAC OUTPUT

Thermodilution measurements of cardiac output (CO) have become exceedingly reliable. The amount of indicator injected divided by the area under the dilution curve can be instantaneously calculated using a bedside computer and translated into a mean indicator transit time reflecting a CO with a reproducibility of ± 10 percent. The averages of three separate determinations are used to assess CO. Several studies have suggested that, because of the dramatic effect that a rapid change in pleural pressure may have on stroke volume, the reliability of thermodilution measurements is substantially altered by random timing of injections of the indicator. Therefore, under conditions of spontaneous or assisted ventilation, the indicator should be injected at the same point in the respiratory cycle, preferably at the time of end expiration. Recently, however, data suggest that the timing of the injection is not important and that the CO does not appreciably change during random injection. Cardiac outputs should be obtained periodically and after therapeutic adjustments. These measurements can be used to calculate derived indexes (e.g., systemic and pulmonary vascular resistance, stroke work), evaluate and optimize cardiac performance, and regulate tissue oxygen delivery.

OXYGEN DELIVERY

The PAC can be used to monitor measurements of mixed venous oxygen tensions ($P\bar{v}O_2$; normal = 36 to 45 mm Hg), the difference between arterial and mixed venous oxygen contents (A-V O_2; normal = 3 to 5 cc per deciliter), as well as oxygen delivery (DO_2; 640 to 1,400 cc of O_2 per minute). In normal individuals, there is little dependency of oxygen consumption on delivery—that is, there is increasing extraction of oxygen with a widening A-V difference as the CO decreases. The extraction ratio $\dot{V}O_2/DO_2$) normally ranges from 20 to 30 percent but may increase to 40 to 50 percent as the CO decreases. It has been suggested that monitoring of PvO_2 can be used to detect reductions in the CO. However, the mean PvO_2 represents a "soup" to which all venous beds contribute and is weighted by the amount of blood flow coming from highly perfused areas. PvO_2 is thus only a rough estimate of the amount of oxygen removed by many vital organs. Furthermore, individual organs have entirely different oxygen extraction ratios. In several critically ill patients, $\dot{V}O_2$ appears to depend on DO_2, with a higher delivery associated with higher oxygen consumption. This translates into a fixed PvO_2 under conditions of changing CO and oxygen consumption, and the PvO_2 value is therefore rarely helpful in estimating changes in CO or vital organ perfusion. However, a very low value (<25 mm Hg) is associated with a poor prognosis and poor cardiac performance. Although continuous monitoring of venous oxygen tension by attachment of a fiberoptic colorimetric analyzer to the PAC adds an additional real-time monitoring parameter, it increases the expense of the PAC and has not been shown to improve patient outcome.

Measurements of $\dot{V}O_2$ and DO_2 have been used to assess clinical progress during therapy. Pushing fluid or vasoactive drugs to elevate a normal or increased DO_2 has not been shown to improve prognosis. In general, a high DO_2 is associated with a better patient outcome, most likely because the presence of a poor cardiac pump worsens patient survival. The documentation of delivery dependence of $\dot{V}O_2$ indicates a poor survival. Correlations between DO_2, lactic acidosis, and outcome are not good except in extreme situations where DO_2 is less than 10 ml per minute per kilogram. Under these circumstances, the failure to augment CO is disastrous.

COMPLICATIONS

Pulmonary Artery Catheters

Complications of PACs are not uncommon and represent a clear patient risk (Table 3). This plus an initial patient charge of approximately $1,000 constitute the major downside to PAC usage. Possibly one of the most important "complications" of the PAC is the long delay in starting necessary treatment that results from waiting for the completion of the catheter insertion and the "truth" to be read from the oscilloscope. We have seen numerous patients who do not receive life-sustaining support because of distractions related to catheter insertion. Besides cognitive delays, inaccurate measurements and false interpretations should also be listed as "complications." In general, major complications occur in approximately 9 percent of patients. Complications occur in 40 to 50 percent of patients, although most of these are minor. Complications can be divided into those associated with (1) central venous cannulation, (2) passage of the catheter through the heart into the pulmonary artery, and (3) the presence of the catheter in the circulation over time.

Venous Cannulation

Problems of insertion are among the most common and serious drawbacks of PAC. Venous access is often mandatory in patient management, however, and once it is established, it reduces the overall risk of PAC usage. One of the most common complications is caused by the need for multiple "sticks" to access a central vessel. Approximately half of the procedures are successful on the very first attempt, with 20 percent requiring three or more attempts. Inadvertent arterial puncture occurs in approximately 8 to 10 percent of patients and infrequently leads to significant sequelae. Hemothorax can be catastrophic if large amounts of blood escape into the pleural space. Because of its anatomic location, the subclavian artery is the most difficult to tamponade. Pneumothoraces occur in only 2 percent of patients, but may also be quite serious. Since an immediate chest x-ray examination may not reveal that the lung has been punctured, one should delay attempts to cannulate central veins on opposite sides of the chest for several hours. Hemomediastinum, although dramatic radiographically, rarely leads to significant physiologic problems.

Passage of the Catheter Through the Heart

Complications of passage of the PAC through the right heart chambers are predominantly those related to arrhythmias. Less than 1 percent of these are serious. Right bundle branch block may occur and, for this reason, catheter

Table 3 Complications of Flow-Directed PACs

Central venous cannulation
 Arterial puncture/hematoma (8%)
 Pneumothorax (2%–4%)
 Hydrothorax (2%)
 Hemothorax, brachial plexus damage, air embolism, phrenic and recurrent laryngeal nerve damage, sheared catheter (<1% each)

Passage of catheter
 Arrhythmias (13%–70%; 1% serious)
 Right bundle branch block (3%)
 Cardiac perforation and tamponade (<1%)

Presence of catheter in circulation
 Infection; colonization-contamination (3%–40%); sepsis (4%–6%)
 Thrombosis - evidence of (66%); clinical thromboembolism (<1%)
 Endocardial damage (36%); valve damage (<1%); aseptic endocarditis (21%);* bacterial endocarditis (0–7%)*
 Pulmonary infarction (<1%–7%)
 Pulmonary artery rupture (<1% each); balloon rupture; knotting

*Seen at autopsy.

insertions should rarely be performed in patients who already have left bundle branch block. The duration of passage of the PAC through the right heart, the length of the catheter inserted, and the failure to completely inflate the balloon (leaving a catheter tip to irritate the ventricular wall) all contribute to the incidence of arrhythmias.

Presence of the Catheter in the Circulation

Among problems related to the presence of the PAC in the circulation, infection is the most common. In several prospective analyses, risk of catheter infection occurred in approximately 1.8 percent of catheters per day. Catheter infection is usually defined by quantitative catheter culture technique since this best correlates with risks of bacteremia. Gram stain of the distal catheter tip is also a reported accurate test for diagnosis of intravascular catheter-associated infection. Additional risk factors associated with catheter infection are (1) frequent manipulations, with or without a protective sheath; (2) inexperience on the part of the inserter; (3) the use of transparent dressings that tend to keep the operative site moist; (4) violations of aseptic technique, such as breaking open a Leur lock to draw blood without prior disinfection of the external catheter surface; (5) the use of multilumen catheters; and (6) inadequate sterilization of reusable pressure transducers. Factors associated with a reduced risk of infection are (1) a team approach to catheter insertion and maintenance, where one team is responsible for the care of all vascular catheters; (2) skin preparation with chlorhexidine gluconate instead of providone-iodine, which may reduce the risk of infection fourfold; and (3) the use of topical antibiotics, especially polymyxin-neomycin-bacitracin ointment (although the risk of *Candida* infection may be increased with this approach). Techniques that have no apparent effect on risk of infection are (1) the use of in-line filters; (2) changing catheters at frequent intervals over guide wires; (3) wearing masks and gowns; and (4) changing intravenous tubing more often than every 72 hours.

The most common organisms infecting PACs are coagulase-negative staphylococci (28 percent), *Staphylococcus aureus* (27 percent), and *Candida* (18 percent). Catheter removal plus prolonged antimicrobial therapy is mandated for *Staphylococcus aureus* and *Candida* infections. Autopsy studies have revealed a frequency of atrial, tricuspid, or pulmonic valve damage of up to 30 percent in dying patients with PACs and may account for the increased risk of endocarditis in this group. Infection clearly relates to how long the catheter remains in place. Risk of infection increases substantially after 3 to 4 days. Recent data suggest that replacement of a catheter over a guide wire at the same insertion site is associated with the same rate of infection as a new catheter inserted at a different site.

Intravascular thrombosis may also be seen at autopsy or by computed tomography in a large percentage of patients, but pulmonary embolism from the PAC appears to be infrequent. Pulmonary infarction or pulmonary hemorrhage from either overinflation of the balloon or wedging of the balloon for prolonged periods occurs rarely. When pulmonary hemorrhage does occur, it is dramatic, difficult to treat, and often fatal.

SUGGESTED READING

Connors AF, Dawson NV, McCaffree R, et al. Assessing hemodynamic status in critically ill patients: do physicians use clinical information optimally? J Crit Care 1987; 2:174–180.

Marini JJ. Hemodynamic monitoring with the pulmonary artery catheter. Crit Care Clinics 1986; 2:551–572.

Matthay MA. Guidelines for pulmonary artery catheterization in the intensive care unit. Pulmonary Perspectives 1987; 4:1–4.

Sharkey SW. Beyond the wedge: clinical physiology and the Swan-Ganz catheter. Am J Med 1987; 83:111–120.

Sise MJ, Hollingsworth P, Brimm JE, et al. Complications of the flow-directed pulmonary-artery catheter: a prospective analysis in 219 patients. Crit Care Med 1981; 9:315–318.

CARDIOVASCULAR THERAPEUTICS

CARDIOGENIC SHOCK

CARL V. LEIER, M.D.

"Cardiogenic shock" is the term used to describe the condition whereby the heart fails as a pump to deliver an adequate amount of blood to the body during rest, with consequent hypoperfusion of organs, tissue, and cells. Basically, the delivery of oxygen (Do_2) and metabolic substrate becomes inadequate to sustain basic cellular function and viability because the heart is not capable of generating an adequate stroke volume and cardiac output. The heart can fail as a pump because of impaired diastolic function, impaired systolic function, or a combination of these impairments. The majority of patients in cardiogenic shock sustain marked depression of ventricular systolic function with a resultant drop in forward stroke volume and cardiac output. In the United States and Europe, the majority of events causing ventricular systolic dysfunction and shock are related to myocardial ischemia-infarction and the complications thereof (e.g., pump failure, ruptured ventricular wall or septum, disrupted papillary muscle). Because of the high prevalence of myocardial ischemia-infarction as the cause of cardiogenic shock, this chapter focuses on the approach and management of this condition.

Approximately 10 to 15 percent of all patients with an acute myocardial infarction experience cardiogenic shock within 1 week of the event. In more than 50 percent, this occurs within the first 48 hours secondary to acute pump failure. Infarction-induced pump failure indicates that at least 40 percent of the myocardium has lost its ability to contract.

Few areas in all of medicine have advanced as dramatically over the past 20 years (even over the past 5 years) as have the therapeutics of myocardial ischemia-infarction. Many of these interventions (e.g., thrombolysis, angioplasty) have a favorable impact on cardiogenic shock by averting myocardial ischemia and infarction, "salvaging" ischemic myocardium, and reducing infarct size in patients with coronary artery disease; all of the interventions are directed at the *prevention* of myocardial loss and dysfunction. Therefore the first step in the approach and management of cardiogenic shock is an "aggressive" approach (e.g., thrombolysis, cardiac catheterization, angioplasty, bypass surgery) to the cardiac ischemic syndromes.

APPROACH AND MANAGEMENT

The main objective in the management of cardiogenic shock is to bring the hemodynamic status of the patient into a physiologically acceptable range to allow definitive diagnostic testing (cardiac catheterization and angiography) and repair (e.g., coronary angioplasty, coronary bypass surgery). If cardiogenic shock is not brought into a hemodynamically acceptable range to allow definitive diagnostic testing and repair, if testing and repair are not pursued, or if angioplastic or surgical repair are not successful or indicated (i.e., the patient does not have a surgically treatable lesion), the overall in-hospital mortality rate associated with cardiogenic shock is more than 80 percent. With proper pharmacologic and mechanical support accompanied by appropriate diagnostic studies and successful intervention (e.g., coronary angioplasty, bypass surgery, valve repair or replacement), the mortality rate decreases to less than 60 percent. Clearly the proper approach and management of these patients can make a difference.

Pharmacologic Intervention

The effectiveness of pharmacologic support in the treatment of cardiogenic shock is related to (1) the prompt recognition of the syndrome with proficient application of therapy and (2) the proper selection of therapy based on the clinical and hemodynamic profile of the patient.

The recognition (and hence the treatment) of cardiogenic shock is often delayed because of misconceptions regarding the shock syndrome in general. The diagnosis of shock is based on evidence of systemic, organ, and/or cellular hypoperfusion. Some of the more established signs of shock, such as hypotension and reduced urine output, may not be present in shock of mild-to-moderate severity or during its early phases; rather, they are usually indications of advanced stages and/or decompensation. It is important to recognize and treat the shock syndrome vigorously at the earliest stage possible.

The recommended pharmacologic interventions, presented in Table 1, are based on the clinical and hemodynamic profile of the patient. The optimal management of cardiogenic shock requires a frequent assessment of systemic, organ, and cellular perfusion via clinical signs (e.g., sensorium, color and temperature of skin) and laboratory data (e.g., urine volume and sodium concentrations, arterial and venous pH, partial pressure of oxygen, carbon dioxide partial pressure, and lactate levels)

Table 1 Recommendations for Initial Pharmacologic Support of Patients Presenting in Cardiogenic Shock Based on the Hemodynamic Profile and Parameters (Clinical and Laboratory) of Systemic/Organ Perfusion

Systemic/Organ Perfusion	Systemic Blood Pressure	LV Filling Pressure	Cardiac Output	Pharmacologic Agents Recommended as Initial Intervention
↓	→ or ↓	↓	→ or ↓	Fluid volume
↓	→ or ↑	→ or ↑	→ or ↓	Vasodilator therapy
↓	↓ (systolic 70–100 mm Hg)	↑	↓	Dobutamine infusion
↓	↓↓ (systolic ≤70 mm Hg)	↑	↓	Dopamine infusion

↓ = decreased; ↑ = increased; ↓↓ = markedly decreased; → = within normal limits.

and of hemodynamics via data attained from a flow-directed pulmonary artery (Swan-Ganz) catheter and a systemic arterial catheter. Pharmacologic and dose choices are made through the evaluation of the state of systemic/organ perfusion, systemic blood pressure, left ventricular filling pressure (assessed indirectly from pulmonary capillary wedge pressure readings), and cardiac output. Other parameters (e.g., heart rate, right atrial pressure) are also important in certain situations.

Low Left Ventricular Filling Pressure, Normal-to-Low Systemic Blood Pressure, Normal-to-Low Cardiac Output, and Systemic Hypoperfusion

It is important to note that 15 to 20 percent of postinfarction shock patients enter with *low* ventricular filling pressures. If this is accompanied by systemic hypoperfusion, the treatment of choice is fluid volume (0.9 N sodium chloride), administered intravenously. The treatment aim is to improve systemic perfusion and generally increase or normalize systemic blood pressure by augmenting stroke volume and cardiac output; this is accomplished via the Frank-Starling mechanism by increasing left ventricular filling pressures from less than or equal to 12 mm Hg to pressures within 15 to 18 mm Hg. In many of these patients, fluid volume administration alone improves and stabilizes the patient's hemodynamics through the acute phase of the infarction and the diagnostic studies, if needed. Fluid must be administered with caution in this setting in order to avoid the development of fluid volume overload and pulmonary edema. It is seldom necessary to drive left ventricular (LV) filling pressures to more than 18 mm Hg.

Some of the patients do not regain an adequate clinical or hemodynamic status after fluid volume therapy has increased the LV filling pressure to 15 to 18 mm Hg. At this point, pharmacologic support is usually needed and is generally guided by the level of systemic blood pressure. Vasodilator therapy (e.g., intravenous nitroglycerin or nitroprusside) is directed at systolic pressures of 100 mm Hg or more, the positive inotrope, dobutamine is used for pressures of 70 mm Hg or more and less than or equal to 100 mm Hg, and dopamine is used for pressures of 70 mm Hg or less. The rationale for these choices is presented below.

Right ventricular infarction is not an infrequent cause of low LV filling pressures, systemic hypoperfusion, hypotension, and reduced cardiac output. Although volume administration is the initial intervention, in my experience, however, it is very difficult to bring LV filling pressures to 15 mm Hg or more despite considerable volume administration (≥ 4 L). Volume administration must therefore often be supplemented by an infusion of dobutamine or dopamine, and occasionally, by the addition of intra-aortic balloon counterpulsation.

Adequate-to-High Left Ventricular Filling Pressure (≥15 mm Hg), Normal-to-High Systemic Blood Pressure (≥100 mm Hg Systolic), Normal-to-Low Cardiac Output, and Systemic Hypoperfusion

While a patient with this hemodynamic profile may be experiencing systemic hypoperfusion, he or she would generally be viewed as having congestive heart failure rather than cardiogenic shock. The basic treatment for such a patient is vasodilator therapy—nitroglycerin (administered sublingually and/or intravenously) or nitroprusside for the initial, more urgent intervention (e.g., moderate-to-marked dyspnea, pulmonary edema), and in less severe and less acute situations, an angiotensin-converting enzyme inhibitor (e.g., captopril, starting at 6.25 mg orally). Concomitant diuretic therapy is also necessary for most of the patients who fall into this general category.

Adequate-to-High Left Ventricular Filling Pressures, Mild-to-Moderate Systemic Hypotension (Systolic Pressures of 70 to 100 mm Hg), Normal-to-Low Cardiac Output and Systemic Hypoperfusion

This clinical-hemodynamic subset makes up the largest portion of those patients who enter the hospital with hemodynamic compromise after an acute myocardial infarction. Generally these patients have symptoms and signs of systemic hypoperfusion with LV filling pressures of 15 mm Hg or more, systemic systolic pressures of 70 mm Hg or more and less than or equal to 100 mm Hg, and decreased stroke volume and cardiac output.

Because the predominant problem in this setting is loss of ventricular contractility and function, the most direct and effective pharmacologic approach is positive inotropic therapy, aimed at improving ventricular contractility. Dobutamine, a synthetic catechol, is the most selective positive inotropic agent available with the fewest undesirable effects. In the presence of depressed ventricular function, high LV filling pressures, mild-to-moderate hypotension, and reduced peripheral perfusion, dobutamine (2 to 15 μg per kilogram per minute) improves ventricular performance, stroke volume, and cardiac output, decreases ventricular filling pressures, normalizes systemic blood pressure (via an increase in stroke volume and pulse pressure), and enhances peripheral perfusion. With proper patient and dose selection, these favorable hemodynamic effects can be attained with little tachycardia, no major changes in blood pressure, and a mild increase or no increase in myocardial oxygen consumption (MV_{O_2}). When dosing is selected to elicit the favorable hemodynamic effects without evoking tachycardia, ventricular ectopy, or major changes in blood pressure, dobutamine has a favorable effect on the MV_{O_2}/O_2 supply ratio; this is particularly important in patients with occlusive coronary artery disease. While positive inotropy is invariably accompanied by an increase in MV_{O_2}, dobutamine offsets this effect by reducing other components of MV_{O_2}; specifically, it decreases ventricular afterload and wall stress (by reducing systemic and pulmonary vascular resistances, ventricular systolic volume, and ventricular filling pressure). By increasing diastolic time (dobutamine decreases the duration of systole) and coronary perfusion pressure (decreased LV filling pressure while diastolic blood pressure remains unchanged or increases), the myocardial oxygen supply tends to increase during dobutamine administration. These points have been proven in animal models and in a variety of human conditions of myocardial ischemia (e.g., myocardial infarction, ischemic cardiomyopathy). It is important to emphasize, however, that the success of positive inotropic therapy (i.e., dobutamine) in this setting depends on proper patient and dose selection. Improper selection of either patients or dose results in the generation of more undesirable (e.g., tachycardia) than desirable effects. The patient must have depressed ventricular function, an adequate-to-high ventricular filling pressure, and mild-to-moderate hypotension, and after an initial dose of 2 to 3 μg per kilogram per minute has been given, doses should be increased by increments of 2 to 3 μg per kilogram per minute every 15 to 30 minutes (at lesser intervals if the patient is unstable and at greater intervals if the patient is generally stable) until the clinical and hemodynamic endpoints are met. Deviation from these guidelines always results in tachycardia (a serious side effect in occlusive coronary artery disease), major pressure changes (decrease or excessive increase), increased LV filling pressures, and symptoms (e.g., angina, dyspnea, tremors, headaches).

Dopamine given in low-to-moderate doses (2 to 6 μg per kilogram per minute) is a reasonable alternative to treatment with dobutamine in this clinical setting. I favor dobutamine because of evidence from experiments with animals and humans suggesting that, in this clinical setting, dobutamine tends to have a more favorable effect on coronary artery resistance, coronary blood flow and myocardial perfusion, ventricular filling pressures, vascular resistances, aortic impedance, stroke volume and cardiac output per change in MV_{O_2}, heart rate, and ventricular ectopy. Increasing dopamine dosing to 8 μg per kilogram per minute or more in an attempt to further improve hemodynamics often elicits an alpha-adrenergic vasoconstricting effect, a potentially detrimental response (increased afterload) for the failing ventricle.

Combination therapy is common in the treatment of patients with cardiogenic shock. Nitroprusside or nitroglycerin may be added to the dobutamine infusion if dobutamine has brought systemic systolic pressure to 100 mm Hg or more, but systemic and organ perfusion will remain depressed. Dopamine (or norepinephrine) may be added to the dobutamine infusion if increasing doses of dobutamine fail to increase the systolic pressure to more than 80 mm Hg.

Dobutamine may augment renal function and urine output in patients whose compromised hemodynamics have resulted in renal dysfunction. Many cardiologists and intensivists have found that renal function can be further improved by the addition of dopamine in doses of 2 to 5 μg per kilogram per minute, which can increase renal blood flow and the glomerular filtration rate by stimulating renal dopaminergic receptors.

Adequate-to-High Left Ventricular Filling Pressures, Marked Hypotension (<70 mm Hg), Depressed Cardiac Output, and Systemic-Organ Hypoperfusion

The patient with this clinical-hemodynamic profile is perceived by most clinicians to be the prototypical cardiogenic shock patient—one whose cardiac dysfunction is severe enough to result in high filling pressures, depressed stroke volume and cardiac output, marked hypotension (systolic pressures <70 mm Hg), and systemic-organ hypoperfusion. The failure to achieve hemodynamic improvement proficiently and advance to definitive diagnostic testing and definitive repair in this population subset sets the stage for a mortality rate of more than 90 percent.

While the most common cause of cardiogenic shock in this setting is loss of myocardial contractility, selective positive inotropic therapy alone is not the optimal first-line pharmacologic approach. Brain, kidney, and myocardium are particularly vulnerable to marked hypotension. This marked hypotension is not reversed in the most efficacious manner by agents like dobutamine. The initial approach should generally include the use of a drug with vasopressor activity. Dopamine, with its combined vasopressor properties (alpha$_1$ receptor agonism) and positive inotropic effects, is the drug of choice. Dopamine, given in an initial dose of 4 μg per kilogram per minute and increased by increments of 3 to 4 μg per kilogram per minute every 10 to 15 minutes as needed generally raises systemic blood pressure to levels acceptable for brain and myocardial perfusion until more definitive intervention (e.g., mechanical assistance device, surgical repair) can be instituted. Cerebral and renal perfusion require systemic systolic pressures of 75 to 80 mm Hg or more, and coronary perfusion requires a systemic diastolic pressure of 60 mm Hg or more (with a LV diastolic filling pressure of 15 mm Hg or less).

If dopamine fails to bring systemic pressure to 80/60 mm Hg or more despite doses of 15 μg per kilogram per minute or more and mechanical assistance has not yet been instituted, the physician must consider the addition of a norepinephrine infusion at a starting dose of 0.02 μg per kilogram per minute with incrementation of dose every 10 to 15 minutes. On the other hand, if dopamine has increased systemic pressures to more than 80/50 mm Hg, further improvement at this stage of hemodynamics is usually best accomplished (for the reasons mentioned above) by the addition of a dobutamine infusion rather than by an increase in the dopamine dosage.

General Overview of Pharmacologic Intervention

At the most fundamental level, the patient in cardiogenic shock can be approached with this basic algorithm:

1. Fluid volume replacement should be given if the LV filling pressure is low.
2. Dopmaine is administered if LV filling pressure is 15 to 18 mm Hg or more and if systemic pressure is markedly depressed at levels of 70/50 or less.
3. Dobutamine (or lower-dose dopamine) is administered if the LV filling pressure is 15 to 18 mm Hg or more and if the degree of hypotension is mild to moderate.
4. A vasodilator (nitroglycerin or nitroprusside) is given if the LV filling pressure is 15 to 18 mm Hg or more and if systemic pressures are greater than 100/70.
5. From a pharmacologic standpoint, any combination of the above may be necessary for the optimal management of the cardiogenic shock patient.

Other Pharmacologic Considerations and Other Support Measures

Many other measures are extremely important in the overall care of the cardiogenic shock patient. Ventilatory support is usually required for the patient whose arterial Po$_2$ remains 60 mm Hg or less while on a high-flow (fractional inspired oxygen > 50 percent) oxygen mask. Diuretic therapy (generally intravenous furosemide) is often indicated to reduce congestion and high LV filling pressures with increasing dose requirements during the development of renal dysfunction and failure. Potassium supplementation may be needed to keep serum K$^+$ levels above 4 mEq per liter, but must be used with caution and/or restricted when renal dysfunction and failure occur. Continuous electrocardiographic monitoring is needed to detect and treat threatening arrhythmias. Hemodynamic values and recordings need to be assessed frequently to ascertain that the proper drugs and doses are being used, that the intravascular volume status is appropriate and optimal, and that the data collected are actually correct. A continuous effort must be directed at preventing the complications of shock (e.g., infection, sepsis, gastrointestinal bleeding) and promptly treating them when they arise. Close "attention to detail" is essential for the optimal management of cardiogenic shock.

Mechanical Assist ("Bridge" Intervention)

Intra-Aortic Balloon Counterpulsation

Intra-aortic balloon counterpulsation (IABC) represents a major advance in the management of cardiogenic shock. When IABC alone is added to pharmacologic support, the in-hospital mortality rate decreases from more than 90 percent to 80 percent. This modest reduction in the mortality rate emphasizes that IABC is not a definitive form of treatment for cardiogenic shock. IABC is a form of "bridge" therapy, providing hemodynamic support until the diagnostic studies and definitive intervention (e.g., angioplasty, bypass surgery) are applied; it is occasionally continued beyond this time. As a bridge to more definitive intervention, IABC becomes an essential part of the pharmacologic-IABC-definitive intervention (thrombolysis, angioplasty and/or bypass surgery) complex, the application of which decreases the in-hospital and short-term mortality rate to less than 60 percent.

IABC is an effective means of improving hemodynamics while reducing MVo$_2$ and increasing the myocardial oxygen supply. The intra-aortic balloon, gated to the electrocardiogram, inflates during diastole. As a result, peripheral perfusion and coronary myocardial perfusion improve during diastole, and LV afterload is reduced. The decrease in afterload then augments LV performance and reduces LV wall stress, diastolic pressure and volume, and MVo$_2$. The prompt application of IABC generally reduces the doses used in pharmacologic support and therefore reduces its undesirable effects.

The intra-aortic balloon is inserted percutaneously (via the femoral artery) and is placed in the descending thoracic-abdominal aorta (above the renal arteries). The two contraindications to IABC are moderate-to-severe aortic valvular insufficiency, which would be greatly exacerbated by diastolic augmentation of aortic pressure, and an aortic aneurysm (dissecting or large saccular).

The timing of the application of IABC is very important. Unfortunately, IABC is often instituted after shock has advanced to severe stages or after the patient has failed to respond to high-dose vasopressors or renal failure has ensued. It is not uncommon to see a "cautious" delay in instituting optimal (albeit invasive) therapy result in death. As soon as it becomes apparent that a patient's clinical and hemodynamic status is refractory to treatment with standard doses of dopamine and/or dobutamine and the decision has been made to pursue the definitive diagnostic/intervention approach, the IABC team should be called and IABC instituted. Hemodynamic stabilization should then be followed by a diagnostic cardiac catheterization, angioplasty, and/or a surgical procedure. Of course, the "aggressive" approach (pharmacologic support-mechanical assistance-definitive intervention) is not indicated for all patients in cardiogenic shock. For the patient in whom this approach is indicated, it is crucial not to delay IABC therapy.

Cardiopulmonary bypass is a reasonable alternative to IABC if the patient is very close (temporally and physically) to undergoing a definitive surgical procedure (e.g., bypass surgery, valve replacement).

Ventricular Assist Devices and the Total Artificial Heart

These modalities require surgical implantation and are applied to the patient who fails to respond to pharmacologic and IABC therapy, and in whom the decision has been made to treat the underlying cardiac condition and cardiogenic shock definitively with cardiac transplantation. As such, these interventions should be regarded as a "bridge" to transplantation and are generally available only at centers performing heart transplants.

Several ventricular assist devices (VAD) are available now. VAD placement may be intrathoracic or extracorporal. Basically, the VAD removes blood from the atrium or ventricle and ejects it into the aorta (pulmonary artery for right VAD). Patients can be managed with a left VAD alone, but often require both right and left VADs (biVAD). To date, most VAD placement has occurred in young patients with a malignant form of acute cardiomyopathy or myocarditis.

The total artificial heart (e.g., Jarvik 7) is an alternative to VAD intervention. However, compared with the biVAD approach, the current total artificial heart units (1989) tend to be associated with more thromboembolic and hemorrhagic complications. In addition, prolonged (>1 month) placement of the total artificial heart makes subsequent surgery (i.e., heart transplant) much more difficult because of mediastinal scarring and perioperative hemorrhage.

"Definitive" Intervention; Coronary Angioplasty, Coronary Bypass Surgery, Valvular Replacement, Cardiac Transplantation

For most patients who enter the hospital in cardiogenic shock, pharmacologic and mechanical assist support is directed at improving and stabilizing hemodynamics to allow the pursuit of definitive diagnostic studies and definitive repair. For most patients, a clear description via cardiac catheterization/angiography of the cardiac pathologic processes makes the selection of a repair procedure a more rational one, its performance easier and considerably better guided, and the eventual outcome more favorable. Preliminary reports indicate that with proper patient selection and preprocedure management, successful coronary angioplasty and bypass surgery are improving inhospital and posthospitalization survival for patients who enter with myocardial ischemia-infarction and cardiogenic shock. It is important to remember that the high intensity of pharmacologic and mechanical support (and the monitoring thereof) should be maintained throughout the diagnostic studies and up to the time the patient receives cardiopulmonary bypass.

While impressive advances have been made over the past two decades to temper the dismal outcome from cardiogenic shock, we have "definitively" solved the problem only to a very limited extent. It is to be hoped that the advances of the next two decades will allow physicians to pull still more shock patients out of death's grip.

SUGGESTED READING

Gunnar RM, Loeb HS. Shock in acute myocardial infarction: evolution of physiological therapy. J Am Coll Cardiol 1983; 1:154.
Leier CV, ed. Cardiotonic drugs. New York: Marcel Dekker, 1986.
Leier CV. Approach to the patient with hypotension and shock. In: Kelley WN, ed. Textbook of internal medicine. Philadelphia: JB Lippincott Co., 1989:393.
Schreiber TL, Miller DH, Zola B. Management of myocardial infarction shock: current status. Am Heart J 1989: 117:435.

ANAPHYLAXIS AND ANAPHYLACTIC SHOCK

MARILYN T. HAUPT, M.D.

Anaphylaxis is a systemic form of immediate hypersensitivity that may progress to a life-threatening crisis. Severe cases are frequently explosive in onset and are associated with sudden death. Involvement of the upper airway, respiratory, and circulatory systems characteristically precede a fatal outcome.

These reactions may be triggered by environmental stimuli (Table 1) that may be antigenic, nonantigenic, or idiopathic. In classic anaphylactic events, antigenic stimuli initiate a sequence of events, mediated by IgE, that results in the release of potent mast cell- and basophil-derived biochemical mediators. Nonantigenic stimuli may also initiate a clinically identical response. In these reactions, also termed *anaphylactoid reactions*, biochemical mediators are released through direct contact of the nonantigenic stimulus with mast cells and basophils. Accordingly, anaphylactoid reactions are not mediated by IgE. Rarely,

Table 1 Agents Implicated in Anaphylactic and Anaphylactoid Reactions

Antibiotics	Diagnostic agents
Penicillin and analogs	Iodinated radiocontrast agents
Cephalosporins	
Sulfonamides	Foods
Tetracycline	Eggs
Erythromycin	Milk and milk products
Streptomycin	Legumes (peanuts, soybeans, kidney beans, chick peas)
Vancomycin	Nuts
Local anesthetics	Fish, shellfish
Procaine	Rice
Lidocaine	Citrus fruits
Cocaine	
	Food additives
Narcotic analgesics	Sulfite preservatives
Morphine	Tartrazine dye
Codeine	
Meprobamate	Venoms
	(Bees, wasps, hornets, snakes, spiders, jellyfish, fire ants)
Nonsteroidal anti-inflammatory agents	
Salicylates	Hormones
Aminopyrine	Insulin
	Adrenocorticotropic hormone
General anesthetics and agents	Pituitary extracts
Thiopental	Vasopressin
Succinylcholine chloride	
Tubocurarine	Enzymes
	Pancreatic enzyme supplements
Other drugs	Acetylcysteine
Protamine	
Chlorpropamide	Extracts of allergens used for desensitization
Parenteral iron, Iodides, Thiazide diuretics	Pollen
Dextrans	Food
Plasmaprotein fraction (Plasmanate)	Venoms
	Animal dander (dog, cat)
Blood products and antisera	Other biologicals
Red blood cell, white blood cell, and platelet transfusions	Semen
	Monoclonal antibodies
Gamma globulin	Antithymocyte globulins
Rabies	Antilymphocyte globulins
Tetanus	
Diphtheria antitoxin	
Snake and spider antivenoms	

Prompt treatment of the patient with anaphylaxis is crucial. Immediate airway control, fluid loading, and pharmacologic support with epinephrine are of proven efficacy. These interventions should be instituted automatically. If they are unsuccessful, additional drugs that modulate the effects of mediators may be tried. However, because the efficacy of these secondary therapeutic modalities in the treatment of anaphylaxis remains unproven, a thorough understanding of the pharmacologic effects, mechanism of action, and toxicity of these modalities must accompany their use. The approach to the use of these secondary drugs should therefore be thoughtful and logical.

ASSESSMENT OF THE PATIENT

Initial assessment of the patient with anaphylaxis should be brief since immediate therapeutic interventions are often required. When the association of the crisis with an offending agent is unclear, conditions that may simulate anaphylactic crises should be considered (Table 2). These conditions include acute cardiac and pulmonary events, vasovagal episodes, carcinoid syndrome attacks, and drug overdoses.

The clinical presentation of the patient with anaphylaxis is characteristically acute but may vary, depending on several factors such as the portal of entry, rate of absorption of the offending agent, and the patient's degree of hypersensitivity. For example, ingestion of a substance associated with anaphylaxis may lead to gastrointestinal symptoms including nausea, vomiting, diarrhea, and abdominal cramps. These symptoms may then progress to generalized systemic manifestations. Skin exposure may be associated with a localized pruritic, cutaneous reaction. Inhalation may initiate nasal coryza, wheezing, hoarseness, stridor, dyspnea, or the sensation of tightness or a lump in the throat. Intravenous injection may immediately progress, without warning, to hypovolemic and circulatory shock. Recent physical activity, ethanol ingestion, and beta-adrenergic blocker therapy appear to exaggerate anaphylactic responses. Although

a thorough clinical evaluation fails to uncover the inciting agent in a patient who has a reaction resembling anaphylaxis. These reactions, which are frequently nocturnal or postprandial, are termed idiopathic anaphylactoid reactions.

Mast cell- and basophil-derived mediators released in anaphylactic, anaphylactoid, and idiopathic anaphylactoid reactions have a variety of pathophysiologic effects. Mediator-induced increases in microvascular permeability and bronchial reactivity are effects that are of major clinical importance because of the association with upper airway obstruction from laryngeal edema, impaired pulmonary gas exchange, and hypovolemic shock. The subsequent activation of the complement and coagulation cascades produces additional adverse systemic effects.

Table 2 Conditions That May Simulate Anaphylaxis

Acute cardiac events
  Supraventricular and ventricular tachycardias
  Acute myocardial infarction

Acute pulmonary events
  Pulmonary embolus
  Asthmatic attack
  Pulmonary edema
  Spontaneous pneumothorax

Carcinoid syndrome attacks

Drug overdose

Insulin shock

Vasovagal episodes

most patients with anaphylaxis respond to initial therapy, some exhibit prolonged persistent reactions despite appropriate therapy. Others exhibit a biphasic anaphylactic reaction, a recurrence of anaphylactic symptoms after an initial favorable response to therapy, usually within 12 to 24 hours.

Physical findings in these patients are highly variable and depend on both the site of antigen introduction and the severity of the reaction. Examination of the skin may reveal diffuse erythema or urticaria. Angioedema may be observed and usually involves the periorbital and perioral areas. Signs of involvement of the upper respiratory tract include edema of the posterior pharynx, uvula, and vocal cords, and inspiratory stridor. Lower respiratory tract involvement may include wheezing, prolonged expiration, and expiratory stridor. Signs of circulatory shock may characterize severe cases of anaphylaxis and include hypotension, tachycardia, oliguria, and alterations of consciousness.

Arterial blood gases are highly variable in anaphylaxis. Nevertheless, significant decreases in oxygen saturation may characterize severe episodes. Ventilation may be impaired. A high anion gap metabolic acidosis from lactic acid accumulation may herald severe perfusion failure. An emergency chest x-ray examination is mandatory if respiratory symptoms are observed. Patients with anaphylaxis are susceptible to acute pneumothoraces and acute pulmonary emphysema, problems produced by forced expiration, especially against a closed, edematous glottis. The electrocardiogram may reveal myocardial ischemia or ventricular irritability. Hemoconcentration is frequently observed and is secondary to the movement of fluid and protein from the intravascular to extravascular space induced by increased microvascular permeability.

INITIAL MANAGEMENT

The initial management of patients with anaphylaxis includes the establishment of a patent airway and adequate gas exchange, the removal of toxin at the site of exposure and/or the reduction of systemic absorption of toxin, pharmacologic support with epinephrine, and the establishment of an adequate circulating blood volume with fluid loading. These interventions should proceed rapidly and, if possible, simultaneously.

All patients with anaphylaxis with systemic symptoms and signs should be admitted to a hospital staffed and equipped to provide emergency airway control and advanced hemodynamic monitoring. A favorable response to the initial therapy should not preclude hospitalization since recurrent symptoms (biphasic reaction) may develop 12 to 24 hours later. The hospitalized patient should be monitored for signs of circulatory shock and respiratory failure. Blood pressure, urine output, and heart rate should be monitored at frequent intervals. Continuous monitoring of the electrocardiogram is important since serious dysrhythmias are characteristic of anaphylactic reactions and may accompany therapy with epinephrine, beta-adrenergic bronchodilators, other catecholamines such as dopamine and levarterenol, and phosphodiesterase inhibitors such as aminophylline and theophylline. If the patient exhibits signs of circulatory shock or if pulmonary edema supervenes after initial therapy, monitoring of intra-arterial pressure, pulmonary artery pressures, and cardiac output should be considered.

In patients who are breathing comfortably but have alterations of consciousness, the head and neck should be positioned so that the airway is not obstructed by the tongue. If laryngeal edema with stridor is present, however, endotracheal intubation should be attempted. If endotracheal intubation fails, it will be necessary to perform an emergency cricothyroidotomy. Supplemental oxygen should be provided, and if spontaneous ventilation is impaired, the patient will require mechanical ventilation.

Retained stingers from Hymenoptera (bees, wasps, yellow jackets, hornets) must be removed completely. If the site of evenomization is an extremity, a proximal constricting band should be applied to delay the absorption of venom. This band should be tightened sufficiently to impair venous flow from the involved area without disrupting arterial flow to the distal extremity. Epinephrine may be injected locally and retards systemic absorption by producing localized vasoconstriction. The removal of sequestered subcutaneous snake venom by suction kits or surgical techniques is controversial. These efforts are unlikely to be helpful if more than 30 minutes has elapsed since the evenomization and may produce additional tissue destruction and/or enhance venom absorption. If the patient has been exposed to an antigen in contact with the skin surface, the involved area should be thoroughly washed without delay.

Epinephrine therapy is of proven efficacy for the treatment of anaphylactic crises. Two concentrations are available: a 1:1,000 solution (1.0 mg per milliliter) and a 1:10,000 solution (0.1 mg per milliliter). Cardiac rhythm should be monitored since this drug may produce life-threatening dysrhythmias and may enhance ventricular irritability. For severe reactions, epinephrine should be given intravenously in a dose of 3 to 5 ml of a 1:10,000 solution (0.3 to 0.5 mg). If an intravenous catheter is not in place, the epinephrine may be injected through a femoral or tongue vein. Epinephrine may also be instilled into the tracheobronchial tree through an endotracheal tube or directly into the trachea by injection through the cricothyroid membrane. The clinician should note, however, that the absorption of epinephrine into the circulation from the tracheobronchial tree is less predictable. For milder reactions, subcutaneous or intramuscular epinephrine may be injected in a dose of 0.3 to 0.5 ml of a 1:1,000 solution (0.3 to 0.5 mg). Several repeated doses of epinephrine may be given at 5- to 10-minute intervals if symptoms persist and if adverse effects have not been observed.

Fluid therapy reverses intravascular volume deficits secondary to mediator-induced increases in permeability. Additionally, fluids counteract the effects of mediator-induced vasodilation on blood pressure by increasing venous return. For mild episodes of anaphylaxis, intravenous fluids may not be required since the abnormalities in vascular permeability and tone may be minor and transient. Prompt volume loading is required, however, for persistent hypotension and/or signs of circulatory shock. Isotonic crystalloidal fluids (e.g., 0.9 percent normal saline, Ringer's lactate) or colloidal fluids (5 percent human serum albumin, 6 percent hydroxyethylstarch, both in normal saline) are preferred since they produce the most rapid expansion of the intravascular space. If hypotension, oliguria, and/or lactic acidosis persist after fluid loading, or if pulmonary edema or acute respiratory failure intervene, the use of advanced hemodynamic monitoring should be considered to further guide fluid therapy.

ADDITIONAL THERAPEUTIC OPTIONS FOR PERSISTENT ANAPHYLAXIS

If the symptoms of anaphylaxis persist after initial therapeutic interventions, the use of additional pharmacologic interventions should be considered. Drugs are available that prevent the release of mediators and inhibit the effects of mediators in experimental conditions that simulate clinical anaphylaxis. These agents may be especially important in preventing or ameliorating the ongoing or recurrent release of mediators that may characterize persistent or recurrent anaphylactic episodes. In general, drugs that increase intracellular cyclic adenosine monophosphate (cAMP) levels or decrease cyclic guanosine monophosphate (cGMP) levels inhibit mediator release (Table 3) and may be beneficial. Conversely, drugs that decrease cAMP and increase cGMP levels are potentially harmful and should be avoided. Bivalent cations, especially calcium, are capable of enhancing mediator release from *in vitro* human basophils. Although the role of calcium in clinical anaphylaxis remains unclear, it seems prudent to avoid calcium administration in this setting.

Aminophylline and Theophylline

Aminophylline and theophylline are methylxanthines that may decrease mediator release by increasing cAMP levels through phosphodiesterase inhibition. Some authorities, however, believe when these agents are used at therapeutic concentrations, this effect on phosphodiesterase is minimal. Nevertheless, these drugs are effective bronchodilators, probably secondary to a direct effect on bronchial smooth muscle, and may thus be useful in the management of patients who continue to exhibit bronchospasm after initial treatment. For adults, a loading dose of 5 to 6 mg per kilogram of aminophylline is infused intravenously over 20 minutes and is followed by a continuous infusion of 0.2 to 0.9 mg per kilogram per hour. Patients with mild bronchospasm who are able to take oral medications may begin anhydrous theophylline, 200 to 400 mg by mouth twice daily. In general, higher doses are required for smokers. Patients with congestive heart failure, cor pulmonale, and liver disease frequently require lower doses. The doses of theophylline and aminophylline should be adjusted to maintain blood levels at 10 to 20 μg per milliliter. The methylxanthines are associated with significant toxic effects, including life-threatening dysrhythmias and seizures.

Corticosteroids

Corticosteroids are recommended by most authorities for severe reactions. These agents may prevent delayed recurrent anaphylactic episodes by inhibiting a secondary wave of degranulation and mediator release by circulating basophils. One hundred to two hundred milligrams of hydrocortisone may be given intravenously, repeated at 4- to 6-hour intervals for 24 hours, and then rapidly tapered.

Inotropic and Vasoactive Agents

Inotropic and vasoactive agents should be considered when signs of circulatory failure persist during aggressive fluid therapy or after the repletion of intravascular volume deficits as determined by hemodynamic parameters and reversal of hemoconcentration. Agents that have been successfully used in anaphylaxis include dopamine (4 to 15 μg per kilogram per minute), norepinephrine (4 to 8 mg in 1 L of normal saline at 4 to 8 μg per minute), and epinephrine (2 to 4 mg in 1 L of normal saline at 2 to 4 μg per minute). These agents have beta-adrenergic activity and, at higher doses, beta- and alpha-adrenergic activity. Alpha-adrenergic effects should be avoided, if possible, since they may produce excessive vasoconstriction and impair systemic perfusion. In addition, alpha-adrenergic stimulation may enhance mediator release (see Table 3). Nevertheless, as circulatory shock progresses, the use of drugs in alpha-adrenergic ranges may be the only means of maintaining arterial pressure and central organ perfusion.

Inhalational Drugs

Inhalational drugs have a limited role in the treatment of anaphylaxis. They may be useful, however, for specific problems. Inhaled beta-agonists may be a useful supplement to aminophylline therapy in patients who exhibit severe or persistent bronchospasm. Metaproterenol, 0.2 to 0.3 ml of 5 percent solution, in 2.5 ml of saline may be administered via nebulization and repeated every 2 to

Table 3 Pharmacologic Modulators of Mediator Release

Inhibit release
 ↑ cAMP:
  Beta-adrenergic drugs
  Phosphodiesterase inhibitors
 ↓ cGMP:
  Anticholinergic drugs

Enhance release
 ↓ cAMP:
  Beta-blockers
  Alpha-adrenergic drugs
 ↑ cGMP:
  Cholinergic drugs

4 hours, if necessary. Ipratropium bromide, an anticholinergic bronchodilator, may also be useful for refractory bronchospasm. Thirty-six micrograms may be inhaled and repeated at 2-hour intervals, as needed. More than 12 inhalations should not be taken over 24 hours. Anticholinergic side effects of these agents are minimal since the inhaled drug is not absorbed systemically. Nebulized racemic epinephrine may be tried for mild laryngeal edema. The localized alpha-adrenergic or vasoconstrictive effects of this drug may reduce laryngeal edema. One-half milliliter of a 2.25 percent solution diluted in 3.5 ml distilled water should be administered by nebulization. The efficacy of this drug is unclear, and it has no role in the treatment of severe laryngeal edema associated with stridor or respiratory distress.

Antihistamines

Antihistamines block the systemic effects of histamine, a mast cell- and basophil-derived mediator, by competitively inhibiting histamine (H_1 and H_2) receptors. These agents may thus have favorable effects on H_1 receptor-mediated increases in vascular permeability and bronchial smooth muscle contraction. These agents may also block histamine-induced cardiac abnormalities (predominantly through H_2 receptors) which include increases in heart rate, dysrhythmias, atrioventricular conduction delays, and coronary vasoconstriction. Despite the theoretical benefits of H_1 and H_2 antagonists, the clinical efficacy of these drugs in the treatment of anaphylaxis remains unclear. However, these agents may be tried in patients who fail to respond to the initial treatment of anaphylaxis, especially those with significant cardiac manifestations. Diphenhydramine, an H_1 antagonist, may be given intravenously or by mouth in doses of 25 to 50 mg at 4- to 6-hour intervals. Three hundred milligrams of cimetidine in 50 ml of normal saline may be given intravenously over 5 minutes and repeated at 6- to 8-hour intervals.

Glucagon and Naloxone

Glucagon, a pancreatic hormone that increases cAMP through the activation of adenyl cyclase, and naloxone, an opiate antagonist that may reverse the effects of endogenous opiates, have been reported to be useful in isolated cases of anaphylaxis. Nevertheless, additional understanding of the physiologic and clinical effects of these drugs in anaphylaxis is required before their routine use can be recommended.

MANAGEMENT AFTER THE ACUTE EVENT

Because of the life-threatening nature of anaphylaxis, acute management must be followed by definitive arrangements for continued medical follow-up by specialists familiar with the management of acute allergic events. Patients who have had anaphylactic episodes may require skin testing and/or immunotherapy. Counseling is required so that repeat episodes may be avoided. Some patients require instruction regarding self-administration of injectable epinephrine at the onset of an anaphylactic reaction, before seeking care at a medical facility. Specialized long-term care is essential for the prevention of recurrent events.

SUGGESTED READING

Cohan RH, Dunnick NR, Bashore TM. Treatment of reactions to radiographic contrast material. AJR 1988; 151:263–270.
Haupt MT, Carlson RW. Anaphylactic and anaphylactoid reactions. In: Shoemaker WC, Holbrook PR, Thompson WL, eds. The society of critical care medicine—textbook of critical care. 2nd ed. Philadelphia: WB Saunders Co., 1989:993.
Perkin RM, Anas NG. Mechanisms and management of anaphylactic shock not responding to traditional therapy. Ann Allergy 1985; 54:202–208.
Serafin WE, Austen KF. Mediators of immediate hypersensitivity reactions. N Engl J Med 1987; 317:30–34.
Valentine MD, Lichtenstein LM. Anaphylaxis and stinging insect hypersensitivity. JAMA 1987; 258:2881–2885.

SEPTIC SHOCK AND OTHER FORMS OF DISTRIBUTIVE SHOCK

CHARLES NATANSON, M.D.
WILLIAM D. HOFFMAN, M.D.

DEFINITION OF DISTRIBUTIVE SHOCK

In all types of shock, body tissues do not receive sufficient oxygen. This lack of oxygen can be caused by decreased blood flow (cardiac output [CO]), decreased perfusion pressure (mean arterial pressure [MAP]), or maldistribution of blood flow (normal or increased flow to areas that may not take up or use the available oxygen, and inadequate flow to areas that may not receive enough oxygen).

In distributive shock, patients have both hypotension and maldistribution of blood flow. In addition, patients with distributive shock frequently develop extravasation of intravascular volume (a capillary leak that causes intravascular volume depletion). Typically, intravascular monitors show decreased MAP, decreased left ventricular filling pressures (pulmonary capillary wedge pressure [PCWP]), increased CO (particularly after fluid resuscitation), and reduced total peripheral resistance (systemic vascular resistance [SVR]). Thus distributive shock is characterized by decreased resistance to flow, maldistribution of flow, and relative hypovolemia.

Sepsis and anaphylaxis are common causes of distributive shock. Septic shock typically occurs over a period of hours to days and is produced when microorganisms (bacteria, fungi, or *Protozoa*) or their toxins are released into the bloodstream and cause host cells (macrophages, leukocytes) to release multiple inflammatory mediators. Anaphylactic shock usually occurs more acutely than septic shock, has a shorter duration, and is produced when foreign substances (e.g., drugs, radiocontrast dyes, insect venom) enter the bloodstream and cause various endogenous mediators to be released. Thus distributive shock, which may be produced by different exogenous and endogenous pathways, has a characteristic hemodynamic abnormality that can be either acute or subacute.

The cardiovascular abnormality of distributive shock is treated by (1) restoring intravascular volume with fluid infusions and (2) increasing peripheral resistance with vasoactive drug infusions. The underlying cause must also be treated. For example, patients with septic shock are given antibiotics, while in patients with anaphylactic shock, the foreign antigen is removed and patients are given histamine-blocking drugs. This chapter discusses treatment of the cardiovascular dysfunction associated with septic shock. Although treatment strategies for anaphylactic shock (and other forms of distributive shock) are similar to those used for septic shock, a detailed discussion of anaphylactic shock and its treatment is discussed elsewhere in this text.

OTHER FORMS OF SHOCK

Many diseases can cause shock (Table 1), most by producing a low CO that leads to hypotension and organ dysfunction (Fig. 1). In cardiogenic shock, myocardial damage results in severely reduced contractile function, a low CO, hypotension, and inadequate systemic perfusion. Massive pulmonary embolus (which obstructs blood flow) and pericardial tamponade (which restricts filling of the heart and thus makes preload inadequate) can cause a low CO, hypotension, and shock. Loss of intravascular volume from hemorrhage, protracted vomiting, or diarrhea causes decreased cardiac filling, low CO, hypotension, and inadequate perfusion.

In contrast to cardiogenic, hypovolemic, and obstructive shock, septic shock produces a normal or increased total blood flow (as measured by CO). Even with normal or increased CO, heart function is not normal. Septic shock uniformly reduces myocardial function, as evidenced by a depressed left ventricular ejection fraction (LVEF, a hemodynamic measure that is relatively independent of preload). In more than 90 percent of patients, the left ventricle (LV) dilates once preload is restored by fluid infusions. LV dilation can increase stroke volume (SV) and CO via the Frank-Starling mechanism. Thus, preload-dependent measures of cardiac function (e.g., SV and CO) can be misleading indicators of LV function. In survivors, the hemodynamic abnormality reverses to normal within 7 to 10 days. In less than 10 percent of patients with septic shock, severe myocardial depression occurs because myocardial function is not compensated by dilation. This condition can be viewed as two coexisting types of shock: (1) cardiogenic shock producing a low CO and (2) sepsis-induced distributive shock (see Fig. 1).

This sepsis-induced cardiovascular abnormality is further complicated by decreased circulating volume. Septic shock mediators (bacterial and host) may cause blood to pool in capillary beds and plasma to leak into the interstitial space, thereby decreasing circulating volume. Thus, relative hypovolemia and maldistribution of blood flow may further exacerbate the hypoperfusion of various tissues and increase the severity of shock. Specifically, certain tissues, such as skeletal muscle, may receive a higher

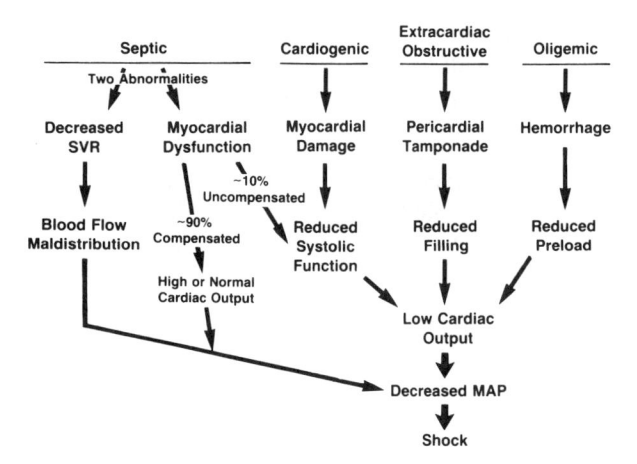

Figure 1 The different pathways of shock. For cardiogenic, extracardiac obstructive, and oligemic shock, hypotension and shock are caused by a low CO. With septic shock, however, a low CO leads to shock in less than 10 percent of patients. The majority of patients with septic shock have a high or normal CO, and their severe decrease in systemic vascular resistance leads to hypotension.

Table 1 Classification of Shock

Distributive
 Septic
 Anaphylactic
 Endocrinologic (e.g., thyroid storm)
 Neurogenic
 Toxic/drug (e.g., anesthetics)

Cardiogenic
 Myopathic (infarction, cardiomyopathy)
 Mechanical (valvular disease, ventricular septal defect, outflow tract obstruction)
 Arrhythmic

Extracardiac Obstructive
 Pericardial tamponade
 Pulmonary emboli (massive)

Oligemic
 Hemorrhage
 Fluid depletion (protracted vomiting, diarrhea)

proportion of blood flow than normal, while other tissues, such as the kidneys, may receive a lower proportion of blood flow. Septic shock therefore results from the following combination of hemodynamic abnormalities: (1) a severe decrease in resistance to blood flow; (2) reversible cardiac dysfunction (which is commonly compensated and CO maintained); (3) relative maldistribution of blood flow; and (4) hypovolemia. Effective treatment strategies for this cardiovascular abnormality should focus on the diagnosis and, specifically, the treatment of the sepsis-induced abnormalities in afterload, preload, and contractility.

SEPTIC SHOCK

Clinical Presentation

Initially, septic shock produces nonspecific symptoms such as malaise, tachycardia, rigors, and fever, and sometimes hypothermia. Other clinical signs may suggest the site of infection (i.e., flank pain and dysuria indicate pyelonephritis; stiff neck and headache indicate meningitis; cough and sputum production indicate pneumonia; and abdominal pain and guarding indicate peritonitis). Infants, the elderly, and immunocompromised patients, however, may have few clinical symptoms. Although many patients with septic shock have an elevated white blood cell count, some patients may have a low white blood cell count, which is a poor prognostic sign. Tachypnea (with or without hypoxia), oliguria, icterus, and mental confusion may suggest that the septic process is far advanced and indicate multiple organ system damage. Thus, this rapidly lethal disease (mortality rate of 50 to 60 percent) is often difficult to diagnose. As septic shock is so rapidly lethal, the clinician should always suspect the disease (particularly in patients at high risk for infection) and treat it early, often well before complete diagnostic and laboratory information is available.

Therapy

Septic shock is a systemic disease involving all organ systems. Optimal treatment of this disease should reverse this generalized process. Three major goals are necessary to treat various stages of the disease (Tables 2 and 3; Fig. 2); (1) eradication of the infection and sterilization of the bloodstream; (2) neutralization of the bacterial toxins and harmful endogenous mediators released in response to these toxins; and (3) providing supportive care for the multiple organ systems (cardiac, pulmonary, and renal) damaged by these toxins.

Eradication of Infection

When septic shock is suspected, the clinician should quickly obtain cultures and then begin antibiotic treatment. The appropriate antibiotic therapy given early can substantially improve the likelihood of survival from septic shock. Even though the source of infection may be apparent, microbiologic identification and antibiotic susceptibility testing takes several days. Initial antibiotic therapy must therefore be empiric, with treatment directed at all likely pathogens of the clinical syndrome and, for nosocomial infections, all probable hospital pathogens. For example, patients with possible intra-abdominal infections should receive antibiotics for gram-positive and gram-negative bacteria, as well as antibiotics that treat anaerobes and *Streptococcus faecalis*, common pathogens found in the bowel. The following minimum empiric antimicrobial therapy is recommended for patients with severe septic shock: (1) administration of one antibiotic for possible gram-positive bacteria; (2) administration of two antibiotics for possible gram-negative bacteria; and (3) when

Table 2 Septic Shock Therapy

Goal 1: Eradicate infection
 Begin empiric antibiotics (broad coverage)
 Attempt to identify source of infection
 Remove focus of infection (remove foreign body, drain abscess)

Goal 2: Neutralize toxins
 Investigational therapy in humans
  Antiserum J-5 *E. coli*
  Immune serum globulin (high titers to common bacterial pathogens)
  Antiendotoxin immunoglobulins
  Corticosteroids

 Beneficial therapy in animals
  Antibodies to tumor necrosis factor
  High-dose naloxone
  Prostaglandin E_1
  Indomethacin
  Lipid-X
  Anticomplement (C5a) antibodies
  Ibuprofen
  Protein C

Goal 3: Provide supportive care
 Intensive care setting
  Full-time critical care nurses, physicians, and technicians
  Intra-arterial monitoring
   Accurate
   Immediate beat-to-beat analysis
   Frequent arterial blood gas sampling
  Right heart catheterization
   Confirmation of diagnosis
   Accurate cardiac filling pressure and flow measurements
  Cardiac rhythm monitoring
   Antiarrhythmic agents
   Electrical cardioversion

 Fluid resuscitation
  Eliminate other causes of cardiovascular depression
   Correct anemia, hypoxemia, acidosis, hypophosphatemia, hypocalcemia, hypoalbuminemia
  If MAP $\leq$ 60, optimize preload
   Volume expansion to PCWP $\geq$ 12-18 mm Hg
   Crystalloids/albumin/synthetic colloids
   Avoid pulmonary edema

 Pressors
  If MAP $\leq$ 60 despite PCWP $\geq$ 12-18 mm Hg, begin pressors (see Table 3 and Fig. 4)

Table 3 Septic Shock Therapy: Goal 3

Pressor	Dose	Cardiac Stimulation	Vasoconstriction	Vasodilatation	Dopaminergic	Indication (MAP ≤60, PCWP ≥12–18)
Dopamine	1–10 μg/kg/min	++	+	++	+++	↑ or normal CO
	10–20 μg/kg/min	+++	+++	+	0	
Norepinephrine	2–8 μg/min	+++	++++	0	0	Dopamine failure
Phenylephrine	20–200 μg/min	0	++++	0	0	Arrhythmias
Epinephrine	1–8 μg/min	++++	++++	++	0	↓ CO, norepinephrine failure
Dobutamine	1–10 μg/kg/min	++++	+	++	0	↓ CO, combine with norepinephrine therapy
Isoproterenol	1–4 μg/min	++++	+	++	0	↓ CO

+ = mild increase; ++ = moderate increase; +++ = large increase; ++++ = very large increase; 0, no significant change

specifically indicated, adminstration of antibiotics for anaerobes, *Staphylococcus epidermidis, S. faecalis*, or fungi. For life-threatening infections, two antibiotics for gram-negative organisms are recommended because these drugs may be synergistic and provide a "safety net" against organisms that may be resistant to a single antibiotic alone. For the critically ill immunocompromised septic patients without a known focus, we commonly prescribe vancomycin, ceftazidime, gentamicin, and clindamycin. Only after the site of infection is determined and the organism is identified should the antibiotic regimen become more selective.

After obtaining all the necessary cultures (urine, blood, sputum, and sites of pus or loculated fluids) and beginning antibiotic treatment, the clinician should search intensely for the sources of infection. When these have been found, infected foreign bodies should be removed and abscesses drained. In some investigations of patients with septic shock, only about 50 percent have an identifiable site of infection or positive blood cultures. Furthermore, patients receiving antibiotics are less likely to have positive cultures. In some cases of septic shock, negative cultures may occur in patients with intermittent bacteremia or no bacteremia (when bacterial products without bac-

TREATMENT OF SEPTIC SHOCK: THREE GOALS

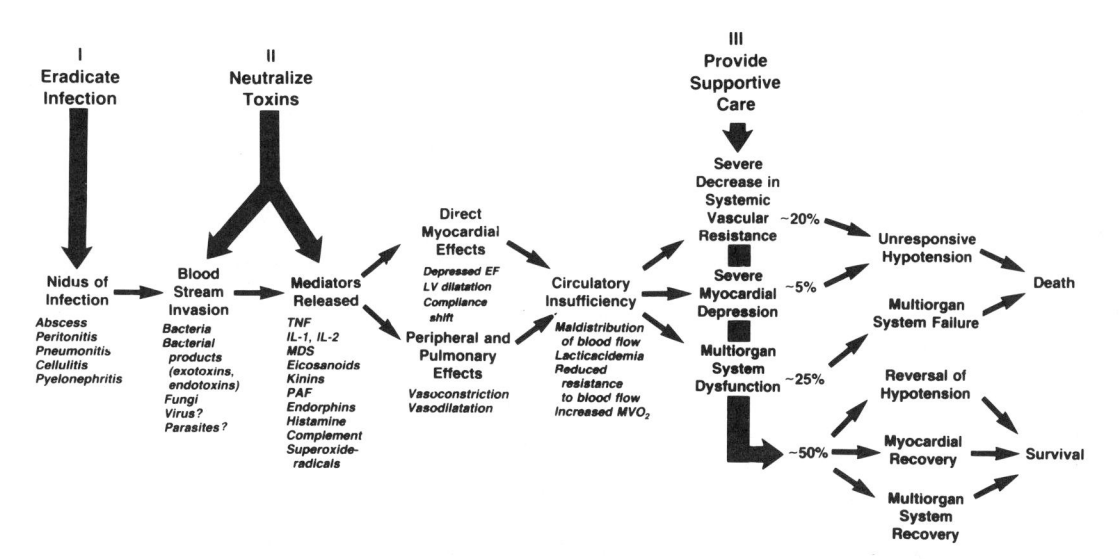

Figure 2 The pathogenesis of septic shock from the nidus of infection to death or survival. In the bloodstream, invading bacteria, fungi, or their products induce the release of endogenous mediators that have direct myocardial effects and that produce peripheral circulatory insufficiency in many organ systems. These substances can produce three distinct syndromes that cause death: (1) refractory hypotension from a low systemic vascular resistance (SVR); (2) refractory hypotension from decreased CO; and (3) multiple organ system failure. Roman numerals I–III are treatment steps in the pathogenesis of septic shock (see Tables 2–4 for more details).

EF = ejection fraction; TNF = tumor necrosis factor; IL-1 and IL-2 = interleukin-1 and -2; MDS = myocardial depressant substance; PAF = platelet-activating factor; MVO_2 = myocardial oxygen consumption.

teria are released into the bloodstream). In addition, neutropenic patients commonly have no identifiable source of infection. For these patients, the source of infection is believed to be microscopic foci (too small to be detected by diagnostic imaging techniques) in the lungs and bowel. Thus some patients with negative blood cultures or no identifiable source of infection can still have septic shock.

Neutralization of Toxins

Even with effective antibiotic regimens and adequate surgical drainage, septic shock remains highly lethal. The high mortality rate is believed to be caused partly by the release of bacterial products and by host factors with toxic effects that are not reversed by antibiotic treatment or by surgical removal of the infection. Available data suggest that these multiple endogenous mediators and bacterial toxins may be responsible for the cardiovascular abnormalities that cause death. In several studies, some antagonists to these mediators have shown promise in the treatment of human septic shock, whereas others have shown improvement only in animal models (see Table 2 and Fig. 2). It is hoped that early therapy with an antagonist to these mediators might block their toxic effects and thereby prevent organ damage and death. Approximately half of the deaths from septic shock are caused by multiorgan system failure that occurs weeks after the onset of hypotension. These deaths are probably caused by the toxic effects of mediators that early in syndrome produce irreversible tissue damage that does not become clinically apparent until much later (see Fig. 2). Two other well-described causes of death in patients with septic shock are a severe decrease in peripheral resistance and a severe myocardial depression, conditions that are probably both related to the acute effects of these toxic mediators (see Fig. 2). Thus, if given early, antitoxins may block or neutralize the toxic effects of these mediators.

Of particular interest is the use of high-dose corticosteroids to treat septic shock. Recently, several large clinical trials have shown that in septic patients, corticosteroids provide no beneficial effects, and in one study, corticosteroids in septic patients with renal failure had harmful effects. In infants with meningitis, however, corticosteroids were found to reduce hearing loss. While current evidence suggests that high doses of steroids are not indicated for the treatment of septic shock, additional studies are necessary to determine the harmful effects versus the beneficial effects of these drugs.

Other antimediator therapies have also been studied in humans and animals. An antiserum for a J-5 *Escherichia coli* mutant with an exposed core endotoxin region has been shown to protect animals against gram-negative infections and improve the course of human septic shock. Although evidence regarding this therapy has been available for more than 7 years, it has not gained acceptance for clinical use. In addition, naloxone has been shown to reverse hypotension in septic animals but has not been shown to be therapeutic in humans. Naloxone has also been associated with harmful side effects (e.g., arrhythmias, pulmonary edema). Antihistamines and eicosanoid antagonists have not been shown to be therapeutically useful in humans. Despite theoretical promise, no therapy to reverse the effects of septic shock mediators has yet gained widespread clinical acceptance. Presently, investigators are performing large clinical trials using monoclonal antibodies to gram-negative bacteria, free radical scavengers, and tumor necrosis factor (a cytokine release from white blood cells). These treatments probably offer the best hope for improving the likelihood of survival of patients with septic shock.

Providing Supportive Care

The optimal management of septic shock and cardiovascular instability requires immediate transfer of patients to a critical care setting (see Table 2). Retrospective studies of patients with septic shock have shown that full-time critical care physicians and nurses, using the monitoring and other technologies available in intensive care units, can significantly increase the survival rate of these patients. The intensive care setting provides the technology to monitor intravascular pressures, the trained personnel to use this equipment, and a place where staff is available to monitor the patient continuously 24 hours per day.

Hemodynamic Monitoring. The treatment of septic shock has also been changed by the introduction of arterial cannulae and pulmonary arterial catheters, which make it possible to give large quantities of fluids and potent cardioselective drugs safely to critically ill patients. Arterial cannulae can be used to obtain an accurate measure of intra-arterial pressure even in shock states. These cannulae also provide beat-to-beat analysis so that decisions regarding therapy can be based on immediate and reproducible blood pressure information. Pulmonary arterial catheters are used to measure right ventricle and left ventricle filling pressures (central venous pressure [CVP] and pulmonary capillary wedge pressure [PCWP], respectively). In addition, these catheters contain right heart infusion ports and a thermistor that allow mixed venous blood sampling and measurement of CO.

Evaluation of these hemodynamic parameters—MAP, CVP, PCWP, and CO—help the clinician diagnose the type of shock (Table 4). In particular, septic shock can be provisionally diagnosed by its unique hemodynamic profile, characterized by low or normal cardiac filling pressures (PCWP), a high or normal CO, a low systemic vascular resistance (SVR), and high mixed venous oxygenation. Pulmonary arterial catheters are used to infuse large quantities of volume safely, because the infusion amount can be based on accurate reproducible cardiac filling pressures and thus avoid fluid overload and pulmonary edema (Fig. 3). In addition, the decision to select a specific pressor agent can be based on measurements of cardiac performance (CO) and filling pressures (PCWP), (i.e., Frank-Starling curves). Data from immediate and repeated measures enable the clinician to monitor the efficacy of treatment and alter therapeutic interventions.

In the intensive care setting, decisions regarding therapy are based on a full hemodynamic profile completed at least every 2 to 4 hours. This hemodynamic profile in-

Table 4 Use of Right Heart Catheterization to Diagnose the Etiology of Shock*

Diagnosis	PCWP	CO	Miscellaneous Comments
Cardiogenic shock			
Myocardial dysfunction	↑↑	↓↓	Usually occurs with evidence of extensive myocardial infarction (>40% of left ventricular myocardium destroyed), severe cardiomyopathy, or myocarditis
Acute ventricular septal defect	↑ or N	↓↓	Oxygen saturation "step-up" occurs at right ventricular level in left-to-right shunt
Acute mitral regurgitation	↑↑	↓↓	V waves in PCWP tracing
Right ventricular infarction	↓ or N	↓↓	Elevated right atrial and right ventricular filling pressures with low or normal PCWP
Extracardiac obstructive			
Pericardial tamponade	↑↑	↓ or ↓↓	Dip and plateau tracing in right and left ventricles. The right atrial mean, right ventricular end-diastolic, pulmonary artery end-diastolic, and pulmonary capillary wedge mean pressures are within 5 mm Hg of one another
Massive pulmonary emboli	↓ or N	↓↓	Usual finding is elevated right heart pressures with normal or low PCWP
Oligemic (hypovolemia)	↓↓	↓↓	
Distributive shock			
Septic	↓ or N	↑↑ or N (rarely ↓)	High mixed venous oxygen saturation
Anaphylactic	↓ or N	↑ or N	

*The hemodynamic profiles summarized in this table refer to patients with the diagnosis listed in the left column who are also in shock (MAP <60 mm Hg).
↑↑ or ↓↓ designates a moderate-to-severe increase or decrease; ↑ or ↓ designates a mild-to-moderate increase or decrease; N = normal.
Modified from Parrillo JE. Septic shock: clinical manifestations, pathogenesis, hemodynamics, and management in a critical care unit. In: Parrillo JE, Aytes SM, eds. Major issues in critical care medicine. Baltimore: Williams and Wilkins, 1984:120.

cludes the PCWP, cardiac index (CI), stroke volume index (SVI), systemic vascular resistance index (SVRI), and stroke work index (SWI). During rapid volume infusions, the PCWP (see Fig. 3) needs to be measured more frequently to prevent fluid overload.

Laboratory Monitoring. Pulmonary and arterial catheters are also used to obtain repeated results of blood gases and other metabolic parameters. In patients with septic shock, so that appropriate treatment interventions can be made, the following must be measured frequently: arterial oxygenation, carbon dioxide, glucose, electrolytes, calcium, magnesium, phosphate, complete blood counts, liver function, renal function, and coagulation parameters (including parameters affected by disseminated intravascular coagulation). In a disease that can produce profound cardiovascular abnormalities, it is crucial to correct possible confounding metabolic abnormalities. Furthermore, measuring serial lactic acid levels can provide information on the severity of shock, adequacy of therapy, and patient course and outcome.

In patients with septic shock, clinical parameters change rapidly. During the first 24 hours, blood tests may be required every 4 hours. If the patient improves, blood sampling can be tapered over 1 to 2 days to every 8 hours and then daily if the patient continues to improve.

Cardiac Rhythm Monitoring. Another important reason for transferring patients with septic shock to an intensive care unit is so that they can undergo continuous cardiac rhythm monitoring. Arrhythmia monitoring is particularly important for septic hypotensive patients who require potent cardiac stimulant drugs and intracardiac catheters. Some patients with septic shock develop serious atrial and ventricular arrhythmias, although this is not common. Treatment of these rhythm disturbances in septic shock should follow the standard practices discussed elsewhere in this text.

Cardiovascular Support. Studies in animals have shown that cardiovascular support and antibiotic treatment are equally important in the treatment of septic shock and that these two therapies work synergistically to improve the likelihood of survival. Specifically, cardiovascular support prolongs survival until the antibiotics become effective. When extrapolated to the clinical settings, these findings emphasize that in patients with this rapidly lethal disease, it is critical to begin both cardiovascular support and antibiotic treatment quickly.

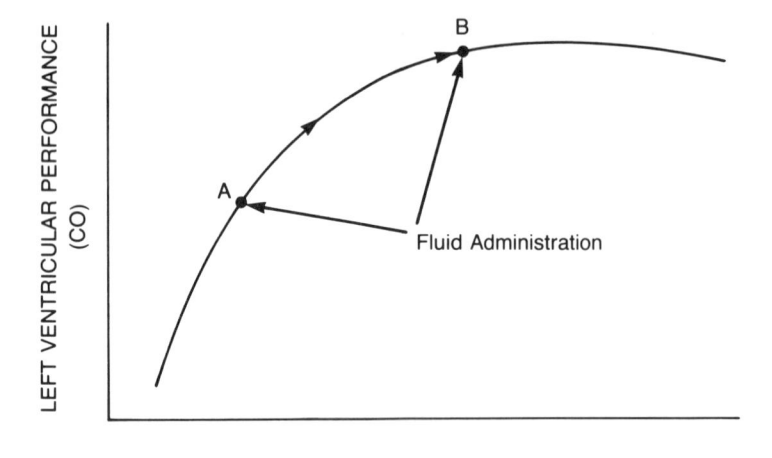

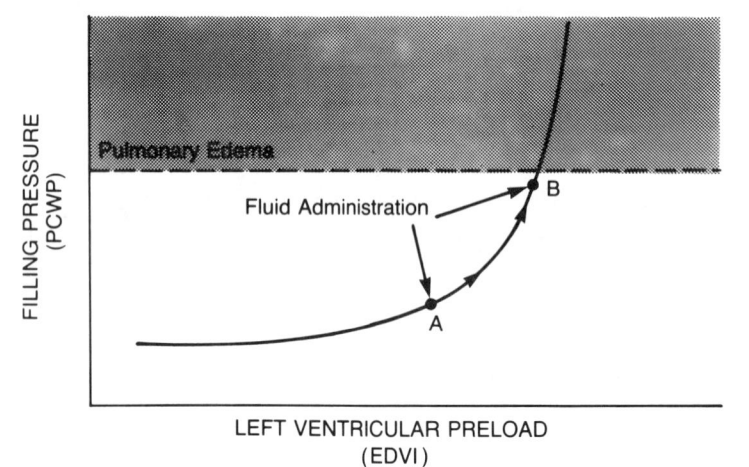

Figure 3 The upper graph shows the Frank-Starling relationship, which is LV performance (CO) vs. preload (PCWP). As preload is increased from point A to B, there is a corresponding increase in LV performance. The lower graph depicts the LV pressure volume relationship in diastole. Increasing preload causes corresponding increases in PCWP. When guided by serial thermodilution pulmonary arterial catheter CO and PCWP measurements, fluid administration can optimize LV performance while avoiding pulmonary edema (shaded area of lower graph). EDVI = end-diastolic volume index.

Volume resuscitation is considered the best initial therapy for the cardiovascular abnormality of septic shock. As an initial goal for fluid support, we recommend an MAP of more than 60 mm Hg and an LV filling pressure (measured by a PCWP) of 12 to 18 mm Hg. The MAP should not decrease to less than 60 mm Hg because coronary perfusion as well as renal and central nervous system blood flow may be reduced as autoregulation becomes compromised. In recent studies of the critically ill, it has been suggested that although a PCWP of at least 12 mm Hg is needed to optimize LV function, a PCWP of greater than 20 mm Hg may produce pulmonary edema. To maintain optimal LV function and avoid pulmonary edema, we therefore suggest a PCWP of 12 to 18 mm Hg.

As soon as the diagnosis of septic shock is made, arterial and pulmonary arterial catheters should be placed while fluid resuscitation is begun. The type of fluid administered is probably less important than the rapid institution of this therapy and whether fluids have been titrated to the appropriate PCWP and MAP. It is not clear that one type of fluid (crystalloids, synthetic colloids, blood products, or albumin) has an advantage over another. Crystalloids are relatively inexpensive and safe. Synthetic colloids, blood products, and albumin are more expensive, but these fluids are more rapid volume expanders. We recommend beginning resuscitation with rapid 500- to 1,000-ml boluses of crystalloid solutions. We also suggest giving packed red blood cells to bring the hematocrit to approximately 35 percent, and giving 25 percent albumin solutions if the serum albumin is less than 2 g per deciliter. It is fairly common for the critically ill septic shock patient to require 10 to 20 L of crystalloids during the first 24 hours of therapy to maintain a near-normal MAP.

Clinicians have long debated whether volume expansion aids the kidneys or hurts the lungs. Septic shock is further complicated by the risk of both the adult respiratory distress syndrome and acute renal tubular necrosis. Both of these sepsis-induced injuries can lead to worsened outcome and organ failure requiring mechanical support. These conditions are also potentially reversible. Some clinicians who desire to "protect the lungs" believe that increasing the PCWP increases lung water and worsens hypoxemia. These clinicians argue that septic patients should be kept "dry" and that pressor drugs should be used mainly to manage blood pressure. Clinicians who want to "protect the kidneys" argue that volume infusion is necessary to maintain renal blood flow, renal tubular flow, and urine output. These clinicians believe that the use of pressors (as opposed to volume infusion) constricts the renal arteries and compromises renal perfusion and function. Because sepsis is a systemic disease, we believe that it is important to maintain perfusion to all organs (including both the lungs and kidneys). In treating septic shock, we believe that cardiac filling pressures (PCWP) of 12 to 18 mm Hg optimize ventricular performance by the Frank-Starling mechanisms, increase blood flow to all body tissues, and does not increase the risk of pulmonary edema. We also believe that if hypotension exists with optimal filling pressures, then using vasopressors to maintain blood flow (by increasing perfusion pressure to all organs) does far more good than harm.

Controversy exists as to whether a pulmonary arterial catheter is required or whether a CVP catheter is sufficient to diagnose and guide the therapy of septic shock. In addition to providing diagnostic information (see Table 4) and determining the efficacy of therapy, the PCWP (as compared with CVP or physical examination) more accurately reflects LV filling. Recent serial studies using sophisticated measures of heart function show severe systolic and diastolic abnormalities during septic shock. Cardiac function changes continuously over the first 10 days. The LVEF during the first 48 hours typically decreases to a nadir less than 20 to 30 percent (with 50 to 60 percent being normal). During this time, the LV dilates, and systolic and diastolic abnormalities occur. Recent studies also show that the LV has a markedly abnormal response to volume infusion. In survivors, this LV abnormality returns to normal within 7 to 10 days. During this period, patients may have received 10 to 20 L of fluids and gained a commensurate amount of weight. With continuously changing LV function and rapid fluid shifts, it is essential to measure left-sided filling pressures to guide the safe and accurate use of fluids, pressors, and diuretics.

If fluid infusion does not rapidly increase the MAP to 60 mm Hg and if the PCWP is not 12 to 18 mm Hg, then vasopressors are indicated. Specific drugs are chosen for their selective vasoconstrictive and inotropic effects (Fig. 4 and Table 3).

Initially, we use dopamine at a low dose (1 to 5 μg per kilogram) because it stimulates the heart, mildly increases blood pressure, increases renal blood flow (a vulnerable organ in septic shock) by stimulating dopaminergic receptors in the kidneys, and has few side effects. If these low doses of dopamine do not increase the MAP to more than 60 mm Hg, we titrate dopamine to a maximal dose of 20 μg per kilogram per minute. At higher doses, dopamine may still have good vasoconstricting properties, but may also commonly produce some adverse side effects such as atrial and ventricular tachycardias. These arrhythmias usually end within minutes after discontinuation of the dopamine infusion.

If high doses of dopamine fail to increase MAP or if they produce arrhythmias, we suggest that norepinephrine be used instead. Norepinephrine is a powerful vasoconstricting agent with less of a tendency to increase chronotropism and produce arrhythmias. In septic shock patients with compensated myocardial dysfunction and a high CO, norepinephrine can increase both total peripheral resistance and blood pressure. Norepinephrine infusion rates of 2 to 10 μg per minute are usually adequate, even in patients who do not respond to fluids and high doses of dopamine.

With norepinephrine infusions, we commonly give low doses of dopamine (1 to 2 μg per kilogram per minute) to improve renal blood flow. Evidence from animal studies suggests that low doses of dopamine increase renal blood flow even when used in conjunction with high doses of norepinephrine. In the past, clinicians were reluctant to use norepinephrine because of its powerful vasoconstricting properties and its ability to produce organ ischemia.

Figure 4 Supportive care of septic shock: Goal 3. Algorithm for selection of vasopressors to achieve an MAP of greater than 60 mm Hg and a PCWP of 12 to 18 mm Hg (see also Table 3).

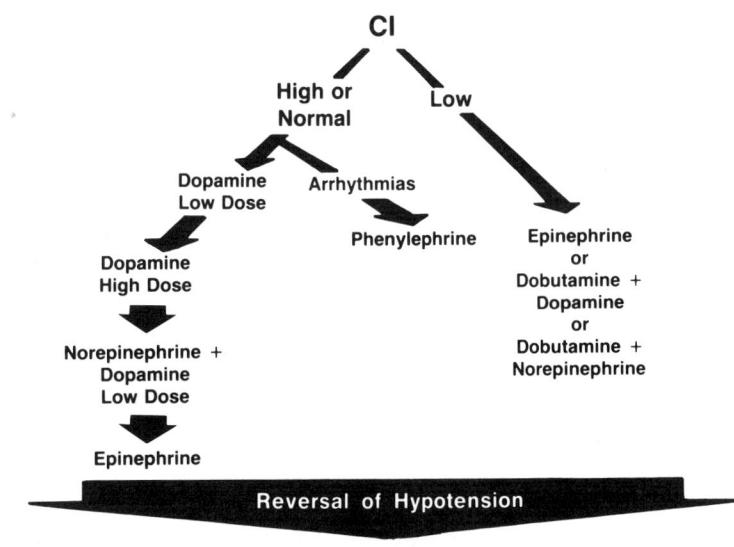

However, several recent clinical studies have shown that norepinephrine can reverse hypotension not responsive to volume infusion or high doses of dopamine without producing significant ischemia. Furthermore, these clinical studies suggest that norepinephrine's inability to produce arrhythmias and its powerful ability to increase MAP make it the ideal drug for treating the severe decrease in peripheral resistance produced during septic shock.

In those rare cases when a patient with a low CO does not respond well to dopamine or norepinephrine, epinephrine may be effective because of its ability to increase both CO and the MAP. In these same patients, the combination of dobutamine and norepinephrine may also be beneficial. However, dobutamine and epinephrine may produce arrhythmias, so these drugs should be administered only when specifically indicated (e.g., if the CO is low).

For patients with serious cardiac arrhythmias, phenylephrine is substituted for norepinephrine. Although the direct cardiac effects of norepinephrine are modest, phenylephrine is a pure vasoconstrictor that produces essentially no direct cardiac stimulation.

Finally, dobutamine or isoproterenol may produce adverse effects when administered alone to patients with septic shock. The vasodilating capabilities of these drugs frequently decrease blood pressure to dangerously low levels. For similar reasons, other vasodilating drugs (e.g., nitroprusside, nitroglycerine) are not readily used to treat septic shock.

SUGGESTED READING

Bone RC, Fisher CJ, Clemmer TP, et al. The methylprednisolone severe sepsis study group: a controlled clinical trial of high-dose methylprednisolone in treatment of severe sepsis and septic shock. N Engl J Med 1987; 317:653–658.

Natanson C, Hoffman WD, Parrillo JE. Septic shock: the cardiovascular abnormality and therapy. J Cardiothorac Anesthesia 1989; 3:215–227.

Parrillo JE. Septic shock in humans: clinical evaluation, pathophysiology, and therapeutic approach. In: Shoemaker WC, Thompson WL, Holbrook P, et al, eds. Textbook of critical care. Philadelphia: WB Saunders, 1989:1006.

Tracey KJ, Fong Y, Hesse DG, et al. Anti-cachectin/TNF monoclonal antibodies prevent systemic shock during lethal bacteremia. Nature 1987; 330:662–664.

Zeigler EJ. Protective antibody to endotoxin core: the emperor's new clothes. J Infect Dis 1988; 58:286–290.

HEMORRHAGIC AND HYPOVOLEMIC SHOCK

ANTHONY F. SUFFREDINI, M.D.

Several common disease processes cause loss or sequestration of blood, plasma, or water and electrolytes, which in turn results in decreased intravascular volume and culminates in circulatory shock (Table 1). A loss of intravascular volume may be a component of other disease states because of decreased vasomotor tone and increased venous capacitance (septic shock, anaphylaxis, and central nervous system blockage occurring after spinal cord injury, anesthesia, or drug intoxication). Therapies of these latter conditions are discussed in other chapters.

The primary pathophysiologic mechanism of hypovolemic shock is cellular and tissue ischemia caused by inadequate perfusion. Several compensatory responses directed toward maintaining selective organ perfusion (heart and brain) and toward conserving the remaining circulatory volume are initiated by the loss of intravascular volume. The effectiveness of these compensatory responses depends in part on the rate and degree of intravascular volume depletion. Intrathoracic and organ-specific (e.g., kidney) baroreceptors are stimulated by loss of intravascular volume, resulting in increased sympathetic nervous system discharge, release of stress hormones (cortisol, catecholamines, and antidiuretic hormone) and activation of the renin-angiotensin-aldosterone system.

The acute loss of intravascular volume results in a low cardiac output due to decreased venous return and cardiac filling pressures. Increased sympathetic nervous system tone results in increased heart rate and systemic vascular resistance, initially allowing maintenance of the perfusion of some organs (cerebral and the coronary circulations) at the expense of others (skin, skeletal, splanchnic, and renal circulations). A patient in this partially compensated state may appear restless, apprehensive, or obtunded, with cool extremities and general pallid skin. Tachypnea, tachycardia, poor capillary refill, and oliguria may be present, and orthostatic changes in blood pressure may be apparent.

Prolonged tissue ischemia may result in lactate production and metabolic acidosis. Ischemic cellular and tissue damage can trigger humoral and cellular inflammatory responses, which can further compromise and exacerbate the circulatory abnormalities. When the compensatory responses are exhausted, life-threatening decreases in organ perfusion occur because of inadequate resuscitation or ongoing losses. Thus the preservation of organ survival is ensured by aggressive fluid resuscitation and an expectant approach to the complications that ensue from decreased intravascular volume

CLINICAL SIGNS

The principles and management of shock, as outlined in *Advanced Trauma Life Support* (Committee on Trau-

Table 1 Causes of Hemorrhagic and Hypovolemic Shock

Hemorrhagic Shock		Hypovolemic Shock	
Traumatic	*Nontraumatic*	*Traumatic*	*Nontraumatic*

Loss of vessel integrity due to direct injury (penetrating wounds, direct impact injury)
 Long bone and pelvic fractures
	Vessel disruption due to:
	   Acid erosion (peptic ulcer disease)
	   Diffuse inflammation of mucosal surfaces (hemorrhagic cystitis)
	   Mechanical disruption (pulmonary arterial rupture)
	   Tumor invasion
	   Atherosclerotic degeneration (aortic aneurysmal rupture)
	   Aorto-enteric fistula
		Burns
		 Reaction to soft tissue injury (edema and inflammation after direct traumatic injury)
			Fluid loss without replacement (excessive vomiting, diarrhea, diabetes insipidis, diabetes mellitus, diuretic excess, pheochromocytoma, adrenal insufficiency, exfoliative dermatitis, excessive perspiration, reaccumulation of ascites)
			 Fluid sequestration (intestinal obstruction, peritonitis, pancreatitis)

ma, American College of Surgeons), are useful guidelines for the evaluation and therapy of traumatic as well as nontraumatic hemorrhagic shock. The clinical presentation of decreased tissue perfusion caused by hypovolemic or hemorrhagic shock is qualitatively similar but nonspecific. Hemorrhagic shock is a more dynamic process because of its potential for rapid blood volume loss and loss of oxygen-carrying capacity. The diagnosis relies on the prompt identification of the signs and symptoms of inadequate perfusion in the appropriate clinical setting. The patient's age, pre-existing medical conditions, severity and type of injury, and the length of time that elapsed before the initiation of resuscitation are factors that can limit the effectiveness of compensatory responses and alter the clinical presentation of patients with hypovolemic-hemorrhagic shock.

Blood volume is approximately 7 percent of the body weight in the adult (i.e., 5 L in a 70-kg patient) and 8 to 9 percent in the child. The clinical signs of increasingly severe blood loss are outlined in Table 2. With increasing blood and fluid loss, the manifestations of heightened sympathetic tone become apparent with increased pulse and respiratory rate, decreased capillary refill, and narrowed pulse pressure (due to increased diastolic tone and maintenance of systolic blood pressure). An altered mental status is usually a late manifestation. A decrease in systolic blood pressure reflects a failure of available compensatory mechanisms to sustain perfusion. In an otherwise un-

Table 2 Hemorrhagic Shock: Clinical Signs and Estimated Fluid and Blood Requirements Based on Initial Presentation (70-kg Male)

	Class I	Class II	Class III	Class IV
Blood loss (ml)	≤750	750–1,500	1,500–2,000	≥2,000
Blood loss (% of blood volume)	≤15%	15–30%	30–40%	≥40%
Pulse rate	<100	>100	>120	≥140
Blood pressure	Normal	Normal	Decreased	Decreased
Pulse pressure (mm Hg)	Normal or increased	Decreased	Decreased	Decreased
Capillary refill test*	Normal	Positive	Positive	Positive
Respiratory rate (breaths/min)	14–20	20–30	30–40	>35
Urine output (ml/hr)	≥30	20–30	5–15	Negligible
Mental status	Slightly anxious	Mildly anxious	Anxious or confused	Confused or lethargic
Fluid replacement (3:1 rule)†	Crystalloid	Crystalloid	Crystalloid and blood	Crystalloid and blood

*The capillary refill test is performed by pressing on the fingernail or the hypothenar eminence. A normal response is for the color to return within 2 seconds. The test is not valid in hypothermic patients.
†The "3:1 rule" derives from the empiric observation that most patients in hemorrhagic shock require as much as 300 ml of electrolyte solution for each 100 ml of blood loss. Applied blindly, these guidelines can result in excessive or inadequate fluid administration. The use of bolus therapy with careful monitoring of the patient's responses can moderate these extremes.
Republished with permission from Committee on Trauma. Advanced trauma life support student manual. Chicago: American College of Surgeons, 1989.

complicated case of hemorrhagic shock, a decrease in the systolic blood pressure suggests a minimum loss of 30 to 40 percent of blood volume or the effective or real loss of at least 2 L (in a 70-kg patient) of blood or intravascular volume. Thus when significant hemorrhage is suspected because of traumatic injury or the presence of large amounts of blood in vomitus or stool, fluid therapy should be initiated immediately, irrespective of the systolic blood pressure.

THERAPY

The clinical approach to the patient with hemorrhagic shock is summarized in Table 3. The mainstay of therapy for patients with hypovolemic-hemorrhagic shock is rapid restoration of circulating volume with blood and crystalloid or colloid fluids as indicated.

Vascular Access

To facilitate the rapid infusion of fluids, two short large-bore intravenous catheters (at least 16- to 18-gauge) should be placed in the upper extremities. Central venous access is not a priority during the initial resuscitation period, and time should not be lost in attempts at central line placement. If the patient's arms are unsuitable for vascular access, then a percutaneous large-bore femoral catheter should be placed. Central venous cannulation or venous cutdown may be considered if these methods fail.

Fluid Therapy

The initial resuscitation fluids used in volume replacement of hypovolemic or hemorrhagic shock are isotonic crystalloid solutions, lactated Ringer's solution (130 mEq Na^+, 109 mEq Cl^-, 4 mEq K^+, 3 mEq Ca^{++}, and 28 mEq lactate per liter), or 0.9 percent saline (154 mEq each of Na^+ and Cl^- per liter). These fluids are inexpensive, readily available, and provide transient intravascular expansion as well as partial correction of electrolyte abnormalities. When signs and symptoms of hypovolemic or hemorrhagic shock are apparent or suspected, administration of 1 to 2 L of crystalloid solution to the adult and 20 ml per kilogram to the child should be undertaken promptly. Because of the equilibration with the extravascular space that occurs after 20 to 30 minutes, only 20 to 25 percent of infused crystalloid volume can be presumed to remain in the intravascular compartment after the infusion (see 3:1 replacement rule in Table 2).

Some controversy persists regarding the use of colloid solutions (hetastarch, or 5 percent and 25 percent albumin) in the acute resuscitation of hypovolemic shock. When used appropriately, colloid and crystalloid solutions are equally effective in the repletion of intravascular deficits. The total volume of crystalloid infused is at least threefold the total volume of colloid because of its rapid distribution into the extravascular compartment. Although excess crystalloid administration is more likely to result

Table 3 Clinical Evaluation of Patient with Hypovolemic-Hemorrhagic Shock

1. Recognition of syndrome

2. Initial physical examination and survey
   Evaluate mental status, skin temperature and color, capillary refill, pulse rate, respiratory rate, pulse pressure, blood pressure, orthostasis

3. Initial resuscitation
   Airway, ventilation, supplemental oxygen, venous access, fluid and blood administration

4. Baseline laboratory studies
   Blood type and cross-match, hemoglobin, hematocrit, platelet count, prothrombin time, partial thromboplastin time, fibrinogen, thrombin time, electrolytes, blood urea nitrogen, glucose, creatinine, arterial blood gas

5. Surgical consultation (hemorrhagic shock)

6. Assessment of initial therapy and re-evaluation
   Need for further fluid resuscitation: central venous, pulmonary arterial or systemic arterial monitoring; inotropic or vasopressor support, as indicated

7. Diagnostic studies
   Imaging techniques (arteriography, computed tomography, nuclear scanning)
   Endoscopic evaluation

8. Definitive therapy
   Surgical intervention
   Endoscopic therapeutic procedures (laser photocoagulation, sclerosing agents)
   Generalized or selective infusion of vasoconstrictor agents (vasopressin)
   Selective embolic therapy
   Mechanical (balloon) tamponade
   Correction of electrolyte abnormalities
   Hormonal replacement therapy (insulin, cortisol)

in peripheral edema, this is rarely associated with any significant morbidity. Colloid solutions are expensive, and some studies suggest that if they are used excessively in patients with increased vascular permeability, prolongation of episodes of respiratory failure will result. In fluid resuscitation of burn patients, colloid solutions are used after 24 hours to minimize the formation of edema that would result from continuing to administer large volumes of crystalloid solutions. Similarly, in the later stages of maintenance fluid therapy of patients who have undergone vigorous crystalloid replacement, colloid solutions are often administered to increase plasma oncotic pressure and mobilize accumulated extravascular fluid once the capillary leak has improved.

Loss of 15 to 30 percent of blood volume (approximately 750 to 1,500 ml in a 70-kg patient) in an otherwise uncomplicated patient can usually be corrected with administration of crystalloid alone. If there is a loss of greater than 30 percent of blood volume (approximately 2,000 ml) both crystalloid and blood products will be required for the adequate restoration of both intravascular volume and oxygen-carrying capacity. A 40 percent blood loss is immediately life-threatening and requires urgent transfusion of red blood cells and crystalloid.

The clinical response to rapid fluid administration should be observed carefully. Is the systolic blood pressure increasing? Is the pulse rate decreasing? Does organ perfusion (capillary refill; mental status; urine output >0.5–1 ml per kilogram in the adult, 1 ml per kilogram in the child, and 2 ml per kilogram in infants) appear to be improved? After clinical reassessment, additional bolus infusions of fluid should be given as indicated. The lactate contained in lactated Ringer's solution does not worsen lactic acidosis and does not affect plasma lactate measurements. Hyperchloremic metabolic acidosis following administration of large volumes of normal saline usually occurs in the setting of renal dysfunction and should not be a major concern during the initial resuscitation period.

Blood Component Therapy

Although blood component therapy is reviewed in another chapter in this text, several basic principles regarding the therapy of hemorrhagic shock deserve particular emphasis. Component therapy is the optimal method for administering blood products. Whole blood is rarely available for the acute resuscitation of the patient with hemorrhagic shock, and it offers no advantage over component therapy. The selection of red blood cell preparations to use during acute hemorrhagic shock depends on the degree of urgency. To fully crossmatch blood takes at least 1 hour. If the patient is stable after initial fluid resuscitation, crossmatched blood should be given. Type-specific blood compatible for ABO and Rh antigens is usually available within minutes and is usually given to those patients who have lost 20 to 40 percent of blood volume or who are still bleeding. If type-specific blood is unavailable, type O Rh-negative blood can be obtained immediately from the blood bank. Its use should be reserved for exsanguinating hemorrhage that requires immediate blood resuscitation. Blood, as well as other resuscitation fluids, can be rapidly infused by pressure infusion devices or hand-infused with large (35 to 60-mL) syringes.

Rapid infusion of blood can be accompanied by hypothermia and the development of a coagulopathy. If available, blood warmers should be used with massive transfusion. The coagulopathy that results from red blood cell replacement is usually caused by the consumption of platelets. Approximately 4 U of platelets should be empirically replaced for each 5 U of packed red blood cells transfused. The goal should be to maintain the platelet count at more than 100,000 per mm^3. Clotting factors should be replaced with approximately 2 U of fresh-frozen plasma per 10 U of packed red blood cells, and prothrombin and partial thromboplastin times should be followed. Fresh-frozen plasma does not have large amounts of factors VIII, V, or fibrinogen and thus, when clinically indicated, cryoprecipitate should be used to replenish these factors. Calcium is not routinely administered unless hypothermia is present and massive transfusion is necessary (i.e., 60 ml/per minute or a transfusion volume exceeding total blood volume).

Re-evaluation After the Initial Resuscitation

Frequent reassessment of the clinical signs of shock assists the clinician in determining the effectiveness of the initial resuscitation efforts. The patient's response to crystalloid alone— rapid improvement, transient stabilization, or no response—permits the clinician to assess the severity and tempo of continuing blood or volume losses. Surgical consultation should be obtained as soon as possible after resuscitation is initiated. If continued fluid or blood needs are apparent after the initial therapy, the clinician should question the adequacy of the fluid resuscitation, the accuracy of the diagnosis (i.e., whether other conditions are present), and whether there are persistent occult losses.

Monitoring of therapy may be facilitated by central venous catheterization. Central venous pressure measurements allow assessment of right ventricular filling pressures. Changes or trends in the central venous pressure measurements after fluid resuscitation are more important than absolute numbers; when associated with improvement in clinical indicators (such as urine output, pulse rate, and blood pressure), these measurements provide a useful means of monitoring complicated cases. It is important to recognize, however, that the initial central venous pressure may be high when the actual intravascular volume is low. This occurs when pneumatic antishock garments are in place, vasopressors are being administered, or when other conditions (such as cardiac tamponade, tension pneumothorax, myocardial ischemia, or mechanical ventilation) complicate the clinical picture of shock.

Placement of a pulmonary artery catheter should be performed under the following circumstances: (1) if the central venous pressure is persistently elevated in the face of shock or pulmonary edema, or (2) if vasopressor agents are needed. This allows assessment of left ventricular filling pressures, mixed venous blood samples, and cardiac output. An arterial catheter, preferably placed in the femoral artery, allows one to make an accurate assessment of arterial pressure and provides convenient access for blood sampling.

Vasopressors (dopamine) and inotropic agents (dobutamine) are not part of the usual initial therapy of hemorrhagic or hypovolemic shock. In the later stages of therapy, these agents may be added if there are complicating conditions such as myocardial infarction, but they are otherwise not indicated. Occasionally patients receive vasopressors to maintain arterial pressure while receiving resuscitation fluids, or vasopressors may be given when the actual diagnosis is unknown or misinterpreted. False elevations of central pressures may occur, misleading the clinician regarding the adequacy of fluid administration. Vasopressors should be titrated as fluid and blood resuscitation is continued. A persistent need for vasopressors or inotropic agents after fluid resuscitation is accomplished should alert the clinician to ongoing losses or to the presence of complicating conditions. In addition to coronary artery disease, myocardial ischemia and pump failure may result from myocardial contusion, aortic dissection, or cardiac tamponade. The clinical presentation and response to therapy should help to discern these conditions.

Laboratory studies should be obtained at the outset. Hematocrit or hemoglobin measurements are slow to reflect an acute blood loss during acute hemorrhage and, except in extreme instances, are not a reliable way to assess the severity of blood loss. If these measurements are low before fluid is administered, pre-existing anemia or severe blood loss is likely. Arterial blood gases may reflect a respiratory alkalosis during the early stages of shock or a metabolic acidosis during the later stages. The presence of a metabolic acidosis may suggest inadequate fluid resuscitation rather than a need for sodium bicarbonate. The latter should be withheld unless the pH decreases to less than 7.2 after adequate fluid repletion.

COMPLICATIONS

Ischemic organ damage that occurs as a result of hypovolemic shock is related to the severity and duration of hypotension. Elderly patients with pre-existing medical conditions are susceptible to cerebral and myocardial ischemia as well as to pulmonary edema caused by systolic and diastolic cardiac dysfunction. The prior chronic use of diuretics or antihypertensive agents may blunt the compensatory responses during the early stages of shock. During extreme hypotension, gut ischemia or necrosis may occur and contribute to the development of septic shock. The development of a consumptive coagulopathy can be controlled in part by rapid treatment of shock and repletion of clotting factors and platelets.

Hypothermia should be evaluated by core temperature measurements using a rectal thermometer or the thermistor of a pulmonary artery catheter. Passive rewarming can usually be accomplished by the use of blood warmers, the warming of crystalloid solutions in microwave ovens, and warming blankets. The clinician should be alert to the development of pulmonary edema caused by excessive fluid resuscitation, heart failure, or adult respiratory distress syndrome. Gastric dilatation should be decompressed with nasogastric suction.

SUGGESTED READING

Committee on Trauma. Advanced trauma life support student manual. Chicago: American College of Surgeons, 1989:57.
Rainey TG, English JF. Pharmacology of colloids and crystalloids. In: Chernow B, ed. The pharmacologic approach to the critically ill patient. Baltimore: Williams and Wilkins, 1988:219.

CARDIAC TAMPONADE

ERNEST WILLIAM HANCOCK, M.D.

Cardiac tamponade is a syndrome of circulatory abnormalities that is caused by an accumulation of fluid in the pericardial space under abnormally increased pressure. The circulatory abnormality is often defined vaguely as "circulatory embarrassment." Many physicians diagnose cardiac tamponade only when the arterial pressure has decreased significantly. However, a decrease in arterial pressure is a late and often preterminal development that is preceded by an increase in the central venous pressure and usually by a decrease in the cardiac output. The decrease in arterial pressure may be regarded as a decompensated stage of cardiac tamponade. Since cardiac tamponade should usually be recognized and treated before decompensation, it is preferable to define the condition as that in which there is a measurable circulatory abnormality, particularly an increase in the central venous pressure, that can be restored by removal of the excessive pericardial fluid.

The pericardium has very little elasticity when it is stretched acutely and therefore has a restraining effect when the heart becomes acutely dilated. When pericardial fluid accumulates rapidly, the pericardium quickly becomes taut and the intrapericardial pressure may rise steeply with as little as 300 ml of fluid. In chronic effusions or with chronic enlargement of the heart the pericardium stretches greatly, so that the restraining effect is no greater than normal; the intrapericardial pressure may be normal even with effusions of 1,000 ml or more.

In most instances, the pericardial space is continuous around all of the cardiac chambers, so that pericardial fluid exerts a similar compressive effect on all four chambers. Adhesions may result in loculated effusion, however, that compresses certain regions of the heart selectively and cause atypical pathophysiologic syndromes. Even when the pericardiotomy incision has been left open at the conclusion of an open heart operation, an accumulation of fluid in a local region of the anterior mediastinum can compress the heart.

The right side of the heart, because of its thinner walls and lower intracavitary pressures, is more readily compressed than the left-sided chambers. If there is left ventricular hypertrophy or elevated left-sided cardiac filling pressures, tamponade can be rather severe while compressing only the right-sided chambers.

Cardiac tamponade can develop with pericardial effusions of any cause; the condition thus encompasses a wide range of medical and surgical disorders. Idiopathic (possibly viral) pericarditis and secondary neoplastic involvement of the pericardium are the two most common causes in a general medical setting. In the setting of the emergency room, hemopericardium caused by trauma or acute ascending aortic dissection is a particularly important cause. In the setting of the intensive care unit, sepsis and postoperative bleeding are particularly important causes. In critically ill patients, several complications of diagnosis and treatment are particularly notable causes of cardiac tamponade (Table 1). Inadvertent perforation of the right atrium by an indwelling catheter used for the administration of total parenteral nutrition is especially likely to cause cardiac tamponade, because the nutritional solution may be infused directly into the pericardial space for some time before the complication is recognized.

CLINICAL RECOGNITION

Except in rare instances of "low-pressure tamponade" that are probably caused by pericardial effusion in the presence of intravascular volume depletion, the central venous pressure should always be elevated in cardiac tamponade. In critical care medicine, the elevation of jugular venous pressure is often difficult to detect because of practical difficulties in examining the neck satisfactorily in both the recumbent and upright positions. Direct measurement of the central venous pressure with an indwelling catheter should be definitive, but the accurate detection of mildly or moderately elevated levels requires careful attention to the zero reference level and to the patient's breathing pattern. Another difficulty is that, in the critical care setting, elevation of the central venous pressure may often be caused by factors such as the amount of intravenous fluid administration, myocardial dysfunction, or mechanical ventilation.

Equalization of right-sided and left-sided filling pressures is expected to be present in typical instances of cardiac tamponade in which the pericardial effusion is not loculated. The equalization need not be perfect, especially when the pulmonary wedge pressure or the pulmonary artery diastolic pressure is used as the measure of left-sided filling pressure. Pulmonary artery wedge pressure varies with respiration to a greater degree than does the right atrial pressure, so that the equilibration should be sought during the end-expiratory phase or, preferably, during a pause between respirations.

Paradoxical pulse is present in most patients with cardiac tamponade who are not receiving mechanically assisted ventilation. However, it is often not detected by palpation of the pulse or by sphygmomanometry. A low mean arterial pressure or pulse pressure, an irregular breathing pattern, or an irregular cardiac rhythm make it difficult to detect. Paradoxical pulse may also be inconspicuous or absent when there is a loculated pericardial effusion that compresses only the right side of the heart or when left ventricular hypertrophy or elevated left-sided filling pressures render the left ventricle incompressible. With the sphygmomanometric method, the degree of respiratory variation in the arterial pressure is often underestimated. The often-cited criterion of 10 mm Hg of variation in systolic pressure frequently corresponds to 15 to 20 mm Hg of variation in the directly recorded arterial pressure. The recording speed and calibration of the direct arterial pressure monitor in the intensive care unit are often designed to reflect the absolute values better than the respiratory variations, which are best appreciated with a slow paper speed and a relatively sensitive calibration.

Echocardiography is the most useful technique for detecting pericardial effusion in the intensive care unit as well as in most other settings. It may fail to detect loculated effusions that compress the right side of the heart. Computed tomography and magnetic resonance imaging are also useful methods and should be used when echocardiography is inconclusive. The determination of whether cardiac tamponade is present should be distinguished from the mere assessment of the presence of pericardial effusion. Certain echocardiographic signs are useful in detecting tamponade. These include reduced size of the right ventricular cavity, persistent distention of the inferior vena cava through all phases of respiration, inward movement ("collapse") of the free wall of the right atrium and right ventricle in early diastole, and exaggerated respiratory variation in the mitral and tricuspid flow velocities. Accurate detection of these signs requires a high level of quality of the echocardiographic recording and of expertise in interpretation.

In the intensive care unit setting, cardiac tamponade should be (at least tentatively) assumed to be present when there is a moderate or large pericardial effusion and if the central venous pressure is elevated to greater than approximately 15 mm Hg. Cardiac tamponade should also be suspected with lower levels of central venous pressure if there are additional signs such as paradoxical pulse or equalization of right-sided and left-sided filling pressures.

Table 1 Complications of Diagnosis and Treatment that Cause Cardiac Tamponade

---

Postoperative hemorrhage with cardiac surgery or by the postcardiotomy syndrome
Anticoagulation
Barotrauma from mechanical ventilation
Esophageal perforation from sclerotherapy
Internal jugular or subclavian vein puncture
Perforation of the heart by indwelling catheter used for pressure monitoring, parenteral nutrition, or pacing
Perforation of the heart by angiographic injections
Perforation of the heart or coronary arteries by balloon angioplasty or valvuloplasty catheters

---

SUPPORTIVE THERAPY

Supportive therapy with drugs and intravenous fluids has a relatively limited role in the management of cardiac tamponade. It may be used during the interim period between the suspicion or recognition of the tamponade and its definitive relief by removal of the fluid. The infusion of additional intravenous fluid in the presence of hypotension is useful in the treatment of cardiac tamponade, but the response should not be expected to be comparable to that seen in conditions such as cardiogenic or septic shock. Unless the tamponade has developed very acutely, the patient has usually had some endogenous compensation by retaining fluid and expanding intravascular volume. Infusions of intravenous fluids are not likely to cause or aggravate pulmonary edema in patients with cardiac tamponade, however, since in patients with this condition, congestion is typically limited to the systemic venous compartment rather than the lungs.

Catecholamines infused intravenously may be helpful in raising the arterial pressure, but this should be a temporary measure only. When there is critical hypotension, such therapy may assist in maintaining the cerebral and coronary blood flow but should not be expected to improve renal and visceral blood flow significantly. Despite speculation that cardiac tamponade may reduce coronary blood flow and induce ischemic myocardial dysfunction, as a rule, the myocardial function appears to be normal in cardiac tamponade

Arterial vasodilators such as nitroprusside are probably not beneficial in the treatment of cardiac tamponade. The elevated left-sided filling pressures are compensatory and need to be maintained rather than reduced. Cardiac tamponade could be rendered critical if the left ventricular diastolic pressure decreased to less than the level of the pressure within the pericardial space. Venodilators and diuretics are also potentially harmful for the same reasons.

DEFINITIVE TREATMENT

The definitive treatment of cardiac tamponade is removal of the fluid. This may be done by pericardiocentesis or by a surgical pericardiostomy. Great variation exists among various medical institutions in the relative use of these two methods. Much of the variation stems from local tradition, but there are several considerations that should influence the choice.

Pericardiocentesis has been used for more than a century, but has never achieved a routine application similar to that of thoracentesis or abdominal paracentesis. This is because of the risks associated with the procedure—in particular, the possibility of puncturing the heart and causing hemopericardium. However, pericardiocentesis has the advantage of being as well tolerated as thoracentesis in most instances, with the capability of relieving cardiac tamponade effectively in approximately two-thirds of cases. It is most effective in large serous effusions, such as those typically found in patients with idiopathic (viral) pericarditis, neoplastic invasion of the pericardium, connective tissue diseases, and dialysis-related pericardial effusion. Diagnostic studies of the pericardial fluid usually give as much information as a pericardial biopsy, since the specific diagnoses are primarily made by bacteriologic smears and cultures and by cytologic studies for neoplasms such as those of breast cancer and lung cancer. Pericardial effusions that recur after a pericardiocentesis can be controlled by leaving an indwelling catheter in the pericardial space; the need for further treatment of recurring effusion can thus be recognized and the treatment carried out with deliberate planning without risking the emergency of recurrent tamponade.

The feasibility and safety of pericardiocentesis is greatly enhanced by performing echocardiography before the procedure is attempted. In general, needle pericardiocentesis should be attempted only if the echocardiogram shows a substantial echo-free space both posterior and anterior to the left ventricle. The presence of echogenic strands within the pericardial fluid should arouse caution about performing pericardiocentesis, since this appearance may indicate that the effusion is organizing and forming loculations.

The subxiphoid point of entry is most frequently used for pericardiocentesis. The needle should be directed upward and laterally, toward the left shoulder. A shallow angle will aim at the retrosternal space anterior to the heart, while a deeper direction will aim at the space between the diaphragm and the posteroinferior surface of the heart. Two-dimensional echocardiography can also be used to select the site of insertion and to guide the passage of the needle; when this is done, an apical or a left parasternal site may appear to be preferable to the subxiphoid site.

Atropine should be used as premedication for pericardiocentesis, because a neurally mediated vasodepressor reaction occasionally occurs. An electrocardiographic recording may be made from the needle, connecting the V-lead electrode to the hub. When the needle makes contact with the ventricular myocardium, a marked elevation of the ST segment is seen. However, this alone should not be relied upon to avoid penetration of the heart. The experienced surgeon can usually detect a characteristic sensation, similar to a grating or scratching, when the needle makes contact with the moving heart. The needle should be withdrawn slightly at this point, even if no elevation of the ST segment has been detected. Failure to record elevation of the ST segment may reflect fibrosis or fatty change in the ventricular myocardium, or contact of the needle with the right atrium rather than the ventricle.

As soon as the pericardial space is entered, and a few milliliters of fluid have been withdrawn, a pressure recording from the needle should be made. This should be done with an electromanometer, if available (otherwise with a saline manometer), as is done during lumbar puncture. Pericardial pressure is normally approximately the same as intrapleural pressure. In cardiac tamponade it is elevated at least to the level of the central venous pressure, and usually several millimeters of mercury higher. Recording such an elevated pressure provides documentation of the presence of cardiac tamponade and of its degree.

If the fluid has the appearance of blood, it must be determined whether it is truly a bloody pericardial effusion, or whether a cardiac chamber has been inadvertently entered. A simple test is to place a drop on a gauze pad; blood will spread out evenly, while a bloody effusion will form an inner circle of darker bloody appearance and an outer halo of much thinner bloody appearance. A phasic electromanometric pressure recording and an injection of a small amount of angiographic contrast material may also be helpful in making this distinction. The fluid should then be withdrawn relatively slowly, either from the needle directly or via an indwelling catheter that is placed within the pericardial space with the use of a flexible guidewire.

When as much fluid as possible has been withdrawn, the intrapericardial pressure should be measured again. In a successful pericardiocentesis, the pressure should decrease to a mean value of approximately zero, with a negative excursion occurring during inspiration. The central venous pressure should also decrease substantially, but not necessarily to normal levels. If the patient has become overloaded with intravascular volume during the period of cardiac tamponade, the central venous pressure may remain moderately elevated until a diuresis has had time to occur. Paradoxical pulse should also diminish substantially, and the mean arterial pressure should increase if it was significantly diminished.

In most patients in whom pericardiocentesis is carried out, a catheter should be left indwelling in the pericardial space. It can be left in safely for up to approximately 4 days. The catheter is closed with a heparin-lock and aspirated approximately every hour to determine the rate of reaccumulation of pericardial fluid. Reaccumulation of pericardial fluid can also be monitored by echocardiography. In special circumstances, it may be useful to instill air in the pericardial space in a volume similar to that of the fluid that was removed, in order to provide air contrast roentgenograms of the pericardial space.

The term "pericardial window" is often used to denote the various surgical procedures that may be performed to remove pericardial fluid and relieve cardiac tamponade. The term is imprecise, however, and is used to indicate disparate kinds of procedures. The most important aspect of the surgical procedure is the creation of an opening in the parietal pericardium, allowing a route for escape of the pericardial fluid. In some instances, a communication into the left pleural space or occasionally the right pleural space may be made, but this is not always essential. It would be preferable to designate the surgical procedure by the site of the incision and the amount and location of the pericardium that is removed. The most frequently used surgical procedure is the subxiphoid pericardiostomy, in which a small area of the inferior parietal pericardium is removed and a temporary external drainage tube is placed. The other common procedure is to remove a moderate amount of the anterolateral parietal pericardium anterior to the left phrenic nerve via a limited left intercostal thoracotomy. In patients with cardiac trauma or after cardiac surgery, hemopericardium is often best managed via a median sternotomy, which permits adequate exposure of the heart for control of sites of active bleeding.

The subxiphoid pericardiostomy is usually well tolerated even in critically ill patients, since it avoids thoracotomy and can even be performed with the patient under local anesthesia, if necessary. It is effective in the treatment of most types of cardiac tamponade. The left lateral parietal pericardiectomy is particularly suited to purulent pericarditis, since the extent of pericardium that can be removed offers better drainage and more certain prevention of constrictive pericarditis.

Surgical drainage of pericardial fluid provides more certain relief of tamponade than does needle pericardiocentesis. Although it is probably at least as safe, since the risk of puncturing the heart by a blind needle entry is avoided, it is associated with the greater morbidity that is inherent in the use of general anesthesia and the creation of a surgical incision. It also provides the opportunity of a pericardial biopsy, which is occasionally more diagnostic than the studies limited to the fluid itself. Tuberculous pericarditis is the most important condition in which the pericardial biopsy has substantially greater diagnostic accuracy.

EFFUSIVE-CONSTRICTIVE PERICARDITIS

If the central venous pressure remains markedly elevated after pericardiocentesis, it is possible that the patient has constrictive pericarditis as well as cardiac tamponade. This condition, termed effusive-constrictive pericarditis, is due to constriction of the heart by a peel on the heart's visceral surface at the same time a substantial pericardial effusion is present. Surgical pericardiectomy is necessary to relieve the constriction due to the visceral peel. Effusive-constrictive pericarditis usually occurs in patients who have a subacute form of pericardial disease that has been in progress for several weeks or longer. It can develop in a few days in some instances, however, particularly with purulent pericarditis or with aggravated instances of the postcardiotomy syndrome after cardiac surgery. In many instances, the fluid is loculated. Effusive-constrictive pericarditis represents a stage in the evolution of subacute or chronic pericardial disease in which the effusion is in a stage of reabsorption and organization that will eventually form a chronic noneffusive constrictive pericarditis.

SUGGESTED READING

Callaham ML. Pericardiocentesis in traumatic and nontraumatic cardiac tamponade. Ann Emerg Med 1984; 13:924–945.

Callahan JA, Seward JB, Nishimura RA, et al. Two-dimension echocardiographically guided pericardiocentesis: experience in 117 consecutive patients. Am J Cardiol 1985: 55:476–479.

Hancock EW. Cardiac tamponade. In: Scheinman MM, ed. Cardiac emergencies. Philadelphia, WB Saunders, 1984:252.

Palatianos GM, Thurer RJ, Kaiser GA. Comparison of effectiveness and safety of operations on the pericardium. Chest 1985; 88:30–33.

CONGESTIVE HEART FAILURE: DIGITALIS THERAPY

RICHARD P. LEWIS, M.D.

Over the past few years, the role of digitalis in the treatment of congestive heart failure (CHF) associated with sinus rhythm has been hotly debated. Although digitalis was once one of the most widely prescribed drugs, its use has declined, especially among younger physicians. Many consider it a "weak" agent that may actually increase risk in patients with ischemic heart disease. However, several recent randomized prospective clinical trials have once again established the safety and efficacy of digitalis for therapy of CHF in patients with sinus rhythm. Furthermore, new alternative oral inotropic agents have been disappointing because of their tolerance or arrhythmogenic effects, and it is unlikely that any such agents will be approved in the foreseeable future. Thus a consensus has been developing since the late 1980s wherein digitalis along with diuretics and vasodilators represents one limb of the so-called "triple therapy" for chronic CHF.

PHARMACOLOGY OF DIGITALIS

Both the inotropic and antiarrhythmic properties of digitalis are caused by inhibition of the cell membrane sodium-potassium ATP'ase enzyme (the "sodium pump"). Binding to the enzyme is enhanced by hypokalemia and is inhibited by hyperkalemia. Inhibition of the sodium pump causes an increase in the intracellular sodium concentration, which in turn activates a sodium-calcium exchange mechanism. This results in increased intracellular calcium, which enhances the contractile performance of the heart. The precise mechanism of this calcium effect is still unclear, but it differs from that of catecholamines or other inotropic agents. Digitalis also causes vascular smooth muscle to contract.

The electrophysiologic effect of digitalis are extremely complex. They are the result of direct effects of the drug, as well as of indirect effects resulting from stimulation or inhibition of the autonomic nervous system. A therapeutic level of digitalis produces an increase in parasympathetic tone and an inhibition of sympathetic nervous system tone. Combined with its direct effects, this causes sinus bradycardia and prolonged A-V nodal conduction, and there maybe possible inhibition of both atrial and ventricular arrhythmias. Toxic levels of digitalis, on the other hand, activate the sympathetic nervous system, which aggravates tachyarrhythmias. The cellular effects of toxic levels of digitalis can lead to "triggered" automaticity, automaticity caused by increased phase 4 depolarization, and ventricular arrhythmias caused by re-entry. Digitalis toxic arrhythmias can consist of bradyarrhythmias caused by sinoatrial or A-V nodal block or tachyarrhythmias. Common tachyarrhythmias include automatic tachycardias (paroxysmal atrial tachycardia with block, nonparoxysmal junctional tachycardia) as well as re-entry and triggered arrhythmias manifest mostly by ventricular arrhythmias.

The two major digitalis preparations available in the United States are digoxin and digitoxin. Although these compounds differ by only one hydroxyl group, they have profound pharmacologic differences because of differences in polarity. Digitoxin is nonpolar and therefore lipid-soluble. It is completely absorbed, has a high level of plasma-protein binding, and a fixed rate of excretion related to hepatic degradation. Digoxin is less well-absorbed, has a lower level of plasma-protein binding, and is excreted as native drug by the kidneys. In patients with normal renal function, the half-life of digitoxin is 5 days, while that of digoxin is 2 days. Many patients with heart failure have impaired renal function, however, which may prolong the half-life of digoxin to up to 4 days. Furthermore, quinidine, verapamil, and amiodarone prolong digoxin half-life by impairing renal elimination. Digoxin absorption is less complete in the presence of bowel edema from congestive heart failure. Approximately 10 percent of patients inactivate digoxin in the gut.

Both digoxin and deslanoside may be used intravenously. Deslanoside has a rapid onset of action (5 to 10 minutes), while the onset of action for digoxin is 25 to 30 minutes. Because the full effect of an intravenous dose is achieved by 1 hour, doses can be repeated hourly. When oral dosing is employed, the onset of action is similar for both digoxin and digitoxin, with the onset of action occurring at 1 to 2 hours and with its peak effect occurring at 4 to 8 hours. The dosages and route of administration of commonly used digitalis glycosides are shown in Table 1.

Digoxin was the first drug for which a radioimmunoassay of serum level of the drug became widely available to monitor therapy. Following the introduction of this assay in 1970, the incidence of digitalis intoxication markedly decreased from nearly 25 percent of hospitalized patients to less than 2 percent. The high incidence of digitalis toxicity before 1970 was also related to the much higher doses employed at that time (when digitalis was the only oral therapy for CHF). The diagnosis of digitalis intoxication depends on the presence of a characteristic arrhythmia; the serum digoxin level is abnormally high in only 80 percent of such cases. Recently, digoxin-specific antibody fragments have been developed that can rapidly bind digoxin in the serum and relieve digitalis toxic arrhythmias within 30 minutes.

Since digitalis exerts its effect by binding to a receptor that has a finite number, there is a finite response to digitalis. It is of interest that the empirically derived recommended digitalis therapeutic blood levels achieve near-maximal effect with minimal risk of toxicity. Administering more than the usual therapeutic amount of digitalis does not result in a substantial increase in effect, but markedly increases the likelihood of toxicity.

Serum digoxin levels are extremely useful for the assessment of digoxin therapy. However, there has been

Table 1 Pharmacologic Parameters of Digitalis Glycosides

Agent	Gastrointestinal Absorption	Peak Effect	Half-Life	Therapeutic Range (ng/ml)	Digitalizing Dose (mg)	Maintenance Dose (mg)
Deslanoside	Intravenous only	10–20 min	42 hours		Initial 0.5 up to 1.0	
Digoxin	Tablets 60%–75%	4–8 hours	44 hours	1–2	1.0–1.5	0.125–0.375
	Digoxin solution in capsules 80%–90%				0.8–1.0	0.05–0.20
	Intravenous	30–60 min			Initial 0.5 up to 1.0	
Digitoxin	Tablets 95%–100%		4–6 days	15–25	0.6–1.2	0.05–0.15
	Intramuscular 95%–100%	4–8 hours				
	Intravenous	1–2 hours			0.6–1.2	

widespread overuse of digoxin levels, in large part reflecting lack of understanding of digoxin pharmacokinetics. Care must be taken to obtain the level at 12 hours after a dose (8 to 10 hours are required for equilibration between serum and the heart after an oral dose). Levels should not be repeated until five half-lives after a dosage change. Daily measurements are seldom indicated. The proper utilization of serum digoxin levels is outlined in Table 2.

CIRCULATORY EFFECTS OF DIGITALIS IN CONGESTIVE HEART FAILURE

The circulatory effects of digitalis in patients with CHF are complex and comprehensive. The inotropic action of digitalis produces an increase in the rate of left ventricular pressure rise (dp/dt), an increase in the ejection fraction, an increase in cardiac output, and a decrease in left ventricular filling pressures. The response of the failing heart is greater than that of the normal heart,

Table 2 Clinical Use of the Serum Digoxin Assay

Diagnosis of digitalis toxicity

Prevention of digitalis toxicity

Validation of dose size

Assessment of patient compliance

Assessment of digoxin absorption in CHF

Assessment of effects of renal failure of drugs which interfere with digoxin elimination

perhaps reflecting the impaired ability of the failing heart to respond to beta-adrenergic stimulation. Although digitalis has been considered a mild agent, experimental studies indicate that the inotropic response is at least 50 percent of that achieved by a maximum tolerable dose of isoproterenol.

Digitalis has a beneficial effect on myocardial energetics. Although positive inotropic agents increase myocardial oxygen consumption (which could be detrimental in ischemic disease), digitalis generally reduces myocardial oxygen consumption and increases myocardial oxygen supply. This is largely achieved by reducing the cardiac rate, which in turn both reduces oxygen consumption (diminished number of contractions) and improves coronary blood flow (prolonged diastolic perfusion time).

Digitalis stimulates arterial baroreceptors, which in many patients with CHF are downregulated. The "blunted" baroreceptors are unable to suppress the adrenergic nervous system and renin-angiotensin-aldosterone system. By enhancing baroreceptor responsiveness, digitalis mitigates the neurohumoral overshoot, thus resulting in both arterial dilation and venous dilation, which reduce preload and afterload. Generally, its effect on preload is more prominent.

Digitalis promotes diuresis by both a direct effect of inhibiting sodium reabsorption and by an indirect effect of increasing renal blood flow. Indeed, Withering's original hypothesis of digitalis action was that it worked on the kidneys.

Digitalis improves atrial contractile function. Many patients with chronic CHF have atrial myocardial failure as well. This is manifested by a loud third heart sound (S_3) gallop and high mean left atrial pressure. By restoring atrial contractile function, the mean atrial pressure is reduced. This is manifested by a re-emergence of an S_4 gallop or by the disappearance of an S_3. In many patients, this may be the major beneficial inotropic effect of digitalis.

When atrial fibrillation is present with a rapid ventricular rate, digitalis improves cardiac efficiency by eliminating ineffectual beats. As noted earlier, slowing the heart rate increases coronary perfusion time and helps relieve chronic subendocardial ischemia, which may be present in patients with advanced ventricular failure.

RECENT CLINICAL TRIALS

Virtually all recent controlled prospective clinical trials of therapy of CHF have shown therapy with digitalis to be significantly better than placebo in patients with sinus rhythm. Digitalis improves signs and symptoms, exercise tolerance, and ejection fraction, and reduces hospital and emergency room visits. Its side effect profile is lower than that of most vasodilators and all other oral inotropic agents. It appears to work best in patients with more advanced CHF. Patients with an S_3 gallop are particularly likely to respond to this treatment.

The short-term studies have shown no increase in the mortality rate, but a long-term study on survival has not yet been performed. Retrospective analysis of one large series of patients with postmyocardial infarction suggested that there is an increased mortality rate when digitalis is used in patients with left ventricular dysfunction and significant ventricular ectopy. However, retrospective analysis of three other large series did not confirm this finding. Nonetheless, longstanding clinical experience suggests that digitalis may aggravate ventricular arrhythmias in some patients with significant ventricular ectopy, and that its use in that setting should be cautious and closely monitored until a prospective study is available.

ESTABLISHING THERAPEUTIC EFFICACY

When atrial fibrillation is present, control of the ventricular rate represents a convenient therapeutic endpoint. In patients with sinus rhythm, bedside clinical evaluation usually provides evidence that a favorable response has occurred, manifested as diminution in an S_3 gallop, diuresis, a decrease in the jugular venous pressure, slowing of the heart rate, and improvement of dyspnea and fatigue. Achievement of a therapeutic steady state serum level provides useful confirmatory evidence. An increase in the left ventricular ejection fraction can be demonstrated by nuclear methods or echocardiography, but this is generally not required. Improvement in exercise tolerance by exercise testing can also be shown, but again is usually not required.

Digitalis may be seen as an ineffective agent in patients with sinus rhythm because of the poor absorption of digoxin resulting in a subtherapeutic serum level. Thus in all patients receiving digoxin, a serum level should be obtained once steady state has been achieved to ensure that a therapeutic level is present. As noted earlier, absorption is generally not a problem when digitoxin is used.

INDICATIONS AND CONTRAINDICATIONS

Atrial Arrhythmias

In most patients with CHF, digitalis is the initial drug of choice for therapy of atrial flutter or atrial fibrillation. It is the only agent which slows A-V conduction and is also a positive inotrope. Doses of digitalis that are higher than is therapeutically necessary should never be given in this setting. If failure to control the ventricular rate occurs after full digitalization, then an oral beta-blocker or verapamil can usually be safely added. In many patients in whom the ventricular rate is not adequately controlled by digoxin, however, the rate can be controlled by digitoxin alone, perhaps because of its longer half-life and more reliable absorption.

Digitalis is often the initial drug of choice for therapy of paroxysmal atrial tachycardia because of its low cost and lack of side effects.

Congestive Heart Failure with Sinus Rhythm

Digitalis causes clinical improvement in the vast majority of patients with frank CHF, especially if an S_3 gallop is present. This is true, however, only if systolic dysfunction is present. It is now recognized that some individuals have CHF with predominant diastolic dysfunction and relatively well-preserved systolic function. This is more commonly seen in the elderly. In this setting, the effects of digitalis are minimal. Echocardiography usually identifies such patients.

In certain acute heart failure states associated with high adrenergic tone, it is difficult to show that digitalis has a beneficial inotropic effect. These acute heart failure states include acute pulmonary edema, acute myocardial infarction, and cardiogenic shock. When atrial fibrillation is present in such patients, digitalis is indicated to control the ventricular rate.

Similarly, in patients with chronic obstructive pulmonary disease with right-sided heart failure, therapy of the underlying pulmonary disease is preferred to digitalis; however, it must be remembered that many such patients have occult left ventricular failure and will benefit from treatment with digitalis. The likelihood of digitalis toxicity is increased in patients with chronic pulmonary disease.

Certain mechanical forms of heart disease producing CHF such as hypertrophic cardiomyopathy, pericardial disease, and aortic and mitral valve stenosis show minimal response to digitalis unless atrial fibrillation supervenes.

Contraindications

Patients with second- or third-degree A-V nodal block should not be given digitalis unless they have a pacemaker. Most patients with first-degree block can receive the agent with careful monitoring. Patients with sick sinus node syndrome may often tolerate digitalis, but some patients develop marked sinus bradycardia or sinus arrhythmia exit block. Thus one must treat these patients with caution.

As noted earlier, patients with significant ventricular ectopy should probably not be treated with digitalis until (or unless) the ectopy is under control. Of interest, perhaps because of its vagomimetic effects, digitalis may reduce ventricular arrhythmias in more than half of these patients.

SUGGESTED READING

Arnold SB, Byrd RC, Meister W, et al. Long-term digitalis therapy improves left ventricular function in heart failure. N Engl J Med 1980; 303:1443–1448.

The Captopril-Digoxin Multicenter Research Group. Comparative effects of therapy with captopril and digoxin in patients with mild to moderate heart failure. J Am Med Assoc 1988; 259:539–544.

DiBianco R, Shabetai R, Kostuk W, et al. A comparison of oral milrinone, digoxin, and their combination in the treatment of patients with chronic heart failure. N Engl J Med 1989; 320:677.

Ferguson DW, Abboud FW, Mark AL. Selective impairment of baroreceptor reflex-mediated vasoconstrictor responses in patients with ventricular dysfunction. Circulation 1984; 69:451–460.

Fisch C, ed. William Withering: an account of the foxglove and some of its medical uses, 1785-1985. J Am Coll Cardiol 1985; 5A:1–123.

Gheorghiade M, St. Clair J, St. Clair C, Beller GA. Hemodynamic effects of intravenous digoxin in patients with severe heart failure initially treated with diuretics and vasodilators. J Am Coll Cardiol 1987; 9:849–857.

Lee DC, Johnson RA, Bingham JB, et al. Heart failure in outpatients: a randomized trial of digoxin versus placebo. N Engl J Med 1982; 306:699–705.

Lewis RP. Digitalis. In: Leier CV, ed. Cardiotonic drugs: a clinical survey. New York: Marcel Dekker Inc., 1987:85.

Ribner HS, Plucinski DA, Hsieh A, et al. Acute effects of digoxin on total systemic vascular resistance in congestive heart failure due to dilated cardiomyopathy: a hemodynamic-hormonal study. Am J Cardiol 1985; 56:896–904.

Smith TA. Digitalis glycosides. Orlando: Grune and Stratton, Inc., 1986:1.

Wenger TL, Butler VP Jr, Haber E, Smith TW. Treatment of 63 severely digitalis-toxic patients with digoxin-specific antibody fragments. J Am Coll Cardiol 1985; 5:118A–123A.

Yusef S, Wittes J, Bailey K, Furberg C. Digitalis—a new controversy regarding an old drug: the pitfalls of inappropriate methods. Circulation 1986; 73:14–18.

CONGESTIVE HEART FAILURE: DIURETIC THERAPY

PHILIP R. LIEBSON, M.D.

Diuretics are used in the treatment of congestive heart failure (CHF) to eliminate excess water and sodium through the kidney, thus decreasing pulmonary congestion and peripheral edema. This must be accomplished while adequate systemic pressure, cardiac output, renal perfusion, systemic acid-base, and electrolyte balance are maintained. Diuretic therapy is of value in both left and right heart failure. The indirect effect of diuretics on cardiac function is to diminish ventricular preload, or end-diastolic volume and pressure. Thus back pressures of the pulmonary and systemic capillaries are reduced. Diuretics can sometimes diminish the sympathetic tone of the arterioles and venules in severe CHF, thus decreasing impedance to contraction to the left ventricle and amplifying diminished preload. Diminished sodium in the arteriolar wall may also decrease vascular tone. It is therefore frequently possible to sustain stroke volume at the same time that preload is reduced. This is most likely to occur with a dilated hypocontractile left ventricle. In CHF associated with a small restricted left ventricle, diuretic therapy is more likely to lead to a decreased stroke volume and blood pressure and must be used more cautiously.

Diuretic therapy in the treatment of CHF has stood the test of time. It is usually administered before vasodilators and, frequently, before digitalis are employed.

Despite their effect of decreasing symptoms of dyspnea in CHF, diuretics do not definitively increase exercise tolerance or enhance cardiac function, nor do they have any demonstrated effect of long-term mortality. There is circumstantial evidence that diuretics may be harmful, producing life-threatening ventricular arrhythmias caused by lowering plasma potassium levels, as suggested by the Multiple Risk Factor Interventional Trial. Participants in that study did not even have CHF; patients with CHF are at still greater risk for life-threatening arrhythmias, indicating the need for meticulous evaluation of electrolyte levels during diuretic therapy.

ACUTE PULMONARY EDEMA

A patient presents to the critical care unit with severe shortness of breath and rales in three-quarters of the chest. Sinus tachycardia at a rate of 120 beats per minute is present. It is clear that the patient has severe pulmonary edema. In this setting, a diuretic, such as furosemide (Lasix), which acts in the renal tubules of Henle's loop (loop diuretic), is likely to produce a rapid beneficial effect on the patient's symptoms. Within 5 to 15 minutes, venous capacitance increases, left ventricular filling pressure and pulmonary capillary pressure decrease, and symptoms are alleviated. The initial effect is therefore caused not by diuresis but by changes in venous capacitance. This may be the result of an indirect effect of loop diuretic on stimulating dilatory prostaglandins. Within 30 minutes of administration, peak urine flow occurs. Within 60 minutes, peak natruresis occurs. Furosemide and other loop diuretics (ethacrynic acid and bumetanide) are so effective that as much as 20 to 30 percent of glomerular filtrate can be excreted in the urine with their usage. These are the only diuretic agents that produce a significant free water clearance despite a natruresis. Thus the effect of a loop diuretic is significant alleviation of clinical signs of CHF within a short period of time. Beyond this initial period, the more definitive use of diuretics can be planned and a variety of classes of diuretics agents can be implemented.

The goal of diuresis is loss of excess fluid, as determined primarily by (1) weight loss, (2) decrease in rales, (3) decrease in peripheral edema or ascites, and (4) clearing of the lung fields on chest x-ray examination. Beyond the initial period of rapid fluid loss, diuretics act as maintenance agents that facilitate the physiologic action for inotropic agents (e.g., digitalis) or vasodilators (e.g., angiotensin-converting enzyme [ACE] inhibitors).

CLASSIFICATION OF DIURETICS

The most practical classification of diuretics is based on their site of action. Diuretics function in four sites in the kidney (Fig. 1): (1) the proximal tubule, (2) the thick ascending limb of Henle's loop, (3) the early portion of the distal tubule, and (4) the late portion of the tubule and collecting duct. It is logical and empirically effective to choose diuretic combinations based on differences in site of action to enhance the efficacy of diuresis.

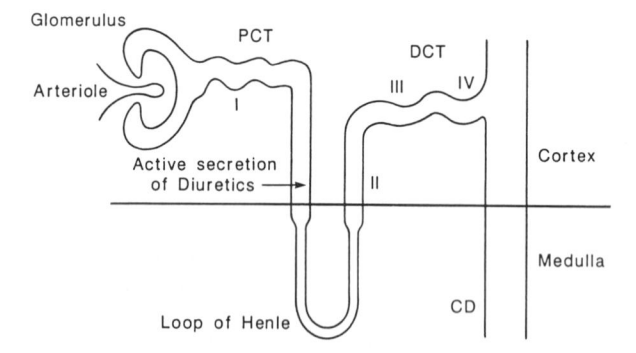

Figure 1 Primary sites of diuretic action in the kidney. Site I = site of action of osmotic diuretics (mannitol) and carbonic anhydrase inhibitor (acetazolamide). Site II = site of action of loop diuretics (furosemide, ethacrynic acid, bumetanide). Site III = site of action of thiazides (hydrochlorothiazide, chlorthalidone), indapamide, and metolazone. Site IV = site of action of spironolactone, triamterene, and amiloride. CD = collecting duct; DCT = distal convoluted tubule; PCT = proximal convoluted tubule.

Site 1: Proximal Convoluted Tubule

This is the site for reabsorption of approximately 65 percent of filtered sodium. Unfortunately, much of the sodium remaining in the lumen is reabsorbed from distal sites, diminishing the diuretic effect. Two agents mildly decrease sodium reabsorption from this site: mannitol, an osmotic diuretic, and acetazolamide (Diamox), a carbonic anhydrase inhibitor. Mannitol may be useful in the treatment of CHF associated with impending acute renal tubular necrosis, especially in conjunction with the use of loop diuretics. Initial diuresis is effected with 50 ml of 25 percent mannitol IV and maintenance with 5 percent mannitol. Mannitol may be prophylactic in CHF when patients are receiving radiocontrast dyes, *cis*-platinum, or amphotericin B. In these situations, low doses of intravenous dopamine (2 to 5 μg per kilogram per minute) can also enhance or maintain diuresis. Cerebral edema is another condition in which osmotic diuretics are useful for the patient with CHF. It is advisable to use other diuretics in combination to avoid an increase in intravascular volume due to its initial action. Thus extreme caution is indicated in the use of mannitol in the treatment of CHF.

Acetazolamide is a rarely used diuretic. During the late 1950s and early 1960s it was frequently used as part of a diuretic "cocktail" with aminophylline and mercurial diuretics to produce the most profound diuresis obtainable in the pre-loop diuretic era. It prevents reabsorption of sodium, potassium, and bicarbonate ions. Its effect is limited because of a decrease in plasma bicarbonate ions. Acetazolamide may promote additional weight loss in patients with normokalemic, hypochloremic alkalosis or in resistance associated with maintenance loop diuretics or spironolactones. It may produce a metabolic acidosis, and it has been used to treat the bicarbonate accumulation of metabolic alkalosis. Used alone, it is a weak diuretic with nonsustained effect after 2 to 3 days of continuous administration. Administration every other day may sustain its weak effect.

Site 2: Ascending Limb of Henle's Loop

This is the site of action of the loop diuretics, furosemide, ethacrynic acid (Edecrin), and bumetanide (Bumex). These agents are bound extensively to albumin. They are secreted in the proximal tubule by an active transport process that competes with lactate, urate, ketone, anions, and drugs such as probenecid, penicillin, and cephalosporins. In addition, bumetanide passively diffuses through the proximal tubule to the lumen. The ascending limb is the only clinically significant site of action for these agents, although they may also have weak activity at Sites 1 and 3. The diuresis is caused by inhibition of an active process that reabsorbs the equivalent of 2 mEq chloride, and 1 mEq each of sodium and potassium. A free water clearance is effected despite the excretion of chloride, sodium, and potassium.

Furosemide is the loop diuretic used predominately. The natruretic effects of furosemide increase linearly with increased dose, but systemic dilatation or arterial resistance increases very little beyond a dose of 20 mg administered intravenously. It is possible that part of the salutary effect of furosemide in pulmonary edema is the redistribution of pulmonary blood flow away from congested alveoli. Increased peripheral arterial resistance that may result from its use is probably secondary to stimulation of the renin-angiotensin system, producing increased angiotensin II levels. Increased angiotensin II may also account for venodilatation, possibly secondary to dilatory prostaglandin release.

Ethacrynic acid, a frequently used agent during the early loop diuretic era, is less commonly used because of its ototoxicity. This side effect can be decreased by infusing intravenous ethacrynic acid over a 5-minute period rather than a bolus. Bolus injection of furosemide can also lead to reversible ototoxicity. This may be synergistic with aminoglycoside antibiotics. Ethacrynic acid may be used in preference to furosemide in sulfonamide-induced interstitial nephritis in patients with CHF.

Bumetanide has a greater potency than furosemide or ethacrynic acid. Bumetanide's greater potency may have some advantage in situations in which competitive transport through the proximal tubule is a consideration, as it is in the case of ketosis and with the use of penicillin or probenecid. Bumetanide may less likely produce adverse effects such as granulocytopenia, thromocytopenia, or ototoxicity because of its decreased dosage. It has a high lipid solubility and accumulates in tubular fluid by passive diffusion across proximal tubule epithelium rather than by active transport, as in the case of furosemide. Bumetanide is absorbed more rapidly in patients with congestive heart failure, and its bioavailability is approximately twice that of furosemide.

Loop diuretics may cause hypokalemia, hypomagnesemia, glucose intolerance, and they may affect plasma lipid levels adversely.

Patients with bowel edema may be refractory to loop diuretics. Frequent dosing or intravenous infusions (0.25 to 0.75 mg per kilogram) of furosemide may overcome resistance with massive edema. Intravenous furosemide may be enhanced in combination with oral metolazone (Zaroxolyn), which acts on the distal tubule. Because of the free water clearance with loop diuretics, hypernatremia can occur. Occasionally, hyponatremia can also develop. This is possibly caused by the effect of potassium depletion on stimulation of antidiuretic hormone. Sodium ion is shifted into cells, leading to hyponatremia. The oral dose of furosemide should be twice the intravenous dose, especially in situations in which gastrointestinal edema is likely. An increase in renal impairment can be encountered by increasing the dose of loop diuretics from two to four times the usual dose (e.g., from 80 to 160 mg furosemide IV). In furosemide intravenous infusion, light shielding is necessary to prevent inactivation of the drug. If furosemide is given orally to patients with CHF, the time lag for effect should be considered. This may be as much as 3 to 4 hours. The oral dose of bumetanide is equal to the intravenous dose. With florid CHF, an increased half-time occurs for absorption of loop diuretics, with decreased peak concentration. The time course of absorption is prolonged. Dosages of loop diuretics are shown in Table 1.

Site 3: Early Portion of Distal Convoluted Tubule

Thiazides and derivatives metolazone and indapamide are active at this site. Thiazides such as hydrochlorothiazides (Hydrodiuril) and chlorthalidone (Hygroton) are effective diuretics, provided that creatinine clearance is greater than 20 to 30 ml per minute. Metolazone remains effective with decreasing renal function. These agents are useful in the treatment of mild CHF and are effective antihypertensive agents, as well. The effects of thiazides and metolazone are not as pronounced as those of loop diuretics (5 to 8 percent of filtered sodium excretion for thiazides and metolazone vs. 20 to 25 percent for loop diuretics).

Thiazides act primarily by inhibiting sodium reabsorption and increasing potassium excretion in the early distal tubule. Thiazides also cause calcium retention with chronic administration as opposed to loop diuretics, which lead to calcium excretion. Clinical deficiency of magnesium is another side effect of these agents, but is probably less likely to occur with thiazides than with diuretics. Metolazone, a quinethazone, produces a prolonged natriuresis and may cause more urinary potassium loss than shorter-acting thiazide diuretics. Metolazone has a renal site of action not only peripheral to furosemide, but also proximal. The proximal action decreases sodium absorption in the proximal convoluted tubule, allowing more filtrate to reach the ascending limb for furosemide action. Distally, metolazone prevents sodium reabsorption, thus increasing the filtrate reaching the collecting duct. Metolazone is poorly absorbed, however, and there may be a response time lag before a synergistic effect is achieved with loop diuretics. On the other hand, the long half-life of metolazone requires complete discontinuation if overdiuresis occurs. Even so, diuresis may persist up to 1 day after the last dose.

Indapamide (Lozol) is structurally related to these diuretics but also has a vasodilatory effect. Its potency for sodium excretion may be greater than that of thiazides. Thiazides may be effective in combination with loop diuretics and may be synergistic.

The potential for increased potassium depletion must be considered in this combination, especially in conjunction with digitalis administration.

Site 4: Late Portion of Distal Tubule and Collecting Duct

Spironolactone (Aldactone) acts as an aldosterone antagonist and decreases Na^+-K^+-H^+ exchange, causing a sodium diuresis with retention of potassium and hydrogen ion. Triamterene (Dyrenium) and amiloride (Midamor) function by a non-aldosterone–dependent mechanism. Both classes of agents are useful for their potassium-sparing effect. Spironolactone requires several

Table 1 Diuretic Dosages and Sites of Action in the Treatment of Congestive Heart Failure

Diuretic	Main Site of Action (see Figure)	Subsidiary	Dosage (mg)	Na+ Excretion (%Δ+)	Onset	Peak	Duration
Loop							
Furosemide	2	1, 3	IV 40–240	20–25	0.1	0.5	2
			PO		0.5	1–2	6
Ethacrynic acid	2	1, 3	IV 50–100	20–25	0.2	0.8	3
			PO		0.5	1–2	6
Bumetanide	2	1, 3	IV 0.5–2.0	20–25	0.2	0.5	4
			PO		0.5	1–3	5–6
Thiazide							
Hydrochlorothiazide	3	1	25–100	5–8	2	4	12
Chlorthalidone	3	1	25–100	5–8	2	6	24–48
Metolazone	3	1	5–10	5–8	1	2–4	12–24
Indapamide	3		2.5–5.0	20–25	1	1–2	12–24
Potassium-sparing							
Spironolactone	4		25–200	2	Gradual	24–72	7 days
Amiloride	4		5–10	2	2	6–10	12–24
Triamterene	4		100–200	2	2	6–8	12–16
Carbonic anhydrase inhibitor							
Acetazolamide	1		IV 500	3–5	1	2–4	8
			PO 250–375				
Osmotic							
Mannitol	1		IV 50–200	5–15	0.1	0.5–1	2–6

1 = proximal tubule; 2 = ascending loop of Henle; 3 = early distal tubule; 4 = late distal tubule and collecting duct; %Δ+ = percentage increase in Na+ excretion effectiveness of diuretic.

days to achieve its maximum effect, whereas the others reach maximal activity within hours. They must be used cautiously in patients with renal insufficiency. Although these agents are relatively weak diuretics, they enhance the diuresis that is promoted by either thiazides or loop diuretics. The effects of the independent use of potassium-sparing diuretics is a less than 2 percent increase in natruresis. Special care should be addressed to combining the use of these diuretics with ACE inhibitors, which also tend to spare potassium excretion. The effects of spironolactone may persist for days after their discontinuation. A mild metabolic acidosis can also be produced by these agents. In the treatment of CHF, they may be useful in combination with thiazide diuretics in situations of chronic obstructive lung disease because there is less of a possibility of diminishing ventilatory drive due to a metabolic alkalosis. Of these agents, triamterene alone inhibits tubular furosemide secretion. Conversely, loop diuretics may diminish the effect of triamterene or amiloride on sodium conductance in the collecting duct. Usages, interactions, and side effects of the various diuretics are summarized in Table 2.

Special Clinical Considerations

Elderly Patients

The potential for diuretic-induced hypokalemia and hypomagnesemia is increased in elderly patients with CHF. In patients 70 years of age and older, the decrease in the glomerular filtration rate is greater than 50 percent. Pharmacokinetic effects attributable to age that influence diuretic dosing include diminished hepatic drug extraction, decreased renal excretion, and decreased volume of distribution. The ensuing increase in plasma levels or the drug may thus produce adverse side effects.

Loop diuretics usually have a shorter duration of action than thiazide diuretics, and thus although a lesser degree of hypokalemia may ensue with the use of loop diuretics in the elderly, hypomagnesemia is common. Potassium-sparing diuretics also retain magnesium and may be used to decrease magnesium loss. Thiazide diuretics alone are rarely responsible for hypomagnesemia. At serum creatinine concentrations of greater than 2 mg per deciliter, the use of loop diuretics may be considered

Table 2 Usage, Interactions, and Side Effects of Diuretics

Diuretic	Usages	Interactions	Side Effects
Loop			
Furosemide	Most common	Increases Ca^{++} excretion	Ototoxicity (esp. with ethacrynic acid)
		Ototoxicity increased with aminoglycosides	Hypokalemia
		Tubule secretion decreased by organic acids, penicillin, probenecid, urates	Hypomagnesemia
Ethacrynic acid	Sulfa allergy		Metabolic alkalosis
			Hypernatremia
Bumetanide	Less dependent on active transport secretion	Cephalosporins increase nephrotoxicity	Arterial vasoconstriction
	Low degree of ototoxicity		Glucose intolerance
Thiazides			
Hydrochlorothiazide	Synergistic with loop diuretic	Not effective with GFR <20 ml/min	Hypokalemia
Chlorthalidone			Hypomagnesemia
			Hyperuricemia
			Decreased glucose tolerance
			Increased LDL cholesterol
			Hyponatremia
Thiazide-related			
Metolazone	Synergistic with loop diuretic	Remains effective with GFR <20 ml/min	
		Pharmacologic half-life up to 7 days in renal sufficiency	
Indapamine	Smooth muscle vasodilator		Extrarenal effects less marked than thiazides
Potassium-sparing			
Spironolactone (aldosterone inhibitor)	Especially in right-sided failure	Caution: Avoid ACE inhibitors Supplemental K^+	Hyperkalemia
			Gynecomastia
			Metabolic acidosis
			Azotemia
Amiloride	Independent of aldosterone mechanisms	Indomethacin (NSAID) may decrease GFR	Hyperkalemia
Triamterene			Azotemia
			Muscle cramps
Carbonic anhydrase inhibitor			
Acetazolamide	Normokalemic, hypochloremic alkalosis	Diuresis decreases with bicarbonate loss	Metabolic acidosis
			Hypokalemia
			Urinary tract calculi
			Hepatic coma
Osmotic			
Mannitol	Impending tubular necrosis	May be used to prevent decrease in GFR after radiopaque dyes, *cis*-platinum, amphotericin B	May increase CHF by fluid mobilization
			Dilutional hyponatremia

GFR = glomerular filtration rate; LDL = low-density lipoprotein.

preferable to that of thiazides. Although, in general, hypokalemia should be treated if the plasma potassium concentration is less than 3 mEq per liter, it is possible that many elderly subjects with CHF who are at risk for hypokalemia-induced ventricular arrhythmia should be treated if the plasma potassium concentration decreases to less than 3.5 mEq per liter. Certainly with concomitant digitalis therapy, one is more likely to replace potassium at the higher level.

In the elderly, other therapies that can enhance potassium loss include glucocorticoids and antibiotics such as amphotericin B and carbenicillin. Although therapy in the critical care setting allows control of medications, one must consider whether the patient will comply with the regimen after being discharged from the hospital. It has been found that direct potassium supplementation and potassium chloride are associated with less patient compliance than are drug combinations that include a potassium-sparing diuretic. The European Working Party in Hypertension in the Elderly study showed a significant reduction in fatal myocardial infarction in patients receiving potassium-sparing diuretics.

Pediatric Patients

Right heart failure rather than left failure is the substrate for the use of diuretic agents in infants and children. Intravenous loop diuretics are effective in infants and are associated with decreased edema, decreased tachypnea, and weight loss. As with adults, combination with thiazides or potassium-sparing agents increase the diuretic effect. Long-term furosemide therapy in premature infants has been associated with the development of renal calcification and nephrolithiasis because of increased calcium excretion. Pediatric dosages of clinically useful diuretics are shown in Table 3.

Drug Response and Side Effects

The possible arterial constricting effects of large doses of furosemide in patients with CHF must be emphasized. Doses of more than 1 mg per kilogram administered intravenously have been found to cause a generalized vasoconstrictor response leading to increased systemic blood pressure with decreased stroke volume index of the left ventricle. This has been associated with an increase in norepinephrine, plasma renin activity, and arginine-vasopressin.

Dilutional hyponatremia has been observed in patients with severe left ventricular hypertrophy treated with thiazide and potassium-sparing diuretics. Institution of an ACE inhibitor or withdrawal of diuretics is effective in resolving hyponatremia. Fluid restriction is also indicated, coupled with moderate salt restriction. Serum sodium concentrations of less than 120 mEq per liter may necessitate administration of 0.9 percent sodium chloride with close monitoring of pulmonary wedge pressures.

Most nonsteroidal anti-inflammatory agents (NSAIDs) decrease renal vasodilatory prostaglandin effects, which tend to maintain renal blood flow. Thus the effects of loop diuretics may be diminished by the simultaneous use of NSAIDs. The effects of NSAIDs are varied in this regard. Sulindac (Clinoril), for example, has little effect on renal prostaglandin synthesis while naproxen (Naprosyn) has been found to produce a 65 percent decrease in prostaglandin synthesis. Triamterene may cause nephrolithiasis and increase renal dysfunction induced by NSAIDs.

Both thiazides and loop diuretics may cause asymptomatic hyperuricemia. Thiazides decrease calcium excretion, and loop diuretics increase calcium secretion, possibly leading to nephrolithiasis in some cases.

In evaluating the effects of diuretics on lung edema, the clinician should appreciate that a significant amount of edema fluid reaches the interstitial spaces of the lungs. Thus even without alveolar involvement (absence of rales), considerable pulmonary edema may occur, decreasing bronchiolar compliance. The absence of rales after diuretic therapy therefore does not indicate the elimination of excessive lung water, and evaluation of serial chest radiographs are helpful in assessing the elimination of extra-alveolar edema.

Glucose intolerance and lipoprotein abnormalities may develop with the chronic use of thiazide or loop diuretics. This is a consideration in acute care units if these agents are initiated in patients with CHF who already exhibit these abnormalities. Indapamide appears to be less likely to produce these abnormalities than other thiazides.

CHF conditions associated with contracted left ventricular diastolic volume in which diuretics may produce a sharp decrease in stroke volume include aortic stenosis, hypertrophic cardiomyopathy, longstanding hypertension with moderately severe left ventricular hypertrophy, and restrictive cardiomyopathies. In these instances, diuretics should be used with great caution, and initial pulmonary wedge pressures should be evaluated along with careful monitoring of the blood pressure, especially when significant diuresis is expected to ensue.

Patients with dilated cardiomyopathy in CHF frequently develop functional mitral regurgitation. Moderate or severe regurgitation can be decreased by decreasing the impedance to forward outflow from the left ventricle by the use of peripheral vasodilators such as ACE inhibitors or nitroprusside in conjunction with diuretics. This is also true in cases of acute CHF associated with acute aortic regurgitation. In general, because diuretics decrease blood volume, they counteract with reflex fluid-retaining effects produced by peripheral vasodilators, presumably

Table 3 Pediatric Dosages of Selected Diuretics

Drug	Initial Dose	Routine Dose	Route and Frequency
Furosemide	2 mg/kg (oral)	6 mg/kg/dose	Oral or IV, 3-4 divided doses
	1 mg/kg (IV)	6 mg/kg/dose	
Ethacrynic acid	1 mg/kg (IV)		Oral or IV
Hydrochlorothiazide	1 mg/kg/24 hrs	2 mg/kg/day	Oral, q12h
Spironolactone	1 mg/kg/24 hrs	3 mg/kg/24 hrs	Oral, 3-4 divided doses
Mannitol	0-5 g/kg/dose	2 g/kg/dose	IV

Adapted from Witte MIC, Stork JE, Blumer JL. Diuretic therapeutics in the pediatric patient. Am J Cardiol 1986; 57:44A-53A.

because of an increase in aldosterone and arginine-vasopressin.

Rotation within the same class of diuretics can occasionally cause diuresis in those refractory to another agent in the same class (Table 4).

The "diuretic cocktail" of acetazolamide/theophylline and mercurial diuretics used during the pre-loop diuretic era was effective because acetazolamide increased plasma chloride, which allowed the mercural diuretic to work more effectively. The same principle holds true with loop diuretics if a hypochloremic alkalosis develops. An ACE inhibitor can serve as a substitute for xanthines in increasing renal blood flow. Theophylline may still have a supporting role with loop diuretics by promoting proximal tubular cell secretions of loop diuretics as well as by enhancing renal blood flow. Low-dose dopamine infusion (2 to 5 μg per kilogram per minute) is also frequently used to sustain or increase renal blood flow.

SUGGESTED READING

Amery A, Brixico P, Clement D, et al. Mortality and morbidity results from the European Working Party on High Blood Pressure in the Elderly Trial. Lancet 1985; 1:1349–1354.

Feig PU. Cellular mechanism of action of loop diuretics: implications for drug effectiveness and adverse effects. Am J Cardiol 1986; 57:14A-19A.

Genton R, Jaffe AS. Management of congestive heart failure in patients with acute myocardial infarction. JAMA 1986; 256:2556–2560.

Narins RG, Chusid P. Diuretic use in critical care. Am J Cardiol 1986; 57:26A-32A.

Sica DA, Gehr T. Diuretics in congestive heart failure. Cardiol Clin 1989; 7:87–97.

Sinoway L, Minotti J, Musch T, et al. Enhanced metabolic vasodilation secondary to diuretic therapy in decompensated congestive heart failure secondary to coronary artery disease. Am J Cardiol 1987; 60:107–111.

Table 4 Treatment of "Refractory" Congestive Heart Failure in Patients Receiving Furosemide

1. Administer furosemide by IV infusion (25–100 mg/hr—Light Shielding)
2. Administer low-dose dopamine infusion to increase GFR (2–5 μg/kg/min)
3. Add metolazone or thiazides
4. Add acetazolamide if hypochloremic alkalosis
5. Administer ACE inhibitors to increase glomerular filtration rate
6. Switch to bumetanide
7. Switch to competing drugs (NSAID, aminoglycosides, probenecid), correct for ketosis

CONGESTIVE HEART FAILURE: VASODILATOR THERAPY

JOHN T. BARRON, M.D., Ph.D.
JOSEPH E. PARRILLO, M.D.

The last decade has witnessed significant progress in the treatment of congestive heart failure (CHF). This progress has been achieved primarily by the introduction of new vasodilators into clinical practice. Vasodilator therapy for treatment of CHF has met with extensive interest because of its theoretical ability to improve left ventricular performance.

Significant impairment of systolic performance of a diseased left ventricle results in diminished cardiac output. As a consequence, several neurohormonal and other compensatory physiologic mechanisms are engaged as a means by which adequate systemic blood pressure and perfusion of vascular beds of critical organs are maintained. Activation of neurohormonal mechanisms results in peripheral vasoconstriction and an increase in total peripheral vascular resistance, a major component of left ventricular afterload. Even in a normal myocardium, ventricular performance is highly sensitive to changes in afterload. With fixed preload, the magnitude of the velocity of contraction (a major index of contractile function) of cardiac muscle diminishes as afterload increases. Thus the increased peripheral vasoconstriction, although initially beneficial in maintaining adequate tissue perfusion, is eventually maladaptive and leads to further left ventricular compromise. Furthermore, increased afterload results in increased myocardial oxygen requirements, possibly leading to relative ischemia of endomyocardial regions, which may contribute to myocardial dysfunction. The primary purpose of vasodilator therapy, therefore, is to interrupt the vicious cycle and augment left ventricular contractile function by altering the loading conditions of the heart without resorting to positive inotropic interventions.

A variety of agents now exist whose action is to induce relaxation of vascular smooth muscle. The selection of agents to be used and the mode of administration (i.e., intravenously or orally) depends in large part on the acuteness and extent of cardiac decompensation. Also, a major consideration is whether a sustained hemodynamic effect of afterload reduction is desired or whether the purpose of vasodilatation is to unload the left ventricle acutely, as might occur in acute pulmonary edema secondary to myocardial infarction. A final consideration in the selection of the vasodilator used, especially in the intensive care unit setting, is the availability of the agent in intravenous form, so that it may be used acutely in patients who cannot take oral medications or in patients in whom rapid reduction of afterload is needed.

INDIVIDUAL AGENTS

The vasodilators used in the treatment of CHF are listed in Table 1.

Nitrates

Nitroglycerin

The vasodilating properties of nitroglycerin have been known for decades. Nitroglycerin acts by increasing the level of cyclic guanylate monophosphate (GMP) in vascular smooth muscle. Although at moderate-to-high doses nitroglycerin relaxes both venous and arterial smooth muscle, at low doses it acts predominantly on venous smooth muscle. Hence, it primarily reduces preload and consistently lowers mean right atrial pressure and mean pulmonary capillary wedge pressure. Whether reduction of preload alone results in augmentation of cardiac output is controversial. In isolated skeletal and cardiac papillary muscle preparations, increasing preload results in an increase in the force of contraction on stimulation of the muscle, which is consistent with the postulates of the sliding filament theory and the Frank-Starling mechanism. With excessive stretch of the muscle (i.e., marked increase in preload), the force of contraction actually decreases and the muscle strip is said to operate on the "descending limb" of the Frank-Starling curve. In intact heart preparations, a descending limb of the Frank-Starling curve is demonstrable only with markedly elevated filling pressures of 40 to 60 mm Hg. Therefore, although preload reduction with nitrates may relieve pulmonary edema, it may not augment forward cardiac output per se. It may be the case that relief of pulmonary edema diminishes the peripheral vasoconstriction that is mediated by the enhanced sympathetic outflow in response to pulmonary edema, resulting in afterload reduction of the left ventricle. Unless the nitrate is present in sufficient doses to decrease systemic vascular resistance, forward cardiac output changes little or increases slightly.

Nitroglycerin is available in several preparations. The intravenous form may be started at 10 to 20 µg per kilogram per minute and titrated upward to as high as 400 to 600 µg per millimeter provided that the systolic blood pressure is greater than 95 to 100 mm Hg. As mentioned, high-

Table 1 Vasodilators Used in the Treatment of Congestive Heart Failure

Agent	Venous Dilatation	Arterial Dilatation	Dose	Comments
Nitroglycerin	+++	++	40–600 µg/min IV	Effective for acute CHF; tolerance develops within 48 to 72 hours
Nitroprusside	+++	+++	0.5–10 µg/kg/min IV	Effective for acute CHF; thiocyanate toxicity may develop
Isosorbide dinitrate	+++	+	20–40 mg q8h or q6h PO	If no effect, either increase or reduce dose or increase interval
Hydralazine	+	++	10–75 mg q6h PO	Beneficial short-term effects; effective in combination with isosorbide dinitrate in chronic CHF
Prazosin	++	++	1–5 mg q8h PO	Beneficial short-term effects; ineffective for chronic CHF
Minoxidil	+	+++	2.5–10 mg q12h PO	Beneficial short-term effects; ineffective for chronic CHF
Nifedipine	+	++	10–30 mg q8h PO	Beneficial short-term effects; ineffective for chronic CHF
Captopril	+	++	6.25–50 mg q8h PO	Effective for chronic CHF
Enalapril	+	++	5–20 mg q12h PO or 0.625–5 mg q6h IV	Effective in chronic CHF; intravenous form also available

dose nitroglycerin may result in afterload reduction and augments cardiac output in patients with severe CHF. Topical nitroglycerin (nitropaste) may be applied 1 to 5 cm every 4 to 6 hours as needed. Several topical transdermal patches are also commercially available in various doses.

It is important to note that sustained high doses of intravenous and topical nitrates have been associated with a loss of hemodynamic efficacy after 24 to 72 hours of administration. Tolerance to the vasodilatory effect of nitrates has been attributed to depletion of cellular stores of cysteine needed for the formation of nitrosothiol groups required for the activation of guanylate cyclase to elevate cyclic GMP. Therefore, the lowest possible dose of nitroglycerin necessary to obtain the hemodynamic effect should be used. If nitroglycerin is still required after 48 to 72 hours, switching to oral preparations such as isosorbide dinitrate should be undertaken as soon as feasible. The issue of nitrate tolerance is also a consideration with the oral preparations. Tolerance may be circumvented by allowing some degree of nitrate-free interval during which cellular cysteine stores may be replenished. Isosorbide dinitrate may be administered in a dose of 20 to 40 mg orally every 8 hours or every 12 hours. If the initial favorable hemodynamic response seems blunted with time, decreasing the dose or using an every-12-hours dosing regimen may be helpful. Recent evidence suggests that a single daily dose of 60 to 80 mg every morning is effective in preventing tolerance in the treatment of angina pectoris. This observation may be applicable to treatment strategies for chronic CHF. The development of nitrate tolerance may partly explain the previously observed lack of clear long-term clinical benefits in patients with CHF treated chronically with oral nitrates. Nitrates in combination with hydralazine, however, have been shown to be effective in the long-term management of these patients.

Nitroprusside

Sodium nitroprusside is a potent vasodilator that relaxes both venous and arterial smooth muscle and thus reduces both preload and afterload. This balanced effect causes a reduction in systemic vascular resistance, a concomitant decrease in systemic arterial and pulmonary venous pressures, and an increase in stroke volume and cardiac output. Its use in the treatment of CHF is ordinarily restricted to patients with particulary severe congestive failure in whom more conservative measures are ineffective in reducing afterload. Patients receiving intravenous nitroprusside ordinarily require placement of a balloon-flotation pulmonary artery catheter and arterial line for close hemodynamic monitoring.

Nitroprusside may be started at 0.5 µg per kilogram per minute and titrated upward to as high as 10 µg per kilogram per minute to achieve a target systemic systolic pressure of 95 to 100 mm Hg. At this pressure, if systemic vascular resistance remains elevated, further small increases in nitroprusside may decrease systemic vascular resistance and augment cardiac output without appreciably decreasing blood pressure further.

As with nitroglycerin, tolerance to the vasodilatory effect of nitroprusside may occur and greater doses may be required subsequently to achieve the desired hemodynamic result. Nitroprusside is metabolized by the liver to thiocyanate which, at sufficient concentrations (10 mg per deciliter), uncouples mitochondrial oxidative phosphorylation. Symptoms of toxicity include confusion, weakness, nausea, and psychosis. Because of compromised oxidative metabolism, an anion gap acidosis may ensue. If these symptoms are manifested or if serum levels are elevated, the nitroprusside infusion should be terminated. Serum thiocyanate levels should be obtained routinely so that incipient toxicity can be prevented. The lowest possible dose of nitroprusside should be used to obtain the desired hemodynamic effect, and therapy with an oral vasodilator should be instituted when feasible so that the patient may be weaned from nitroprusside.

Hydralazine

Hydralazine directly dilates vascular smooth muscle. Apparently, the effect of hydralazine is relatively specific for arterial smooth muscle and has only a modest effect on venous capacitance vessels. It therefore primarily reduces afterload. Reflex tachycardia is frequently seen in patients treated with this agent for hypertension, but less frequently in patients with chronic CHF. Because of its marked afterload reducing effect, hydralazine may be administered emergently at doses of 10 to 40 mg intravenously in patients with fulminant cardiogenic pulmonary edema, if intravenous loop diuretics and nitrates are insufficient. Intravenous hydralazine may be instituted and repeated as necessary, provided that the systolic blood pressure is at least 110 to 120 mm Hg.

The oral form of hydralazine has been used for the treatment of chronic CHF. The bioavailability of hydralazine correlates with the acetylator phenotype and is greater for slow acetylators than it is for fast acetylators. Accordingly, patients who are slow acetylators are more prone to develop untoward side effects, especially if high doses are used. The most serious side effect is drug-induced lupus, occurring in 15 to 20 percent of patients who receive high doses chronically.

Some patients develop reflex tachycardia with the use of hydralazine, as noted previously. Also there is a tendency for enhanced activation of the renin-angiotensin system and for increased salt and fluid retention. These observations and others have been used to explain the lack of sustained hemodynamic benefit and the development of tolerance to this agent in patients with chronic CHF. Indeed, several well-controlled clinical trials using hydralazine as a single vasodilator in the treatment of chronic CHF have failed to demonstrate long-term improvement in symptoms or improved exercise tolerance. Nevertheless, the combination of hydralazine and oral nitrates has been shown to improve New York Heart Association functional class and increase the lifespan of patients with chronic CHF.

Prazosin

Prazosin is a specific postsynaptic alpha$_1$ receptor blocker that antagonizes the tonic vasoconstrictor effect of endogenous catecholamines. CHF is ordinarily characterized by the elevation of endogenous catecholamines and other neurohormonal agonists that serve to maintain perfusion pressure by elevating systemic vascular resistance. A rational approach to blunt peripheral vasoconstriction, therefore, is to inhibit the vasoconstrictive action of endogenous catecholamines. Prazosin produces initial improvement in symptoms and hemodynamic variables in CHF patients. These initial favorable effects are commonly short-lived, and tolerance to the action of prazosin frequently develops within days to weeks of treatment. The development of tolerance has been attributed to centrally mediated enhancement of neurohormonal sympathetic stimulation as well as to increased activity of the renin-angiotensin system. A multicenter clinical trial assessing the efficacy of prazosin has failed to demonstrate that it has a favorable chronic effect on symptoms, left ventricular function, or survival. The use of this agent in the treatment of chronic CHF therefore does not seem to be supported by the available investigations. Prazosin may be useful, however, in the short-term management of CHF. The starting dose is 1 mg orally two to three times daily and may be increased to a total of 15 mg daily. Since orthostatic hypotension frequently occurs with the initial dose, patients must be cautioned regarding rapid changes in position during initiation of prazosin.

Minoxidil

Minoxidil is another agent that has direct vasodilating properties that result in increases in cardiac output and decreases in systemic vascular resistance at rest and during exercise. Its mechanism of action is similar to that of hydralazine—that is, it has a direct smooth muscle dilating effect. Although minoxidil can produce salutory short-term hemodynamic effects, there is presently a lack of clinical evidence indicating that this agent has any benefit over placebo in the long-term treatment of CHF. Like prazosin, it may be useful for the short-term management of CHF. Minoxidil may be started at a dose of 2.5 to 5 mg twice daily and increased to a dose of 10 mg twice daily. Fluid retention is commonly noted with its use, and adding or increasing the dose of diuretic is often necessary. A well-known side effect of chronic minoxidil administration is hirsutism. Pericardial effusion rarely occurs.

Calcium Channel Blockers

Nifedipine is the prototype agent that directly blocks entry of Ca^{++} into vascular smooth muscle, causing vasodilation. Compared with other Ca^{++} blockers such as diltiazem and verapamil, nifedipine has the least myocardial depression and, therefore, has been studied for use in CHF. Nifedipine has been shown to have beneficial hemodynamic effects when administered acutely. It acutely decreases systemic vascular resistance and mean blood pressure and increases cardiac index. After long-term treatment, these initial effects are negated, perhaps because of the development of reflex tachycardia and fluid retention and perhaps also because of direct, albeit slight, myocardial depression. At present, no significant survival benefit has been documented for the treatment of chronic CHF with nifedipine.

Because nifedipine can produce acute hemodynamic benefit and is available in liquid form (contained within a capsule), oral nifedipine has been used to produce acute vasodilation and thus acutely lower blood pressure in patients with hypertensive emergencies. It also has been used in patients with cardiogenic pulmonary edema to unload the left ventricle and thereby relieve pulmonary edema when other measures such as diuretics or nitrates are not sufficient. This mode of acute afterload reduction should be used only when the systolic blood pressure is greater than 100 to 110 mm Hg because untoward hypotension may ensue. Ten milligrams may be administered orally by puncturing the capsule with a needle and having the patient swallow the liquid or chew and then swallow the capsule whole. Ten to twenty minutes is usually required for appreciable changes to be seen in blood pressure and amelioration of pulmonary edema.

Angiotensin-Converting Enzyme Inhibitors

The theoretical and experimental appeal of these agents has been confirmed in clinical practice. A plethora of information now exists indicating that angiotensin-converting enzymes (ACE) inhibitors produce acute and chronic improvement in hemodynamic variables and left ventricular function. Furthermore, ACE inhibitors improve New York Heart Association functional class and significantly reduce mortality rates. Tolerance does not seem to develop as readily as it does with other vasodilators, making this class of drugs ideal for use in the management of CHF.

By inhibition of the formation of angiotensin II (AII), the pronounced vasoconstriction typical of CHF is relieved and the production of aldosterone is attenuated. Thus, afterload of the left ventricle is diminished, peripheral and renal blood flow is augmented, and salt and fluid retention is ameliorated. Also, because reduced AII seems to modulate sympathetic outflow, circulating catecholamine levels are diminished. This property may explain why the reflex tachycardia seen with other vasodilators is not produced by ACE inhibitors. AII has also been implicated in the local tissue elaboration of vasoactive prostaglandins that may be importantly involved in the regulation of the microcirculation.

The prototypical ACE inhibitor is captopril. In patients receiving diuretics, the starting dose is 6.25 mg by mouth. If this dose does not produce unacceptable hypotension, it may continue to be given every 8 hours. The dose is then doubled daily until a dose of 50 mg every 8 hours is achieved. Since AII has some vasoconstrictor effect on venous capacitance vessels, patients who are mildly dehydrated are particularly prone to hypotension with the use of ACE inhibitors. The presence of hyponatremia presages accentuated activation of the renin-angiotensin system; caution should therefore be exercised in administering ACE inhibitors under these circumstances. If hypotension occurs, it usually responds to intravenous fluid boluses or to placing the patient in the Trendelenburg position.

Another principal adverse reaction is renal insufficiency. Marked deterioration in renal function may be seen in the presence of renal artery stenosis. With withdrawal of captopril, renal function usually normalizes. Mild renal dysfunction may also be seen in patients without renal artery stenosis. In these instances, it has been ascribed to the initial decrease in the glomerular filtration rate (GFR) attributable to the withdrawal of AII-dependent vasoconstriction of the postcapillary arterioles. Ordinarily, postcapillary vasoconstriction is a compensatory mechanism in CHF to maintain an adequate GFR. With improved cardiac output and renal blood flow with ACE inhibitors, the GFR improves and azotemia usually resolves. Thus, because the deterioration in renal function is usually short-lived, it is prudent not to discontinue captopril at the first sign of azotemia.

Because they prevent the elaboration of aldosterone, ACE inhibitors may produce hyperkalemia, especially in patients with renal impairment. Extra caution, therefore, should be undertaken in patients taking concomitant K^+ supplementation. Serum electrolyte tests should be obtained routinely in these patients. Angioedema is another serious side effect of ACE inhibitors that is usually manifested after the first one or two doses. If this occurs, the drug should be immediately discontinued.

PREFERRED AGENT

Presently, three ACE inhibitors are available for clinical use (captopril, enalapril, and lisinopril) but which of these is the preferred agent remains controversial. A direct comparison of captopril with enalapril in patients with CHF indicated that captopril produces greater and more sustained hemodynamic improvement than does enalapril. Furthermore, symptomatic hypotension occurred more frequently and there was a greater decline in renal function and K^+ retention in patients treated with enalapril. These differences were attributed largely to the long duration of action of enalapril as opposed to the short duration of action of captopril. On the other hand, a recent comparison of the long-acting lisinopril indicated that lisinopril is superior to captopril. Nevertheless, for the treatment of chronic CHF, our preference is captopril. This is based primarily on the greater flexibility one has in controlling the dose of captopril. Patients with CHF are usually treated with diuretics concomitantly, and the administration of ACE inhibitors in this setting may result in severe hypotension. The peak effect of the long-acting ACE inhibitors (enalapril and lisinopril) occurs in 6 to 7 hours, whereas that of captopril occurs within 30 to 90 minutes. Also, the duration but not the magnitude of the hemodynamic effect of captopril is dose dependent. Therefore if symptomatic hypotension occurs, it becomes manifest and is maximal within approximately 1 hour of administration of the first dose and is usually short-lived, depending on the starting dose used. By contrast, the peak hemodynamic effect of enalapril or lisinopril occurs at about 4 to 6 hours, having a prolonged duration of action because of a longer half-life.

An ancillary benefit of captopril that is unrelated to its ACE inhibition and not shared by other ACE inhibitors is its action as a scavenger of free oxygen radicals. The generation of free oxygen radicals has been experimentally implicated in potentiating myocardial cell injury during an acute myocardial infarction. Myocardial infarction size has been reduced in experimental animals pretreated with captopril. The sulphydryl moieties present on captopril (but not on other ACE inhibitors) may impart the free oxygen radical scavenging property.

Enalaprilat, the active metabolite of enalapril, has recently been made available for intravenous use. Although used primarily as an antihypertensive agent, we have used this agent for afterload reduction in patients with decompensated chronic CHF who are unable to take oral medications. The starting dose is 0.625 mg every 6 hours, and the dose may be increased to 5 mg every 6 hours, as needed. The peak effect occurs within 4 hours after dosing and the half-life is 11 hours. Adjustment in dosing must be made in patients with renal insufficiency.

INDICATIONS FOR VASODILATOR THERAPY

The intravenous form of nitrates and hydralazine and oral nifedipine have great utility for reducing acute afterload in patients who have acute cardiogenic pulmonary edema, provided that systemic arterial blood pressure is adequate. But because of the relatively rapid development of tolerance to their hemodynamic action, the use of vasodilators other than the ACE inhibitors for the long-term treatment of chronic CHF is, in our opinion, not supported by available evidence. On the other hand, the combination of oral isosorbide dinitrate and hydralazine has been shown in a multicenter study to prolong life and marginally improve left ventricular performance. Interestingly, the doses of isosorbide dinitrate (40 mg every 6 hours) and hydralazine (75 mg every 6 hours) used in this study should have induced tolerance to the hemodynamic effects of these drugs, at least theoretically. For these reasons, we recommend the use of the isosorbide dinitrate–hydralazine combination if ACE inhibitors are not tolerated because of hemodynamic instability or unacceptable side effects.

From the results of large clinical trials, it is clear that ACE inhibitors are indicated for patients with New York Heart Association functional class IV CHF. Not only was 2-year survival improved, but there was significant improvement in functional class. An ACE inhibitor is also indicated for patients who remain symptomatic with treatment with digoxin and diuretics alone. Recent evidence suggests that captopril is an acceptable alternative to digitalis for patients in whom digitalis is not tolerated. Indeed, other recent evidence suggests that captopril may be an effective first-line agent in CHF and may be indicated in patients with asymptomatic left ventricular dysfunction. It is our practice to initiate therapy with an ACE inhibitor in any patient with evidence of significantly diminished left ventricular systolic function (i.e., ejection fraction <35 percent) (Table 2).

Coronary vasodilating drugs such as nifedipine and isosorbide dinitrate are, of course, indicated in CHF if there is co-existing coronary artery disease, especially if ischemia contributes to myocardial dysfunction. In addition, we have occasionally seen patients with idiopathic dilated cardiomyopathy but no coronary artery disease respond favorably to the administration of isosorbide dinitrate for the relief of noncoronary chest pain.

It is unclear whether vasodilator therapy for afterload reduction is beneficial in CHF patients with normal systolic left ventricular function but abnormal diastolic function, as might occur in restrictive cardiomyopathy or severe left ventricular hypertrophy. In these instances, the compliance abnormality of the left ventricle leads to elevated filling pressures and pulmonary edema. Venous vasodilators such as nitroglycerin may reduce ventricular filling pressures and thereby relieve symptoms. Negative inotropic and lusitropic agents such as beta-blockers and verapamil may be the more appropriate agents for chronic therapy, but controlled clinical trials are needed to determine this.

Table 2 Indications for Vasodilator Therapy in Chronic Congestive Heart Failure

Indications:
1. Patient has New York Heart Association functional class IV. ACE inhibitor is the preferred agent. Second-line regimen is combination of isosorbide dinitrate + hydralazine.
2. Patient remains symptomatic receiving treatment with diuretics and digoxin alone. ACE inhibitor is the preferred agent.
3. Digoxin is not tolerated. ACE inhibitor is acceptable alternative to digoxin.

Controversial indications and usages:
1. ACE inhibitor as first-line agent in place of digoxin
2. ACE inhibitor used for asymptomatic left ventricular dysfunction (EF <35%)

SUGGESTED READING

Chatterjee K. Vasodilator therapy for heart failure. In: Cohn JA, ed. Drug treatment of heart failure. Secaucus NJ: Advanced Therapeutics, Communications International, 1988:199.

Cohn JA. Drugs used to control vascular resistance and capacitance. In: Hurst JW, Shlant RC, eds. The heart. New York: McGraw-Hill, 1990:1673.

Packer M. Vasodilator and inotropic drugs for the treatment of chronic heart failure: distinguishing hype from hope. J Am Coll Cardiol 1988; 12:1299–1317.

CONGESTIVE HEART FAILURE: INOTROPIC AGENTS

ALAN J. BANK, M.D.
SPENCER H. KUBO, M.D.

Patients with congestive heart failure (CHF) frequently require the use of intravenous inotropic agents to improve symptoms and overall hemodynamics. This chapter focuses on many practical aspects of the use of inotropic agents in the intensive care unit, including patient selection, hemodynamic monitoring, and therapeutic endpoints. It also discusses the indications and uses of the drugs available for inotropic support, including their different hemodynamic profiles.

PATIENT SELECTION

The most common indication for the use of inotropic drug therapy in patients with heart failure admitted to an intensive care unit is the treatment of low cardiac output syndrome. Patients with this syndrome may have symptoms of somnolence, fatigue, or obtundation. Common clinical findings include hypotension, pulmonary congestion with hypoxemia, Cheyne-Stokes respiration, weak peripheral pulses with evidence of poor distal extremity perfusion, and oliguric renal failure. In more severe cases, lactic acidosis and occasionally multiorgan system failure can occur. In these cases with severe hypotension and critical reduction in perfusion of vital organs, potent vasoconstrictor agents may be required in addition to inotropic drug therapy for hemodynamic stabilization.

Not all patients with CHF should be given inotropic therapy. Patients with pulmonary congestion but normal blood pressure may be better treated with vasodilators, such as nitroprusside and diuretics. Other patients may have decompensated "heart failure" without significant underlying left ventricular systolic dysfunction and hence do not require inotropic therapy. For example, inotropic therapy is contraindicated in patients with heart failure resulting from high output syndromes such as thyrotoxicosis or beriberi, or in patients with severe diastolic dysfunction. Thus, strict attention to the findings of the physical examination and to abnormalities of cardiac output and cardiac filling pressures identified during invasive monitoring is often required.

PRECIPITATING CAUSES

The initial evaluation of the patient with decompensated heart failure admitted to the intensive care unit should focus on the potential precipitating factors of his or her condition (Table 1), since therapy directed at reversing many of these causes may be associated with prompt recovery and may lessen the need for inotropic drug support. For example, in a patient with borderline compensated heart failure, the hemodynamic deterioration associated with the onset of an atrial tachyarrhythmia should be aggressively treated with antiarrhythmic therapies designed to restore sinus rhythm. Similarly, the hypotension associated with an infectious or thromboembolic complication may be temporarily supported with inotropic agents but effective reversal requires either antibiotic or antithrombotic therapy. We have occasionally seen patients present with severe hypotension caused by overdiuresis in combination with an intensive vasodilator regimen who respond to the judicious use of saline infusion and the temporary discontinuation of diuretic and vasodilator therapy. Finally, the possibility of myocardial ischemia and associated mechanical complications such as a ventricular septal defect or papillary muscle rupture clearly require additional support and intervention.

THE ROLE OF INVASIVE MONITORING

It is our strong preference to use invasive hemodynamic monitoring, including balloon-tipped right heart catheters and intra-arterial cannula, in patients who require the use of inotropic agents for the management of severe heart failure. Although estimates of cardiac output and right and left heart filling pressures can frequently be inferred from the physical examination and laboratory testing, precise data are critical for the accurate titration of therapy to desired endpoints and to avoid the undesirable effects of excessive doses. Furthermore, hemodynamic monitoring may assist in determining the need to use other more invasive interventions, such as intra-aortic balloon pumps or ventricular assist devices. We believe that invasive hemodynamic monitoring optimizes therapy and avoids unnecessary (and potentially lethal) guesswork and that these benefits outweigh the low risk of infection, arrhythmias, and thrombosis. Finally, however, the initial treatment of the decompensated patient should not be delayed while one is awaiting catheter placement. Treatment should be started based on clinical evaluation and then adjusted once hemodynamic data are available.

"THERAPEUTIC ENDPOINTS"

There are no standard therapeutic endpoints that can be established to guide therapy for all patients. Specific criteria for drug efficacy must be tailored to the needs of each patient, based on the appropriate clinical, laboratory, and hemodynamic features. For example, in a patient with a previous blood pressure of 150/90, a blood pressure of 90/70 may be associated with acute circulatory shock after myocardial infarction, but it can also be the typical blood pressure of a patient with chronic left ventricular failure. Likewise, a patient with multiorgan failure may require a total cardiac output of more than 5 liters per minute to optimize cerebral, renal, and myocardial perfusion. One must therefore carefully examine the entire spectrum of clinical (mental status, peripheral perfusion, urine output, symptoms), laboratory (renal function, oxygenation, liver function) and hemodynamic (cardiac output, cardiac filling pressures, arterial pressure) endpoints to measure the efficacy of inotropic agents.

SPECIFIC INOTROPIC AGENTS

The nonglycoside inotropic drugs available for intravenous therapy in the intensive care unit (Table 2) increase contractility and cardiac output through one of two mechanisms: (1) beta-adrenergic stimulation, (2) phosphodiesterase (PDE) III inhibition. The beta-agonists bind to myocardial beta$_1$ receptors and increase cyclic adenosine monophosphate (cAMP) formation. By contrast, the PDE III inhibitors block cAMP degradation similar to the actions of the methylxanthines. In both cases, the resultant increase in cAMP levels leads to activation of several protein kinases that ultimately cause increased delivery of calcium to the contractile proteins and increased inotropy.

DOBUTAMINE

Dobutamine is the drug of choice for the majority of patients with heart failure requiring inotropic support. It is a synthetic catecholamine that has been in general use since 1978. Dobutamine produces increases in myocardial contractility through stimulation of myocardial beta$_1$-adrenergic receptors. Thus its major physiologic effect is to increase cardiac output by increasing stroke volume. Compared with dopamine and isoproterenol, dobutamine has a smaller chronotropic effect, although the heart rate will increase with higher infusion rates of the agent. Dobutamine is actually a racemic mixture of L- and D-isomers. The D-isomer stimulates peripheral vas-

Table 1 Common Precipitating Causes of Heart Failure

Dietary sodium intake
Medication noncompliance
Infection
Arrhythmias
Thromboembolism
Anemia
Volume depletion; excessive diuresis
Myocardial ischemia
Mechanical complications
    Ventricular septal defect
    Papillary muscle dysfunction

Table 2 Intravenous Inotropic Agents

Agent	Alpha₁ (Peripheral Vasoconstriction)	Beta₂ (Peripheral Vasodilation)	Beta₁ (Positive Inotropy)	Other	Physiologic Response
Dobutamine	+	+	+++		↑ CO MAP—no change ↓ PCWP
Dopamine	+++	+	+++	DA₁ and DA₂ stimulation	↑ CO ↑ RBF ↑ PCWP (or no change) ↑ MAP
Amrinone				PDE III inhibition	↑ CO ↓ MAP (or no change) ↓ PCWP
Digitalis				Na⁺-K⁺ ATPase inhibition	↑ CO (slight)
Norepinephrine	+++		+++		↑ CO (or no change) ↑ MAP ↑ PCWP
Epinephrine	+++	++	+++		↑ CO ↑ MAP

CO = cardiac output; MAP = mean arterial pressure; PCWP = pulmonary capillary wedge pressure; RBF = renal blood flow.

cular beta₂- adrenoceptors, thereby causing vasodilation, while the L-isomer stimulates alpha₁-adrenoceptors, thereby causing vasoconstriction. These competing effects usually result in little change in blood pressure. Calculated systemic vascular resistance decreases during dobutamine therapy, which is likely related to improved cardiac output and reflex withdrawal of sympathetic tone. Unlike dopamine, dobutamine reduces left ventricular filling pressure, probably secondary to a combination of improved left ventricular systolic performance and mild venodilation. Urine flow and sodium excretion frequently increase as a result of improved cardiac output and not as a result of effects on renal vascular receptors.

Dobutamine infusion is usually started at a dose of 2.5 μg per kilogram per minute administered intravenously. There is generally a good correlation between dobutamine dose, plasma levels, and hemodynamic changes. The dose can be increased every 15 to 30 minutes by increments of 2.5 μg per kilogram per minute until the desired hemodynamic effect is obtained. In most patients, 7.5 to 15 μg per kilogram per minute is an adequate maintenance dose, but on rare occasions, doses greater than 20 μg per kilogram per minute are required.

The onset of action of dobutamine is rapid and occurs within 2 to 3 minutes of starting an infusion. The peak effect occurs at approximately 10 minutes. In patients with heart failure, the half-life of dobutamine is approximately 2.5 minutes, enabling rapid up and down titration. Dobutamine is metabolized by catechol-o-methyltransferases and excreted in the kidney.

Drug tolerance to infusions of dobutamine continued for more than 72 hours has been reported, and is possibly related to beta receptor downregulation produced by prolonged exposure to the agonist. However, we have been able to treat many patients with this agent for extended periods, sometimes by slightly increasing their maintenance dose.

The most common adverse effects of dobutamine are related to its beta agonist activity and include tachycardia, hypertension, and the provocation of atrial and ventricular arrhythmias. Other less common side effects include nausea, headache, nonspecific chest pain, shortness of breath, palpitations, tremor, and anxiety. These adverse effects are usually dose-related and can be treated by decreasing the dose of drug. Rarely must the drug be discontinued.

DOPAMINE

Dopamine is a naturally occurring catecholamine precursor of norepinephrine. Its physiologic action is highly dependent on the dose. At low doses (<3 to 4 µg per kilogram per minute), dopamine activates dopamine$_1$ (DA$_1$) postsynaptic receptors in renal mesenteric, cerebral, coronary, and other vascular beds, resulting in vasodilation. The most important clinical effects of DA$_1$ stimulation are diuresis and natriuresis, which may result from a direct effect of dopamine on the renal tubule or to a redistribution of intrarenal blood flow. At doses of 4 to 8 µg per kilogram per minute, beta$_1$-adrenoceptors are activated, resulting in increased cardiac contractility and cardiac output. At doses greater than 8 µg per kilogram per minute, there is vasoconstriction due to activation of alpha$_1$ receptors in the peripheral vasculature.

The dosage used in CHF is thus based on the physiologic response desired. In the majority of patients, the use of low doses of dopamine (<3 to 4 µg per kilogram per minute) improves renal blood flow and natriuresis. This can be very useful in patients with pulmonary congestion and edema who also require large doses of diuretics. When compared with dobutamine, however, dopamine produces a smaller decrease or occasionally an increase in left ventricular filling pressure. This effect is more prominent when dopamine is given at higher doses (>8 µg per kilogram per minute) but may also occur when the dose is kept in the beta range due to some alpha-mediated vasoconstriction causing increased left ventricular afterload. Dopamine's potential to increase afterload and, at times, to increase pulmonary capillary wedge pressure makes it less desirable than dobutamine for most patients with severe heart failure. In patients with marked hypotension, however, dopamine is more advantageous.

The most frequent serious adverse effect of dopamine is ventricular tachyarrhythmias. This complication is usually dose-related and can frequently be treated by decreasing the dose of dopamine without initiating antiarrhythmic therapy. Other side effects include angina, nausea, vomiting, and tachycardia. These effects are also dose-related and are initially treated by decreasing the dose or discontinuing the drug, when necessary. Gangrene has been reported after extravasation of the drug, especially in patients with severe peripheral vascular disease. If a patient develops ischemia of the extremities, phentolamine, an alpha-adrenergic blocker, should be injected locally into the subcutaneous tissue at a dose of 5 to 10 mg in 15 ml of saline.

AMRINONE

Amrinone, an inhibitor of PDE III, has both inotropic and vasodilating actions. Its hemodynamic profile is characterized by increased contractility and increased cardiac output, as well as by decreased ventricular filling pressures. When compared with other inotropic agents, amrinone has a more prominent direct vasodilating action that may decrease blood pressure. However, mean arterial pressure is not uniformly decreased because of the associated increase in cardiac output. The combined inotropic and vasodilating activity of amrinone causes improved hemodynamics without increasing myocardial oxygen demand, which may be of particular benefit in patients with ischemic cardiomyopathy.

Amrinone is administered in a loading dose of 0.75 mg per kilogram over 2 to 3 minutes, followed by a maintenance infusion of 5 to 10 µg per kilogram per minute. Patients may be given additional bolus injections of 0.75 mg per kilogram if the desire clinical effect is not maintained. The total daily dose should not exceed 10 mg per kilogram.

Amrinone has a rapid onset of action of 5 minutes. The half-life of amrinone is variable. In normal subjects, the half-life is about 2.5 hours, but this can be prolonged to 12 hours in patients with heart failure, thus making rapid dose titration difficult. Because the major route of excretion is via the kidney, with as much as 40 percent of the drug excreted unchanged in the urine, the dose may have to be adjusted in cases of renal failure.

Side effects associated with amrinone include arrhythmias (3 percent), thrombocytopenia (2.4 percent), nausea, vomiting, abdominal pain (0.4 to 1.7 percent), fever (0.9 percent), and liver function test abnormalities (0.2 percent).

DIGITALIS

The inotropic action of digitalis is related to inhibition of the sodium-potassium adenosine triphosphatase, which increases intracellular sodium and, subsequently, intracellular calcium via the sodium-calcium exchange. While its inotropic action has been shown to increase the ejection fraction and improve clinical symptoms in patients with stable, relatively mild heart failure, its hemodynamic activity in CHF is probably modest. Furthermore, since most patients have already been taking this drug as maintenance therapy before the development of decompensation, its value in the acute management of hypotensive patients with low cardiac output syndrome is limited.

NOREPINEPHRINE

Norepinephrine is a potent agonist of both alpha$_1$ and beta$_1$ receptors. It therefore increases contractility as well as blood pressure and left ventricular impedance. This vasoconstrictor response greatly limits the utility of norepinephrine as an inotropic agent for patients with left ventricular dysfunction. Norepinephrine is therefore generally reserved for the treatment of cardiogenic shock, when blood pressure has been reduced to a level less than the critical perfusion pressure.

EPINEPHRINE

Epinephrine also has alpha$_1$ and beta$_1$ agonist activity. Unlike norepinephrine, however, epinephrine has peripheral beta$_2$ agonist activity that counteracts some of the alpha$_1$ vasoconstrictor action. Like norepinephrine, epinephrine is a useful agent in cases of profound circulatory collapse, particularly in patients who have progressive hemodynamic deterioration while they are receiving treatment with dobutamine. Given its chronotropic effect and arrhythmogenic potential, epinephrine should be initiated at a low dose of 0.1 µg per kilogram per minute and slowly titrated to a maximum dose of 4 µg per kilogram per minute.

COMBINATION INOTROPIC DRUG THERAPY

The beta-adrenergic pathway may be desensitized in patients with heart failure, and further desensitization can result from the exogenous administration of beta agonist drugs. Therefore, many patients may not sustain the hemodynamic benefits from beta-adrenergic agonists. Since the myocardial response to cAMP is intact, it may be anticipated that the maximal responses to a beta agonist can be increased by the concomitant administration of a PDE inhibitor. This augmented hemodynamic response has been demonstrated with the combination of dobutamine and amrinone, as well as dobutamine and milrinone, an experimental PDE inhibitor. This approach may permit the use of lower doses of each drug, thereby limiting the severity and incidence of adverse effects that can occur when a single drug is used in high concentrations.

MAINTENANCE THERAPY AND CHANGE TO ORAL THERAPY

After initiating therapy and achieving the desired hemodynamic and clinical responses, we generally maintain inotropic therapy for at least 2 to 3 days. The exact duration of therapy is dependent on the clinical response as well as on the underlying etiology and severity of ventricular dysfunction. Although there are no standard protocols for the discontinuation of these agents, we recommend reducing the medication dose over several hours during continuous hemodynamic monitoring. While the dose is being tapered, oral vasodilator medication can be initiated. At present, although several orally active inotropic agents are under investigation, digitalis is the only inotropic agent available for oral administration in patients with heart failure.

OTHER INTERVENTIONS

Inotropic drug therapy is not the final intervention to consider for a patient with left ventricular dysfunction and persistent low output heart failure; additional measures include intra-aortic balloon pump, left ventricular assist device, and cardiac transplantation. Intra-aortic balloon pumping decreases afterload and increases cardiac output, which may add to the action of the intravenous inotropic agents. Most importantly, the augmentation of diastolic blood pressure improves coronary perfusion, which may reduce myocardial ischemia in patients with underlying coronary artery disease. This is especially important in patients with significant hypotension in whom reduced aortic diastolic pressure and increased left ventricular end-diastolic pressure lead to markedly reduced coronary perfusion. However, these pumps are invasive, require the use of heparin, and are associated with infections, thrombosis, thrombocytopenia, and occasionally, reductions in blood flow to the leg. Since they cannot be used for prolonged periods of time, they are generally indicated for reversible processes, or for temporary support before surgery. However, they can still be employed for the temporary support of selected patients with chronic heart failure and superimposed acute decompensation. Left ventricular assist devices are generally reserved for cardiac transplantation candidates who have low-output heart failure that is refractory to intravenous inotropic therapy and intra-aortic balloon counterpulsation. These devices require thoracotomy and are associated with serious infections because of external connections, but in the future may be totally implantable. Finally, although the nationwide shortage of appropriate donor organs continues to limit the total number of cardiac transplants performed, urgent transplantation can still be managed in some cases with temporary support maintained by many of the previously discussed therapies. This may require early transfer to a center experienced in urgent transplantation. Exclusion criteria are somewhat variable, but generally patients older than 60 years of age or those with a pulmonary resistance of more than 6 Wood units, irreversible renal dysfunction, malignancy, or active infection are not considered optimal candidates for transplantation.

SUGGESTED READING

Chatterjee K, et al. Dobutamine: A ten-year review. New York: NCM Publishers Inc., 1989.

Colucci WS, Wright RF, Braunwald E. New positive inotropic agents in the treatment of congestive heart failure. N Engl J Med 1986; 314:290–299.

Francis G. Inotropic agents in the management of heart failure. In: Cohn JN, ed. Drug treatment of heart failure. 2nd ed. Secaucus, NJ, Advanced Therapeutics, Communications International, 1988:179.

Leier CV, Unverferth DV. Dobutamine. Ann Intern Med 1983; 99:490–496.

Mancini D, LeJemtel T, Sonnenblick E. Intravenous use of amrinone for the treatment of the failing heart. Am J Cardiol 1985; 56:8B–15B.

SUPRAVENTRICULAR ARRHYTHMIA

RICHARD P. LEWIS, M.D.

Supraventricular arrhythmia is extremely common in the intensive care unit. Although it is usually not life-threatening, it can produce hypotension and low cardiac output, especially if underlying cardiovascular disease is present. Furthermore, prolonged periods of uncontrolled rapid heart rate from supraventricular tachycardia may eventually produce ischemic dysfunction of the left ventricle. This is a consequence of shortening of diastole (when most left ventricular myocardial blood flow occurs) and increased myocardial oxygen consumption from the tachycardia. Thus, failure to control supraventricular tachycardia may contribute to adverse outcome in critically ill patients in the intensive care unit.

Supraventricular arrhythmia consists of both bradycardia and tachycardia. Traditionally, atrioventricular junctional arrhythmia (A-V) is considered supraventricular arrhythmia even though the junctional pacemaker site probably resides in the ventricles near the bundle of His. Generally patients with supraventricular arrhythmia have underlying conduction disease either as an isolated process or secondary to some form of cardiac disease. However, severe metabolic derangements (particularly hypokalemia, hypomagnesemia, hypoxia, increased adrenergic tone, and drugs) may be responsible for supraventricular arrhythmia in patients with no organic heart disease.

The majority of supraventricular tachycardias are caused by re-entry mechanisms. Re-entrant tachycardia is always initiated by a premature atrial impulse and can be terminated by overdrive pacing or DC countershock. Automatic tachycardia is caused by an independent focus. Such arrhythmias have a gradual onset and gradual offset and may be quite persistent. Automatic tachycardia is almost always related to metabolic derangements or drugs and may respond only to correction of the underlying metabolic derangement. Increased adrenergic tone is invariably present in supraventricular tachycardia and may aggravate the arrhythmia by increasing automaticity or facilitating A-V nodal conduction. This is the rationale for the use of beta-adrenergic blocking agents in these patients.

Right or left bundle branch blocks may accompany supraventricular tachycardia, resulting in a "wide complex tachycardia" that may be extremely difficult to distinguish from ventricular tachycardia (which is the most common cause). Such blocks may be transient. Identifying a wide complex tachycardia as supraventricular in origin is critical for therapy. If the tachycardia is rapid and the patient is unstable, DC countershock should be performed in the absence of a clear-cut diagnosis. All wide complex tachycardias should be regarded as ventricular tachycardia until proven otherwise.

Identification of atrial activity is the key in making the distinction between supraventricular and ventricular tachycardia. Tracings from monitor leads are frequently inadequate to make this distinction. Thus a high-fidelity 12-lead electrocardiogram with three simultaneous leads should always be obtained to define atrial activity. If the diagnosis is still unclear, then a vagal maneuver (generally carotid sinus massage) should be performed with electrocardiographic monitoring. If the diagnosis is still unclear, insertion of an esophageal lead will nearly always identify atrial activity.

The use of carotid sinus massage is a simple and generally effective bedside method for evaluating or terminating supraventricular tachycardia. Care must always be taken to exclude significant obstructive carotid artery disease, and both carotid arteries should be stimulated separately. If initially no response occurs from carotid sinus massage (or other vagal maneuvers), the maneuver should be repeated after the institution of the drug or after other types of therapy (e.g., after digitalis administration).

It must be remembered that most antiarrhythmic drugs are negative inotropes (beta-blockers, verapamil, class I antiarrhythmic agents). This is of minimal concern in patients with good ventricular function, but may lead to worsening hemodynamics in patients with heart disease, especially when the agent is administered intravenously.

Fortunately, the antiarrhythmic actions of beta-blockers occur at relatively low doses. Recently, the cardioselective beta-blocking agent metoprolol, which can be given both orally and intravenously, has gained acceptance as the beta-blocking agent of choice for arrhythmias in the intensive care setting. It can be given to patients with pulmonary disease in the absence of bronchospasm (no beta-blocker should be given to a patient with active bronchospasm). The short-acting agent esmolol hydrochloride is less useful, since sustained control of an arrhythmia is usually required. Propranolol, a nonselective agent, has been the traditional intravenous beta-blocking agent of choice but may be less well tolerated in patients with pulmonary disease.

Digitalis, beta-blocking agents, and verapamil have additive effects on the sinoatrial (SA) and A-V nodal tissue which can produce excessive bradycardia in patients with underlying conduction system disease. Atropine, digitalis specific antibodies, isoproterenol, or occasionally, a temporary pacemaker may be required. Because quinidine and amiodarone impair digoxin excretion, the digoxin dose should be halved when it is used in combination with these agents.

The characteristics and therapy of supraventricular tachycardia are summarized in Table 1. The dosages for commonly used antiarrhythmic agents are summarized in Table 2.

SINUS TACHYCARDIA

Sinus tachycardia is the most common supraventricular tachycardia seen in the intensive care unit. In younger patients it can be extremely rapid (>200 beats per minute). The P wave generally closely resembles the pa-

Table 1 Characteristics and Therapy of Supraventricular Tachycardia

Arrhythmia	Usual Atrial Rate (beats/min)	P Wave Morphology	Carotid Sinus Massage	Therapy
Sinus tachycardia	100–160	Normal	Transient slowing	Treatment of underlying disease
Atrial flutter	200–300	Flutter waves	Transient abrupt slowing of ventricular rate	Digitalis (oral or IV) Beta-blocker (oral or IV) Verapamil (oral or IV) Cardioversion or overdrive pacing Class I-A antiarrhythmic
Atrial fibrillation	300–450	Fibrillation waves	Transient slowing of ventricular rate	Digitalis (oral or IV) Beta-blocker (oral or IV) Verapamil (oral or IV) Cardioversion Class I-A antiarrhythmic Heparin/warfarin
Multifocal atrial tachycardia	100–160	Three or more P wave morphologies, variable PR interval	No response or AV block	Treatment of underlying disease DC theophylline Metoprolol (oral or IV) Verapamil (oral or IV)
Sinus node re-entry	100–140	Normal	Terminates	Digitalis (oral) Beta-blocker (oral) Verapamil (oral) Class I-A antiarrhythmic (oral)
Re-entry atrial tachycardia	100–150	Abnormal	A-V block only	Class I-A antiarrhythmic (oral)
Automatic atrial tachycardia	120–300	Abnormal	A-V block only	DC digitalis* Treatment of underlying disease Beta blocker (oral or IV) Verapamil (oral or IV)
Paroxysmal atrial tachycardia—dual AV node pathway	150–200	Retrograde, not visible in two-thirds	Terminates or no response	Verapamil (IV) Beta-blocker (IV) Digitalis (IV) Cardioversion Procainamide (IV)
Paroxysmal atrial tachycardia—via retrograde accessory pathway	150–220	Retrograde in ST segment or T segment	Terminates or no response	Same as 8 but consider procainamide (IV)
Nonparoxysmal junctional	80–170	Retrograde or normal if A-V block	No response	DC digitalis* Rx underlying disease Beta-blocker (oral or IV)
Wolff-Parkinson-White syndrome with atrial fibrillation or flutter	200–300	Flutter or fibrillation	No response	Procainamide (IV) Cardioversion

*If digitalis is suspected cause.

tient's normal morphology. Carotid sinus massage causes transient slowing. Commonly, sinus node re-entry tachycardia and automatic atrial tachycardia may resemble sinus tachycardia.

SICK SINUS SYNDROME

Sick sinus syndrome is extremely common among the elderly and is usually caused by degenerative changes in the conduction system (which may involve more than the sinus node), and patients with significant symptoms often have more than simple sinus node dysfunction. Re-entrant atrial tachycardia is commonly associated ("tachycardia-bradycardia" syndrome), related to the conduction system disease. If there is impaired responsiveness of the junctional pacer, termination of a supraventricular arrhythmia may result in a prolonged period of asystole. Finally such patients may also have ventricular tachycardia as a cause of the symptoms of this condition.

Table 2 Dosage and Route of Administration of Antiarrhythmic Agents Employed in the Intensive Care Unit

Drug	Dosage
Digoxin	IV—0.5 mg IV bolus and 0.25 mg q1–2h up to
Deslanoside	1.25 mg
Metoprolol	IV—5 mg bolus up to 15 mg
	Oral—25–50 mg q4h
Esmolol	IV—loading infusion 500 mg/kg/min
	maintenance infusion up to 300 µg/kg/min
Propranolol	IV—1–3 mg (slowly) up to 10–15 mg
	Oral—10–40 mg q4h
Verapamil	IV—5 mg (slowly) up to 10–15 mg
	Oral—80–120 mg 3–4 times daily
Procainamide	IV—10–15 mg/kg at 50 mg/min, then 4 mg/min infusion
Quinidine	Oral—200–300 mg 3–4 times daily
Disopyramide	Oral—100–150 mg 3–4 times daily

Patients with sick sinus syndrome are unusually sensitive to cardioactive drugs such as digitalis, beta-blockers, calcium channel blockers, and other antihypertensives. If recurrent supraventricular tachycardia is a problem, a pacemaker insertion may be required for the patient to tolerate antiarrhythmic drugs.

In a patient with sick sinus syndrome admitted for syncope, an electrophysiologic study should be performed if monitoring reveals no obvious arrhythmic cause of the syncope other than sinus bradycardia.

ATRIAL FLUTTER

Atrial flutter is an arrhythmia that is extremely common in the intensive care unit, particularly in patients with decompensated pulmonary disease or acute myocardial infarction and in those who have undergone operation. Also, it may well be the most commonly misdiagnosed arrhythmia. Atrial flutter has a uniquely large re-entry loop involving most of the right atrium. This produces characteristic large amplitude flutter waves seen in leads II, III, and aVF. The flutter wave is remarkably constant in morphology from patient to patient, but in the presence of conduction system disease or drugs, it may be slower and of lower amplitude. In the absence of A-V node disease there is usually a conduction ratio of 2/1. Since the usual flutter rate is 300, the usual ventricular rate is 150 per minute. This is an unusual rate for most other forms of supraventricular tachycardia. Thus, any supraventricular tachycardia with a rate of 150 per minute should be considered atrial flutter until proven otherwise.

Usually carotid sinus massage transiently slows the ventricular response and allows the flutter waves to be clearly seen. Occasionally there is an irregular ventricular response to flutter, reflecting varying degrees of A-V nodal block, and the flutter may therefore resemble atrial fibrillation.

Atrial flutter is an unstable rhythm that usually reverts spontaneously to either atrial fibrillation or sinus rhythm. Control of the ventricular response to atrial flutter is often difficult, partly because of excessive adrenergic tone which facilitates A-V conduction. There is a tendency for the rate to abruptly change up or down (i.e., the conduction ratio may change from 2/1 to 4/1 or vice versa).

Since atrial flutter is often produced by transient hemodynamic or metabolic abnormalities, attempts to convert the arrhythmia to sinus rhythm may not be successful until the underlying abnormalities are corrected. It is therefore generally prudent to slow the ventricular rate and stabilize the patient before instituting definitive treatment. A-V node conduction can be prolonged by digitalis, beta-blockers, or verapamil. Beta-blockers and verapamil have more rapid onset of action than digitalis (usually 1 to 3 minutes), but both have negative inotropic properties. In patients with underlying left ventricular dysfunction, the initial drug of choice is intravenous digoxin. An intravenous digoxin dose reaches maximum effect within 30 to 60 minutes. Thus doses of 0.25 mg can be repeated hourly until a total dose of 1 to 1.5 mg is achieved. More than a digitalizing dose should never be given. If the flutter rate is not controlled by a digitalizing dose, either a beta-blocker or verapamil can be added, usually given orally.

In many patients, simply controlling the rate eventually results in reversion to sinus rhythm. If the flutter persists, overdrive pacing with a right atrial wire or DC cardioversion with low-level electrical energy (usually <50 J) can be performed. Overdrive pacing is useful when sedation or anesthesia are undesirable, but the technique must usually be performed in the electrophysiology laboratory. A third alternative is to begin an oral class I antiarrhythmic agent (quinidine or disopyramide). Class I agents should never be added until the ventricular rate is controlled, as most such agents enhance A-V node conduction and accelerate the ventricular rate.

ATRIAL FIBRILLATION

Atrial fibrillation, like atrial flutter, can occur as an isolated arrhythmia ("lone" atrial fibrillation), or it may be secondary to chronic cardiac disease. Atrial fibrillation is manifested by high-frequency and variable amplitude fibrillatory waves on the scaler electrocardiogram. When extensive atrial disease is present, the oscillations become less obvious and may be seen only on a high-fidelity electrocardiograph tracing. In the absence of A-V node disease, the ventricular response to atrial fibrillation varies from 110 to 200 beats per minute, in part depending on the state of adrenergic tone. The ventricular response is "irregularly irregular" even at rapid heart rates. Determination of the irregularity may require caliper measurement. Carotid sinus massage transiently slows the ventricular rate.

Approximately three-fourths of patients with acute atrial fibrillation revert to sinus rhythm within 24 hours after receiving an intravenous digitalizing dose of digoxin. As noted earlier, digoxin is the drug of choice for patients with underlying heart disease because of its positive inotropic properties. Furthermore, atrial fibrillation often has a hemodynamic basis (acute left atrial dilatation from left ventricular failure) which may be improved by digitalis. As with atrial flutter, if a full digitalizing dose administered over 24 hours has not adequately controlled the ventricular response, either a beta-blocker or verapamil (usually oral) can be added. In patients with pulmonary disease, verapamil is the initial drug of choice.

Certain patients may have both flutter and fibrillation present simultaneously in the atria, which is manifest as "atrial flutter-fibrillation" on the electrocardiogram. In these patients, control of the ventricular rate is often extremely difficult because the ventricular response may be alternatively controlled by either a flutter or fibrillation mechanism. The ventricular rate of such patients is going either "too fast" or "too slow." If the rhythm cannot be reverted to sinus rhythm, a pacemaker is often required for control of the heart rate.

Once the ventricular response is controlled, the issue of reversion of the arrhythmia to sinus rhythm must be addressed. Attempts to convert the patient to sinus rhythm are not indicated when atrial fibrillation is associated with marked left atrial dilatation or when it is clear that extensive atrial conduction disease is present and there is a history of inability to maintain sinus rhythm. Although there are clearly benefits to sinus rhythm in terms of improved atrial transport function and better heart rate control, chronically diseased atria are unable to provide effective transport function and attempts to maintain sinus rhythm may not be cost effective.

It has been known for many years that cardioversion of atrial fibrillation is associated with a 1 to 2 percent incidence of systemic embolization. Although this is more likely to occur in high-risk patients (e.g., those with mitral valve disease or cardiomyopathy) it can occur in any patient with atrial fibrillation of more than a few days' duration. Although it is generally accepted that attempts to revert to sinus rhythm should be performed only after anticoagulant therapy has been instituted, the nature and duration of such therapy is still controversial. For most patients admitted with new onset atrial fibrillation, it is prudent to begin therapeutic doses of heparin at the time of admission. If the arrhythmia does not convert within 1 to 2 days, warfarin therapy should be started. It is currently recommended that no attempts to revert the rhythm be made until after 2 weeks. Of interest, no data exist indicating whether either spontaneous reversion or reversion induced by drugs is as likely to produce an embolic event as cardioversion. Therefore, one should probably not begin class I agents until a 2-week anticoagulant period is completed, since many will revert with the addition of a class I agent alone.

Most cardioversions should be performed while the patient is receiving a class I agent to ensure maintenance of sinus rhythm. It is not necessary to stop digitalis before cardioversion if the patient is not toxic. Discontinuing digitalis before cardioversion may cause the heart rate to increase inappropriately and may diminish the likelihood of success.

ATRIAL TACHYCARDIA
Multifocal Atrial Tachycardia

Multifocal atrial tachycardia (MAT) (sometimes called chaotic atrial tachycardia) is an unstable arrhythmia that occurs almost exclusively in the intensive care unit setting, usually in the elderly or in patients with decompensated pulmonary disease. It may be a precursor to atrial fibrillation. Patients with this arrhythmia are often critically ill. The arrhythmia is characterized by multiple P wave morphologies and variations in the PR interval and in ventricular rate. The average heart rate is usually 100 to 130 beats per minute.

MAT can be produced (or aggravated) by theophylline, with electrolyte abnormalities and hypoxemia often contributing. Since this is not a re-entrant tachycardia, it does not respond to electroversion. In most cases, if one simply treats the underlying metabolic derangements and discontinues theophylline, spontaneous disappearance of the arrhythmia will result. If the arrhythmia persists, metoprolol has been shown to be the most effective therapy. Verapamil has had limited success in the treatment of this disorder, and the arrhythmia does not respond to digitalis or class I agents.

Sinus Node Re-entry Tachycardia

This arrhythmia accounts for 5 to 10 percent of atrial tachycardias and occurs mostly in elderly patients with underlying heart disease. The average rate is 120 to 140 beats per minute. The P wave morphology is normal and there may be A-V block. The arrhythmia may be abolished by carotid sinus massage. It may be eliminated by digitalis, beta-blockers, or verapamil, although occasionally a class I agent is required. This arrhythmia may easily be confused with sinus tachycardia and determining its paroxysmal nature is critical.

Re-entry Atrial Tachycardia

Re-entry atrial tachycardia occurs mostly in patients with underlying heart disease and often is nonsustained. The P wave morphology is abnormal and it is unresponsive to vagal maneuvers. The arrhythmia is usually less than 150 beats per minute. A class I antiarrhythmic agent is the most effective for control.

Automatic Atrial Tachycardia

This is a heterogeneous group of arrhythmias, most of which are related to drug or metabolic abnormalities. The most classic form is "paroxysmal atrial tachycardia with block," which is caused by digitalis intoxication but which can also occur in the absence of digitalis in patients with decompensated pulmonary disease. The atrial rate is generally 150 to 200 beats per minute, and the P wave morphology is abnormal, frequently a small pointed deflection seen best in lead V_1. There are variable degrees of A-V block. When the atrial rate is fast it may resemble atrial flutter ("atypical" atrial flutter), although the baseline is not truly undulating and the atrial activity is best seen in the precordial leads rather than in leads II, III, and aVF. Carotid sinus massage produces A-V block but does not affect the atrial activity. Because these are automatic tachyarrhythmias, cardioversion is unsuccessful. Treatment of underlying metabolic derangements and/or withdrawal of digitalis or other stimulatory drugs is generally highly useful. If digitalis is not discontinued, lethal ventricular arrhythmias may result. In digitalis toxicity, potassium (and usually magnesium) may terminate this arrhythmia even if the initial serum levels are normal. Beta-blockers or verapamil may slow the ventricular rate when the atrial rate is extremely rapid and no A-V block is present.

Paroxysmal Atrial Tachycardia

Classic paroxysmal atrial tachycardia (PAT) consists of two separate re-entry mechanisms that involve tissue below the atria. Approximately two-thirds are caused by A-V nodal re-entry and one-third involve a "concealed" accessory pathway between the atrium and ventricle, which conducts only in a retrograde fashion.

A-V nodal re-entrant tachycardia may be caused by a variety of anatomic variants, but essentially it involves "dual" pathways in the A-V node region. One pathway conducts rapidly and one pathway conducts slowly. Generally the slow pathway conducts antegrade whereas the rapid pathway conducts retrograde. A premature atrial beat sets up a re-entry loop. Because the atrium is depolarized in a retrograde fashion via the rapid pathway, the P wave is inverted in leads II, III, and aVF, and is usually buried in the QRS complex. In approximately one-third of the patients, the P waves are seen just beyond the QRS complex. The usual atrial and ventricular rates are 150 to 200 beats per minute.

This arrhythmia occurs mostly in young patients with no underlying heart disease. Syncope or severe hemodynamic dysfunction is unusual. Vagal maneuvers including the Valsalva maneuvers often terminate the arrhythmia and should be tried first. Intravenous verapamil (5 to 10 mg IV) terminates the arrhythmia in nearly all patients within a few minutes. If this is unsuccessful, intravenous propranolol (up to 5 mg) may be tried. If this is unsuccessful, either intravenous digitalization, DC cardioversion, or overdrive intracardiac pacing should be considered, depending on the hemodynamic status. In patients with hemodynamic compromise, cardioversion or digitalis should become the initial treatment of choice. Class I antiarrhythmic agents may also terminate this arrhythmia, but generally cardioversion should be performed before these agents are used.

PAT due to re-entry over a concealed accessory pathway resembles the previously discussed form of PAT in most respects. However, because the retrograde depolarization of the atria occurs over the accessory pathway, the RP interval is longer and the inverted P wave is usually seen in the ST segment or T wave. A prolonged RP interval suggests this mechanism of tachycardia. If the patient is known to have an accessory pathway that conducts *only* in a retrograde fashion, treatment is identical to that just described for A-V nodal re-entry tachycardia. However, patients with Wolff-Parkinson-White (WPW) syndrome can exhibit this arrhythmia while still maintaining the ability to conduct antegrade in a rapid fashion over an anomalous pathway. As will be discussed below, administration of digitalis and verapamil may be dangerous in such a patient. PAT due to concealed accessory pathway is often faster than PAT from a dual A-V node pathway and should be considered as the etiology if the heart rate exceeds 200 beats per minute.

NONPAROXYSMAL A-V JUNCTIONAL TACHYCARDIA

This automatic tachycardia is commonly caused by digitalis intoxication, but it may also be associated with acute myocardial infarction, decompensated pulmonary disease, or the early postoperative period in open heart surgery patients. Occasionally it is a chronic arrhythmia in an otherwise healthy individual and can present great difficulty in therapy. Atrial activity consists of retrograde P waves (accompanied by large V waves in the jugular venous pulse) if A-V conduction is intact. If A-V block is present, atrial activity is independent and occasional atrial capture may occur. Characteristically there is no response to carotid sinus massage. Therapy of the underlying disease is the treatment of choice, although a beta-blocking agent or class I agent may be used if the arrhythmia is persistent. A particularly subtle form of this arrhythmia can occur in patients with atrial fibrillation and digitalis intoxication. The arrhythmia is heralded by the appearance of a regular ventricular response, generally with a rate of 70 to 90 beats per minute. If frequent ventricular ectopy accompanies this arrhythmia (or PAT with block), digoxin-specific antibody fragments should be considered. Cardioversion is contraindicated.

PRE-EXCITATION SYNDROME (WPW SYNDROME)

A variety of anomalous atrioventricular pathways have been described, but the majority are manifest as the "delta wave" of classic WPW syndrome. Patients with this syndrome may have a variety of atrial and ventricular arrhythmias. The most common arrhythmia is re-entry supraventricular tachycardia employing retrograde conduction over an anomalous pathway, as described earlier in this chapter. When this form of PAT occurs, the QRS complex does not show the delta wave. Patients with WPW syndrome are also uniquely predisposed to develop atrial fibrillation or flutter which may represent a life-threatening situation when the anomalous pathway is capable of conducting antegrade. If the anomalous pathway has a short refractory period, it can conduct impulses to the ventricle at a rate of up to 300 beats per minute from either atrial flutter or fibrillation. This rapid supraventricular stimulation can result in ventricular fibrillation.

When atrial flutter or fibrillation is conducted over the anomalous pathway, the QRS complex is widened. As the arrhythmia becomes more rapid, the QRS complex becomes more bizarre, since nearly all ventricular excitation occurs via the anomalous pathway. The superficial resemblance to ventricular tachycardia is therefore very great. Because in most such patients there is significant hemodynamic compromise, initial treatment should consist of prompt DC cardioversion.

It is crucial to remember that the standard drugs for therapy of PAT (digitalis, beta-blockers, verapamil) may be dangerous in patients capable of rapid antegrade conduction over an anomalous pathway. Digitalis shortens the refractory period of the anomalous pathway, and verapamil and beta-blockers may favor conduction over the anomalous pathway by slowing conduction through the A-V node. Both verapamil and digitalis have been reported to cause cardiac arrest when used for the treatment of atrial flutter or fibrillation. Initial pharmacotherapy for a supraventricular tachycardia in which a delta wave is present consists of a class I agent, usually intravenous procainamide. It can be argued that in a patient with known or suspected WPW syndrome, all supraventricular tachycardias should be initially treated with procainamide until an invasive electrophysiologic study has been performed to define the antegrade conduction characteristics of the anomalous pathway. As noted above, DC cardioversion frequently is also performed as initial treatment. Since these patients are amenable to surgical or catheter ablation therapy, they are always candidates for an invasive electrophysiologic study.

SUGGESTED READING

Akhtar M, Shenasa M, Jazayeri M, et al. Wide QRS complex tachycardia: reappraisal of a common clinical problem. Ann Intern Med 1988; 109:905–912.
Byrd RC, Sung RJ, Marks J, et al. Safety and efficacy of esmolol (ASL-8052: an ultrashort-acting beta-adrenergic blocking agent) for control of ventricular rate in supraventricular tachycardias. JACC 1984; 3:394–399.
Gillette PC, Smith RT, Garson A Jr, et al. Chronic supraventricular tachycardia: a curable cause of congestive cardiomyopathy. JAMA 1985; 253:391–395.
Gulamhusein S, Ko P, Carruthers SG, et al. Acceleration of the ventricular response during atrial fibrillation in the Wolff-Parkinson-White Syndrome after verapamil. Circulation 1982; 65:348–354.
Klein GH, Bashore TM, Secler TB, et al. Ventricular fibrillation in the Wolff-Parkinson-White Syndrome. N Engl J Med 1979; 301: 1080–1085.
Leier CV, Johnson T, Lewis RP. Uncontrolled ventricular rate in atrial fibrillation. Br Heart J 1979; 42:106–109.
Scher DL, Arsura EL. Multifocal atrial tachycardia: mechanisms, clinical correlates, and treatment. Am Heart J 1989; 118:574–580.
Weiner P, Bassan MM, Jarchovsky J, et al. Clinical course of acute atrial fibrillation treated with rapid digitalization. Am Heart J 1983; 105:223–227.
Wellens JJH, Brugada P, Heddle WF. Value of the 12 lead electrocardiogram in diagnosing type and mechanism of a tachycardia: a survey among 22 cardiologists. JACC 1984; 4:176–179.

VENTRICULAR ARRHYTHMIA

THOMAS A. BUCKINGHAM, M.D.
JOSEPH E. PARRILLO, M.D.

A variety of ventricular arrhythmias can occur in the intensive care unit setting. These include frequent premature ventricular contractions (PVCs) and repetitive forms, such as couplets and nonsustained ventricular tachycardia. More serious ventricular arrhythmia syndromes such as sustained ventricular tachycardia, torsades de pointes, and ventricular fibrillation may occur as well. Although more serious ventricular arrhythmias tend to occur in the presence of significant underlying heart disease, this is not always the case. The mechanisms causing malignant ventricular arrhythmias are still the subject of much debate. However, there is some agreement that re-entry may be the cause of sustained ventricular tachycardia in many cases, particularly in the setting of coronary artery disease with left ventricular dysfunction. Patients with scar tissue from prior myocardial infarctions may form a focus around which re-entry can occur. *Torsades de pointes* is a ventricular tachycardia with a characteristically electrocardiographic appearance occurring in the setting of QT prolongation and may be related to bradycardia-dependent early after depolarizations. Torsades de pointes also appears to be related to regional imbalances in autonomic influences on the heart. The etiology of ventricular fibrillation is multifactorial; among the various causes of this condition are electrolyte imbalances, hypoxia, acidosis, and ischemia. Electrical storm is defined as incessant or recurrent sustained ventricular arrhythmias despite aggressive treatment with antiarrhythmic drugs and repeated cardioversion or defibrillation. This condition may occur in the setting of acute ischemia or commonly as a manifestation of a proarrhythmia effect of an antiarrhythmic drug.

APPROACH TO THE PATIENT

In approaching a patient in the intensive care unit with malignant ventricular arrhythmia, the physician should always first determine whether the arrhythmia is immediately life-threatening. In a case of tachycardia with hemodynamic compromise, immediate therapy may be required and most commonly consists of cardioversion or defibrillation. Synchronous cardioversion can be used in sustained monomorphic ventricular tachycardia, whereas an unsynchronized defibrillation is used in torsades de pointes or ventricular fibrillation. If the patient's arrhythmia does not require immediate therapy, the physician can direct his attention to obtaining further diagnostic information. If possible, a 12-lead electrocardiogram of any tachycardia should be recorded. This allows later retrospective review of the tachycardia and a possible diagnosis of its mechanism. A work-up of possible precipitating reversible factors should also be initiated. Such factors include ischemia, myocardial infarction, reperfusion, hypoxia, acidosis, hypercapnia, hypokalemia, hyperkalemia, hypocalcemia, drug toxicity, and the proarrhythmic effect of antiarrhythmic drugs (Table 1). Those arrhythmias seen in the intensive care unit may also be catheter induced. The initial work-up may consist of a 12-lead electrocardiogram, and measurements of cardiac enzymes, arterial blood gas, electrolytes, and drug levels. If the patient has an indwelling catheter such as a Swan-Ganz catheter, a chest radiograph should be obtained to confirm that the catheter is in the proper position and not misplaced in the right ventricle.

THERAPEUTIC APPROACHES

Antiarrhythmic Drugs

In the intensive care unit setting, it is important to be familiar with the use of antiarrhythmic drugs by the intravenous route. Drugs available by intravenous route include lidocaine, procainamide, bretylium, phenytoin, and beta-blockers (Table 2). The use of the intramuscular route is not popular because it may produce a rise in myocardial enzymes. There are more drugs that can be given orally. These drugs can also be useful in the treatment of the acutely ill patient.

Lidocaine

Lidocaine is the mainstay of treatment of ventricular arrhythmia in the intensive care unit. This drug is available only in the intravenous form, is easy to administer and has a low incidence of serious side effects. It is effective in treating acute episodes of sustained ventricular tachycardia and in suppressing frequent ventricular ectopy. In the setting of acute myocardial infarction, lidocaine reduces the incidence of episodes of ventricular fibrillation during the first 24 to 48 hours. Lidocaine undergoes extensive first-pass metabolism in the liver and therefore cannot be taken orally. Its metabolites cause both therapeutic and toxic effects. The half-life is approximately 2 hours. Because of its extremely short half-life, careful attention to loading and maintenance dose is required. The most common toxic effects come from the central nervous system and include circumoral numbness, drowsiness, speech disturbance, confusion, and seizures. Extremely elderly patients seem to be more susceptible to these side effects, which are also enhanced by cimetidine. Clinical significant hemodynamic effects are rarely noted. The drug is most commonly given intravenously but may also be given intramuscularly. Lidocaine has little effect on atrial arrhythmia. The prophylactic use of lidocaine during the early myocardial infarction can be performed as follows: a loading dose of 1 mg per kilogram is administered as a bolus and is repeated 10 minutes later; while the first bolus is being administered, one should initiate an infusion of 2 to 3 mg per minute to be continued for 24 to 48 hours. The same dosage and approach may be used to treat acute arrhythmias as well.

Procainamide

This is another useful class I antiarrhythmic drug. Procainamide has an active metabolite N-acetyl procainamide (NAPA), which has antiarrhythmic and proarrhyth-

Table 1 Potentially Reversible Causes of Sustained Ventricular Arrhythmia

Ischemia
Hypoxia, hypercapnia
Acidosis
Hypokalemia
Hypocalcemia
Hypomagnesemia
Hyperthyroidism
Catecholamines (endogenous or exogenous)
Drug toxicity
Digitalis toxicity
Intracardiac catheters

Table 2 Doses of Selected Intravenous Antiarrhythmic Drugs

Drug	Loading Dose	Maintenance Dose
Lidocaine	1 mg/kg bolus; repeat 10 min later	2–4 mg/min infusion
Procainamide	1,000 mg load given slowly over 30 min	2–6 mg/min infusion
Bretylium tosylate	5–10 mg/kg over 10–20 min; may repeat 1 hr later	0.5–2 mg/min infusion
Phenytoin	250 mg given over 10 min; later may give 100 mg every 5 min as needed	100 mg q6–8h
Metoprolol	5 mg IV every 5 min × 3	PO maintenance
Esmolol	500 µg/kg/min over 1 min	50–200 µg/kg/min
Propranolol	1–3 mg load or 0.15 mg/kg	PO maintenance
Adenosine	6-mg bolus; may repeat treatment with 12-mg bolus	Not used

mic effects that are different from the parent compound. Procainamide may depress myocardial contractility, and high doses may result in peripheral vasodilatation. Elimination half-time for procainamide is 3 to 5 hours, with 50 percent eliminated by the kidney and 30 percent by the hepatic metabolism. Procainamide may be given by oral, intravenous, or intramuscular routes. A dose of 25 to 50 mg can be given intravenously over a 1-minute period, and then be repeated every 5 minutes until the arrhythmia is controlled, hypotension results, or the QRS complex is prolonged by more than 50 percent. Intravenous administration of procainamide requires close monitoring of the electrocardiogram and the patient's vital signs. The total loading dose should be about 1,000 mg. This must be given slowly over a 30-minute period with careful monitoring of the blood pressure and electrocardiogram. After the loading dose, an infusion of 2 to 6 mg per minute is used to maintain therapy. Oral procainamide is administered at intervals of 3 to 4 hours, with the total daily dose being 2 to 6 g. There is a slow-release form of procainamide which is given at 6-hour intervals. The intramuscular route is avoided because it may produce a rise in skeletal muscle enzymes. Procainamide is useful for treating both supraventricular and ventricular arrhythmias and has a range of efficacy similar to that of quinidine. In the electrophysiology laboratory, procainamide typically slows the rate of induced ventricular tachycardia. It prevents reinduction of the sustained ventricular tachycardia in approximately 20 percent of patients who were previously inducible. Adverse effects include skin rashes, myalgias, and Raynaud's phenomenon. Central nervous system side effects occur less frequently than with lidocaine, but procainamide may cause hallucinations and depression. In toxic concentrations, procainamide diminishes myocardial performance and causes hypotension. Procainamide may cause prolonged QT intervals and polymorphic ventricular tachycardia with a torsadelike pattern. Fever and thrombocytopenia may be caused by a hypersensitivity reaction. Arthritis, fever, pleuropericarditis, and hemorrhagic pericardial effusion with tamponade have been described in a syndrome similar to systemic lupus erythematosus. The incidence of this appears to increase with chronic use.

Bretylium Tosylate

This drug was initially introduced as an antihypertensive and its antiarrhythmic potential was recognized later. This drug is concentrated in sympathetic ganglia and postganglionic nerve terminals. After initially causing norepinephrine release, bretylium tosylate prevents norepinephrine release from sympathetic nerve terminals without depressing nerve conduction. Bretylium tosylate does not depress myocardial contractility, but after the initial increase in blood pressure, the drug may cause significant hypotension. The drug is effective orally as well as parenterally but is poorly absorbed from the gastrointestinal tract. The elimination half-life is 5 to 10 hours without a wide variability. Renal clearance accounts for almost all elimination. Bretylium tosylate is approved for parenteral administration only and can be given intravenously in a dose of 5 to 10 mg per kilogram of body weight diluted in 50 to 100 ml of 5 percent dextrose in water and administered slowly over 10 to 20 minutes. The dose can be repeated in 1 hour if the arrhythmia persists. The total daily dose should not exceed 30 mg per kilogram. The maintenance intravenous infusion dose is 0.5 to 2 mg per minute. The drug may be used intramuscularly with a similar initial dose which is undiluted. The drug is used for patients in the intensive care unit who have life-threatening or recurrent ventricular arrhythmia that does not respond to treatment with lidocaine, quinidine, or procainamide. The most significant side effect is hypotension, which is usually orthostatic. Transient hypertension, sinus tachycardia, or proarrhythmia may follow initial drug administration.

Phenytoin

Phenytoin was originally used to treat seizure disorders and was subsequently noted to abolish ventricular tachycardia in dogs. Its role as an antiarrhythmic is limited to use in patients with digitalis toxicity. The drug has a variable oral absorption, and 90 percent of the drug is protein-bound in the plasma. Intramuscular administration is not advised as it is associated with pain, muscle necrosis, and variable absorption. The elimination half-time is about 24 hours, with elimination occurring primarily in the liver. To achieve a therapeutic plasma concentration rapidly, 100 mg of phenytoin should be administered every 5 minutes until the arrhythmia is controlled, adverse side effects occur, or approximately 1 g has been given. Generally 700 to 1,000 mg controls the arrhythmia. A large central vein should be used to avoid causing pain and the development of phlebitis. The most common manifestations of any toxicity are the central nervous system effects of drowsiness, stupor, and coma.

Beta-Adrenergic Receptor Blocking Agents

A variety of beta-blocker drugs are available for use in the United States. In general, these drugs are useful in preventing sudden death after myocardial infarction and can be used to treat patients with long QT intervals and torsades de pointes. These drugs may be subdivided into cardioselective beta-blockers, which block beta$_1$-receptors more than they block beta$_2$-receptors and nonselective beta-blockers. It should be noted, however, that high doses of the beta$_1$-blockers also block beta$_2$-receptors. Some beta-blockers have intrinsic sympathomimetic activity and slightly activate the beta-receptor. These drugs have a direct membrane stabilizing action on the myocardium in His-Purkinje cells. They depress automaticity and block catecholamine-induced increase in the sodium current. Hemodynamically, they exert significant negative inotropic effects and may precipitate or worsen congestive heart failure. In the intensive care unit, the intravenous route is desirable. Several beta-blockers available in this form include metoprolol, esmolol, and propranolol. These drugs may be used to treat digitalis-induced arrhythmias as well as long QT interval and torsades de pointes. In addition, there are data indicating that the use of beta-blockers in the treatment of acute myocardial infarction reduces the incidence of ventricular fibrillation. Beta-blockers are contraindicated in the presence of congestive heart failure, asthma, or A-V block.

Quinidine

Quinidine is an isomeric alkaloid isolated from cinchona bark. Quinidine decreases peripheral vascular resistance and may cause hypotension because of its alpha-adrenergic blocking effects. The concomitant administration of vasodilating drugs may exaggerate hypotension. No significant direct myocardial depressant action occurs unless large intravenous doses are given rapidly. Eighty percent of quinidine is protein bound. Both the liver and the kidneys remove quinidine. The elimination half-life is 5 to 8 hours after oral administration. Quinidine is not used commonly in the intravenous form because of hypotension. The usual oral dose of quinidine sulfate for an adult is 300 to 600 mg four times daily. A loading dose of 600 to 1,000 mg produces an earlier effect and may be used. The intravenous dose of quinidine gluconate is approximately 10 mg per kilogram and is given at a rate of about 0.5 mg per kilogram per minute with careful monitoring of blood pressure and electrocardiographic parameters. Oral doses of the gluconate form are approximately 30 percent greater than those of the sulfate form. A new extended-release quinidine preparation is available. Quinidine has a broad range of action against both supraventricular and ventricular tachycardia. The most common adverse effects of chronic oral quinidine therapy are gastrointestinal and include nausea, vomiting, diarrhea, abdominal pain, and anorexia. Central nervous system toxicity includes tinnitus, hearing loss, visual disturbances, confusion, delirium, and psychosis. Allergic reaction may include rash, fever, thrombocytopenia, and a hemolytic anemia. Quinidine may produce QT prolongation and torsades de pointes. Quinidine may elevate serum digoxin concentrations by decreasing the total body clearance, decreasing the volume of distribution, and displacing digoxin from tissue receptors.

Disopyramide

Disopyramide has electrophysiologic effects similar to those of quinidine and procainamide. It is a class I antiarrhythmic and acts by blocking the sodium channels and depressing phase 0 of the action potential. It also has marked vagal side effects. Hemodynamically, disopyramide reduces blood pressure and has significant negative inotropic effects. Eighty to 90 percent of disopyramide is absorbed, and the mean elimination half-time is 8 to 9 hours. This half-time is longer in patients with heart failure or renal insufficiency. This drug is available only in the oral form, and the typical dose is generally 100 to 200 mg every 6 hours, with a range of 400 to 1,200 mg per day. The drug has a range of efficacy similar to that of quinidine and procainamide against supraventricular and ventricular arrhythmias. Adverse reactions to disopyramide include effects related to its parasympatholytic properties, including urinary retention or constipation, blurred vision, glaucoma, and dry mouth. Disopyramide may also produce ventricular tachyarrhythmia commonly associated with QT prolongation and torsades de pointes.

Mexiletine

Mexiletine is a local anesthestic with anticonvulsant properties approved by the Food and Drug Administration for the oral treatment of ventricular arrhythmias and which has electrophysiologic action similar to that of lidocaine. It has no major adverse hemodynamic effects and does not depress myocardial performance. It is absorbed rapidly and completely after oral ingestion, and the elimination half-life is 10 to 17 hours. Seventy percent of the drug is protein bound, and the drug is metabolized by the liver. The recommended starting dose is 200 mg administered orally every 8 hours, and the dose may be increased or decreased by 50 to 100 mg every 2 to 3 days. The drug is better tolerated when given with food. The total daily dose should not exceed 1,200 mg. The drug is useful for the treatment of ventricular tachyarrhythmia. Its adverse effects include tremor, dizziness, paresthesia, confusion, anxiety, nausea, and vomiting.

Tocainide

Tocainide is an amine analog of lidocaine with electrophysiologic effects similar to those of lidocaine. The drug is rapidly and completely absorbed, having a mean elimination half-life of 11 hours. The oral dose is 400 to 600 mg every 8 hours, and the dose is not increased more often than every 3 days. It is useful in treating ventricular arrhythmia. The adverse effects are dose related and include nausea, vomiting, anorexia, loss of memory, rash, perspiration, dizziness, and anxiety. Hematologic disorders include agranulocytosis, leukopenia, bone marrow depression, hypoplastic anemia, and thrombocytopenia with an incidence of 0.18 percent.

Flecainide

Flecainide is an antiarrhythmic drug initially approved for the treatment of ventricular arrhythmia. The Cardiac Arrhythmia Suppression Trial (CAST) study recently showed that this drug increased the incidence of sudden death and arrhythmic events in patients after myocardial infarction with frequent ventricular ectopy. Since the publication of the CAST results, many authorities have restricted the use of flecainide to patients with malignant ventricular arrhythmia. Flecainide exhibits marked depressant effects on the rapid sodium channel. Hemodynamically, flecainide depresses left ventricular function, and therefore caution should be exercised in its use in patients with heart failure. In patients with arrhythmia, the elimination half-life is 20 hours, with 85 percent of the drug excreted in the urine. Proarrhythmic effects are among the most important adverse effects of flecainide and may occur in 5 to 25 percent of patients. This agent may also produce incessant ventricular tachycardia, which is refractory to therapy and associated with a high mortality rate.

Encainide Hydrochloride

Electrophysiologically, encainide hydrochloride resembles flecainide. It appears to have a lesser myocardial depressant effect. Its elimination half-life is 3 to 4 hours. However, the existence of several active metabolites permits a longer interval between doses. In the CAST study, this agent was also shown to have proarrhythmic effects and is now considered to be of limited usefulness in the treatment of malignant ventricular arrhythmia. Adverse effects includes dizziness, parasthesia, leg cramps, and a metallic taste in the mouth.

Amiodarone

Amiodarone is an unusual drug that was introduced more than 15 years ago as a smooth muscle relaxant and coronary vasodilator. Its antiarrhythmic actions were noted subsequently. Amoidarone prolongs action potential duration and refractoriness as well as blocks the sodium channels. Amiodarone also prolongs the QT interval; however, it appears less likely to produce torsades de pointes than quinidine, disopyramide, or procainamide. It is known to have mild direct negative inotropic effects. Amiodarone has a slow, variable, and incomplete oral absorption. Elimination takes place by hepatic excretion to bowel with some enterohepatic recirculation. The drug and its metabolites accumulate in all body tissue, and the drug is highly protein bound. Elimination half-life is multiphasic, with an initial reduction in plasma concentration of 50 percent 3 to 10 days after drug termination followed by a terminal half-life of 26 to 107 days. Because of these unusual pharmacokinetics, an optimal dose schedule that can be used for all patients has not been determined. One recommended approach is to administer 800 to 1,600 mg daily for 1 to 3 weeks, reducing the dose to 800 mg daily for the next 2 to 4 weeks, then to 600 mg daily for 4 to 8 weeks, and finally after 2 to 3 months of treatment, administering a maintenance dose of 400 mg per day. This drug is not yet available in the intravenous form. It has a wide range of efficacy against both supraventricular and ventricular arrhythmias that exceeds that of all other antiarrhythmic agents. Because of its long half-life it is difficult to start another antiarrhythmic drug and to assess patient response. This and its side effect profile make amiodarone a "last ditch" antiarrhythmic agent. Of its noncardiac adverse reactions, pulmonary toxicity is the most serious. This consists of pulmonary fibrosis with an unknown mechanism. An asymptomatic elevation of liver enzymes is found in most patients. Hypothyroidism or hyperthyroidism are also common. Cardiac side effects include symptomatic bradycardia and occasional proarrhythmic effects.

Invasive Approaches

Invasive approaches to the management of ventricular arrhythmia include pacing, cardioversion, defibrillation, surgery, and catheter ablation.

Pacing

Occasionally, pacing may be used in the intensive care setting to treat or prevent ventricular tachyarrhythmia. Sustained monomorphic ventricular tachycardia can be treated directly by pacing. It is important to have a defibrillator available during this technique. Pacing wires are placed in the right ventricular apex and the heart is paced at a rate slightly faster than that of the ventricular tachycardia for 10 to 15 beats. Often this results in reversion of ventricular tachycardia to sinus rhythm. Sometimes, however, these rhythms may worsen, and ventricular fibrillation or faster ventricular tachycardia may result. This approach is generally used in patients who have a hemodynamically stable ventricular tachycardia. Patients who have intermittent episodes of torsade de pointes in the setting of sinus bradycardia or other bradyarrhythmia respond to measures that increase heart rate. These measures may include atropine, isoproterenol infusion, or ventricular pacing. Pacing is typically carried out at a rate of 90 beats per minute.

Cardioversion and Defibrillation

These are standard and successful approaches for treating malignant ventricular arrhythmia. They may be used emergently with hemodynamically unstable rhythms or electively. In synchronized cardioversion, the electrical impulse is synchronized to the R wave. This is used for sustained monomorphic ventricular tachycardia. The usual starting dose is 100 J. Synchronous cardioversion of ventricular tachycardia requires less energy than defibrillation and there is a slightly lower risk of reinducing malignant ventricular rhythms. An unsynchronized shock (defibrillation) is used to treat ventricular fibrillation or torsades de pointes. The usual dose is 200 to 360 J. (A detailed discussion of cardiopulmonary resuscitation is given elsewhere in this book.)

Surgery

A surgical approach may be used to treat ventricular tachycardia, particularly in patients with ischemic heart disease or in those who require other cardiac surgery. With this approach, the focus of origin of ventricular tachycardia is mapped in the operating room and either directly excised or destroyed by cryoablation. This surgery carries an 80 percent success rate and a 10 percent mortality rate when performed on an elective basis.

Catheter Ablation

For patients with ventricular tachycardia, catheter ablation (fulguration) may be attempted. The purpose of catheter ablation is to destroy myocardial tissue by delivering electrical energy to the heart by a catheter electrode. This procedure requires an electrophysiologic mapping procedure to locate the focus of ventricular tachycardia. Complications include pump failure, electromechanical dissociation, and vascular accidents. This procedure is generally reserved for patients who do not respond to other forms of therapy and has a 50 percent success rate.

SPECIFIC ARRHYTHMIAS

Premature Ventricular Contractions

PVCs occur in patients with normal hearts as well as in those with diseased hearts. In patients with poor left ventricular function, PVCs are associated with an increased risk of sudden death and arrhythmic events. However, it is not yet clear whether treatment of the arrhythmia reduces the risk of death. During the acute phase of myocardial infarction, it is not clear that PVCs should be treated. It is argued by many that prophylactic lidocaine should be used because ventricular tachycardia and ventricular fibrillation often occur in this setting without preceding arrhythmias. However, the rapid availability of resuscitation in most coronary care units makes the prevention of ventricular fibrillation less important. In addition, the use of lidocaine increases costs and is associated with some side effects. For these reasons, this issue remains controversial. The occurrence of frequent PVCs in the setting of acute myocardial infarction cannot be used as a reliable predictor of ventricular fibrillation or ventricular tachycardia.

Ventricular Tachycardia

Ventricular tachycardia is defined as the occurrence of three or more PVCs in a row at a rate of 100 beats per minute or greater. Accelerated idioventricular rhythm (AIVR) is defined as a ventricular rhythm occurring at a rate of 50 to 100 beats per minute. This rhythm, which is common with myocardial infarction, may be well tolerated and may not require treatment. If it occurs in the presence of an inferior myocardial infarction, it may be an escape rhythm and can be treated by acceleration of the underlying sinus rate with atropine. Longer runs of ventricular tachycardia associated with hypotension, ventricular tachycardia lasting more than 30 seconds, or ventricular tachycardia requiring cardioversion are considered *sustained* ventricular tachycardia. This form of ventricular tachycardia requires treatment.

Sustained ventricular tachycardia requires immediate treatment, depending on the degree of hemodynamic compromise. In the most severe cases, immediate cardioversion is warranted. If the blood pressure is stable, intravenous antiarrhythmic drugs or burst pacing in the right ventricle may be attempted to terminate the arrhythmia. The first drug used should be lidocaine. If this fails, then intravenous procainamide followed by intravenous bretylium tosylate may be used. These drugs may be administered during an acute episode of ventricular tachycardia and to prevent further attacks. If these measures fail, then cardioversion may be attempted. Potentially reversible causes of ventricular tachyarrhythmia should always be looked for and corrected (see Table 1).

In an intensive care unit patient who develops a wide QRS tachycardia, it is not always clear whether it is ventricular tachycardia or aberrant supraventricular tachycardia. If the patient has underlying coronary artery disease with left ventricular dysfunction, it is best to assume that the rhythm is ventricular tachycardia and act accordingly. Otherwise, electrocardiographic criteria exist that can be used to differentiate these tachycardias. If the patient's condition permits, a 12-lead electrocardiogram should be obtained. The criteria favoring a diagnosis of ventricular tachycardia are as follows:

1. QRS interval greater than 0.14 seconds (without prior bundle branch block).
2. Capture or fusion beats (evidence of A-V dissociation.
3. Left axis deviation.
4. Monophasic or biphasic QRS in V_1.
5. S wave greater than the R wave in V_6.

Intravenous verapamil should never be used to treat a wide QRS tachycardia. This drug is associated with a high complication rate in such patients. When verapamil is inadvertently given to a patient with ventricular tachycardia, a decrease in blood pressure commonly occurs and there is often an increased need for vasopressors and cardioversion. Recent evidence suggests that the use of intravenous adenosine may be successful in treating supraventricular tachycardia without carrying the same risk that it does for the patient with ventricular tachycardia.

Torsades de Pointes

This is a form of polymorphic ventricular tachycardia with a characteristic electrocardiographic pattern. Torsades de pointes has the appearance of twisting around the isoelectric line with a varying QRS axis and morphology. This explains its name, which in French means "twisting of the points." Table 3 lists the causes of torsades de pointes. If it is sustained, immediate cardioversion is required. Attention is then directed to predisposing factors, which should be removed whenever possible. In many cases, this rhythm responds to measures that increase the sinus rate—for example, treatment with atropine or isoproterenol. Pacing can also be used to prevent recurrences of torsades de pointes. In addition, magnesium therapy has been

Table 3 Causes of Torsades de Pointes

Drugs
   Procainamide
   Quinidine
   Disopyramide
   Tricyclic antidepressants
   Phenothiazines

Electrolyte abnormalities
   Hypokalemia
   Hypomagnesemia
   Hypocalcemia

Bradycardia
Myocarditis
Ischemic heart disease
Subarachnoid hemorrhage
Liquid protein diet
Organophosphate poisoning
Congenital disorders

described as useful in the treatment of this syndrome, even if the magnesium level is normal. This syndrome is associated with a prolonged QT interval. The above therapeutic approach applies to cases of acquired long QT syndromes. Cases with congenitally prolonged QT intervals respond better to beta-blockade.

Ventricular Fibrillation

Ventricular fibrillation results in immediate hemodynamic collapse and requires prompt defibrillation. With the initial onset of ventricular fibrillation, the characteristic electrocardiographic pattern is said to be *coarse* ventricular fibrillation. As time progresses and the patient remains in ventricular fibrillation, the amplitude of chaotic electrocardiographic activity diminishes and the patient is said to be in *fine* ventricular fibrillation. Treatment is more effective when instituted early with coarse ventricular fibrillation. Treatment consists of immediate defibrillation with 200 to 360 J of DC current. Repeated defibrillations may be required, along with correction of acidosis and adequate ventilation.

SUGGESTED READING

Jackman WM, Friday KJ, Anderson JL, et al. The long QT syndromes: a critical review, new clinical observations, and a unifying hypothesis. Prog Cardiovasc Dis 1988; 31:115–172.
Zipes DP. Management of cardiac arrhythmias: pharmacological, electrical, and surgical techniques. In: Braunwald E, ed. Heart disease: a textbook of cardiovascular medicine. Philadelphia: WB Saunders Co., 1988; 621
Zipes DP. Specific arrhythmias: diagnosis and treatment. In: Braunwald E, ed. Heart disease: a textbook of cardiovascular medicine. Philadelphia: WB Saunders Co., Philadelphia, 1988; 658.

ATRIOVENTRICULAR BLOCK IN THE CRITICALLY ILL

THOMAS A. BUCKINGHAM, M.D.

The term "atrioventricular (A-V) block" refers to the interference of conduction of the electrical impulses from the atria to the ventricles. It is a general term that refers to the lack of A-V conduction and not to the anatomic location of the block. Anatomically, A-V block may be located in the A-V node, bundle of His, or may involve block of both right and left bundle branches. The anatomic location of the block is important in determining prognosis and the need for pacemaker therapy. A block below the A-V node (infranodal) carries a worse prognosis than a block at the level of A-V node itself. A-V block has many causes (Table 1). In adults, common causes include coronary artery disease, drug toxicity, and degenerative processes that damage the A-V node and conduction system. A-V block may be divided into varying degrees of severity by its electrocardiographic appearance.

FIRST-DEGREE A-V BLOCK

On a surface electrocardiogram, this type of block is characterized by an appearance of a prolonged PR interval greater than 0.20 seconds. If this pattern occurs in combination with a bundle branch block pattern, it may indicate infranodal disease. Transient first-degree A-V block may be caused by changes in autonomic tone acting on the upper part of the A-V node. A-V block may also occur in a small percentage of the patients with normal hearts. Many of the conditions listed in Table 1 cause first-degree A-V block. This condition by itself requires no therapy. If any reversible causes are detected, however, they should be addressed.

SECOND-DEGREE A-V BLOCK

This type of A-V block is divided into two subcategories: Mobitz type I and Mobitz type II second-degree A-V block. Mobitz I A-V block (Wenckebach) refers to an electrocardiographic pattern with a progressive lengthening of the PR interval with successive complexes until a QRS complex is dropped. Mobitz II A-V block refers to the intermittent failure of A-V conduction without a progressive prolongation of the PR interval. If a patient has continuous 2/1 A-V block, it cannot be classified by this system. However, 2/1 A-V block is usually associated with infranodal block. Mobitz type 1 block is generally associated with block at the upper levels of the A-V node and is responsive to changes in autonomic tone or manipulation of the autonomic nervous system. Mobitz type II A-V block is located lower and carries a worse prognosis. Mobitz type II A-V block may be infranodal in nature, particularly if a wide QRS complex accompanies it. For Mobitz type II A-V block, which is more often progressive, permanent pacing is recommended. Type I second-degree A-V block does not require pacing unless more advanced conduction defects or symptoms occur.

THIRD-DEGREE A-V BLOCK

Third-degree A-V block is characterized by the complete loss of A-V conduction. Unless there is retrograde conduction, there is no relationship between the P waves and the QRS complexes on these surface electrocardio-

Table 1 Causes of A-V Block in Adults

Common causes
    Drug toxicity
    Coronary artery disease
    Degenerative diseases (Lev's disease and Lenegre's disease)

Less common causes
    Vagal hyper-responsiveness
    Cardiac tumors
    Infectious causes
        Chagas disease
        Endocarditis
    Infiltrating processes
        Hemochromatosis
        Amyloidosis
    Electrolyte imbalances (hyperkalemia)
    Hypoxia
    Thyrotoxicosis
    Myxedema
    Congenital heart disease
    Congenital heart block
    Valvular heart disease (calcific aortic stenosis)
    Myocarditis
    Collagen vascular disease
        Sclerodema
        Ankylosing spondylitis
    Granulomatous disease (sarcoidosis)
    Cardiomyopathy
    Trauma
    Surgery
    Progressive muscular dystrophy

grams. Generally a ventricular or fascicular escape rhythm is present. These escape rhythms have variable QRS widths and rates. In general, the slower escape rhythms have wider QRS complexes and represent idioventricular escape rhythms. Escape rhythms with wider QRS complexes and slower rates are less reliable and indicate a worse prognosis. Third-degree A-V block can involve various anatomic locations, the upper or lower A-V node, bundle of His, or a combination of blocks in the right and left bundle branches.

A-V DISSOCIATION

AV dissociation should be distinguished from A-V block. In A-V dissociation, there is loss of the relationship between the P waves and QRS complex on the surface electrocardiogram. This can occur when the sinus node slows to a rate less than that of a nodal escape rhythm; the nodal rhythm takes over the pacing of the heart and A-V dissociation occurs. Alternatively, there may be an acceleration of the nodal rhythm, with its rate increased in comparison with that of the sinus rhythm, causing the same phenomenon. These two situations can occur without the presence of A-V block; however, if third-degree A-V block is present, A-V dissociation is also present.

BUNDLE BRANCH BLOCK

Bundle branch block occurs in 1 percent of adults. Right bundle branch block can occur in asymptomatic healthy individuals with normal hearts. The presence of left bundle branch block is usually associated with underlying heart disease. Bundle branch block is generally a chronic condition; however, it may occur acutely in the intensive care setting—for example, in the setting of an acute myocardial infarction. Acute right bundle branch block can occur with the sudden onset of cor pulmonale.

Acute right bundle branch block may also be induced by catheter trauma to the right side of the interventricular septum. This may occur with Swan-Ganz catheters or pacing catheters placed while the patient is in the intensive care unit. If a patient has chronic left bundle branch block great care should be taken in putting catheters in the right side of the heart. The production of a right bundle branch block with pre-existing left bundle branch block may produce sudden third degree A-V block. Temporary pacing equipment should be available if right heart catheters are used in such patients.

A-V BLOCK IN THE SETTING OF ACUTE MYOCARDIAL INFARCTION

Inferior Myocardial Infarction

Inferior myocardial infarctions are caused by occlusion of the right coronary artery and less frequently by occlusion of the left circumflex coronary artery. The A-V nodal artery arises from the right coronary artery in 90 percent of patients; in 10 percent, it arises from the circumflex. For reasons that are not clearly understood, ischemic injury to the A-V node is rarely permanent. Inferior myocardial infarctions are usually associated with transient A-V block which may be limited to first-degree A-V block or Mobitz type I second-degree A-V block. In most cases, there is an escape rhythm with a narrow QRS complex. Third-degree A-V block is rare. The escape rhythm in this type of A-V block is usually stable with a narrow QRS complex and occurs at a rate of 50 beats per minute. If the right ventricle is involved in the inferior myocardial infarction, the likelihood of A-V block is greater. This is because right ventricular infarctions may be associated with obstruction of the right coronary artery near its origin. In the setting of an inferior myocardial infarction, A-V block usually responds to drug therapy. This may consist of atropine in doses of 0.5 mg IV, which may be repeated at 5-minute intervals until a maximum dose of 2 mg is achieved. Isoproteronol may be given as an infusion of 2 to 20 μg per minute. Temporary pacing should be used only if A-V block fails to respond to medication and is associated with symptoms or compromised cardiac output. Occasionally, bradycardia with a rate of less than 40 beats per minute may be associated with ventricular tachycardia, congestive heart failure, or cardiogenic shock. These are all indications for temporary pacing. Rarely, A-V block persists after inferior myocardial infarction and requires permanent pacing.

Anterior Myocardial Infarction

Anterior myocardial infarction is caused by occlusion of the left anterior descending coronary artery. This vessel supplies anterior and lateral portions of the left ventricle and the anterior two-thirds of the septum. A-V block is produced by ischemic destruction of the conducting structures below the A-V node. This may include the bundle of His, the bundle branches, and the Purkinje tissue that passes through the septum. Therefore, A-V block in the setting of anterior myocardial infarction is located at a lower level than A-V block in the setting of inferior myocardial infarctions. Escape rhythms come from the ventricle at a much slower rate (about 30 beats per minute). This escape rhythm has a wide QRS complex and is less reliable than that seen in inferior myocardial infarctions. Concomitant administration of antiarrhythmic drugs such as lidocaine may worsen the problem by suppressing potential ectopic pacemakers. The occurrence of A-V block in the setting of anterior myocardial infarction may be sudden in onset and the escape rhythm unreliable or slow to become established. Occasionally, a warning is given in the form of a conduction disturbance, such as right bundle branch block and left anterior hemiblock occurring acutely. If this occurs, complete A-V block follows in about 50 percent of cases. The new onset of left bundle branch block or the new onset of Mobitz type II second-degree A-V block also portends the development of third-degree A-V block. A-V block in the setting of an acute anterior wall myocardial infarction is less likely to respond to atropine or sympathomimetics, although these drugs may be used in an emergency. Anterior myocardial infarction with A-V block therefore requires temporary pacing. In addition, when A-V block occurs in the setting of anterior myocardial infarction, it is a sign that a large part of the left ventricle and septum have been damaged by infarction. These patients often have cardiogenic shock and a poor prognosis. Occasionally in the setting of acute anterior myocardial infarction, one is uncertain whether a conduction disturbance is acute or chronic. In such cases, it is best to assume that the conduction disturbance is new. Thus the development of bundle branch block pattern during an acute anterior wall infarction is a serious sign and calls for the insertion of a temporary pacemaker. If the patient has acute anterior myocardial infarction, I prefer a transvenous pacemaker with any manifestation of A-V block. In anterior infarction with transient second-degree or third-degree infranodal A-V block, permanent pacing is indicated after the patient's condition becomes stable.

HIS BUNDLE RECORDING

The technique of recording the His bundle potential is useful for determining the anatomic location of A-V block. In this technique, an electrode catheter is passed into the right atrium across the tricuspid valve in the region of the bundle of His. Direct recording of atrial, His, and ventricular activation can then be obtained. If A-V block occurs above the bundle of His, one will see an atrial activation without a His bundle activation or ventricular activation. If block occurs below the bundle of His, one will see atrial activation and His activation without ventricular activation. In addition, one may sometimes see split His potentials, which indicate intra-Hisian block. As already stated, intra-Hisian or infra-Hisian block is more serious and usually warrants permanent pacing. The occurrence of trifascicular block is also an indication for pacing in an asymptomatic patient. Trifascicular block can be defined as the occurrence of bifascicular block with first-degree A-V block or alternating right and left bundle branch block. Table 2 lists the causes of bundle branch block. Electrocardiographic recordings of A-V block in association with the patient's symptoms are important in determining and documenting the need for a permanent pacemaker.

TEMPORARY TRANSVENOUS PACING

The following is my method for temporary transvenous pacing. It is usually best to put in a temporary pacemaker through the right internal jugular or left subclavian vein. These sites are chosen because they provide the most direct route to the right ventricular apex and require that the catheter make only one curve. The left internal jugular or right subclavian veins, on the other hand, require that the catheter take an S-shaped curve and make it slightly more difficult to place the catheter in the right ventricular apex, but they can be used if necessary. After the site is selected, the patient is placed in the Trendelenburg position and the Seldinger technique is used to insert an introducer sheath into the vein. A bipolar catheter (temporary pacing lead) is passed through this introducer and fluoroscopy is used to position the catheter in the right ventricular apex. Passage across the tricuspid valve is easier if a small curve is created in the last 5 cm of the catheter. This can be done by hand before the catheter is inserted into the sheath or by creating a loop in the catheter inside the right atrium and then rotating it across the tricuspid valve. Once the tricuspid valve is crossed, the catheter is manipulated down to the right ventricular apex. Smaller-size catheters (5-Fr) have a lower incidence of cardiac perforation, however, these catheters are some-

Table 2 Causes of Bundle Branch Block

Coronary artery disease
Hypertensive heart disease
Valvular heart disease (aortic stenosis)
Degenerative disease of the conduction system
Myocarditis
Cardiomyopathy
Muscular disorders
Congenital heart disease
Cardiac surgery

what more difficult to manipulate. The danger of perforation is greatest when the catheter is in the right ventricular outflow tract. The risk is greater in elderly women with a small habitus. Before insertion of the lead into the sheath, an expandable plastic cover may be placed over the lead. This allows later manipulation of the catheter with less chance of contamination. When the catheter is placed in the right ventricular apex, a curve should be left on the catheter. The catheter should be sutured and taped into position to reduce the likelihood of accidental dislodgement. Temporary wires may be also be placed in the right atrium, although these are less stable and have a higher incidence of dislodgement than right ventricular wires.

Swan-Ganz catheters with an extra lumen allowing passage of a pacing wire are available. These catheters have a disadvantage in that the opening for the pacing wire is fixed in position on the catheter. There are also Swan-Ganz catheters available with electrodes incorporated as part of their design. These catheters have a similar disadvantage in that when the catheter is in the proper position for pulmonary capillary wedge pressure readings, the pacing electrodes may be out of position. I prefer to use a separate pacing wire and Swan-Ganz catheter in patients that need both. In patients with pre-existing left bundle branch block who need both catheters, the pacing wire should be placed first.

After the pacing wire is placed in position, threshold measurements are taken. The heart is paced at a rate faster than its intrinsic rhythm and the current is adjusted. Most temporary pacing devices are battery powered and use a pulse width of a 0.5 ms with adjustable current. The threshold is usually less than 1 mA, but this may vary slightly from patient to patient.

In addition, the catheter should be observed under fluoroscopy to determine its stability. Normally the tip of the catheter moves with each heart beat and with respirations. It is useful to have the patient take a deep breath and cough several times to make sure that the tip of the catheter is stable in the right ventricular apex and that there is sufficient slack left in the lead to allow for these movements. The lead is taped and sutured into position and connected to the temporary pacing device. Generally the output of the device is set to three to four times the threshold to allow an adequate safety margin. In addition, sensitivity is checked. This is done by setting the pacing rate below the intrinsic rate and adjusting the sensitivity setting up until the failure of sensing is seen. This is the point at which the pacemaker fails to sense and is the R wave amplitude (measured in mV). The pacemaker is then set to a setting half of the R wave or less to allow a safety margin for sensing. The threshold and sensitivity should be checked two to three times per day and the results recorded on the chart. A sudden increase in threshold or a decrease in the R wave amplitude suggests lead dislodgement. This should be checked by chest roentgenography. Chest roentgenography should be performed daily in patients with temporary pacemakers to review the lead position. In general, the pacing wire should be changed every 3 days to reduce the chance of infection.

In patients who are recovering from cardiovascular surgery, temporary epicardial wires are often left in place by the surgeon. These allow temporary pacing of the atria and ventricles. These wires can be connected to temporary pacing devices with measurement of threshold and sensing in the same manner.

When temporary atrial pacing is desired, the use of the transesophageal route is helpful. With the transesophageal route, one can successfully pace the left atrium using a pulse width of approximately 2 to 10 ms with an output of 20 mA. Unfortunately, conventional transvenous pacing devices do not provide this level of current. A variety of commercial electrodes are now available and typically use an interelectrode spacing of 2 to 4 cm. These electrodes are passed through the nasopharynx after coating with local anesthetic. The lead is advanced 50 cm and then withdrawn until the pacing commences.

In recent years, external cardiac pacing has become a useful approach for temporary pacing of the ventricles. Research has shown that an increase in the surface area of stimulating electrodes reduces the cardiac threshold and the degree of skeletal muscle stimulation. The combination of large surface electrodes and improved conducting media between the electrode and the skin reduces cutaneous nerve stimulation and patient discomfort. Electrodes used for this purpose have a surface area of approximately 100 square cm. The external pacing device uses a pulse width of 20 to 40 ms with outputs of 140 to 200 mA. This device may be useful for patients who are at low risk for developing A-V block or for patients who have a contraindication to the insertion of a temporary pacemaker. Such patients include those with abnormal bleeding tendencies, such as those who have received thrombolytic agents. This technique is not a substitute for temporary transvenous pacing when this is required for prolonged periods of complete heart block. This form of pacing is uncomfortable to the patient because it causes contraction of the skeletal muscles. External pacing may be used as a temporary measure while a temporary transvenous pacemaker is being inserted or while equipment and personnel are assembled for this purpose.

SUGGESTED READING

Barold SS, ed. Modern cardiac pacing. Mt Kisco, NY: Futura, 1985.
Frye RL, Collins JJ, DeSanctis RW, et al. Guidelines for permanent cardiac pacemaker implantation, May 1984: a Report of the Joint American College of Cardiology/American Heart Association Task Force on Assessment of Cardiovascular Procedures (Subcommittee on Pacemaker Implantation). J Am Coll Cardiol 1984; 4:434..

UNSTABLE ANGINA PECTORIS

GARY L. SCHAER, M.D.

Unstable angina is one of the most common reasons for which patients are hospitalized in the United States. It is also one of the most serious. Patients with unstable angina are at risk for acute myocardial infarction, hemodynamic instability, congestive heart failure, malignant cardiac arrhythmias, and sudden cardiac death. This disorder is of particular importance to the critical care physician because optimum management requires admission of the patient to the critical care unit for careful monitoring and aggressive medical treatment.

Patients with unstable angina typically present with severe angina of recent onset, a marked worsening in the pattern of their previous symptoms, or angina at rest. Unstable angina is part of a spectrum of acute coronary syndromes which also includes non-Q and Q wave myocardial infarction. These disorders are related because they share a common pathophysiologic event: rupture of a coronary atherosclerotic plaque. The consequence of plaque rupture includes platelet aggregation, thrombus formation, and coronary vasoconstriction (caused in part by the release of platelet-derived vasoconstrictors). These events substantially narrow the coronary artery lumen, reduce coronary blood flow, and diminish myocardial oxygen supply. Thus myocardial ischemia results despite a stable myocardial oxygen demand. If the thrombotic obstruction to coronary blood flow progresses to complete occlusion, myocardial infarction results.

INITIAL APPROACH TO THE PATIENT

Once the diagnosis of unstable angina is made and electrocardiography is performed, therapy should be instituted promptly. As intravenous access is obtained, therapy should begin with nitroglycerin, 0.2 mg sublingual (which may be repeated as needed provided that the systolic blood pressure is greater than 100 mm Hg) and aspirin, 325 mg orally or chewed (see below). Although it is helpful to treat anxiety with benzodiazepines, analgesics should be withheld in an attempt to monitor the response of angina to specific anti-ischemic therapy. In addition, factors that might be exacerbating myocardial ischemia (by augmenting myocardial oxygen demand) should be sought for and treated. Such factors include anemia, marked hypertension, supraventricular arrhythmias, congestive heart failure, and thyrotoxicosis.

MEDICAL MANAGEMENT IN THE CRITICAL CARE UNIT

The goals of medical therapy include (1) relief of ongoing myocardial ischemia; 2) prevention of further episodes of ischemia; and 3) stabilization and initial healing of the ruptured atherosclerotic plaque prior to more definitive coronary revascularization by coronary angioplasty or bypass surgery. Agents commonly used include aspirin and heparin, nitrates, calcium antagonists, and beta-blockers (Table 1).

Aspirin and Heparin

The presence of a fresh, partially obstructing thrombus in the coronary arteries of patients with unstable angina has been demonstrated by recent angioscopic and pathologic studies. These findings provide the rationale for the use of anticoagulant drugs in the management of unstable angina. Both aspirin and heparin have been shown to have independent benefits in several randomized clinical trials and have therefore become standard agents in the medical management of unstable angina. Although controversy exists about precisely how and when these agents should be utilized, it is my practice to begin therapy with aspirin (325 mg chewed or swallowed) promptly after the diagnosis is made. Administration of aspirin is then continued on a daily basis. The major adverse effect of aspirin is the increased risk of bleeding, particularly in patients requiring surgical revascularization. However, the risk is outweighed by the benefits of aspirin in reducing ischemic episodes and the risk of infarction.

Heparin for systemic anticoagulation may be given in addition to aspirin in patients with angina at rest who also demonstrate ischemic ST segment or T wave changes on the electrocardiogram. Heparin should also be used in those patients with recurrent angina despite the use of aspirin, nitrates, and calcium antagonists (see below). Although the combination of aspirin and heparin has not been proven to be superior to aspirin alone, it is a reasonable approach in these patients, who are at highest risk for infarction. Because bleeding complications may be increased in patients receiving both aspirin and heparin, they

Table 1 Therapeutic Approach to Unstable Angina Pectoris

Therapy	Purpose
Aspirin	Cause platelet inhibition, reduce progression to thrombotic occlusion
Heparin	Diminish propagation and encourage dissolution of intracoronary thrombus
Nitrates (intravenous nitroglycerin)	Coronary vasodilation, reduce preload (reduce left ventricular wall stress)
Calcium blockers (e.g., diltiazem)	Coronary vasodilation, prevent coronary spasm, reduce myocardial oxygen demand (decreased heart rate and inotropy)
Beta-blockers (e.g., propranolol)	Reduce myocardial oxygen demand (decrease heart rate and inotropy)
Coronary revascularization (PTCA or CABG)	Definitive therapy for recurrent ischemia or severe coronary disease

CABG = coronary artery bypass grafting; PTCA = percutaneous transluminal coronary angioplasty.

should be observed closely. Heparin should be administered as an intravenous bolus of 5,000 U, followed by 1,000 U per hour by constant infusion. The dose should be titrated to achieve a partial thromboplastin time of 1.5 to 2 times control.

Nitrates

Nitrates are very useful agents in the management of unstable angina, with intravenous nitroglycerin being the preferred preparation. Nitrates are beneficial because they reduce preload by vasodilating capacitance vessels, thereby diminishing myocardial oxygen demand. They also improve myocardial oxygen supply by coronary artery vasodilation, counterbalancing local coronary vasoconstriction at the site of the ruptured atherosclerotic plaque. The critical care unit is ideally suited for careful administration of intravenous nitroglycerin. The advantages of intravenous rather than topical or oral nitrates include that its onset is immediate, its duration of effect is short, and titration is precise. The drip should be started at 10 μg per minute and can be increased as needed to eliminate angina completely. Systolic arterial pressure should be reduced by 10 to 20 mm Hg but should not be allowed to decrease to a level much less than 100 mm Hg. Doses as high as 200 to 400 μg per minute may be needed in some cases. Frequent blood pressure monitoring is important, as an occasional patient becomes hypotensive during even low-dose infusions. Nitrate-induced hypotension is usually caused by vasodilation and can be rapidly corrected with intravenous boluses of normal saline (100 to 200 ml). For patients with hemodynamic instability, however, especially in the presence of signs of heart failure (i.e., pulmonary rales), direct measurement of the pulmonary capillary wedge pressure and cardiac output is recommended.

In addition to hypotension, tachyphylaxis is an important adverse effect of intravenous nitroglycerin. It is manifested by a reduction in antianginal efficacy despite a constant drug infusion. This condition can be managed by increasing the infusion rate by about 10 percent every 24 hours to ensure continued efficacy. In general, it is best to continue administration of intravenous nitroglycerin for several days after the last bout of angina. This provides a period of maximal therapy to permit stabilization of the involved coronary artery. After several angina-free days, intravenous nitroglycerin can be discontinued and topical nitrates (Nitropaste) begun at a dose of 1 to 2 inches every 6 hours.

Calcium Antagonists

Calcium antagonists such as nifedipine, diltiazem, and verapamil are beneficial in most patients with unstable angina because they are potent coronary vasodilators. These agents may therefore prevent periodic coronary vasoconstriction resulting from platelet-derived products (i.e., thromboxane A_2, serotonin) released at the site of the ruptured atherosclerotic plaque. By preventing this transient reduction in coronary blood flow, ischemic episodes are prevented. In addition, calcium antagonists reduce myocardial oxygen demand by decreasing afterload and left ventricular wall stress. Diltiazem and verapamil also reduce myocardial oxygen demand by decreasing the heart rate.

For most patients with unstable angina, diltiazem is the preferred agent. It should be started along with intravenous nitroglycerin at a dose of 30 to 60 mg by mouth every 6 to 8 hours. Although a long-acting preparation (Cardizem SR) is now available, it should not be used in the critical care setting. The strategy of using short-acting rather than long-acting agents should be followed because the dose of short-acting drugs can be more readily titrated upwards (or downwards) as the clinical situation dictates. Nifedipine is a potent arteriolar vasodilator but has the disadvantage of reflexively increasing the heart rate (and thus the myocardial oxygen demand) in patients not concurrently receiving beta blockers. Diltiazem is also less likely than nifedipine to produce significant hypotension. Verapamil shares with diltiazem a beneficial effect on the heart rate, but has the disadvantage of being a more potent negative inotrope. However, because diltiazem also possesses negative inotropic properties, it should be used with caution (if at all) in patients with signs of congestive heart failure.

Beta-Blockers

Beta-blockers are another class of agents useful in the management of unstable angina. These agents are beneficial because they reduce myocardial oxygen demand by decreasing heart rate and arterial pressure. Although beta-blockers are recommended by some physicians as first-line therapy in the management of unstable angina, I prefer to administer them to patients with anginal symptoms inadequately controlled by aspirin, intravenous nitroglycerin, and diltiazem. Beta-blockers are particularly beneficial in those patients with a persistently rapid heart rate that is not caused by volume depletion or reduced cardiac output.

Beta-blocker therapy should be instituted with the short-acting agent propranolol, 20 mg by mouth every 6 hours, and then titrated to a resting heart rate of 55 to 60 beats per minute. An alternative oral beta-blocker is the beta$_1$ selective agent metoprolol, which can be started at a dose of 25 mg by mouth every 6 hours and increased to up to 100 mg by mouth twice per day. In patients in whom more rapid beta-blockade is desired, metoprolol can be given intravenously at a dose of 5 mg intravenously every 5 minutes $\times$ 3, followed by the above dosing regimen.

Although beta-blockers have distinct benefits, they also have several important potentially adverse effects. Because beta-blockers possess negative inotropic effects, they should generally not be administered to patients with signs of congestive heart failure or with moderate-to-severe depression of left ventricular function. It is strongly recommended that one obtain an echocardiogram to assess left ventricular function before beginning beta-blocker therapy in those patients suspected of having depressed left ventricular function. Caution should also be exercised in patients with a resting bradycardia (<55 beats per minute) and in those with a history of obstructive lung disease or asthma.

Thrombolytic Therapy

Although our current understanding of the pathophysiology of unstable angina (i.e., ruptured atherosclerotic plaque with associated intracoronary thrombus) suggests that thrombolytic therapy may be beneficial, this approach has not yet been adequately studied. Several multicenter, randomized trials in progress will address this important question. However, until data are available, routine administration of intravenous thrombolytic therapy is not recommended.

INVASIVE EVALUATION AND REVASCULARIZATION STRATEGIES

Intra-Aortic Balloon Counterpulsation

This mode of therapy is highly effective in reducing myocardial ischemia and is indicated in unstable angina patients with chest pain or hemodynamic instability refractory to other forms of medical management. However, intra-aortic balloon counterpulsation should be viewed as a temporary measure only, useful in stabilizing patients before or during coronary angiography, coronary angioplasty, or coronary artery bypass surgery. This is because prolonged balloon pumping is associated with an increased risk of limb ischemia, thromboembolism, and infection.

The intra-aortic balloon pump is generally inserted percutaneously via the femoral artery and is positioned within the descending thoracic aorta. The procedure is usually performed under fluoroscopic guidance in the cardiac catheterization laboratory or critical care unit, but the device can also be inserted without fluoroscopy if necessary. The mechanism by which intra-aortic balloon counterpulsation reduces myocardial ischemia is believed to be caused by its favorable effect on the myocardial oxygen supply-demand relationship. Myocardial oxygen supply is facilitated because the balloon inflates during diastole, thereby increasing diastolic pressure and augmenting myocardial perfusion. Myocardial oxygen demand is reduced because the balloon deflates during systole, thereby unloading the left ventricle and reducing myocardial wall stress.

Coronary Angiography

The vast majority of patients with unstable angina should undergo coronary angiography soon after they have been stabilized medically. The goals of this procedure are to determine the lesion responsible for the unstable syndrome (the "culprit" lesion) and to clarify the extent of disease in the remainder of the coronary vasculature. The results are helpful in deciding further management. In the 10 to 20 percent found to have insignificant coronary artery disease, coronary artery spasm or noncardiac (i.e., gastrointestinal) cause of chest pain should be strongly considered. Coronary artery bypass surgery is clearly indicated in the 10 percent of patients in whom significant left main disease is demonstrated. For the rest of the patients, the decision to proceed with coronary angioplasty, coronary artery bypass grafting or medical therapy can be carried out on an individual basis.

In those patients whose angina persists or recurs despite maximal therapy with nitrates, calcium blockers, aspirin, and heparin, coronary angiography should be performed immediately. Based on these findings, this highly unstable subset of patients should promptly undergo a revascularization procedure, either coronary angioplasty or coronary artery bypass grafting. Placement of an intra-aortic balloon pump in the catheterization laboratory is extremely helpful in stabilizing these patients and decreasing the risks associated with revascularization.

Percutaneous Transluminal Coronary Angioplasty

Coronary angioplasty has been shown to be an effective treatment for many patients with unstable angina. Although reported success rates range from 85 to 94 percent, several studies have documented a higher complication rate in unstable angina than with elective coronary angioplasty. This is probably due to the presence of intracoronary thrombus. The procedure is indicated for those patients with single- or double-vessel disease in whom the "culprit" lesion is amenable to balloon dilatation. Patients with more extensive multivessel disease, left main disease, or significantly depressed left ventricular function may be better candidates for bypass surgery. As is the case for patients with stable angina, the major disadvantage of coronary angioplasty is the risk of restenosis, which ranges from 25 to 40 percent depending on the site of balloon dilatation.

The optimum timing of coronary angioplasty has been a matter of debate, but I prefer to administer systemic heparin (in addition to aspirin, nitrates, and calcium blockers) for 3 to 5 days before balloon dilatation. This may encourage resolution of associated coronary thrombus and permit initial healing of the ruptured atherosclerotic plaque. This approach appears to reduce the incidence of angioplasty-associated acute complications (e.g., abrupt closure, distal embolization, myocardial infarction, and the need for emergency bypass surgery), particularly in those patients in whom intracoronary thrombus has been identified on the initial coronary angiogram. If significant thrombus continues to be apparent angiographically when the patient returns for angioplasty, intracoronary administration of the thrombolytic agent such as tPA (20 mg) or urokinase (250,000 U) may be beneficial.

Coronary Artery Bypass Grafting

Bypass surgery is also an effective revascularization strategy for patients with unstable angina and is indicated for significant left main disease (>50 percent diameter narrowing), and in most patients with severe triple vessel coronary disease. Surgical revascularization is also indicated for patients with less extensive coronary disease when lesions are unsuitable for coronary angioplasty. Preoperative placement of an intra-aortic balloon pump is helpful in stabilizing these patients by augmenting coronary blood flow and reducing myocardial oxygen demand.

SUGGESTED READING

de Feyter PJ, Serruys PW. Percutaneous transluminal coronary angioplasty for unstable angina. In: Topol EJ, ed. Textbook of interventional cardiology. Philadelphia: WB Saunders Co., 1990;254.

Fuster V, Badimon L, Cohen M, et al. Insights into the pathogenesis of acute ischemic syndromes. Circulation 1988; 77:1213–1220.

Sherman CT, Litvack F, Grundfest W, et al. Coronary angioscopy in patients with unstable angina pectoris. N Engl J Med 1986; 315:913–919.

Theroux P, Ouimet H, McCans J, et al. Aspirin, heparin, or both to treat acute unstable angina. N Engl J Med 1988; 319:1105–1111.

ACUTE MYOCARDIAL INFARCTION

EDWARD L. PASSEN, M.D.
GARY L. SCHAER, M.D.

Myocardial infarction is a medical emergency requiring prompt evaluation and treatment. In recent years, treatment has changed from a passive supportive approach to an active interventional approach aimed at restoring blood flow to ischemic myocardium.

PATHOPHYSIOLOGY

In 1912 James B. Herrick first proposed that acute myocardial infarction was caused by the thrombotic occlusion of a coronary artery. However, it was not until the angiographic studies by DeWood and co-workers were reported in 1980 that coronary thrombosis was firmly established as the primary event causing acute myocardial infarction. This knowledge has led to a revolution in the management of acute myocardial infarction by stimulating the development of interventional therapy directed toward reperfusion of the occluded coronary artery.

Atherosclerotic coronary artery disease is typically the precursor of thrombotic coronary occlusion. Lipid-laden atherosclerotic plaques gradually narrow the lumen of the coronary artery, eventually preventing myocardial oxygen supply from meeting myocardial oxygen demand. This imbalance results in transient myocardial ischemia and angina pectoris. However, spontaneous ulceration or rupture of these atherosclerotic plaques suddenly expose collagen, smooth muscle, and lipids to blood. A cascade of adverse events results, including platelet aggregation, release of platelet-derived vasoconstrictors, and activation of the coagulation systems. These events lead to a diminished coronary flow with formation of occlusive thrombus within the coronary artery. If coronary blood flow is not promptly restored, myocardial necrosis results.

DIAGNOSIS

The diagnosis of myocardial infarction has traditionally been based on the patient's history, electrocardiogram (ECG), and cardiac enzymes. In the present era of rapid intervention to salvage myocardium, only the history and ECG are immediately available. These must therefore be obtained and interpreted rapidly and accurately to make the correct diagnosis and initiate appropriate therapy with minimal risk.

History

The recognition of an acute myocardial infarction depends on obtaining an adequate history and correctly interpreting the patient's symptoms. Chest pain caused by myocardial infarction usually resembles angina but is more severe and prolonged. Some patients, particularly diabetics, the elderly, and those with hypertension may have atypical symptoms. Other patients present with severe and/or prolonged chest pain that may have noncardiac causes (gastrointestinal, musculoskeletal) or other cardiovascular disease (pericarditis, aortic dissection). The characteristics of the chest discomfort along with the patient's past medical history and risk factors for coronary artery disease suggest the diagnosis of myocardial infarction. Noting the time of onset of chest pain is important because it permits estimation of the likelihood of myocardial salvage with reperfusion therapy. Once the initial history is obtained, subsequent interviews with the patient are helpful in determining the patient's response to therapeutic agents.

Physical Examination

In patients with myocardial infarction, the physical examination may be normal or may provide clues to underlying atherosclerosis (e.g., peripheral vascular disease) or may reveal coronary risk factors (e.g., hypertension). During the initial physical examination, it is important to obtain accurate information on baseline vital signs, identify potential complications of infarction (e.g., cardiogenic shock, right ventricular infarction, congestive heart failure), exclude other cardiac problems (e.g., aortic stenosis, other valvular disease, hypertrophic cardiomyopathy, pericarditis) and exclude other noncardiac ailments that may cause chest pain (e.g., aortic dissection, pulmonary embolism, pneumothorax, peptic ulcer disease).

Electrocardiography

The ECG is usually quite helpful in the diagnosis of acute myocardial infarction and should be obtained immediately at the time of the patient's presentation. Initial ECG changes depend on the time the ECG is first recorded in relation to the onset of symptoms. Acute myocardial infarction should not be excluded on the basis of an initially normal ECG, since changes may be delayed or intermittent. Repeating the ECG (once or more often) increases the diagnostic yield and is particularly important if the diagnosis is in doubt. Minor changes in the ST segment or T wave should not be overlooked. It is ST segment elevation that is most suggestive of acute myocardial infarction, however, and it frequently identifies the location of myocardial ischemia (i.e., anterior, inferior, lateral). Other causes of ST segment elevation should be considered, especially Prinzmetal's angina, ventricular aneurysm, pericarditis, and early repolarization. A pathologic Q wave is not usually present if the ECG is obtained soon after the onset of discomfort, but it may develop later. Although the development of pathologic Q waves usually suggests a completed infarct, if significant chest pain and ST segment elevation persist, the infarct may still be evolving and amenable to myocardial salvage with reperfusion. In Q wave infarctions (generally caused by complete thrombotic occlusion), the ECG evolves a decrease in R wave voltage, return of the ST segment to baseline, symmetric inversion of the T waves, and pathologic Q waves. In non-Q wave infarctions (caused by subtotal or intermittent coronary occlusion by thrombus and/or spasm), the ECG usually evolves ST segment depression and/or T wave inversions in the area overlying the infarction.

Cardiac Enzymes

Enzyme diagnosis of acute myocardial infarction is precise, widely available, and easy to interpret, but the results are not usually available until after treatment has been initiated. Irreversibly injured myocardial tissue releases creatine kinase (CK) into the blood. The MB isoenzyme of CK is most specific for myocardial necrosis and should be obtained immediately and serially for 24 to 36 hours. Lack of elevation of CK or its MB fraction excludes infarction. Plasma CK usually exceeds normal levels 4 to 6 hours after the onset of infarction, peaks at two to ten times normal levels within 24 hours, and returns to baseline within 4 days. When thrombolytic therapy successfully opens the occluded coronary artery, the rates of enzyme release from the heart are altered, usually resulting in a high and rapid peak of CK.

Echocardiography

The echocardiogram may be helpful in the diagnosis of myocardial infarction by identifying regional wall motion abnormalities consistent with ischemia. The echocardiogram is also useful when the history and/or ECG are not diagnostic of infarction, and it can be used to look for evidence of pericardial, valvular, or aortic root disease.

INITIAL THERAPEUTIC APPROACH

An assessment of the probability of myocardial infarction based on the history and ECG should be made within the first 10 minutes of presentation. Baseline vital signs and physical findings should also be obtained during this time and used to formulate the management plan, particularly the need for thrombolytic therapy.

General Care

Although the initial diagnostic and therapeutic maneuvers usually take place in the emergency room of most hospitals, the patient should be transferred to the critical care unit as soon as possible. Complete bed rest is mandatory during the acute period. ECG monitoring for arrhythmias should begin immediately and peripheral intravenous access should also be obtained (preferably with an 18-gauge catheter). The patient should receive nothing by mouth until medically stable. To prevent hematoma formation if thrombolytic therapy or anticoagulation is used, intramuscular injections should be avoided. Supplemental oxygen should be administered by nasal prongs (2 to 4 L per minute). Cutaneous oximetry may be used to ensure an adequate systemic oxygen saturation, especially if the patient has a history of pulmonary disease, dyspnea, or signs of heart failure. Routine arterial blood gases, invasive arterial pressure monitoring, central lines, and pulmonary artery catheters should be avoided unless specifically indicated by respiratory distress or hemodynamic instability.

Analgesia and Sedation

The best analgesic is reperfusion of the occluded coronary artery. Even before thrombolytic therapy is begun, however, analgesic agents are recommended to reduce discomfort and diminish myocardial oxygen demands. Morphine sulfate (2 to 5 mg IV) is the analgesic of choice because it is potent, rapidly acting, and has favorable hemodynamic effects (venodilation). In addition, if adverse effects occur (e.g., hypotension, respiratory depression), morphine can be rapidly reversed by naloxone hydrochloride (Narcan, 0.4 to 1 mg IV). Sedation with benzodiazepines (e.g., diazepam, 5 mg by mouth four times per day, as necessary) may also be useful to reduce myocardial oxygen demand in anxious patients. Analgesics and sedatives should be carefully titrated to avoid respiratory depression and hemodynamic instability. This is particularly true in the treatment of the elderly.

Aspirin

Early administration of aspirin to patients with acute myocardial infarction has become standard practice. Unless contraindicated by an allergic history, aspirin (160 to 324 mg chewable or orally) should be given promptly to the patient with presumed infarction. Chewable aspirin is recommended for the first dose because it accelerates absorption. The Second International Study of Infarct Survival (ISIS-2) recently demonstrated that chewable aspirin (160 mg per day) reduces the rates of reinfarction and mortality in patients with acute infarction; furthermore, these benefits were in addition to those derived from thrombolytic therapy. The mechanism of aspirin's beneficial effect is platelet inhibition. Aspirin irreversibly inactivates platelet cyclooxygenase, thereby impairing platelet aggregation and reducing the release of platelet-derived vasoconstrictors (thromboxane A_2, serotonin). The main toxicity of aspirin is manifested as dose-related gastrointestinal symptoms. Subsequent doses may be given as an enteric-coated preparation (e.g., Ecotrin) to minimize abdominal symptoms. A mild bleeding tendency may result, but this is usually not clinically significant unless there are co-existing coagulation abnormalities.

Nitrates

Nitrates are useful agents in the management of myocardial infarction and should be instituted immediately at the time of presentation. Unless contraindicated by hypotension (systolic blood pressure < 90 mm Hg), therapy should begin with sublingual nitroglycerin (0.4 mg). Although this dose may be repeated again in 5 to 10 minutes, it is best to continue therapy with intravenous nitroglycerin. Intravenous nitroglycerin may be started at 5 to 10 µg per minute and increased in increments of 5 to 10 µg per minute every 5 minutes. There is no fixed optimum dose, and therapy must be individualized based on symptoms and blood pressure. Titration to pain resolution may not be practical or possible in the treatment of acute myocardial infarction. A 10 to 20 percent reduction in systolic blood pressure is a reasonable target for titration, but the systolic blood pressure should not be permitted to decrease to less than 100 mm Hg.

Nitrates have several beneficial effects in the treatment of acute myocardial infarction. In the initial treatment of severe chest pain and ST segment elevation, nitrates occasionally dramatically reduce myocardial ischemia in patients with vasospastic (Prinzmetal's) angina. For patients with thrombotic occlusion of a coronary artery, nitrates are beneficial because they reduce myocardial oxygen demand by venodilation and preload reduction. Nitrates may also improve myocardial oxygen supply by increasing collateral blood flow to the ischemic region.

The major adverse effect of nitrates is hypotension, which is more likely to occur in patients who are volume depleted or in those patients with right ventricular infarction (discussed later in this chapter). Nitrate-induced hypotension may also be associated with a reflex tachycardia that further worsens myocardial ischemia by increasing myocardial oxygen demand. Sinus tachycardia and hypotension should be avoided through careful titration of the dose. If volume depletion is suspected, intravenous boluses of normal saline should be administered as needed. Headache is also common and may be treated with a mild analgesic.

Heparin

Although routine systemic anticoagulation with heparin has not been shown to improve survival independently in the emergent treatment of acute myocardial infarction, its major value is as an adjunct to thrombolytic therapy to diminish reocclusion after successful reperfusion (see below). In addition, systemic heparin has been shown to reduce the incidence of left ventricular mural thrombi and systemic embolism in patients with a large anterior myocardial infarction. Heparin should be administered as a 5,000-U bolus followed by a maintenance infusion of 1,000 U per hour and titrated to keep the partial thromboplastin time (PTT) 1.5 to 2 times control. It is generally continued for the initial 2 to 5 days postinfarction. If the patient is not yet ambulatory when systemic heparin is discontinued, it should be administered subcutaneously (5,000 U every 12 hours) to prevent deep venous thrombosis. Bleeding complications are the most common adverse effect of systemic heparinization.

Beta-Blockers

The early use of beta-blockers in acute myocardial infarction has been shown to reduce the incidence of ischemic pain, nonfatal reinfarction, cardiac arrest, and death. Their mechanism of action involves a dose-dependent competitive binding to beta receptors. The heart contains primarily $beta_1$ receptors, which cause an increase in the heart rate and myocardial contractility when stimulated. By inhibiting cardiac beta-adrenergic receptors, beta-blockers cause a reduction in heart rate, blood pressure, and contractility, all of which reduce myocardial oxygen demand. Left ventricular wall stress is also reduced, decreasing the risk of myocardial rupture. Additionally, the threshold for ventricular fibrillation is raised. Beta-blockers appear to be most useful in patients with continued ischemic discomfort and sympathetic hyperactivity manifested by tachycardia or systemic arterial hypertension. Beta-blockers should be avoided in patients with signs of heart failure by physical or chest x-ray examination, hypotension (systolic pressure < 90 mm Hg), bradycardia (heart rate < 60 beats per minute), severe first-degree atrioventricular (A-V) block (PR > 240 msec), and second- or third-degree A-V block. Caution is also advised for those with obstructive lung disease, or peripheral vascular disease.

For patients with acute myocardial infarction in whom no contraindications exist, beta-blockers should initially be administered intravenously to achieve immediate beta-blockade, and then be administered orally. We recommend beginning therapy as soon as possible with metoprolol, 5 mg IV, to be repeated twice at 2- to 5-minute intervals. If the patient appears to have tolerated the total 15-mg intravenous dose (as assessed by physical examination, ECG, and measurement of blood pressure), oral therapy should follow 15 minutes later with administration of metoprolol tablets in a dose of 50 mg by mouth every 6 hours for 48 hours and thereafter in a dose of 100 mg orally twice daily. Propranolol, atenolol, and esmolol are other potential choices for intravenous beta-blockade. Metoprolol or atenolol are preferred because they are $beta_1$-selective agents and have been proven to be beneficial in clinical trials of acute myocardial infarction. Because of its brief half-life, esmolol may be advantageous in situations in which precise control of the heart rate is necessary or if the need for rapid drug withdrawal is anticipated if adverse effects develop. The major adverse consequences of beta-blocker therapy include exacerbation of heart failure, hypotension, and A-V conduction abnormalities. Careful physical examination and close monitoring of the blood pressure and heart rate are important during initial treatment with beta-blockers.

Antiarrhythmic Therapy

Premature ventricular contractions, couplets, and nonsustained ventricular tachycardia are common during the initial 12 to 24 hours of acute myocardial infarction and may increase substantially with reperfusion (reperfusion arrhythmias). Primary ventricular fibrillation may also occur without warning during this time. We recommend prophylactic lidocaine for all patients with proven or suspected acute myocardial infarction. Lidocaine is administered as an intravenous bolus (1 mg per kilogram) followed by a maintenance infusion of 1 to 3 mg per minute. A second bolus of 0.5 mg per kilogram IV should be given 5 minutes after the initial bolus to maintain blood levels. The bolus dose and infusion rate should be reduced by one-half in elderly patients and those with severe heart failure, hypotension, or liver disease. Toxic manifestations primarily involve the central nervous system (lethargy, confusion) and should prompt one to reduce the dose or discontinue the drug.

INTERVENTIONAL THERAPY

Several major clinical trials have clearly demonstrated that expeditious coronary reperfusion decreases the mortality rate and improves left ventricular (LV) function. The major mechanism responsible for these beneficial effects is restoration of coronary blood flow, which results reduction in myocardial infarct size. Prompt reperfusion may be achieved with thrombolytic agents, coronary angioplasty, or coronary artery bypass surgery; however, thrombolytic therapy should be viewed as the first-line approach for the majority of patients.

Thrombolytic Therapy: Indications and Contraindications

The prompt institution of thrombolytic therapy should be considered in all patients presenting with suspected acute myocardial infarction. It is essential that treatment be instituted as soon as possible, preferably within 4 hours of symptom onset, because the longer the delay to reperfusion, the less the potential for myocardial salvage.

Specific indications and contraindications for thrombolytic therapy are listed in Table 1. Good candidates for thrombolytic therapy include those patients with chest pain persisting for more than 30 minutes but less than 6 hours, associated with ST segment elevation of at least 1 mm (0.1 mV) in at least two contiguous leads. In addition, there should be no contraindications to thrombolytic therapy (see below). Patients with intermittent chest pain for more than 6 hours should also be considered for thrombolytic therapy, provided that ST segment elevation persists. By contrast, thrombolytic therapy has not been proven to be beneficial when the ECG demonstrates other than ST segment elevation (e.g., ST segment depression, T wave abnormalities). Before administering a thrombolytic agent, the clinician should weigh the potential benefits, estimated by the duration of ischemia and the amount of myocardium in jeopardy, versus the risks, estimated by the patient's age, the presence of other medical problems, and potential bleeding complications. Although the elderly seem to derive the most benefit from thrombolytic therapy, they are also more likely to have complications. We recommend that there not be a strict age cut-off for the use of a thrombolytic agent. Rather, the overall status of the patient should be considered.

Absolute contraindications to thrombolytic therapy include active internal bleeding, known bleeding diathesis, history of cerebrovascular accident, intracranial neoplasm, arteriovenous malformation or aneurysm, recent intracranial or intraspinal surgery or trauma, recent major surgery, and severe uncontrolled hypertension. Relative contraindications include prolonged cardiopulmonary resuscitation, recent invasive procedures, poorly controlled hypertension, hemorrhagic ophthalmic conditions (i.e., diabetic proliferative retinopathy), and postpartum or menstruating women. A history of a prior allergic reaction (particularly with streptokinase) should also be considered, but should not preclude the use of another thrombolytic agent. Approximately one-third of patients presenting with an acute myocardial infarction are eligible to receive thrombolytic therapy using the above-mentioned guidelines.

Choice of a Thrombolytic Agent

Several thrombolytic agents are presently approved by the Food and Drug Administration (FDA) for intravenous or intracoronary administration for acute myo

Table 1 Indications and Contraindications of Thrombolytic Therapy for Acute Myocardial Infarction

Indications	Contraindications
Ischemic chest pain of >30 minutes and <6 hours duration ST segment elevation ≥ 1 mm in two contiguous ECG leads (e.g., leads II, aVF, or leads V_3, V_4)	History of cerebrovascular accident, transient ischemic attacks Severe uncontrolled hypertension Active internal bleeding Recent gastrointestinal bleeding (within 10 days) Major surgery within 10 days Prolonged cardiopulmonary resuscitation Recent (within 2 months) intracranial or intraspinal surgery or trauma Intracranial neoplasm, arteriovenous malformation or aneurysm Known bleeding diathesis

cardial infarction. The intravenous route is preferred because it facilitates rapid treatment, thereby accelerating time to reperfusion. The intracoronary route is less often often used because of the intrinsic delay in performing emergency catheterization and because these invasive facilities may not be routinely available. Thrombolytic agents may be generally classified as fibrin selective or nonselective. Fibrin-selective agents (e.g., t-PA) locally activate the plasminogen-fibrin complex, cause less systemic fibrinogen breakdown, and achieve a higher 90-minute patency rate. Nonselective agents (e.g., streptokinase, urokinase, APSAC) cause extensive systemic fibrinolysis and a systemic lytic state. In addition, the resulting elevation in fibrin-split products produce platelet inhibition, which may be beneficial by reducing the incidence of reocclusion following successful reperfusion. Despite the systemic lytic state produced by the nonselective agents, the incidence of bleeding complications does not appear to be significantly different than that observed with the fibrin-selective agents.

Tissue Plasminogen Activator (t-PA)

Alteplase, or t-PA is a serine protease enzyme produced by vascular endothelial cells and commercially produced by recombinant DNA technology. It is a fibrin-selective agent with a marked affinity for the plasminogen-fibrin complex. Multicenter clinical trials have demonstrated that t-PA is the most effective thrombolytic agent available for achieving prompt reperfusion of the occluded coronary artery. The mean patency rate at 90 minutes is 76 percent, whereas streptokinase (see below) achieves a mean 90-minute patency rate of 51 percent. More importantly, clinical trials have demonstrated that t-PA reduces the mortality rate and improves LV function. The currently recommended dosing regimen is a 10-mg intravenous bolus administered over 2 minutes, followed by a 50-mg infusion administered over the first hour, a 20-mg infusion administered over the second hour, and another 20-mg infusion over the third hour. Thus patients receive a total of 100 mg over 3 hours. In patients weighing less than 65 kg, a lower total dose of 1.25 mg per kilogram should be used. A variety of other dosing regimens to improve vessel patency rates and decrease the incidence of reocclusion are currently under investigation. As with all thrombolytic agents, bleeding complications are the major adverse consequence of t-PA therapy; however, because of the short half-life of this agent, bleeding complications are less prolonged. An additional disadvantage of t-PA is its high cost. The advantages of t-PA over other agents include the lack of allergic and hypotensive reactions and the higher rate of early reperfusion associated with this drug.

Streptokinase

A product of beta-hemolytic streptococci, streptokinase is a non-fibrin-selective thrombolytic agent. Multicenter clinical trials have demonstrated that with this drug, the mean 90-minute infarct-related artery patency rate is 51 percent, considerably lower than that seen with t-PA. However, the patency rate at 24 hours increases to 85 percent, which is comparable to that of t-PA. This agent has also been clearly shown to reduce the mortality rate and improve LV function in patients with myocardial infarction. Streptokinase is administered as a 1.5 million-U intravenous infusion over 1 hour. Adverse effects occur more frequently with this agent than with t-PA and include allergic reactions, hypotension, and bleeding. The allergic reactions include fever, rash, urticaria, serum sickness, or vasculitis. Hypotension occurs in 5 to 10 percent of patients and appears to be caused by kinin and complement activation. It is also partially related to the rapidity and magnitude of the dose administered. Streptokinase-induced hypotension is best treated by slowing the rate of drug infusion and by cautious administration of intravenous boluses of normal saline to increase intravascular volume. Bleeding complications occur because of extensive fibrinogenolysis and a systemic lytic state. Fibrinogen levels are frequently reduced to 20 percent of baseline and may take more than 24 hours to recover. Therefore, if bleeding complications occur, they may be more difficult to control because of this sustained lytic effect. The advantages of streptokinase are its low cost and a lower incidence of reocclusion of the reperfused coronary artery.

APSAC

Anistreplase, or APSAC (Anisoylated Plasminogen Streptokinase Activator Complex) is an anisoylated derivative of streptokinase that results in greater persistence of fibrinogenolytic activity and improved thrombolytic patency compared with streptokinase given in equivalent doses. Although APSAC also produces a systemic fibrinolytic state, it may be somewhat more fibrin-selective than streptokinase. This is suggested by data from several clinical trials that have demonstrated a mean 90-minute patency rate of 77 percent. This is far superior to the mean 90-minute potency rate of streptokinase and comparable to that of t-PA. APSAC has also been shown to reduce the mortality rate and improve LV function in patients with myocardial infarction. APSAC is administered as a 30-U intravenous bolus over 2 to 5 minutes and thus has a distinct advantage over other thrombolytic agents which must be infused over a longer period of time. The adverse effects of APSAC are similar to those of streptokinase, including allergic reactions and bleeding complications. Although it costs less than t-PA, it is still eight to ten times more expensive than streptokinase.

Urokinase

Although urokinase is FDA-approved for intracoronary use, it is not presently approved for intravenous administration in patients with acute myocardial infarction. However, recent clinical trials have shown that intravenous urokinase (2 million- to 3 million-U bolus) is an effective therapy, having 90-minute patency rates of 60 to 67 percent. Advantages of urokinase include bolus administration, an absence of allergic reactions or hypotension, and a lower incidence of vessel reocclusion. Disadvantages include bleeding complications similar to those associated with other thrombolytic agents and its high cost as compared with t-PA. Further studies are in progress to determine the effects of this agent on mortality and LV function after intravenous administration for myocardial infarction.

Adjunctive Medical Therapy

Aspirin is probably the most important agent to combine with thrombolytic therapy because it has been demonstrated to further reduce the mortality rate and decrease the rate of reinfarction after successful thrombolysis. Administration of aspirin (160 to 325 mg by mouth daily) should probably be continued indefinitely after myocardial infarction.

The precise role of heparin as an adjunct to thrombolytic therapy has not yet been completely defined. At the present time, we recommend that heparin (as a 5,000-U bolus followed by 1,000 U per hour by continuous infusion) be administered 1 hour after beginning thrombolytic therapy. It should be continued for 2 to 5 days, with the partial thromboplastin time (PTT) maintained at 1.5 to 2 times control. The major purpose of heparin is to prevent reocclusion of the newly reperfused coronary artery.

Beta-blockers should be administered early and intravenously in all patients receiving thrombolytic therapy, provided that there are no contraindications. Immediate beta-blockade has been shown to decrease significantly the incidence of recurrent ischemia, reinfarction, cardiac rupture, and intracerebral hemorrhage in this patient population.

Although no randomized controlled studies have investigated the benefits of nitrates in patients treated with thrombolytic therapy, nitrate therapy was demonstrated to reduce the mortality rate in infarction patients during the prethrombolytic era. We therefore recommend that intravenous nitroglycerin be administered in an attempt to improve myocardial blood flow and reduce myocardial oxygen demand. Although calcium blockers are excellent coronary vasodilators, there are insufficient data regarding the use of these agents in thrombolysis-treated acute myocardial infarction patients to support their routine use.

Indications for Invasive Procedures Post-Thrombolysis

Invasive procedures such as placement of central venous or arterial lines, pulmonary artery catheters, and diagnostic cardiac catheterization are not routinely indicated during the acute period following thrombolytic therapy. For patients who are hemodynamically stable and who do not have recurrent chest pain during the early post-thrombolytic period, it is best to avoid the added bleeding complications associated with these invasive procedures. Indeed, clinical trials have shown that acute cardiac catheterization with immediate coronary angioplasty of the newly reperfused infarct-related artery is associated with an increased incidence of vessel reocclusion, a greater need for bypass surgery, major bleeding necessitating transfusion, and a greater overall mortality rate. Thus, this invasive approach should not be routinely performed in stable patients after thrombolytic therapy.

Patients with persistent or intermittent chest pain and continued ST segment elevation during the early hours of thrombolytic therapy should be considered for emergency cardiac catheterization. Even after thrombolytic therapy with t-PA, currently the most effective thrombolytic agent, coronary angiography in these patients frequently demonstrates total occlusion of the infarct-related artery. Many of these patients should be considered for "rescue" coronary angioplasty aimed at reperfusing the occluded infarct-related vessel. If coronary angiography demonstrates significant left main or triple vessel disease, or if the anatomy is otherwise unsuitable for coronary angioplasty, patients should be considered for emergency bypass surgery.

Whether or not diagnostic cardiac catheterization should be performed before hospital discharge is currently a matter of debate. We recommend that cardiac catheterization be performed in those patients who spontaneously develop rest or exertional angina and in those patients in whom angina is provoked by a submaximal exercise test. In addition, we recommend diagnostic cardiac catheterization for patients at hight risk for ischemic complications postdischarge, such as patients with significant left ventricular dysfunction, extensive infarct territory (particularly anterior infarction), complex ventricular arrhythmias, and in younger patients (younger than 55 years of age).

Primary Coronary Angioplasty: Reperfusion Without Thrombolysis

When patients with acute infarction present with absolute or relative contraindications to thrombolytic therapy, an invasive approach should be strongly considered. Provided that catheterization and angioplasty facilities are readily available, these patients should undergo emergent diagnostic catheterization so that the infarct-related vessel can be defined. If technically feasible, primary (or direct) angioplasty of the infarct-related vessel should then be performed to restore coronary blood flow. This invasive approach is also valuable in patients in whom the diagnosis is in doubt, such as patients with typical ischemic chest pain without ST segment elevation or in patients with atypical symptoms. A medical catastrophe may result if thrombolytic therapy is administered to a misdiagnosed patient with aortic dissection or acute pericarditis. Thus, when the clinical findings and ECG do not "fit" entirely with acute infarction, it is best to withhold thrombolytic therapy and immediately proceed with coronary angiography and possible angioplasty.

COMPLICATIONS

Postinfarction Angina

The recurrence of chest pain after completed infarction should prompt an aggressive approach because these patients have an increased risk of reinfarction and sudden death. This is particularly true after thrombolytic therapy or in patients with non-Q wave myocardial infarction. Although the infarct-related artery is likely to be patent, the culprit lesion is unstable, probably associated with thrombus, and prone to reocclude.

Patients with postinfarction angina should be immediately transferred to a monitored bed in the critical care unit. Aspirin (325 mg by mouth), nitroglycerin (preferably intravenous), and a calcium antagonist (preferably diltiazem) should be administered. Systemic heparinization should be strongly considered. Virtually all patients with postinfarction angina should undergo diagnostic cardiac catheterization followed by coronary angioplasty of the culprit lesion in most cases of single- and double-vessel disease. Coronary artery bypass surgery is indicated for patients with more extensive coronary artery disease or if angioplasty is not technically feasible. If postinfarction angina is severe and persistent or is accompanied by hemodynamic instability, an intra-aortic balloon pump should be inserted at the time of cardiac catheterization or, in the event of catheterization delay, inserted in the critical care unit before catheterization.

Cardiogenic Shock

This is a dramatic complication of acute myocardial infarction, carrying a high mortality rate. It is typically the result of an extensive infarction involving greater than 40 percent of the LV mass. Clinically, cardiogenic shock is present when the systolic blood pressure decreases to less than 90 mm Hg in association with pulmonary congestion and diminished peripheral perfusion. Unless these patients are treated immediately and aggressively, the mortality rate is staggering (60 to 90 percent).

Recent clinical investigation suggests that prompt reperfusion of the occluded coronary artery is the only way to reduce the mortality rate associated with cardiogenic shock. We therefore recommend that all patients with cardiogenic shock immediately receive thrombolytic therapy (preferably t-PA) in addition to aspirin and heparin. Inotropic and/or vasopressor agents (e.g., dobutamine, dopamine, norepinephrine) may be needed for hemodynamic support, and mechanical ventilation should be instituted for respiratory distress. Agents that could potentially further decrease the blood pressure (vasodilators, morphine) should be withheld.

In centers where cardiac catheterization facilities are available, patients should be immediately transported to the cardiac catheterization laboratory for diagnostic cardiac catheterization and placement of a pulmonary artery catheter (to monitor cardiac filling pressures and cardiac output) and an intra-aortic balloon pump (to enhance coronary flow and reduce myocardial oxygen demands). If coronary angiography demonstrates total or subtotal occlusion of the infarct-related vessel (present in approximately 25 percent of patients treated with t-PA), "rescue" coronary angioplasty should be immediately performed to restore coronary blood flow. After catheterization, patients should be transported to the critical care unit where intra-aortic balloon counterpulsation and inotropic agents can be weaned, as clinically indicated. In centers without catheterization facilities, consideration should be given to immediate transport of the patient to a hospital capable of performing rescue angioplasty.

Right Ventricular Infarction

In a patient with an inferior infarction, the appearance of hypotension and poor peripheral perfusion should raise the possibility of right ventricular (RV) infarction. Although they may appear to be in cardiogenic shock, patients with RV infarction have a better prognosis. In addition, a different therapeutic approach is indicated. RV infarction results in right heart failure with inadequate filling of the LV. This explains the typical clinical features of this disorder: systemic hypotension, elevated jugular venous pressure, and clear lung fields. The diagnosis is made by identifying ST segment elevation in lead V_4R

(right precordial lead in V_4 position) or by characteristic hemodynamic findings on right heart catheterization (elevated right atrial mean and RV end-diastolic pressure, normal-to-low pulmonary capillary wedge pressure, and low cardiac output). Echocardiography frequently demonstrates depressed RV contractility.

In addition to prompt treatment with thrombolytic therapy (if indicated), patients with RV infarction should receive normal saline (e.g., 200-ml intravenous boluses, as needed) to increase LV preload and inotropic therapy (dobutamine 5 to 10 μg per kilogram per minute IV) to stimulate contractility of the RV.

Congestive Heart Failure

Congestive heart failure that develops soon after presentation with acute myocardial infarction results from depression of LV contractility and is often exacerbated by ischemia-induced increased diastolic stiffness (decreased compliance). Provided that the patient's blood pressure is stable, therapy should be directed toward reducing LV preload. This can be accomplished with diuretic agents (e.g., furosemide 20 to 40 mg IV) and/or nitrates. A thermodilution pulmonary artery catheter is useful for monitoring the pulmonary capillary wedge pressure, which should be reduced to 15 to 18 mm Hg for optimum cardiac performance. If cardiac output is depressed and the blood pressure is stable, afterload reduction with nitroprusside should be considered. The drug should be administered by continuous intravenous infusion under constant arterial pressure monitoring, beginning with a dose of 10 μg per minute and increasing the dose by 5-μg increments every 3 to 5 minutes to reduce the pulmonary capillary wedge pressure to 15 to 18 mm Hg. The average therapeutic starting dose is 1 to 2 μg per kilogram per minute. Arterial pressure should not be permitted to decrease to much less than 100 mm Hg. If hypotension occurs, the infusion can be reduced or discontinued.

As congestive heart failure improves over the initial 48-hour period postinfarction, the patient should be weaned from intravenous medications and started on an oral regimen consisting of digoxin, furosemide, and an angiotensin-converting enzyme inhibitor (captopril or enalarpril). Most of these patients should also undergo diagnostic cardiac catheterization during their hospital course. This is particularly true for those patients with severe heart failure.

Myocardial Rupture and Mechanical Causes of Cardiogenic Shock

Sudden rupture of the LV free wall or the interventricular septum is a dramatic complication of acute myocardial infarction. These catastrophic events typically appear 3 to 5 days after infarction. Although earlier reports suggested an incidence of myocardial rupture as high as 20 percent, these complications appear to be less common with the routine use of thrombolytic therapy, since smaller, nontransmural infarcts are much less likely to rupture. In addition, the increased early use of beta-blockers and more aggressive treatment of hypertension postinfarction has also contributed to the decreased incidence of myocardial rupture.

Rupture of the left ventricular free wall usually presents with sudden severe hypotension and evidence for pericardial tamponade from hemopericardium. If this condition is not recognized and treated immediately, these patients progress rapidly to electromechanical dissociation with cardiac death. The diagnosis can frequently be made on clinical grounds, but echocardiography can be extremely helpful. Treatment should involve emergency pericardiocentesis, intravenous fluids, vasopressor support (with dopamine and/or norepinephrine), ventilatory assistance (if indicated), and rapid transfer of the patient to the operating room for definitive surgical repair.

Rupture of the interventricular septum frequently presents with the appearance of a new harsh holosystolic murmur best heard at the lower left sternal border, which is associated with rapidly progressive biventricular heart failure. The diagnosis can be confirmed during right heart catheterization by demonstrating a step-up in oxygen saturation from right atrium to RV (left to right shunt), or it can be confirmed noninvasively by 2D echocardiography with doppler. Although afterload reduction with nitroprusside is helpful in decreasing the left to right shunt, vasopressors may also be needed to maintain the systolic blood pressure at greater than 90 mm Hg. An intra-aortic balloon pump should be considered to stabilize these patients. Emergency cardiac catheterization and urgent surgical repair of the defect are usually necessary.

Rupture of a papillary muscle is another serious mechanical complication that commonly presents 3 to 5 days postinfarction. In the diagnosis, it can sometimes be confused with an acute ventricular septal defect because of the appearance of a loud, holosystolic murmur in association with respiratory distress. However, the murmur of papillary muscle rupture is caused by severe mitral regurgitation and is more commonly apical in location. In addition, right heart catheterization fails to demonstrate a "step-up" in oxygen saturation from right atrium to right ventricle. Rather, large "V" waves are present in the pulmonary capillary wedge tracing. The diagnosis can also be confirmed by doppler echocardiography. Treatment is similar to that for acute ventricular septal defect, including afterload reduction with nitroprusside and vasopressor support (if needed). Likewise, placement of an intra-aortic balloon pump is extremely beneficial in severe cases. Cardiac catheterization and definitive surgical repair should be performed as soon as possible after the diagnosis is made.

SUGGESTED READING

DeWood MA, Spores J, Notse R, et al. Prevalence of total coronary occlusion during the early hours of transmural myocardial infarction. N Engl J Med 1980; 303:897.

ISIS-2 (Second International Study of Infarct Survival) Collaborative Study Group. Randomized trial of intravenous streptokinase, oral aspirin, both, or neither among 17,187 cases of suspected acute myocardial infarction. Lancet 1988; 2:349-360.

TIMI Study Group. The Thrombolysis in Myocardial Infarction (TIMI) Trial: Phase I findings. N Engl J Med 1985; 312:932-936.

TIMI Study Group. Comparison of invasive and conservative strategies after treatment with intravenous t-PA in acute myocardial infarction: results of the TIMI Phase II Trial. N Engl J Med 1989; 320:618-627.

Topol EJ, Califf RM, George BS, et al. A randomized trial of immediate versus delayed elective angioplasty after acute myocardial infarction. N Engl J Med 1987; 317:581-588.

PULMONARY EMBOLISM

RONALD N. RUBIN, M.D.
SOL SHERRY, M.D.

The management of acute pulmonary embolism has three basic goals: (1) rapid support for the morbid disturbances associated with the event; (2) prevention of recurrence(s) that contribute to the morbidity and mortality associated with this disorder; (3) removal of the anatomic obstruction and its hemodynamic consequences.

Optimal treatment of the patient also requires an understanding of the source of the disorder and the role played by each type of intervention; it should be noted that pulmonary embolism is a complication of an underlying thrombus, most frequently a deep vein thrombosis in the lower extremity. Thus adequate management should also take into consideration the most effective treatment for the entire problem so as to avoid any undesirable long-term consequences.

Immediate supportive care is directed at alleviating the hypoxemia with oxygen, allaying the often-associated apprehension with nonrespiratory depressing analgesics (e.g., demerol), and if hypotension and reduced cardiac output are present, treatment usually with pressor agents.

Prevention of recurrence can be undertaken with anticoagulants or by an interventional procedure (inferior vena caval interruption or placement of a filter).

In the more seriously ill patients, prompt relief of the obstruction and pulmonary hypertension also requires either thrombolytic therapy or pulmonary embolectomy.

PREVENTION OF RECURRENCE

This therapeutic approach is not directed at the embolic episode or its consequences (recovery is dependent on physiologic responses and native mechanisms for resolution); it is aimed at the source of the problem. Nevertheless, prophylaxis against recurrence is an essential and necessary part of the treatment. By itself it is usually entirely adequate if the following criteria are met:

1. There is no significant hemodynamic aberration or if the initial hemodynamic disturbances subside rapidly while the patient is receiving supportive therapy, without evidence of persisting pulmonary hypertension (i.e., disappearance of accentuated second pulmonic sound, right ventricular heave, right axis deviation on electrocardiogram, or gallop rhythm.
2. The total of the perfusion defect does not exceed 25 percent of the total lung volume.
3. No significant underlying cardiac disease or clinically evident deep vein thrombophlebitis (obvious leg swelling) is present.

Under these circumstances, prophylaxis alone is satisfactory because spontaneous resolution of the obstruction takes place progressively over the next few weeks, alleviating any remaining hemodynamic abnormalities and leaving little residue of the previous event.

Anticoagulant Therapy

In the absence of contraindications, anticoagulation is the preferred method of therapy for the prevention of thrombus growth and recurrent pulmonary embolism. It is initiated with heparin therapy systemically and then followed with orally active anticoagulants.

Heparin

Heparin preparations are available as calcium and sodium salts. The preponderance of data indicate that because these two forms of preparations have essentially comparable efficacy and toxicity, cost considerations favor the latter. The porcine intestinal preparation of heparin is usually the preferred form because its use is associated with a lower incidence of thrombocytopenia. Heparin has a half-life of approximately 60 minutes, and clearance is more rapid in the setting of pulmonary embolism than in deep vein thrombosis alone. Thus patients with pulmonary embolism require a higher heparin dose initially. Heparin can be given either intravenously by bolus or by continuous infusion through the use of an infusion pump, or it may be administered subcutaneously. In the critical care setting, control rendered by a continuous infusion of heparin is preferred. The anticoagulant effect of heparin is monitored by the prolongation of in vitro thrombin-induced clotting times. The most commonly used and widely available test in North America is the activated partial thromboplastin time (APTT).

Traditional contraindications to heparin therapy are listed in Table 1. The major lethal complication is cerebral

Table 1 Contraindications to Anticoagulant Therapy

Recent neurosurgery or ocular surgery
Diastolic hypertension greater than 110 mm Hg
Central nervous system hemmorhage
Major active bleeding sites
Recent major surgery or trauma
Recent CVA or transient ischemic attack
Gastrointestinal bleeding
Bacterial endocarditis
Coexistent hemorrhagic diathesis
Severe comorbid conditions with impaired hemostasis
  (e.g., renal or hepatic failure)

---

bleeding; if an increased risk for such an event exists, interruption of the vena cava or placement of a filter (see below) is indicated. When, on the basis of clinical judgment, heparin is used in patients with relative contraindications (increased risk of bleeding at other sites), very carefully controlled, well-monitored heparin therapy is essential.

The recommended regimen begins with a loading dose of 5,000 U followed by a sustaining infusion of 15 to 25 U per kilogram per hour. This results in dosages of 1,000 to 1,750 U per hour in a 70-kg man. Because of the more rapid clearance of heparin in pulmonary embolism, it is not unusual that higher doses are required, especially early in the course of the disease. Approximately 4 to 6 hours after initiation of therapy, the APTT is repeated. The goal is to give sufficient heparin to effect a prolongation to 1.5 to 2.5 times the baseline APTT. Early and aggressive heparin in amounts adequate to achieve an APTT in this therapeutic range is the key to successful therapy; the result is prevention of new thrombus formation and propagation, with a decrease in the rate of recurrent embolization to less than 5 percent. If the initial APTT is not within the therapeutic range, the 24-hour dose is increased by 2,000 to 4,000 U and the APTT is repeated after 4 to 6 hours. Conversely, if the APTT is in excess of 2.5 times control, the 24-hour heparin dose is decreased by 2,000 to 4,000 U followed by a repeat APTT after 4 to 6 hours. Such maneuvers usually quickly result in an appropriate heparin regimen. Thereafter, a daily APTT usually suffices. Heparin therapy is continued for at least 7 days.

Oral Anticoagulants

In patients able to tolerate oral medication, oral anticoagulants can be started as early as the second day after the initiation of heparin therapy to allow for an effective 4 to 5 days' overlap with the heparin. Once appropriate anticoagulation has been stabilized by the oral agents (steady state of prothrombin (PT) times of 1.4 to 2 times the baseline), heparin can be discontinued. Oral anticoagulants are continued for 3 to 6 months after pulmonary embolism unless there are persisting risk factors; under the latter circumstance, more extended therapy may be advisable. Warfarin is the most commonly used oral anticoagulant. Because of variations in patient response to this agent and various drug interactions, careful titration of the dose is required initially. Subcutaneous heparin (usually in a dose of 7,500 U twice daily but with evidence of prolongation of the APTT) can be used as an alternative to long-term prophylaxis against recurrence.

PREVENTION OF PULMONARY EMBOLISM BY INTERRUPTION OF THE VENOUS SYSTEM

In selected patients who have sustained and survived a major embolic episode, interruption of the venous system can be an important adjunctive procedure designed to prevent a second, possibly fatal embolism from occurring during the acute period. Interruption procedures are indicated for the following reasons: (1) there is an approximate incidence of recurrent pulmonary embolism of 2 to 5 percent even when adequate anticoagulation or thrombolytic therapy is carried out; and (2) because of the known linkage between pulmonary embolism and proximal deep vein thrombosis of the legs.

A variety of techniques are available to interrupt the inferior vena cava below the renal veins (interruptions of the saphenous vein, femoral vein, or ileac vein are not recommended since they may be distal to the site of the thrombotic source and ineffective; they may also enhance the thrombotic process in the lower extremity). Procedures available include surgical ligation or plication and transvenous placement of a variety of filters. Nonsurgical transvenous filter placement by a vascular surgeon or invasive radiologist, avoiding the use of anesthesia, is less dangerous in critically ill patients and is rapidly becoming the procedure of choice. Although the advantage of transvenous filter placement has lessened the morbidity and mortality rates of surgical interruption of the vena cava, their use requires clinical judgment, including appropriate diagnostic studies of the presence of pulmonary embolism in the lung and thrombosis in the vena cava distal to the renal veins. Morbidity rates within the range of 1 to 2 percent should be expected when the clinician is experienced. An exception to filter placement is septic emboli, since foreign materials should probably be avoided.

Specific indications for vena cava interruption include the following:

1. Pulmonary embolism in patients in whom anticoagulants are absolutely contraindicated (e.g., those with active bleeding, those in the immediate postoperative state, the neurosurgical patients).
2. Documented recurrent pulmonary embolism in patients adequately anticoagulated (anticoagulant failures are uncommon when cases of inadequate anticoagulation are excluded).
3. Patients surviving a massive pulmonary embolism who are unstable hemodynamically and might not survive a recurrence.

4. Patients undergoing pulmonary embolectomy.
5. Patients with septic pulmonary emboli from the lower extremity or pelvic veins who have not had a very favorable and clinical response within 24 hours after the initiation of antibiotic and anticoagulant therapy. Vena cava interruption in the latter four groups should be accompanied by anticoagulation with heparin, when possible, for maximal prevention of further thromboembolism, thrombus extension in the lower extremity, and long-term adverse effects (postphlebitic venous insufficiency).

SPECIFIC THERAPY

Because anticoagulation or interruption of venous flow does not address the problem of the acute embolic episode directly, more severe cases of pulmonary embolism will benefit from rapid relief of the acute occlusive event and the avoidance of any long-term consequences (e.g., increased pulmonary vascular resistance and persistent pulmonary hypertension that are further aggravated by effort or exercise).

Thrombolytic Therapy

Thrombolytic therapy is an effective medical treatment for rapidly dissolving pulmonary emboli and reducing associated morbidity—especially that associated with large, centrally located emboli. In our experience, it results in effective thrombolysis with excellent reperfusion in 90 percent of patients. It also has the advantage of lysing the originating source of the embolus and reducing the likelihood of the long-term consequences of the deep vein thrombosis (persisting venous hypertension in the affected lower extremity).

Spurious arguments have been offered against the use of thrombolytic therapy—for example, that there is no evidence that it reduces mortality and that there is a high incidence of bleeding complications. The largest trial, the Urokinase Pulmonary Embolism Trial, had only 160 patients (78 of whom received heparin, and 82 of whom received urokinase) and was not designed as a mortality trial; rather it was undertaken to demonstrate the superior ability of urokinase as compared with heparin in lysing pulmonary emboli, and to improve perfusion and alleviate the hemodynamic disturbances. Evidence of a reduction in the mortality rate would require that thousands of patients participate in the trial since most patients who die of a pulmonary embolism either die quickly before therapy can be instituted or are undiagnosed. If the diagnosis is made and the patient survives for several hours, the mortality rate is low and is frequently associated with other underlying diseases. However, rapid reduction of acute morbidity from massive emboli by thrombolytic therapy has been demonstrated in several studies.

In several studies, serious bleeding complications have been shown to be markedly diminished to an acceptable level (almost similar to that seen with full-dose heparin therapy) when the treatment is carried out with minimal invasive procedures, careful technique, and attention to contraindications (see below).

Currently there are multiple agents available. Streptokinase, a product of hemolytic streptococci, and urokinase, produced by human fetal kidney tissue cell cultures, have FDA approval for the treatment of pulmonary embolism. Produced by recombinant technology, t-PA also has been used in pulmonary embolism subsequent to its widespread use in myocardial infarction. Although clinically insignificant febrile reactions are more common with streptokinase, in our opinion, cost considerations render it the primary choice since efficacy and *major* toxicity (i.e., bleeding) data are essentially identical among all agents. Dosage for these agents is as follows. For *streptokinase*, a loading dose of 250,000 U is administered over 30 to 60 minutes to bind and neutralize pre-existing inhibiting antibodies and to initiate a thrombolytic state. A sustaining infusion of 100,000 U per hour is then administered for a 24-hour period. Longer therapy, up to 72 hours, can be used if the deep vein thrombosis of an extremity is also being addressed. For *urokinase*, a loading dose of 4,400 U per kilogram is administered over 10 minutes, which is then followed by a maintenance infusion of 4,400 U per kilogram per hour for 12 hours. Since most of the lysis of pulmonary emboli takes place within the first few hours of therapy, current interest is in investigating treatment of shorter duration in which higher doses are used, much like that used for acute myocardial infarction. For *t-PA*, 100 mg given intravenously over 2 hours has been used, although precise dosage regimens need to be clarified; similar studies are being carried out with urokinase and streptokinase.

The classical indication for the use of thrombolytic agents is "massive" pulmonary embolism defined as embolism resulting in (1) angiographic evidence of occlusion of greater than or equal to 40 percent of the pulmonary vasculature; (2) hypotension with systolic pressure less than 90 mm Hg; and (3) syncope. Thrombolytic agents are much more effective than heparin in addressing these acute hemodynamic abnormalities. Some clinicians, including ourselves, also consider thrombolytic therapy for patients with less extensive pulmonary embolism, especially those with pre-existing significant underlying heart or lung disease. This view is based on the findings of residual anatomic and physiologic abnormalities in cases treated with anticoagulants alone.

Thrombolytic agents work best on fresh clots; if there has not been a delay in initiating therapy, this is not an important issue, since the onset is usually acute and symptomatic. For minimizing bleeding complications, important considerations include patient selection, avoidance of nonessential invasive procedures, and attention to contraindications. Absolute contraindications include active bleeding lesions; history of active intracranial disease, such as tumor or cerebrovascular accident (CVA) or arteriovenous (AV) malformations; and severe uncontrolled hypertension (e.g., diastolic blood pressures >110 mm Hg). Relative contraindications include pregnancy (only because of lack of experience with such patients); deep closed biopsy within 10 days; general surgical procedures within 7 to 10 days; and other contraindications to anticoagulation such as the presence of bleeding disorder, uremia, and liver failure.

While the patient is receiving thrombolytic agents, procedures such as multiple blood gas analysis and placement of lines should be avoided since there will be bleeding from these iatrogenic wounds. For the initial blood gas analysis, puncture of the radial artery rather than the femoral artery is recommended because hemostasis can be more readily accomplished with pressure dressings.

If the patient has undergone pulmonary angiography and the catheter is in place, lytic therapy can be given through it. However, although this allows for a repeat angiogram, it actually offers no added efficacy compared with peripheral intravenous infusion. Separate catheter placement merely for local drug administration should be avoided.

Before therapy is initiated, baseline hemoglobin and coagulation studies should be obtained. Our preference is plasma fibrinogen to monitor the lytic state, and the APTT for eventual change-over to heparin. If streptokinase is the agent employed, hydrocortisone sodium succinate in a dose of 100 mg or its equivalent is given intravenously, and this reduces the incidence of febrile and allergic reactions to less than 5 percent. After the sustaining infusion has been in place for 2 to 4 hours, fibrinogen is again checked as an indicator of the presence of a plasma thrombolytic state. With streptokinase, the plasma fibrinogen should be decreased significantly, often to far less than 50 percent of pretreatment levels. Lesser degrees of hypofibrinogenemia, on the order of a 25 percent, are seen with urokinase and t-PA. Once the presence of a plasma thrombolytic state is demonstrated, therapy should continue at standard doses for the previously noted treatment period. No titration of dosage is required since, in contrast to heparin therapy, studies have shown that neither the efficacy nor the toxicity of thrombolytic therapy are affected by attempts to target specific levels of change in coagulation parameters. After completion of the thrombolytic infusion, after a waiting period of 3 to 4 hours, coagulation tests are repeated. If the APTT remains elevated within heparin's therapeutic range, 1.5 to 2.5 times the baseline, a sustaining infusion of heparin, without a loading dose, is started and maintained. If the APTT exceeds 2.5 times that of the control, one should wait another 2 to 3 hours, repeat the APTT, and as soon as it is in the therapeutic range for heparin, start heparin as described above. If the APTT is less than 1.5 times that of the control, a small bolus of heparin is given followed by a sustaining infusion. Heparin and oral anticoagulants should then be administered as described above.

Pulmonary Embolectomy

With the advent of thrombolytic therapy, there has been very little need for pulmonary embolectomy. Currently, those patients for whom this heroic procedure is indicated include: (1) those in total collapse and who will die quickly unless there is immediate relief; (2) those in persistent shock with massive embolism and in whom thrombolytic therapy is contraindicated; and (3) those in persistent shock who are unresponsive to 4 hours of thrombolytic therapy. When pulmonary embolectomy is indicated, excessive delay to the point of a cardiovascular collapse has been reported to result in a mortality rate of more than 90 percent. In experienced hands, however, properly timed embolectomy in critically ill patients can be expected to be associated with a 50 percent survival rate.

SUGGESTED READING

Sherry S, Bell WR, Duckert FH, et al. Thrombolytic therapy in thrombosis: a National Institute of Health consensus Development Conference. Ann Intern Med 1980; 93:141–144.

Greenfield, LJ. Current indications for and results of Greenfield filter placement. J Vasc Surg 1984; 1:502–504.

Wilson J, Lampman J. Heparin therapy: a randomized prospective study. Am Heart J 1979; 97:155–158.

Sharma GV, Cella G, Parisis AF, et al. Thrombolytic therapy. N Engl J Med 1982; 306:1267–1274.

ACUTE MYOPERICARDITIS

ROBERT E. CUNNION, M.D.

In approaching a patient with suspected myopericarditis, it is useful to decide whether the inflammatory process involves predominantly the pericardium, the myocardium, or a combination of the two (Table 1). The symptoms and signs of pericarditis, which may be either constant or intermittent, usually include pleuritic precordial pain, fever, and a pericardial friction rub. Characteristically, the leukocyte count and the erythrocyte sedimentation rate (ESR) are elevated, and in many cases a pericardial effusion is demonstrable on the echocardiogram or suggested by the chest film. Pericarditis frequently occurs alone, without concomitant clinically overt myocarditis. When pericarditis is accompanied by superficial myocarditis (epicarditis), rhythm disturbances and electrocardiographic changes may be seen: classically, ST-segment elevation, followed within a few days by T-wave inversion. Myocarditis, while often subclinical, may become apparent when nonspecific signs of inflammation are accompanied by recent-onset conges-

Table 1 Clinical Features of Pericarditis and Myocarditis

Diagnostic Category	Common Findings
Pericarditis	Pleuritic chest pain Fever Pericardial friction rub Leukocytosis Elevated ESR Pericardial thickening or effusion on echocardiogram
Pericarditis and superficial myocarditis (epicarditis)	All of the above, plus: Electrocardiographic abnormalities Arrhythmias
Pericarditis with diffuse myocarditis	All of the above, plus: Congestive heart failure Evidence of impaired systolic function on echocardiogram or radionuclide gated blood pool scan Conduction disturbances Systemic emboli Myocardial uptake on gallium scan Leukocytic infiltration of the myocardium or myocardial immunoglobulin deposition on endomyocardial biopsy

tive heart failure, ventricular arrhythmias, atrioventricular fascicular conduction abnormalities, or systemic emboli. Clinical myocarditis is usually acute in onset and typically occurs in the setting of a recent viral syndrome. Myocarditis can also be chronic; histologic myocarditis has been reported in a subpopulation (recent estimates ranging from 4 percent to 15 percent) of patients with dilated cardiomyopathy (see chapter on Dilated Cardiomyopathy). However, myocarditis remains a poorly understood disease in the sense that its clinical diagnosis correlates poorly with its histologic diagnosis, and it is often unclear which, if either, to rely upon. Furthermore, even though consensus does exist regarding conventional therapy of myocarditis (directed at palliation of symptoms), there is longstanding controversy regarding the use of immunosuppressive therapy (directed at the presumed etiologic mechanism). The histologic distinction between active inflammatory myocarditis and idiopathic dilated cardiomyopathy may prove to be an important one if controlled studies currently in progress prove that immunosuppressive therapy is beneficial.

DIAGNOSIS OF PERICARDITIS

Idiopathic inflammatory pericarditis is typically a benign, self-limited disease process. Many patients report an antecedent upper respiratory infection (commonly due to an influenza virus or an enterovirus), and some patients have an influenza-like syndrome of fever, malaise, and myalgias concomitant with pericarditis. Acute pericarditis may present with or without effusions; the most common lesion is fibrinous inflammation without clinically recognizable fluid. Only a minority of patients will develop large effusions or tamponade. Although symptoms may be absent, acute pericarditis is usually heralded by anterior chest pain, which is usually sharp and sudden in onset. The pain is distinguished from that of angina pectoris by its prolonged duration, pleuritic quality, and absence of association with effort. The pathognomonic physical sign, the pericardial friction rub, may wax and wane but is usually detectable if sought carefully. When the history and physical examination are diagnostic, echocardiography is probably not routinely needed. Pericarditis can have several serious complications that should be kept in mind: tamponade, severe debilitating chest pain, and the late development of constrictive pericarditis (especially in patients with recurrent bouts of pericardial inflammation). Atrial fibrillation or flutter occurs in 5 percent to 10 percent of patients.

Although inflammation of the pericardium usually is idiopathic, it can be caused by a wide variety of identifiable processes: infections, neoplasms, renal failure, the postcardiac injury syndrome, collagen-vascular disease, hypothyroidism, and drug hypersensitivity reactions (especially to procainamide and hydralazine). It is important to identify such processes because specific therapies are available.

TREATMENT OF PERICARDITIS

A general approach to treatment of pericarditis is outlined in Table 2. Initial therapy depends on the clinical stage of the disease and the severity of symptoms. Many patients with acute pericarditis have only a 1- to 3-day bout of mild chest pain; in such episodes, it is reasonable to give no therapy and to allow the process to subside by itself.

Ibuprofen. If symptoms are prolonged or moderately severe, the nonsteroidal anti-inflammatory agent ibuprofen (400 to 600 mg orally every 6 to 8 hours) may decrease fever and relieve chest pain, or at least decrease pain to a tolerable level. Most patients who are going to benefit from ibuprofen note alleviation of their symptoms within 48 hours. Some clinicians prefer aspirin over ibuprofen, but aspirin causes protracted impairment of platelet function and is best avoided in critically ill patients. If therapy with ibuprofen is successful, a 2-week course should be given to minimize the chance of recurrence of symptoms when therapy is stopped.

Indomethacin. Patients who do not respond to ibuprofen adequately within 48 hours should be given indomethacin, starting at a dose of 25 to 50 mg orally every 8 hours. Although indomethacin has more side effects than ibuprofen, it appears to have superior analgesic and anti-inflammatory efficacy. In addition to ameliorating fever and chest pain, indomethacin often decreases the ESR and reduces the amount of pericardial fluid. Many patients obtain relief after the first few doses, but several

Table 2 Therapy for Inflammatory Pericarditis

Manifestation	Treatment Regimen
Uncomplicated pericarditis	Ibuprofen, 500–600 mg PO q6h–q8h for 48 hours; if effective, continue for 2 weeks If ibuprofen ineffective: indomethacin, 25–50 mg PO q8h Avoid anticoagulants if possible
Atrial arrhythmias	Antiarrhythmics (digoxin, verapamil, beta blockers, and/or type Ia agents) Indomethacin, 25–50 mg PO q8h If antiarrhythmics and indomethacin ineffective: prednisone, 60 mg PO daily for 5–7 days, then taper
Severe unresponsive chest pain	Prednisone, 60 mg PO daily for 5–7 days, then taper
Pericardial tamponade	Percutaneous or surgical drainage Prednisone, 60 mg PO daily for 5–7 days, then taper

days may be needed before the full effect is seen. If effective, therapy should be continued for 2 weeks to prevent recurrences.

Most patients taking indomethacin retain sodium and water, which may precipitate or exacerbate congestive heart failure. Patients should be examined frequently and weighed daily. Other side effects include headache, dysphoria, and gastrointestinal intolerance, which can be minimized by giving indomethacin with food or antacids. Both ibuprofen and indomethacin inhibit platelet aggregation and prolong the bleeding time. In patients who are already receiving heparin or warfarin, this platelet inhibition could result in generalized bleeding or bleeding into the inflamed pericardial sac. In general, anticoagulant therapy is relatively contraindicated in patients with idiopathic pericarditis. Warfarin and heparin should be withheld except in the presence of strong indications (e.g., pulmonary embolism). In patients with idiopathic pericarditis who are not receiving anticoagulants, ibuprofen and indomethacin do not appear to increase the incidence of hemorrhage into the pericardium. If ibuprofen and indomethacin must be administered to patients who are receiving warfarin or heparin, then the prothrombin time or partial thromboplastin time should be maintained carefully in a low therapeutic range.

Indomethacin should be considered as initial therapy for patients whose pericarditis is accompanied by epicarditis with atrial arrhythmias; its anti-inflammatory potency can help to prevent further atrial arrhythmias. The atrial arrhythmias should also be treated with appropriate antiarrhythmic agents such as digitalis, verapamil, beta-blockers, and/or type Ia agents.

Corticosteroids. Corticosteroids are highly effective in controlling the manifestations of pericarditis, but there is anecdotal evidence that the use of corticosteroids as initial empiric therapy for pericarditis increases the likelihood of subsequent relapse. Further, corticosteroids have potentially serious side effects and therefore should be reserved for the following indications: (1) severe, persistent, debilitating chest pain that has been unresponsive to nonsteroidal agents, (2) arrhythmias that are refractory to indomethacin and antiarrhythmic therapy, and (3) pericarditis with pericardial tamponade. Corticosteroid therapy usually produces rapid relief of pain, a decrease in the ESR, and resorption of pericardial fluid; however, occasional failures do occur. Corticosteroids also can correct arrhythmias that have been refractory to antiarrhythmic agents and other less potent anti-inflammatory drugs; this probably is attributable to abolition of arrhythmogenic foci of inflammation in the epicardium.

When indicated, prednisone, the corticosteroid of choice, should be started at an oral dose of 60 mg daily for 5 to 7 days. If rapid relief of symptoms occurs, prednisone can be tapered by 5 to 10 mg per day so that the course of therapy lasts approximately 2 weeks. Such a short course does not produce suppression of the pituitary-adrenal axis, so that the patient will not require coverage with corticosteroids for future episodes of physiologic stress. However, a 2-week course sometimes is insufficient to control pericarditis, and exacerbations may occur during steroid withdrawal. If these exacerbations are mild, they may be controlled with indomethacin, but a significant recrudescence of symptoms necessitates reinstitution of prednisone therapy in higher daily doses. Under these circumstances, the prednisone should be tapered slowly to an alternate-day regimen. Once the dosage of 60 mg every other day is achieved, the alternate-day regimen can be maintained for several months if necessary, with fewer side effects than from daily doses of corticosteroids. Eventually, the alternate-day regimen can be tapered by 5-mg decrements every other day, while one observes carefully for evidence of relapse. Indomethacin can sometimes be used on the "off" day to keep symptoms under control.

Recurrences

A recurrence of pericarditis should prompt the clinician to reconsider the possibility of an occult systemic connective tissue disease. If the recurrence remains idiopathic, it should be treated in the same manner as the first episode. In general, therapies that have been successful in the past should be reinstituted. However, if one can substitute a nonsteroidal agent for prednisone therapy, then the side effects of corticosteroids can be avoided. An occasional patient may have recurrent bouts of pericarditis refractory to long courses of corticosteroids. Pericardiectomy is sometimes efficacious; however, cases of recurrent pericarditis after total pericardiectomy have been reported and presumably result from visceral pericarditis. A few of these patients have been controlled successfully with cytotoxic therapy (cyclophosphamide or azathioprine at 1 to 2 mg per kg body weight per day).

Specific Pericarditides

Other forms of pericarditis may require specific therapies. Purulent pericarditis (which usually occurs in association with endocarditis, bacteremia, or contiguous intrathoracic infection) is fatal unless recognized and treated with appropriate antibiotics and surgical drainage. Uremic pericarditis usually responds to intensified dialysis; if possible, dialysis should be performed with regional heparinization to minimize the risk of intrapericardial hemorrhage. Malignant pericarditis may respond to appropriate chemotherapy or radiotherapy; recurring malignant pericardial effusions sometimes can be ameliorated by intrapericardial instillation of sclerosing agents, but often pericardiectomy becomes necessary. Tuberculous pericarditis requires antimicrobial chemotherapy and often leads to pericardiectomy. The postcardiac injury syndrome (a term encompassing postpericardiotomy syndrome, postmyocardial infarction syndrome, and postcardiac trauma syndrome) is treated in much the same way as idiopathic inflammatory pericarditis. Particular attention should be paid to surveillance for tamponade, avoidance of anticoagulation, and careful exclusion of conditions such as pulmonary embolism and coronary ischemia, which may cause symptoms mimicking postcardiac injury syndrome.

DIAGNOSIS OF MYOCARDITIS

The clinical presentation of myocarditis ranges from a benign self-limited illness, in which neither congestive heart failure nor important arrhythmias develop, to a serious illness, in which life-threatening derangements occur. Patients in the latter group frequently find their way to critical care units. Serious myocarditis is manifested most commonly as unexplained congestive heart failure. Causes of heart failure such as ischemic, hypertensive, or valvular disease should be excluded before arriving at a presumptive diagnosis of myocarditis. The cause of myocarditis usually is not discernible, despite exhaustive evaluation. On the basis of epidemiologic findings and serologic tests, these bouts of myocarditis often are presumed to be sequelae of viral infection.

Several lines of evidence suggest that myocarditis has an immune pathogenesis: (1) Myocarditis often is associated with signs of inflammation and immune abnormalities (elevated ESR, leukocytosis, and circulating antimyocardial antibodies), (2) bouts recur in many individuals, suggesting recrudescence of a hypersensitivity phenomenon, (3) endomyocardial biopsy specimens from these patients sometimes show leukocytic infiltration or immunoglobulin deposition, and (4) empiric treatment with immunosuppressive drugs has been associated in some cases with clinical improvement.

Nonetheless, a strong argument can be made that endomyocardial biopsy should not be performed routinely, outside of a research context, for clinically suspected myocarditis. Establishing a histologic diagnosis of myocarditis conveys no clearcut therapeutic or prognostic implications, and endomyocardial biopsy carries risks. Even though a theoretical rationale exists for immunosuppressive therapy, benefit from immunosuppression has not been shown in controlled clinical trials, and in some animal models immunosuppression exacerbates myocarditis. Accordingly, in suspected myocarditis endomyocardial biopsy should be restricted to two settings: (1) when the clinician needs to exclude infiltrative cardiomyopathies such as amyloidosis; and (2) when the clinician has decided beforehand that if histologic myocarditis is found, the patient will be given empiric immunosuppression, in spite of its unproven efficacy, or will be enrolled in a randomized clinical trial.

Radioisotope imaging of the heart with gallium-67 has been advocated as an initial noninvasive screening test for myocardial inflammation. It has not proved specific, but some investigators believe that a positive gallium scan may enhance the likelihood that a subsequent endomyocardial biopsy will reveal inflammation. Whether or not controlled studies eventually establish a role for endomyocardial biopsies in the management of myocarditis, they clearly are useful in evaluating transplant rejection, anthracycline cardiotoxicity, amyloidosis, sarcoidosis, hemochromatosis, and cardiac hypereosinophilia, and for excluding myocardial disease prior to pericardiectomy in patients with restrictive hemodynamic findings.

TREATMENT OF MYOCARDITIS

Conventional Treatment

Conventional treatment of myocarditis is directed at palliation of congestive heart failure, suppression of arrhythmias, and prevention of embolic complications (Table 3). Patients with myocarditis should be kept at bed rest during the acute phase of the illness; strenuous physical exercise has been shown to exacerbate the severity of acute myocarditis in experimental animals. For congestive heart failure, diuretics are the main pharmacologic therapy. Digoxin is administered almost universally to patients with dilated cardiomyopathy, although (in sinus rhythm) most evidence suggests that its effect on contractility is only modest. Vasodilator agents are often beneficial.

Even though controlled studies of the efficacy of prophylactic anticoagulation in these patients have not been conducted, warfarin certainly should be administered in any of the following situations: (1) if left ventricular thrombus is seen on echocardiography, (2) if the patient is in atrial fibrillation, or (3) if the patient has had systemic embolic events. Anticoagulants should be withheld when pericarditis coexists, to minimize the risk of hemorrhage into the pericardium. Symptomatic ventricular tachycardia mandates treatment with antiarrhythmic agents (see Table 3). Asymptomatic ventricular tachycardia probably should be treated if runs of 30 or more consecutive beats are documented. Even though patients with shorter runs of

Table 3 Therapy for Myocarditis

Manifestation	Treatment Regimen
Congestive heart failure	Bedrest Diuretics Digitalis Vasodilators
Atrial arrhythmias	If unstable, electrical cardioversion Digoxin If necessary for rate control, verapamil or beta blockers (may exacerbate congestive heart failure) For pharmacologic cardioversion, type Ia or Ic agents If refractory to pharmacologic therapy, elective electrical cardioversion
Symptomatic or sustained ventricular arrhythmias	If unstable, electrical cardioversion Acutely, IV lidocaine, procainamide, or bretylium Chronically, PO procainamide, quinidine, encainide, or amiodarone
Intracardiac thrombus; clinical embolism; atrial fibrillation	Acutely, IV heparin Chronically, PO warfarin
Worsening congestive heart failure (despite intensive conventional therapy) or cardiogenic shock	Parenteral inotropic agents (dobutamine and/or amrinone) Consider mechanical circulatory support (intra-aortic balloon counterpulsation and/or left-ventricular assist device) Consider cardiac transplantation (?) Immunosuppressive agents

asymptomatic ventricular tachycardia conceivably could benefit from the administration of antiarrhythmic drugs, it should be borne in mind that these drugs also can induce or aggravate arrhythmias and that no evidence exists that antiarrhythmic drugs can decrease the incidence of sudden death in patients without symptomatic arrhythmias.

Acute myocarditis occasionally develops into a fulminant disease marked by intractable pulmonary edema or cardiogenic shock. As a general rule, myocarditis should always be regarded as a potentially reversible condition, since spontaneous remissions are common. These patients warrant a very aggressive management approach, sometimes necessitating high-dose inotropic agents, intra-aortic balloon counterpulsation, and even insertion of left-ventricular assist devices. If heart failure is intractable and a donor organ can be located, transplantation carries an 85 percent prognosis for 1-year survival.

Immunosuppressive Agents

The efficacy of immunosuppressive therapy in myocarditis is unresolved, although many clinicians have adopted the view that such therapy is helpful. A number of small, uncontrolled series have shown that corticosteroids alone or corticosteroids with azathioprine can decrease signs of myocardial inflammation and improve ventricular function. One difficulty in evaluating these series lies in the highly variable natural history of acute myocarditis; there is evidence that most adult patients recover spontaneously. Another difficulty with these anecdotal reports is the lack, until recently, of standardized histologic criteria for the diagnosis of myocarditis in endomyocardial biopsy specimens.

Currently underway is the Myocarditis Treatment Trial, a randomized controlled study designed to assess an immunosuppressive regimen of cyclosporine and low-dose prednisone in patients meeting the "Dallas Criteria" for myocarditis (i.e., unequivocal leukocytic infiltration and myocyte necrosis on endomyocardial biopsy). Pending the outcome of the Myocarditis Treatment Trial, the routine use of immunosuppressive therapy, even for patients with histologically documented myocarditis, cannot yet be endorsed. If a patient is potentially a candidate for cardiac transplantation, the clinician should take into account that many centers are reluctant to transplant chronically immunosuppressed patients.

Immunosuppressive therapy is reasonable as a last resource for a patient with histologically proven myocarditis, progressive worsening of heart function despite intensive conventional therapy, and contraindications to transplantation. The choice of immunosuppressive regimen is problematic, and explicit recommendations are impossible. Daily doses of prednisone, administered in a controlled trial for dilated cardiomyopathy, produced improvements in ventricular function that were only modest in magnitude and that disappeared when prednisone was tapered to an alternate-day schedule. Cyclosporine is widely given to prevent transplant rejection, but there is very little experience with cyclosporine for myocarditis, even though it was chosen for use in the Myocarditis Treatment Trial. Most published cases of immunosuppression for myocarditis have involved a combination of azathioprine (typically 2 mg per kg body weight per day) and corticosteroids (in varying dosages and durations). Azathioprine must be used carefully; it produces leukopenia and can cause hepatitis. Daily blood counts should be performed during the first few weeks of therapy, with appropriate adjustments in dosage. In general, changes in leukocyte counts lag 7 to 10 days behind dosage adjustments, and the total leukocyte count and absolute neutrophil count should be maintained above 3,000 and 2,000 per cu mm, respectively.

If immunosuppressive therapy is to be given, baseline ventricular size and function should be assessed by echocardiography and/or radionuclide gated blood pool scanning. Serial measurements of ventricular size and function, together with serial endomyocardial biopsies, can then be performed to gauge response to therapy. It is reasonable to obtain the first set of follow-up studies 6 to 8 weeks into therapy; if no evidence of improvement is seen, immunosuppression may be assumed to be ineffective and should be discontinued. If the patient has improved, follow-up studies can be obtained at 3-month intervals and efforts made to withdraw immunosuppression after 6 to 12 months of therapy.

SUGGESTED READING

Aretz HT, Billingham ME, Edwards WE, et al. Myocarditis: a histopathologic definition and classification. Am J Cardiovasc Pathol 1986; 1:3–14.

Hawkins JW, Vacek JL. What constitutes definitive therapy of malignant pericardial effusion? "Medical" versus surgical treatment. Am Heart J 1989; 118:428–432.

Lie JT. Myocarditis and endomyocardial biopsy in unexplained heart failure: a diagnosis in search of a disease. Ann Intern Med 1988; 109:525–528.

Mason JW, O'Connell JB. Clinical merit of endomyocardial biopsy. Circulation 1989; 79:971–979.

Spodick DH. The normal and diseased pericardium: current concepts of pericardial physiology, diagnosis and treatment. J Am Coll Cardiol 1983; 1:240–251.

DILATED CARDIOMYOPATHY

ROBERT E. CUNNION, M.D.

Dilated cardiomyopathies are diseases of the ventricular myocardium that result in chamber dilatation and diminished contractility. The usual presenting symptoms are exertional dyspnea and fatigue, although occasionally the first manifestation is an arrhythmia or an arterial embolism. Some patients, despite severely depressed left ventricular function, have well-preserved exercise tolerance, so that dilated cardiomyopathy is occasionally discovered incidentally in an asymptomatic patient. The prognosis of dilated cardiomyopathy is variable. Some patients pursue a relentless downhill course leading to transplantation or death in weeks to months, while others live for years without progression of symptoms; rarely, a patient may spontaneously recover normal ventricular function. Approximately one half of deaths are sudden and one half are due to progressive congestive heart failure.

It is important clinically to distinguish dilated cardiomyopathy (in which left and right ventricular contractility are reduced, ventricular wall thicknesses are normal, and ventricular cavity sizes are increased) from hypertrophic cardiomyopathy (in which left ventricular contractility is normal or increased, the left ventricular walls are very thick, and left ventricular cavity size is normal or reduced) and from restrictive cardiomyopathy (in which left and right ventricular contractility are normal or mildly reduced, ventricular walls are moderately thick, and ventricular cavity sizes are usually normal). The signs and symptoms of dilated cardiomyopathy are primarily a result of systolic dysfunction, whereas those of hypertrophic and restrictive cardiomyopathies are primarily a result of diastolic dysfunction and are discussed in separate chapters.

The diagnosis of dilated cardiomyopathy is often assigned loosely both to primary cardiomyopathies, in which the pathologic process lies within the myocardium itself, and to secondary cardiomyopathies, in which myocardial dysfunction is the result of hypertensive, valvular, or coronary artery disease (Table 1). Here, dilated cardiomyopathy will refer only to patients with primary dilated cardiomyopathies, in whom secondary causes of cardiomyopathy have been excluded.

Some cases of dilated cardiomyopathy have discernible causes; the most prominent example is alcoholic cardiomyopathy. It is well established that some individuals, with even moderately heavy chronic alcohol use, are susceptible to development of biventricular dilatation and hypocontractility, and that abstinence from alcohol often leads to significant reduction in heart size and improvement in contractility. Another cause is anthracycline cardiomyopathy, which typically occurs in patients who have received large cumulative doses of adriamycin chemotherapy. Still another, less common example is the dilated cardiomyopathy of hemochromatosis, caused by iron deposition in the myocardium. This diagnosis can be inferred from serum iron studies and documented by endomyocardial biopsy; chelation therapy to remove iron can reverse myocardial dysfunction. Dilated cardiomyopathy appears with somewhat increased frequency in the third trimester of pregnancy and in the puerperium, but this so-called postpartum cardiomyopathy is not clearly distinguishable clinically from idiopathic dilated cardiomyopathy. Most cases of dilated cardiomyopathy do not have discernible causes. There are several lines of evidence suggesting that viral infections, particularly with Coxsackie B virus, can initiate an immune-mediated process that eventually leads to dilated cardiomyopathy. Unfortunately, by the time symptoms appear and dilated cardiomyopathy is diagnosed, it is almost always impossible to establish a specific etiologic diagnosis.

Patients with dilated cardiomyopathy often require management in critical care units for severe congestive

Table 1 Etiologies of Dilated Cardiomyopathy

Primary Dilated Cardiomyopathies
    Alcoholic cardiomyopathy
    Hemochromatosis
    Inflammatory cardiomyopathies (rheumatic myocarditis, viral myocarditis)
    Anthracycline cardiomyopathy
    Peripartum cardiomyopathy
    Idiopathic dilated cardiomyopathy

Secondary Causes of Dilated Cardiomyopathy
    Valvular lesions (severe aortic stenosis, aortic regurgitation, or mitral regurgitation)
    Coronary artery disease (ventricular aneurysm, chronic recurrent ischemia and infarction)
    Uncontrolled hypertension

heart failure, atrial and ventricular arrhythmias, or pulmonary or systemic emboli. In addition, an occasional patient may require monitoring for suspected myocardial infarction. Even though most dilated cardiomyopathy patients do not have significant coronary artery disease, approximately one fourth have atypical chest pain; the source of this pain is unclear but may be related to spasm of the small vessels or to abnormal coronary vasodilator reserve.

DIAGNOSIS OF DILATED CARDIOMYOPATHY

In the initial approach to the patient, it is important to consider the differential diagnosis of potentially treatable conditions that can resemble idiopathic dilated cardiomyopathy (Tables 1 and 2). Left ventricular pressure overload, due to severe aortic stenosis, and left ventricular volume overload, due to severe aortic or mitral regurgitation, can present clinically with ventricular enlargement and systolic impairment. The pathognomonic cardiac murmurs and other physical findings may be masked by severe heart failure; therefore, as a general rule, all patients with newly diagnosed heart failure should undergo echocardiography.

Because of severe generalized ischemia and multiple infarctions, some patients with advanced coronary artery disease have dilated, globally hypocontractile hearts that may be confused with those in idiopathic dilated cardiomyopathy. Others may have large ventricular aneurysms, caused by prior myocardial infarctions, that have resulted in heart failure. In patients with heart failure, if the history is ambiguous concerning prior myocardial infarction, the existence of coronary artery disease can usually be inferred from echocardiography. Patients with coronary artery disease typically have regional left ventricular wall motion abnormalities, rather than the global ventricular hypocontractility characteristic of idiopathic dilated cardiomyopathy. Some of these patients may benefit from transluminal coronary angioplasty, surgical revascularization, or aneurysmectomy. Left-sided cardiac catheterization and coronary arteriography need not be performed in every patient with dilated cardiomyopathy, but patients should be studied if they have chest pain syndromes, multiple risk factors for atherosclerosis, electrocardiographic infarct patterns, or echocardiographic regional wall motion abnormalities.

Severe, longstanding hypertension in its end stages can cause ventricular dilatation and diminished contractility. This can readily be differentiated from idiopathic dilated cardiomyopathy by history and by the finding of thickened ventricular walls on echocardiography. End-stage hypertensive cardiomyopathy usually cures hypertension, but the administration of vasodilators may produce dramatic improvement in ventricular function.

Right-sided cardiac catheterization and thermodilution measurement of cardiac output yield valuable diagnostic, therapeutic and prognostic data in dilated cardiomyopathy and should be performed in all newly diagnosed

Table 2 Diagnostic Evaluation of Dilated Cardiomyopathy

In All Patients
  History
    Alcohol use
    Recent viral syndrome
    Rheumatic fever
    Coronary artery disease
    Hypertension
    Family history of cardiomyopathy
    Geographic exposure (Chagas' disease)
  Physical examination
    Blood pressure
    Cardiac murmurs or gallops
    Signs of heart failure
    Pericardial rub
  Laboratory studies
    Routine chemistries
    Iron and iron-binding capacity
    Thyroid function tests
  Electrocardiogram
    Rhythm disturbances
    Conduction disturbances
    Chamber hypertrophy or enlargement
    Pseudoinfarction pattern
  Chest film
    Pulmonary vascularity
    Chamber enlargement
  Echocardiography
    Chamber sizes
    Left and right ventricular contractility
    Valvular structure and movement
    Pericardial effusion
    Intracardiac thrombus
  Right-sided cardiac catheterization and measurement of cardiac output

In Selected Patients
  Radionuclide ventriculography, when precise assessment of left ventricular ejection fraction is needed
  Left-sided heart catheterization with coronary arteriography, to exclude coronary artery disease when suspicion exists
  Transvenous endomyocardial biopsy, to exclude infiltrative cardiomyopathies (e.g., amyloidosis) when suspicion exists

patients. Some right-sided cardiac catheterizations will unexpectedly reveal a restrictive profile of filling pressures and alert the clinician to the presence of an infiltrative cardiomyopathy or a constrictive pericardial process. In the therapy of dilated cardiomyopathy, since symptoms and physical findings do not consistently correlate well with invasively measured filling pressures, right-sided cardiac catheterization is very useful in deciding the initial aggressiveness of diuretic and vasodilator therapies. Prognostically, multivariate analyses have consistently shown right atrial pressure and pulmonary artery wedge pressure to be among the most reliable factors in predicting which patients will die or will require heart transplantation.

Radionuclide ventriculograms can be obtained if there is a need for precise quantitation of left ventricular ejection fraction—e.g., if a new therapy is being started and serial measurements of ejection fraction will be used to guide therapy. However, in most patients, estimation of ejection fraction from the echocardiogram is sufficient for all practical purposes, and radionuclide ventriculography is unnecessary.

Acute myocarditis may be suspected clinically in the patient with recent-onset heart failure of unknown cause, particularly when associated with pericarditis or a recent viral prodrome. Although it is tempting to use clinical criteria as a basis for diagnosing myocarditis, many patients with clinical myocarditis do not have histologic myocarditis on endomyocardial biopsy, and vice versa. At present, the routine use of endomyocardial biopsy cannot be recommended for acute or chronic dilated cardiomyopathy for two reasons: (1) Although some cases of myocarditis may respond favorably to immunosuppressive therapy, no randomized, controlled study has yet proved that such therapy is beneficial. (2) Even if immunosuppressive therapy were proven beneficial, the prevalence of myocarditis among patients with dilated cardiomyopathy has been consistently low (no more than 15 percent) when strict diagnostic criteria for histologic myocarditis are applied.

MANAGEMENT OF DILATED CARDIOMYOPATHY

Treatment of Heart Failure

Initial Approach in the Critical Care Unit. If a patient with dilated cardiomyopathy has heart failure severe enough to require management in a critical care unit, then an aggressive approach is clearly warranted. Invasive hemodynamic monitoring should not delay initiation of therapy, but a radial artery catheter should be placed for continuous blood pressure monitoring and serial blood gas analysis; a thermodilution pulmonary artery catheter helps to eliminate guesswork. Parenteral medications are often needed initially, but a transition to oral agents should be made as soon as possible. Although acute hemodynamic responses to diuretics and vasodilators are not absolutely predictive of chronic responses, it is reasonable to titrate the initial oral regimen to an optimal hemodynamic response while the pulmonary artery catheter is still in place.

Diuretic Therapy. The initial therapy for severe heart failure, in the absence of hypotension, is to give 40 mg of furosemide intravenously; if the patient has previously required higher doses, more than 40 mg can be given. Furosemide produces a transient direct reduction in afterload, and the diuretic action of furosemide reduces preload, thereby relieving pulmonary congestion and improving oxygenation. Intravenous furosemide usually triggers copious urine output within 30 to 45 minutes, and its diuretic effects persist for several hours. Failure to effect a prompt diuresis in the face of persistent pulmonary edema warrants repeated bolus injections of higher doses of furosemide until a response becomes apparent. Its kaliuretic effects necessitate careful surveillance and supplementation of serum potassium. Once stabilized, the patient should be treated with appropriate doses of oral furosemide, typically 40 mg daily. Bumetanide and ethacrynic acid may be used in place of furosemide; metolazone (5 to 10 mg orally) will often produce a diuretic effect even in patients with renal insufficiency who are refractory to furosemide. The thiazide and potassium-sparing diuretic agents do not have a principal role in acute therapy of heart failure, although they are useful chronically in the management of mild heart failure. A more detailed discussion of this subject is given elsewhere in this text.

Digoxin Therapy. When patients with dilated cardiomyopathy present in sinus rhythm with severe heart failure, there is no compelling reason to administer digoxin immediately. However, when rapid atrial fibrillation is present, parenteral digoxin is indicated to control the ventricular response rate. Although the role of digoxin in chronic heart failure has been a subject of controversy, several recent studies document its efficacy in increasing left ventricular ejection fraction (albeit modestly) and in ameliorating symptoms (at least in some patients). When digoxin is used, the serum potassium level should be maintained above 4 mg per dl and the serum digoxin level should be assayed periodically. A discussion of dosing regimens and side effects is given elsewhere in this text.

Vasodilator Therapy. The goals of vasodilator therapy are to improve cardiac output by reducing unnecessarily high levels of afterload and to reduce elevated filling pressures and thereby relieve pulmonary congestion. The use of vasodilator agents in patients with dilated cardiomyopathy and other forms of heart failure has yielded substantial benefits, both acutely and chronically. When a patient is admitted to a critical care unit with severe heart failure, the administration of nitroprusside, a balanced arterial and venous vasodilator, can result in dramatic relief of symptoms and improved hemodynamics. Before nitroprusside is started, the patient should have a mean arterial pressure of at least 60 mm Hg or a systolic blood pressure of at least 90 mm Hg, and an arterial catheter should be in place for continuous arterial pressure monitoring. In addition, a thermodilution pulmonary artery catheter is almost essential in this setting. Once the baseline pulmonary artery wedge pressure, cardiac output, and arterial blood gases have been measured, nitroprusside can be started intravenously at 20 μg per minute. The infusion can be gradually increased every few minutes until the pulmonary artery wedge pressure falls to 15 mm Hg. Great caution must be exercised to avoid decreasing the mean arterial pressure to less than 55 mm Hg. Should excessive hypotension occur, the nitroprusside drip can be discontinued, and its hypotensive effects will disappear within 5 to 10 minutes. However, as a precaution, another intravenous access site should be available to infuse normal saline should the need arise. An adverse effect of prolonged high-dose nitroprusside therapy is cyanide toxicity; symptoms include weakness, nausea, confusion, and psychosis, and are usually associated with a metabolic acidosis, an increased mixed venous oxygen saturation, and an elevated thiocyanate level. Accordingly, it is important to taper the nitroprusside and to begin therapy with an oral vasodilator drug as soon as the patient is stable. Other available parenteral afterload-reducing agents (such as hydralazine and enalapril) generally have no advantages over nitroprusside for treatment of heart failure in the critical care unit. Parenteral nitroglycerin, a predominantly venous vasodilator, is useful if cardiac output is normal but filling pressures are high.

Among the multitude of oral vasodilators, angiotensin-converting enzyme inhibitors (e.g., captopril) have two advantages: (1) Like nitroprusside, they are balanced vasodilators, exerting effects on both resistance and capacitance vessels. (2) In the chronic management of patients with heart failure they have been shown to produce sustained improvement in exercise tolerance and functional class, and, more importantly, to reduce mortality. Captopril should be started cautiously, at a dose of 6.25 or 12.5 mg orally every 6 to 8 hours and increased, if tolerated, to 25 to 50 mg orally every 6 to 8 hours. The maximal hemodynamic response to captopril usually occurs within 2 hours; should hypotension occur, it usually can be reversed with intravenous normal saline. After angiotensin-converting enzyme inhibitors, the second choice in oral therapy is with a combination of isosorbide dinitrate (20 to 40 mg orally every 6 hours) and hydralazine (50 to 100 mg orally every 6 hours). These agents should be started in low doses and then titrated upward to obtain the desired hemodynamic response. A more detailed discussion is given elsewhere in this text.

Therapy with Inotropic Agents. If a patient with dilated cardiomyopathy is receiving appropriate diuretic and vasodilator agents but remains dyspneic or has a persistent low cardiac output syndrome, then dobutamine should be given. A continuous infusion is started at 5 mcg per kg body weight per minute and can be increased as required every 10 minutes to a maximum of 20 mcg per kg per minute. Once the desired cardiac output has been achieved, the dosage of vasodilator agents should be readjusted to maintain a pulmonary artery wedge pressure of 15 to 18 mm Hg. Once therapy with dobutamine is initiated, it usually is continued for 24 to 72 hours and then tapered off gradually. For patients with chronic dilated cardiomyopathy who are severely limited by their symptoms, the intermittent administration of 48- to 72-hour infusions of dobutamine sometimes produces symptomatic relief lasting as long as 4 to 6 weeks. Unfortunately, however, such intermittent infusions have failed to reduce mortality.

An alternative parenteral inotropic agent is the phosphodiesterase inhibitor amrinone, which can be used in place of or in addition to dobutamine. Relative to dobutamine, amrinone has the disadvantages of a relatively long half-life and a somewhat unpredictable hemodynamic effect. Digoxin remains the only proven oral inotropic agent, although clinical trials with new oral agents are ongoing.

Therapy of Shock. Patients with dilated cardiomyopathy who develop shock are difficult to manage and have an exceedingly poor prognosis. The most likely cause of shock in these patients, end-stage heart failure, is intractable, but other potentially reversible factors must be considered. Excessive diuretic or vasodilator therapy can reduce preload to a degree that compromises cardiac output. In such patients, the pulmonary artery wedge pressure will be low (usually below 10 mm Hg), and therapy should aim at increasing left ventricular preload by administering normal saline and by reducing vasodilator dosage. Also, shock creates a vicious circle in which hypoxia and acidosis can further depress myocardial contractility. Arterial blood gases should be monitored frequently and derangements corrected. Another potentially treatable etiology of shock in these patients is septic shock. Some may be at increased risk for infection because of immunosuppressive therapy, indwelling catheters, or general debility. If sepsis is suspected, empiric broad-spectrum antibiotic coverage should be initiated, and appropriate vasopressors should be administered.

For patients with cardiomyopathy and shock, the initial vasopressor of choice is dopamine, which is capable of augmenting myocardial contractility and cardiac output while causing moderate peripheral vasoconstriction. In addition, at low doses of 2 to 4 μg per kg body weight per minute, dopamine improves renal perfusion. The primary goal of vasopressor therapy in this setting is to raise the mean arterial pressure above 60 mm Hg. If the pulmonary artery wedge pressure is above 20 mm Hg and the arterial pressure has stabilized on dopamine, nitroprusside can be carefully added to maintain a pulmonary artery wedge pressure of 15 to 18 mm Hg.

If the arterial pressure remains below 60 mm Hg despite a dopamine infusion of 20 μg per kilogram per minute, then a more potent vasopressor agent is required. In this setting, norepinephrine should be started at 20 μg per minute and increased every few minutes until a mean arterial pressure of 60 mm Hg is restored. When norepinephrine is started, the dopamine infusion can be tapered to 2 μg per kilogram per minute to minimize norepinephrine-induced renal vasoconstriction.

Mechanical Circulatory Assist Devices. When cardiogenic shock or intractable pulmonary edema develops in a patient with dilated cardiomyopathy, pharmacologic interventions represent temporizing measures. Death will very likely occur unless some form of mechanical assistance is provided to the failing heart. Unlike the patient with coronary or valvular disease, the patient with dilated cardiomyopathy cannot hope to be helped by revascularization or valve replacement. Instead, the patient must hope to survive long enough with an intra-aortic balloon pump or a left ventricular assist device (e.g., a Thoratek pump) to receive a cardiac transplant. Insertion of such devices into patients who are not candidates for transplantation is unwarranted.

Role of Heart Transplantation. Heart transplantation should be considered when patients with dilated cardiomyopathy are severely limited by symptoms of heart failure despite optimal pharmacologic therapy with digoxin, diuretics, and vasodilators. Generally it is unwise to delay transplant referral until the patient is near death. More than one-half of patients undergoing heart transplantation in the United States have dilated cardiomyopathy as the cause of heart failure. The current 1-year survival rate after cardiac transplantation is about 85 percent. Most centers restrict cardiac transplantation to patients under 60 years of age, with pulmonary vascular resistances of less than 8 Wood units, and no serious coexisting illnesses. Patients with both cardiomyopathy and pulmonary hypertension may be candidates for combined heart-lung transplantation.

Immunosuppressive Therapy. As noted earlier, current evidence does not support routine performance of endomyocardial biopsies in patients with dilated cardiomyopathy, insofar as histologic myocarditis is infrequently found and it has not yet been shown that immunosuppressive therapy for myocarditis is beneficial. A recent randomized, controlled study of prednisone in patients with dilated cardiomyopathy (only a few of whom had histologically diagnosed myocarditis) documented that prednisone produced modest improvement in left ventricular ejection fraction in certain subgroups of these patients. However, the study concluded that prednisone was only marginally beneficial and did not recommend its use as standard therapy.

Treatment of Arrhythmias

Patients with dilated cardiomyopathy often have arrhythmias, particularly atrial fibrillation, which occurs in 10 to 20 percent of cases. The immediate management of rapid atrial fibrillation associated with severe heart failure is electrical cardioversion. However, in the more stable patient, the initial aim is to reduce the ventricular response rate with intravenous digoxin. If the fibrillation has been chronic, the patient should be anticoagulated for 2 weeks and then cardioversion attempted pharmacologically or electrically. Verapamil and beta-blockers, which have negative inotropic effects, are potentially dangerous in patients with dilated cardiomyopathy and should be used only with caution. For a detailed consideration of this topic, see the chapter Atrial Arrhythmias.

The therapeutic approach to ventricular arrhythmias in dilated cardiomyopathy is somewhat controversial, especially since antiarrhythmic agents can have proarrhythmic effects. One approach to this difficult problem is to treat aggressively all patients with symptomatic ventricular tachycardia as well as asymptomatic patients with sustained ventricular tachycardia (more than 30 beats), withholding antiarrhythmic therapy from asymptomatic patients with nonsustained ventricular tachycardia (less than 30 beats). In the acute setting, the agent of choice is intravenous lidocaine, with procainamide and bretylium as alternative intravenous agents. Once the arrhythmia has been suppressed, oral therapy may be started with procainamide, quinidine, mexiletine, or amiodarone. Agents with significant negative inotropic effects, such as disopyramide, encainide, and flecainide, are contraindicated. The role of invasive electrophysiologic studies in selecting antiarrhythmic agents and assessing their suppressive efficacy in dilated cardiomyopathy has not been established. The management of these problems is presented elsewhere in this text.

Indications for Anticoagulation

It seems reasonable to administer long-term prophylactic anticoagulant therapy to patients with dilated cardiomyopathy who have chronic or paroxysmal atrial fibrillation, or intracardiac thrombi documented by echocardiography, or who have had embolic events. In the absence of controlled clinical trials, the practice of routinely anticoagulating all patients with dilated cardiomyopathy is open to question. It is not clear in this disease that anticoagulation reduces the likelihood of embolic events; furthermore, prothrombin times in patients with dilated cardiomyopathy often fluctuate unpredictably because of congestive hepatopathy.

SUGGESTED READING

Keogh AM, Freund J, Baron DW, Hickie JB. Timing of cardiac transplantation in idiopathic dilated cardiomyopathy. Am J Cardiol 1988; 61:418–422.

Parrillo JE, Cunnion RE, Epstein SE, et al. A prospective, randomized, controlled trial of prednisone for dilated cardiomyopathy. N Engl J Med 1989; 321:1061–1068.

Poll DS, Marchlinski FE, Buxton AE, Josephson ME. Usefulness of programmed stimulation in idiopathic dilated cardiomyopathy. Am J Cardiol 1986; 58:992–997.

Popma JJ, Cigarroa RG, Buja LM, Hillis LD. Diagnostic and prognostic utility of right-sided catheterization and endomyocardial biopsy in idiopathic dilated cardiomyopathy. Am J Cardiol 1989; 63:955–958.

Rahimtoola SH. The pharmacologic treatment of chronic congestive heart failure. Circulation 1989; 80:693–699.

HYPERTROPHIC CARDIOMYOPATHY

JOHN MICHAEL CRILEY, M.D.
ROBERT J. SIEGEL, M.D.

Hypertrophic cardiomyopathy (HCM) is frequently, but not invariably, familial with an autosomal dominant inheritance pattern. HCM is a condition of unknown etiology in which there is an inordinate degree of hypertrophy, principally involving the left ventricle with a small ventricular cavity. The morphologic criteria for diagnosis are summarized in Table 1. By definition, this is a condition in which there is no demonstrable cause for the hypertrophy such as aortic stenosis or systemic hypertension. Excessive regional wall thickness of the upper interventricular septum occurs in two-thirds to three-fourths of reported cases of HCM. Less commonly, hypertrophy is concentrically distributed, whereas another variant is characterized by inordinate apical hypertrophy.

The histologic findings, while not specific for HCM, consist of myocyte hypertrophy and fiber disarray. The latter finding, first described by Teare, consists of a crisscrossing of myofibers detectable by light and electron microscopy. Abnormal thickening of the intramural coronary arteries primarily in the interventricular septum has also been described. Patchy fibrosis and evidence of prior myocardial infarctions may be found in the absence of coronary arterial obstructions.

The pathophysiology of HCM is summarized in Table 2. The systolic function of the left ventricle is usually characterized by a pattern of emptying that is rapid and complete; the ejection fraction is frequently in the range of 80 to 95 percent (normal, 55 to 75 percent). Early descriptions of this disease focused on a functional or "dynamic obstruction" of the ventricular outflow tract, characterized by a pressure gradient within the left (and/or right) ventricle. Subsequently this gradient was detected in only one-fourth to one-third of patients with HCM, and its presence has not been found to correlate with morbidity, mortality, or extent of hypertrophy. The significance of this "obstruction" has therefore been the subject of long-standing debate. There is, however, general agreement that interventions that diminish the filling pressure ("preload") or arterial impedance ("afterload") or that increase the contractile state of the ventricle lead to reductions in cardiac output and systemic arterial pressure and therefore should be avoided or used with extreme caution.

Mitral valve function is often abnormal in HCM. The valve and enlarged papillary muscles are crowded in the small diastolic cavity, and the rapid and excessive systolic ventricular emptying results in distortion of the mitral complex. As a consequence, mitral regurgitation and systolic anterior motion (SAM) of the valve apparatus are frequently present, leading to characteristic murmurs and echocardiographic features (Tables 2 and 3). The left atrium may be enlarged because of the combination of mitral regurgitation and impaired emptying.

The diastolic function of the left ventricle is often impaired, as manifested by high filling pressures and the inability to tolerate tachycardia or the loss of atrial transport function in atrial fibrillation. The degree of diastolic dysfunction has been shown to be related to the extent of hypertrophy. It is critical to recognize the primacy of diastolic dysfunction in the pathophysiology of HCM: the stroke volume is limited by impaired filling and not by impeded emptying. What gets into the affected ventricle,

Table 1 Pathologic Anatomy of Hypertrophic Cardiomyopathy*

Idiopathic primary ventricular hypertrophy
    Usually asymmetric
        Left ventricle > right ventricle
        Septum > free wall
        Regional variants (including apical)
    Nondilated ventricular cavities
    "Crowded" and traumatized mitral valve
        Disproportionate elongation of leaflets
        Thickened leaflets
        Impact endocardial lesions (plaques)
            Septal (opposite anterior leaflet)
            Mural (beneath posterior leaflet)
        Calcified annulus

Atrial dilatation (left atrium > right atrium)

Microscopic features
    Focal myofiber disarray
    Myocyte hypertrophy
    Interstitial fibrosis
    Thickened intramural coronary arteries

*Adapted from Siegel RJ, Pelikan PCD, Allen HN, Criley JM. Echo-Doppler in HCM. In: Shapira J, Harold J, eds. Two-dimensional echocardiography and cardiac Doppler. Baltimore: Williams and Wilkins, 1990.

Table 2 Pathophysiology of Hypertrophic Cardiomyopathy*

Systolic features
   "Hyperdynamic" ventricular contractions
      Increased ejection fraction (degree of emptying)
      Increased rate of ventricular emptying
         Ventricle "empty" by midsystole
         Aortic valve "preclosure"
      Sustained contraction (after emptying)
      Intracavitary pressure gradients
      Brisk aortic upstroke (increased dP/dT)
   Mitral valve dysfunction
      Mitral regurgitation
         Holosystolic
         Late systolic augmentation
      Systolic anterior motion

Diastolic features
   Delayed rate of isovolumic relaxation
   Decreased diastolic compliance
   Increased atrial transport function ("atrial kick")

*Adapted from Siegel RJ, Pelikan PCD, Allen HN, Criley JM. Echo-Doppler in HCM. In: Shapira J, Harold J, eds. Two-dimensional echocardiography and cardiac doppler. Baltimore: Williams and Wilkins, 1990.

Table 3 Echocardiographic Characteristics of Hypertrophic Cardiomyopathy*

Hypertrophic, nondilated left ventricle in the absence of inciting cause (e.g., aortic stenosis, hypertension, coarctation, etc.)

Abnormal thickening of left ventricular wall in the absence of myocardial infarction:
   Asymmetric septal hypertrophy (ASH)
   Disproportionate upper septal thickening (DUST)
   Apical hypertrophy
   Other regional
   Concentric

Hyperdynamic left ventricle with obliteration of submitral cavity
   Increased percentage of fractional shortening
   Increased inward excursion of posterior left ventricular wall
   "Sessile" interventricular septum (by M mode)

Mitral valve
   Prolonged diastolic septal apposition
   M mode: reduced e to f slope and prominent b shoulder
   Anterior position of mitral valve apparatus
   Systolic anterior motion (SAM) with or without SAM-septal contact
      "Hockey stick"
      "Crossed swords"
      Thickened leaflets
      Annular calcification

Aortic valve
   Systolic fluttering
   Systolic preclosure
   Reduced diastolic slope (M-mode) of aorta

Left atrial enlargement

*Adapted from Siegel RJ, Pelikan PCD, Allen HN, Criley JM. Echo-Doppler in HCM. In: Shapira J, Harold J, eds. Two-dimensional echocardiography and cardiac doppler. Baltimore: Williams and Wilkins, 1990.

gets out, and reduced cardiac output and elevated venous pressure are related primarily to impaired filling.

CONSEQUENCES OF HYPERTROPHIC CARDIOMYOPATHY

Many subjects with HCM have no symptoms. In symptomatic patients the major clinical manifestations of HCM (see Table 2) can be attributed to the pathologic ventricular hypertrophy and function.

Dyspnea is the most frequent symptom and results from elevated left atrial pressure, which is due to impaired transport into the hypertrophic left ventricle. As with mitral stenosis, in which there is impeded emptying of the left atrium, tachycardia or the presence of mitral regurgitation will further amplify the left atrial and the pulmonary venous hypertension.

Dyspnea is frequently related to obligate increases in either cardiac output or heart rate, or both—e.g., exertion, fever, pregnancy, anemia, thyrotoxicosis, or tachyarrhythmias. Increased cardiac output increases left atrial filling, and tachycardia shortens the available atrial emptying time. A superimposed myocardial supply-demand imbalance in the hypertrophic left ventricle will further diminish the ability of the ventricle to relax, owing to ischemia.

This form of "congestive heart failure" should *not* be treated with inotropic or arteriolar dilating agents, as these may worsen the tachycardia and ischemia, further limiting ventricular filling and stroke volume. Therefore, the cornerstone of management of this form of cardiac decompensation is to facilitate the filling of the left ventricle.

For example, acute episodes of *tachycardia* should be rapidly alleviated, and atrial transport function (which is lost in atrial fibrillation or flutter) must be restored, if at all possible. It should be recognized that tachycardia begets tachycardia through enhanced adrenergic drive when vital organs and baroreceptors are underperfused. Therefore, *beta-adrenergic blockade* is a mainstay in the management of sinus or supraventricular tachycardias. We recommend intravenous propranolol, in doses of 1 to 2 mg, to a maximum of 15 mg in the setting of an acute supraventricular tachycardia. Because verapamil may cause vasodilation or hypotension and may be hazardous in patients with pulmonary congestion, we believe that this agent should be avoided in this setting. Electrical cardioversion is appropriate for poorly tolerated recent-onset atrial fibrillation or flutter or other supraventricular tachycardias.

The chronic use of antiarrhythmic agents is indicated in patients with HCM who are subject to episodic arrhythmias and should be selected on the basis of the specific arrhythmia(s) present. Atrial arrhythmias can be controlled or prevented by propranolol or verapamil or in combination with type Ia drugs (quinidine, procainamide, or disopyramide). If atrial fibrillation occurs despite adequate doses of type Ia agents, amiodarone has been very effective. Patients with established or paroxysmal atrial fibrillation should undergo chronic anticoagulation because of the propensity for the large fibrillating atrium to embolize. In this regard, HCM is similar to mitral stenosis, as both have large atria with impeded emptying—the former because of an incompliant ventricle, the latter because of an obstructed mitral valve.

Ventricular arrhythmias may provide a substrate for *sudden cardiac death* in patients with HCM and should be sought for by ambulatory electrocardiographic monitoring in all newly diagnosed patients. Symptomatic or potentially life-threatening rhythm disturbances should be treated, if present, with effective doses of appropriate agents. We do not advocate invasive electrophysiologic testing in patients with HCM because of the nonspecificity of inducible ventricular tachyarrhythmias in this condition and concern that iatrogenically induced arrhythmias may not respond readily to standard resuscitative measures. Acute management with intravenous lidocaine or procainamide is usually effective for frequent ventricular premature beats or salvoes of ventricular tachycardia. Although a discussion of chronic treatment is beyond the scope of this chapter, the reader is reminded that type Ia agents and amiodarone have been used effectively. Amiodarone has been shown to reduce the risk of sudden cardiac death in patients with HCM with documented ventricular tachycardia. Because of the drug's potential toxicity, its use should be closely monitored.

Dyspnea at rest in the absence of tachycardia should be managed by the judicious use of diuretics, while one bears in mind that a low filling pressure may place the patient in greater jeopardy than a high filling pressure. The hypertrophic left ventricle requires a higher than normal filling pressure to achieve adequate ventricular filling, cardiac output, and coronary perfusion. Overt *pulmonary edema* is often precipitated by secondary factors such as fever, infection (especially pneumonia), thyrotoxicosis, or tachycardia.

Primary measures to slow the heart rate, preserve atrial transport function (sinus rhythm), and improve oxygenation should be undertaken. If the chest film demonstrates an obvious volume overload of the pulmonary circuit, relatively low doses of intravenous diuretics (e.g., 5 to 10 mg of furosemide) should be titrated to produce a moderate diuresis and relief of pulmonary congestion without overshooting to the point of producing an inadequate filling pressure for the left ventricle.

Exertional dyspnea should be managed by beta-adrenergic blockade, if this is not contraindicated or poorly tolerated. In patients with concurrent asthma or bronchospasm, calcium-channel blocking drugs may be effective. Echocardiographic dimensional changes, Doppler measurements of inflow velocity patterns, and radionuclide and contrast ventriculography have been used to quantitate diastolic function and to evaluate therapeutic interventions.

Low to moderate doses of propranolol (60 to 120 mg per day) will slow the heart rate and thus prolong *filling time* but do not demonstrably increase filling rate. Higher doses of propranolol (above 5 mg per kilogram or about 400 mg per day) may enhance filling indices by decreasing the isovolumic relaxation time as measured by M-mode echocardiography. Although the other available beta-blocking agents have not been studied as extensively as has propranolol, our experience with the cardioselective agents atenolol and meteprolol has been favorable. Rough dose equivalents for atenolol would be 100 to 200 mg per day; for metroprolol, 100 to 400 per day in one to two divided doses, and for nadolol, 100 to 400 mg per day. If dyspnea persists after administration of maximal doses of beta-adrenergic blocking agents, it can often be alleviated by low doses of loop diuretics, e.g., 20 mg of furosemide three times per week with additional doses as needed. The patient should be weighed daily, and in the event of a 1-kg weight gain, additional 20 mg doses of furosemide should be prescribed ad lib.

Calcium-channel blockers have also been demonstrated to enhance filling parameters in HCM. Acute administration of verapamil also shortens isovolumic relaxation time indices by echocardiography, and chronic administration is associated with favorable effects on exercise tolerance and on diastolic function demonstrable by radionuclide angiography. Other calcium-channel blocking drugs can be used effectively, but have been less well studied than verapamil. Both diltiazem and nifedipine improve filling parameters, but the reflex tachycardia usually induced by nifedipine may require concomitant treatment with a beta blocker. Diltiazem is better tolerated by some older patients because of its relative freedom from the constipation encountered with the use of verapamil and the edema, hypotension, and tachycardia encountered with nifedipine.

Verapamil has been effective in doses of 40 to 120 mg three times per day and diltiazem, 30 to 90 mg three times per day. Nifedipine is a more potent arterial dilator, making it less desirable as a single therapy. However its relative lack of negative chronotropism renders it the safest agent to use when beta blocking drugs are administered concomitantly.

Chest pain, on the basis of a myocardial supply-demand imbalance, is commonly present in HCM. The hypertrophic myocardium has a high demand for nutrients because of its bulk and increased contractile performance, and this demand is heightened by tachycardia. The supply side of the equation may be adversely affected by low coronary arterial perfusion pressure, elevation of the left ventricular diastolic pressure, and the need for the nutrient arteries to traverse hypertrophied and hypercontractile myocardium. Coronary arteriography has shown that septal perforator branches may be "milked" as a result of systolic thickening of the surrounding septal muscle and may exhibit reversal of the direction of flow. This is compelling, albeit subjective, evidence that coronary blood flow is impeded on its passage through the myocardium in HCM.

Our management of the presumed supply-demand imbalance inherent in patients with HCM and angina consists of reduction of the demand side through the use of beta-blocking agents, which decrease heart rate and the inotropic state of the left ventricle; or calcium-channel blockers if the beta-blockers are ineffective or intolerable; and/or disopyramide, which exerts a powerful negative inotropic effect on the left ventricle and may be effective in controlling angina in HCM. The antiatrial arrhythmic properties of disopyramide may also be useful in patients who are prone to atrial fibrillation. We have employed disopyramide in doses of 100 to 200 mg three to four times per day, starting with low doses and increasing gradually if it is tolerated with good effect.

The *asymptomatic* patient with HCM poses a challenge, since it is in this type of patient that sudden cardiac death may be the first clinical manifestation. Although there are no data to support the superiority of any form of therapy in the asymptomatic patient, the knowledge that HCM is one of the major causes of unexpected sudden death in young athletes compels us to counsel all patients with HCM, regardless of symptoms or lack thereof, to avoid competitive or strenuous exercise. Asymptomatic HCM may be found by the detection of the characteristic physical findings or overt electrocardiographic or echocardiographic features, often as a result of a family survey following the detection of HCM in a first-degree relative. In the latter instance, a family history of sudden death portends a greater risk for other family members with HCM; careful scrutiny for latent arrhythmias should be undertaken and repeated at least yearly.

It has been found that some family members of patients with HCM may appear normal during childhood and later manifest the characteristic echocardiographic features after adolescence. This observation complicates the already expensive and problematic task of family screening, which we nevertheless believe should be undertaken on all first-degree relatives of patients known to have HCM.

Bacterial endocarditis prophylaxis is indicated in all patients with HCM undergoing procedures that may introduce bacteria into the bloodstream. Most patients with HCM have mitral regurgitation, which is well tolerated but puts them at risk for endocarditis. The infected valve may in turn worsen the degree of mitral regurgitation and precipitate the need for valve replacement.

Operative intervention (septal myotomy, myectomy, and or mitral valve replacement) has been advocated by many investigators because of their conviction that *outflow tract obstruction* plays a primary role in the disease. Because pathologic degrees of hypertrophy frequently occur in patients with HCM in the absence of intracavitary pressure gradients (hemodynamic evidence of obstruction), and symptomatic patients without pressure gradients in many cases have a worse prognosis than those who do, we do not believe that a convincing argument has been made for this high-risk operative intervention. On the other hand, most patients with HCM *are* responsive to medical therapy, albeit with individual tailoring of the approach to each patient. We have found that changing beta-blockers, or changing from beta- to calcium-channel blocking agents, or adding disopyramide is often desirable or necessary, as noted above.

Finally, we believe that patients with HCM and their responsible relatives should be informed and reassured about their heart condition and its implications. Most HCM patients have a normal or near-normal lifespan, so that it is not justified to focus needlessly on the remote potential for a fatal outcome unless the individual is determined to indulge in strenuous exercise against medical advice, has arrhythmias, or a family history of sudden death associated with HCM. Patients with HCM in the latter two categories warrant extraordinary interventions such an implantable cardioverter-defibrillators. We provide our patients and their families with a clear explanation of the pathophysiology of HCM so that they can understand the need to maintain effective control of their heart rate and avoid or block deleterious adrenergic stimuli.

SUGGESTED READING

Bonow RO, Dilsizian V, Rosing DR, et al. Verapamil-induced improvement in left ventricular diastolic filling and increased exercise tolerance in patients with hypertrophic cardiomyopathy: short and long-term effects. Circulation 1985; 72:853–854.

Braunwald E, Lambrew CT, Morrow AG, et al. Idiopathic hypertrophic subaortic stenosis. Circulation 1964; 30, IV:1–213.

Criley JM, Siegel RJ. Has "obstruction" hindered our understanding of hypertrophic cardiomyopathy? Circulation 1985; 72:1148–1154.

Epstein SE, Rosing DR. Verapamil: its potential for causing serious complications in patients with hypertrophic cardiomyopathy. Circulation 1981; 64:437–441.

Goodwin JF. The frontiers of cardiomyopathy. Br Heart J 1982; 48:1–18.

Maron BJ, Bonow RO, Cannon RO III, et al. Hypertrophic cardiomyopathy: interrelations of clinical manifestations, pathophysiology and therapy. N Engl J Med 1987; 316:780–789, 844–851.

RESTRICTIVE CARDIOMYOPATHY

ERNEST WILLIAM HANCOCK, M.D.

Restrictive cardiomyopathy can be defined broadly or narrowly. The term "restrictive" refers to heart disease in which impairment of diastolic filling of the heart is a major feature. Constrictive pericarditis is a condition that does not involve the heart itself but typifies the entity of restrictive heart disease. Those forms of myocardial disease that resemble constrictive pericarditis most closely are the most aptly termed restrictive cardiomyopathy. In such instances the cardiac chambers are neither dilated nor hypertrophied and appear to have normal systolic contractile function. The abnormality appears to reside solely in the diastolic function of the heart, in the form of impaired relaxation or diminished passive compliance in diastole.

Idiopathic restrictive cardiomyopathy occurs rarely in the United States. Endomyocardial fibrosis as part of an eosinophilic syndrome is also seen occasionally, and presents a form of restrictive-obliterative cardiomyopathy that is similar to the African endomyocardial fibrosis. Specific myocardial diseases such as amyloidosis are more frequent causes of the restrictive cardiomyopathy syndrome in the United States, although these are not cardiomyopathies in the strictest sense of the term. Patients with hypertrophic cardiomyopathy also present diastolic abnormalities that are similar to those of restrictive cardiomyopathy in some instances. Indeed, a pattern of restrictive physiology is seen in advanced forms of almost all forms of heart disease, illustrating the ubiquity of diastolic functional abnormalities in heart disease even when the systolic contractile abnormalities are clearly earlier and more important.

Clinical recognition of the restrictive cardiomyopathy pattern requires measurements of both the intracardiac pressures and the dimensions of the cardiac chambers. The ventricular filling pressures are elevated, and the pressure wave forms typically show the early diastolic dip and later the diastolic plateau pattern that signifies relatively normal filling in early diastole but restricted filling later in diastole. The imaging studies should show normal dimensions of the ventricular cavity and normal systolic wall motion, thus giving a normal ejection fraction.

In the purest forms of the restrictive cardiomyopathy pattern, the picture closely resembles constrictive pericarditis. Because constrictive pericarditis is correctable by surgery, while restrictive cardiomyopathy can only be palliated by nonspecific therapy for congestive heart failure, the differential diagnosis between the two is vital. Indeed, the principal justification for distinguishing restrictive cardiomyopathy from the broad spectrum of cardiomyopathy is to call attention to this differential diagnosis and to ensure that patients with constrictive pericarditis are not overlooked.

Several clinical points serve to differentiate constrictive pericarditis from restrictive cardiomyopathy:

1. Many patients with constrictive pericarditis will have a history of acute pericarditis in the recent or remote past, or will have a predisposing condition such as connective tissue disease, chronic renal failure, past radiotherapy, or past open heart surgery.
2. The electrocardiogram in restrictive cardiomyopathy frequently shows atrioventricular or intraventricular condition defects, such as right or left bundle branch block, that are rare in constrictive pericarditis.
3. Patients with constrictive pericarditis often have a sharp early diastolic sound in diastole (pericardial knock), while in restrictive cardiomyopathy there may be an S_3 that is lower pitched and later than the pericardial knock, or there may be an S_4. S_4 is rarely, if ever, present in constrictive pericarditis.
4. Right and left atrial enlargement are often present in restrictive cardiomyopathy but are generally not present in constrictive pericarditis. The absence of S_4 and of atrial enlargement in constrictive pericarditis relates to the fact that the pericardial process constricts the atria as well as the ventricles and impairs the contractile function of the atria.
5. Paradoxical pulse is often present in constrictive pericarditis but is generally not present in restrictive cardiomyopathy. A corollary finding is exaggerated variation in the mitral and tricuspid flow velocities during the phases of respiration, detectable by pulsed wave Doppler recordings.
6. While echocardiographic evidence of thickening of the pericardium is not a very reliable method of distinguishing the two conditions, the greater precision of computed tomographic (CT) scans and of magnetic resonance imaging studies (MRI) does provide useful evidence. A normal thickness of the pericardium in a CT or MRI scan goes far to rule out constrictive pericarditis.
7. Endomyocardial biopsy is usually normal in constrictive pericarditis or shows only a mild degree of myocardial fibrosis, whereas in restrictive cardiomyopathy there are likely to be myopathic changes or a greater degree of fibrosis, if not a specific form of disease such as amyloidosis.

One form of the restrictive cardiomyopathy that deserves special mention is the obliterative endomyocardial fibrosis variant. In this condition it may be possible to remove surgically the core of restrictive fibrous tissue from the cavity of the left ventricle. These patients can be recognized by the distortion and partial obliteration of the left ventricular cavity that is seen in the left ventricular cineangiogram. They also usually have significant mitral and tricuspid valvular regurgitation.

MEDICAL MANAGEMENT

The broad principles of management of congestive heart failure generally apply to patients with restrictive cardiomyopathy as they apply to patients with dilated cardiomyopathy or congestive heart failure of any of the usual causes (see chapters regarding these topics). Yet some principles have emerged that suggest differences in the therapeutic approach.

Digitalis and other inotropic drugs are thought to improve only systolic impairment of the heart; therefore, it may not be wise to use inotropic drugs in patients with only diastolic dysfunction. Certainly these agents should not be considered the prime or initial mode of therapy in patients with relatively pure forms of restrictive cardiomyopathy. In amyloid heart disease digitalis has traditionally been considered to be particularly likely to induce toxic arrhythmias and conduction defects, an additional reason for caution in its use.

Diuretics are undoubtedly useful in the right-sided congestive heart failure that is characteristically seen in restrictive cardiomyopathy. In the critical care setting, however, diuretics should be used with particular caution in patients with restrictive cardiomyopathy because it may not be physiologic to lower the filling pressure of the heart in such patients. In the more common forms of heart disease with congestive heart failure, the elevated filling pressures follow secondarily after the diminished systolic function and the consequent sodium and water retention, while in restrictive cardiomyopathy this is closer to the primary abnormality.

Vasodilator drugs have assumed great importance in the management of congestive heart failure in general and may be considered the routine and first-choice treatment in many circumstances. However, restrictive cardiomyopathy presents a special circumstance in which vasodilator therapy may be less appropriate. The rationale for vasodilator therapy includes the concept that systolic function of the heart is impaired and that reducing the load against which the systolic contraction is working should lead to improved systolic function. If the systolic function is unimpaired, the rationale for this therapy is weakened. Unless the systemic arterial pressure is distinctly elevated, vasodilators should be used cautiously in patients with restrictive cardiomyopathy, preferably only under the cover of hemodynamic monitoring.

Calcium-channel blocking drugs, particularly verapamil, tend to be contraindicated in most patients with congestive heart failure, because their negative inotropic effect is additive to the basic inotropic defect. In restrictive cardiomyopathy, however, the calcium blockers may be helpful in that they may have a direct relaxing effect upon the myocardium in diastole. Indeed, the diastolic abnormality may be related to the sequestration of inappropriate amounts of calcium in the myocardial cells. This phenomenon has been best studied, both experimentally and clinically, in patients with hypertrophic cardiomyopathy, where restrictive features are often prominent. It is reasonable to carry out a cautious clinical trial of a calcium blocker in restrictive cardiomyopathy, especially in the intensive care unit setting, where its hemodynamic effects can be immediately observed.

Beta-adrenergic blocking agents, also generally contraindicated in congestive heart failure, may be given special consideration in restrictive cardiomyopathy. One action that might be beneficial is to slow the heart rate and allow a longer time for diastolic filling. Conversely, however, some patients with restrictive cardiomyopathy may have a severely limited stroke volume and may require a particularly rapid heart rate in order to maintain the cardiac output. Beta-blockers should therefore be used cautiously, in small doses initially and with careful monitoring.

Restrictive cardiomyopathy has in common with hypertrophic cardiomyopathy the enhanced importance of the atrial contribution to ventricular performance. Atrial fibrillation, or other arrhythmias in which the atrioventricular sequence is disturbed, can be particularly deleterious to the hemodynamics of such patients. In the critical care setting there may be a place for atrial or atrioventricular dual pacing as a temporary means of optimizing the atrial contribution to ventricular performance.

Despite the fact that the ventricle is not dilated, there is a risk of mural thrombosis and systemic arterial embolism in patients with restrictive cardiomyopathy, similar to the risk in dilated cardiomyopathy. Prophylactic anticoagulation should probably be considered to be similarly indicated, therefore.

Cardiac transplantation is the therapy of last resort for patients with congestive heart failure due to dilated cardiomyopathy, and the same is true in the idiopathic forms of restrictive cardiomyopathy. The fact that the left ventricle is not dilated and that the ejection fraction is normal should not be taken as necessarily favorable for the future if there is a severe refractory congestive heart failure due to restrictive cardiomyopathy. Patients with amyloidosis or sarcoidosis of the heart have only rarely been subjected to cardiac transplantation because of the expectation that the primary disease would develop in the transplanted heart; this has not always occurred, however, and further trials of transplantation in the specific myocardial diseases are appropriate.

SUGGESTED READING

Benotti JR, Grossman W. Restrictive cardiomyopathy. Annu Rev Med 1984; 34:113.

Child JS, Perloff JK. The restrictive cardiomyopathies. Cardiol Clin 1988; 6:289.

Shabetai R. Pathophysiology and differential diagnosis of restrictive cardiomyopathies. In: Shaver JA, ed. Cardiomyopathies: clinical presentation, differential diagnosis, and management. Philadelphia: FA Davis, 1988.

Topol EJ, Traill TA, Fortuin NJ. Hypertensive hypertrophic cardiomyopathy of the elderly. N Engl J Med 1985; 312:277.

SEVERE AORTIC OR MITRAL VALVULAR REGURGITATION

JOHN T. BARRON, M.D., Ph.D.

The major hemodynamic derangements seen in acute mitral or aortic regurgitation result from volume overload of the left ventricle. Volume overload from regurgitant blood results in distention of the left ventricle and, depending on the compliance state of the left ventricle, a marked rise in interventricular pressure and left ventricular wall tension. Excessive wall tension compromises myocardial contractile function and depresses forward stroke volume, which lead to dilatation of the left ventricular cavity, a further rise in interventricular pressure and consequent pulmonary edema. As forward flow diminishes, compensatory vasoconstriction ensues as a means by which adequate blood pressure is maintained. The increased peripheral vascular resistance imposes an additional load on a myocardium that is already failing. The unfavorable loading conditions of the heart depress myocardial systolic function even more, setting up a "vicious circle." In the case of mitral regurgitation, dilatation of the left ventricular cavity results in dilatation of the mitral valve annulus, limiting coaptation of the mitral leaflets and leading to further mitral insufficiency.

Acute severe valvular insufficiency almost invariably requires urgent surgical replacement of the incompetent valve. Medical management is directed toward hemodynamic stabilization of the patient until the definitive surgical procedure is performed. Acute severe valvular regurgitation poses much greater concern than chronic regurgitation because there is insufficient time for the compliance of the left ventricle and left atrium to increase to accommodate the marked and sudden increase in intrachamber volume. Consequently, intracardiac chamber pressures in acute regurgitation rise much more precipitously.

A strategy of medical management for hemodynamic stabilization applies as well to the management of severe, decompensated chronic regurgitation. However, the degree of hemodynamic instability is typically not so severe because of the greater compliance of the usually chronically dilated cardiac chambers, which can accommodate large volumes of regurgitant blood without a precipitous rise in interchamber pressure. The benefits of surgical intervention are less well defined and depend in large part on the functional state of the left ventricle.

ACUTE VALVULAR REGURGITATION

Pathophysiology, Features, Diagnosis

Mitral Regurgitation. The mitral valve may be made suddenly incompetent by rupture of a papillary muscle or chordae tendineae or by accretion of a vegetation that occurs in acute or subacute endocarditis. Abscess formation on the valve apparatus may also cause perforation of a valve leaflet.

Salient auscultatory features of the cardiac examination are a diminished S_1 and a holosystolic murmur that is loudest at the apex with radiation to the axilla and infrascapular area. Not uncommonly, the murmur may be heard throughout the precordium. An S_3 or S_4 (in sinus rhythm) may also be present.

The auscultatory and other physical findings in acute valvular regurgitation may differ from those of chronic regurgitation and may be confused with other cardiac pathophysiologic states. Therefore, noninvasive diagnosis is most reliably made by echocardiography and Doppler color flow mapping of the regurgitant jet. Echocardiography may also define valvular and cardiac anatomy, provide an assessment of left ventricular function, and detect vegetations if endocarditis is the cause of valvular regurgitation. Flailed mitral leaflets is a particularly ominous sign, indicating severe regurgitation. Before definitive surgery, complete right- and left-sided cardiac catheterization with coronary angiography should also be performed in stabilized patients if coexisting coronary artery disease is suspected, especially in patients more than 40 years of age. Right-sided cardiac catheterization with oximetry runs will also detect any coexisting intracardiac shunts, which are frequently associated with valvular abnormalities.

The pulmonary capillary wedge pressure tracing obtained at catheterization typically demonstrates prominent "v" waves indicative of regurgitation of blood into a relatively noncompliant left atrium. The magnitude of a significant "v" wave is usually at least 10 mm Hg greater than the mean pulmonary capillary wedge pressure (PCWP), which is ordinarily elevated in severe acute mitral regurgitation.

Aortic Regurgitation. Causes of acute regurgitation include bacterial endocarditis, inflammatory aortitis, and dissection tears of the aorta and valve structure. Severe aortic regurgitation is accompanied by a blowing diastolic murmur heard along the left sternal border. Because of the elevated left ventricular pressure at the end of diastole causing close apposition of the mitral leaflets, S_1 may be soft. The second heart sound may also be soft or absent, owing to the incomplete closure of the incompetent aortic valve. An apical diastolic rumble, known as the Austin-Flint murmur, is also common in severe acute regurgitation. It represents antegrade flow across a narrowed mitral valve opening caused by the close apposition of the mitral leaflets resulting from the rapidly rising left ventricular diastolic pressure from aortic regurgitation.

Echocardiography and Doppler ultrasonography will confirm the presence of aortic regurgitation. Premature diastolic closure of the mitral valve detected by two dimensional (2D) guided M-mode echocardiography is indicative of severe aortic regurgitation and is a consequence of the markedly elevated left ventricular end-diastolic pressure (LVEDP). Fluttering of the anterior leaflet of the mitral valve caused by impingement of the regurgitant jet in diastole on the opened leaflet is also frequently seen.

As is the case for mitral regurgitation, complete right- and left-sided cardiac catheterization is indicated in appropriate patients prior to surgery to define coronary anatomy and to exclude other cardiac pathology.

Management (Table 1)

Preload and Afterload Reduction. Among the major determinants of myocardial contractile function are ventricular preload and afterload. The mainstay of therapy in valvular heart disease, therefore, is reduction of left ventricular preload and afterload using peripheral vasodilators to ameliorate the pronounced peripheral vasoconstriction typical of severe heart failure and to reduce ventricular filling pressures, thereby augmenting forward cardiac output and reducing pulmonary edema (Table 1). Vasodilation therapy may be carefully initiated first, provided that the systolic blood pressure is greater than 95 to 100 mm Hg. Placement of a balloon-floatation pulmonary artery catheter and an arterial line is recommended to optimize the monitoring of changes in cardiac performance with adminstration of vasodilators and to follow systemic blood pressure closely.

Preload and afterload reduction of the left ventricle is best achieved and controlled with the use of nitrates by constant intravenous infusions. Nitrates are preferred primarily because of their rapid onset of action and short half-life. We prefer initially to use intravenous nitroglycerin over sodium nitroprusside. Nitroglycerin is primarily a venodilator and hence reduces preload; at moderate doses it dilates arterial smooth muscle as well. Its major advantage over nitroprusside is that prolonged use of nitroprusside is accompanied by accumulation of the thiocyanate metabolite, a metabolic poison. Also, unlike nitroprusside, nitroglycerin will not produce a coronary steal syndrome in patients with coexisting coronary artery disease. The major advantage of nitroprusside over nitroglycerin is that it is a more potent arterial vasodilator. As such, should nitroglycerin at high doses fail to improve hemodynamic status significantly, nitroprusside should be administered. Nitroglycerin should be administered beginning at 20 μg per kilogram body weight per minute and titrated aggressively upward in increments of 10 to 20 μg every 5 to 10 minutes, to as high as 40 to 600 μg per kilogram per minute to maintain a systolic blood pressure of 90 to 100 mm Hg. At this target blood pressure, further increases in nitrates may continue to improve cardiac output without depressing blood pressure, especially if the systemic vascular resistance and mean pulmonary capillary wedge pressure (PCWP) remain elevated. If nitroprusside is used, the starting dose is 0.5 μg per kilogram body weight per minute and titrated to 10 μg per kilogram per minute. Serum thiocyanate levels should be obtained daily; should the level exceed 10 mg per dl, nitroprusside should be discontinued. It is important to note that after 24 to 48 hours of intravenous nitrate therapy, the initial favorable hemodynamic response may be attentuated, owing to tolerance of vascular smooth muscle to the dilating effect of nitrates. It is often then necessary

Table 1 Treatment of Acute Severe Valvular Regurgitation

	Agent	Dose
Acute Mitral Regurgitation		
Hemodynamic stabilization		
• IV diuretics and nitrates for preload and afterload reduction	Furosemide	20–80 mg IV
	Nitroglycerin	40–60 μg/min
	Nitroprusside	0.5–10 μg/kg/min
• Inotropes if low forward cardiac output or hemodynamic instability persists	Dobutamine	5–20 μg/kg/min
	Amrinone	0.75 mg/kg/load, then 5–20 μg/kg/min
• Pressors if hypotension refractory to inotropic intervention	Dopamine	10–25 μg/kg/min
	Norepinephrine	2–8 μ/min
• Intubation and mechanical ventilation and placement of intra-aortic balloon pump if cardiogenic shock		
Valve replacement surgery		
• Surgery performed as soon as possible		
• If endocarditis and patient stabilized, sterilize blood with antibiotics and normalize temperature and WBC count before surgery		
Acute Aortic Regurgitation		
Hemodynamic stabilization		
• Treatment as for mitral regurgitation, except intra-aortic balloon pump contraindicated		
Valve replacement surgery		
• Treatment as for mitral regurgitation		

to increase the dose of nitrate to achieve the same effect at previously smaller doses.

Under normal conditions, the mean PCWP satisfactorily reflects the filling pressure of the left ventricle, or LVEDP. In severe mitral regurgitation, however, the mean PCWP is usually greater and does not faithfully reflect the true LVEDP because of the contribution of the prominent "v" wave to the value of the mean PCWP. Therefore, the optimal range at which the mean PCWP should be maintained should be determined empirically, based on the response of the cardiac output and systemic vascular resistance to drugs and other interventions. The mean PCWP in aortic regurgitation ideally should be kept at 15 to 20 mm Hg, or at a value at which cardiac output and urine output is normal yet pulmonary edema is minimal.

The administration of diuretics concomitantly with vasodilators is usually necessary to maintain adequate urine output (at least 60 ml per hour) and relieve pulmonary edema. Furosemide in doses of 20 to 80 mg intravenously every 6 to 8 hours is usually sufficient to induce a brisk diuresis. Patients who do not respond to furosemide will occasionally respond to bumetinide (Bumex), a loop diuretic (1 mg of bumetinide is equivalent to approximately 40 mg of furosemide). Alternatively, ethacrynic acid may be administered at a dose of 50 to 100 mg intravenously every 6 to 8 hours. We have found that the combination of ethacrynic acid with either furosemide or bumetinide may be effective, whereas either diuretic alone is ineffective. Rarely, if the diuresis is still inadequate, oral metalozone at 5 to 10 mg daily may be added. The doses of diuretics may be adjusted as needed to match the hydration state of the patient. At high doses of potent loop diuretics there is greater risk of nephrotoxicity (and ototoxicity) and routine serum renal function tests should be followed closely.

Low-dose dopamine (2 to 4 μg per kilogram body weight per minute) is often a useful adjunct to achieve diuresis. It does so by increasing renal blood flow by dilatation of the renal vascular bed mediated by dopaminergic smooth muscle receptors.

Inotropic Intervention. Frequently, in young and otherwise healthy patients, the regimen of preload and afterload reduction with vasodilators and diuretics is sufficient to maintain adequate cardiac output and urine output and to relieve pulmonary edema. Often, however, in patients with pre-existing left ventricular dysfunction or in patients with particularly severe ("wide open") regurgitation, positive inotropic intervention is required. The decision to use inotropes should be made relatively early in the course of management of these patients and should be based on the patient's prior cardiac history and on the lack of an unequivocal improvement in hemodynamic status using vasodilators and diuretics alone. Dobutamine, a beta-1-adrenergic agonist with modest arterial dilating proprieties, augments myocardial contractility at doses starting at 5 μg per kilogram per minute, up to 20 μg per kilogram per minute as required. Dobutamine has minimal chronotropic properties. Since beta-adrenergic agonism can frequently provoke ventricular ectopy, patients must be closely monitored for ventricular arrhythmias. With prolonged infusion (72 hours) of dobutamine, the positive inotropic response may be attenuated because of downregulation of beta-1-cardiac receptors. If malignant ventricular arrhythmias supervene or if the initial favorable response seems blunted, even at high doses, amrinone may be substituted. Because it is a phosphodiesterase inhibitor, amrinone has both positive inotropic and direct vasodilating properties. An initial loading dose of 0.75 mg per kilogram intravenously over 10 to 20 minutes is required, followed by constant infusion of 5 to 15 μg per kilogram per minute. Because amrinone can cause ventricular arrhythmias, monitoring is required. Thrombocytopenia and elevation in serum liver transaminases are not uncommon, and platelet counts and liver function tests should be determined periodically. We have occasionally used a combination of both dobutamine and amrinone with good response, when the response to either drug alone seemed inadequate.

The role of digitalis in the management of heart failure is controversial. Certainly, digitalis is very effective in controlling some supraventricular tachyarrhythmias, especially atrial fibrillation. On the other hand, its positive inotropic actions are modest and the benefit-to-toxicity ratio is narrow. We recommend the use of digitalis to control ventricular rate in supraventricular tachycardia and also to add additional inotropic support if dobutamine and amrinone are deemed insufficient. In the case of atrial fibrillation, for rapid control of fast ventricular rates, 0.5 mg of digoxin intravenously may be given initially (in patients not previously on digoxin) followed by an additional 0.5 to 1.0 mg in divided doses over the next several hours. For inotropic support, there is ordinarily no need to rapidly digitalize patients, and a daily maintenance dose of 0.125 to 0.25 mg intravenously or orally may be started. Since virtually any arrhythmia can occur with digoxin, it is our practice to obtain a serum digoxin level after digitalization, especially in patients with deterioration in renal function.

Arrhythmias. Unless there is evidence of hemodynamic compromise during episodes of complex ventricular ectopy or salvoes of nonsustained ventricular tachycardia, it is not our practice to treat these arrhythmias with antiarrhythmic agents. Rather, correction of possible underlying acidosis, hypokalemia, or hypomagnesemia is undertaken, especially if diuresis is a cause of the electrolyte disorder. Even if serum magnesium is not depressed, we have often observed reduction in ventricular ectopy with administration of 2 to 4 g of magnesium sulfate intravenously, especially if a brisk diuresis has been induced by loop diuretics.

Sustained ventricular tachycardia (greater than 15 to 30 seconds in duration), with or without hemodynamic compromise, should be aggressively treated with intravenous lidocaine, starting at a loading dose of 75 to 225 mg, followed by a drip of 1 to 4 mg per minute, as required. If lidocaine at reasonably high doses fails to control malignant arrhythmias, or if unacceptable side effects of lidocaine supervene, intravenous procainamide may be substituted. Also, procainamide is the preferred initial agent if there is coexisting supraventricular tachycardia. Procainamide may be administered at a 1-g load intravenously over 1 hour, followed by constant infusion of 1 to 4 mg per minute. Hypotension may occur with procainamide during the loading period, in which case the rate of infusion should be decreased. With either supraventricular or ventricular tachycardias, should hemodynamic compromise ensue, immediate electrical cardioversion should be performed.

Issues In Critically Ill Patients

The use of vasopressors in patients with valvular regurgitation should be avoided if possible. As noted previously, there is usually intense pre-existing peripheral vasoconstriction, which increases afterload and contributes to the pathophysiology of valvular regurgitation. Thus, the utilization of pressors defeats the purpose of the strategy of afterload reduction with vasodilators. Therefore, if borderline hypotension is initially present (systolic blood pressure of 85 to 95 mm Hg), it is advisable to attempt to elevate blood pressure by augmenting forward cardiac output with inotropes such as dobutamine. Nevertheless, when profound hypotension is present, vasopressors are indicated to maintain perfusion of coronary and systemic vascular beds. Dopamine, beginning at doses of 5 to 10 μg per kilogram body weight per minute, exerts both pressor and inotropic effects. It may be titrated to as high as 20 to 30 μg per kilogram per minute to achieve a systolic blood pressure of 90 to 100 mm Hg or a mean pressure of approximately 60 mm Hg. The role of intravenous nitrates under these circumstances is to decrease the left ventricular filling pressure or preload. Since dopamine has chronotropic properties, sinus tachycardia may occur at higher doses. Atrial tachyarrhythmias may occasionally occur as well. If hypotension persists or if heart rate is unacceptable, norepinephrine, predominantly an alpha-1-adrenergic agonist, may be used, beginning at 5 to 10 μg per minute and increased as required to restore blood pressure.

In the rapidly deteriorating patient with fulminant pulmonary edema and respiratory failure, endotracheal intubation and mechanical ventilation are indicated. Mechanical ventilation corrects hypoxemia and acidosis and often results in stabilization of the patient's hemodynamic status by decreasing the work of breathing, thereby lessening the portion of the cardiac output that would otherwise be distributed to the respiratory muscles. On occasion, we have obviated intubation of a patient with fulminant pulmonary edema by performing the age-old procedure of phlebotomy. Phlebotomy may be performed by inserting a phlebotomy line into an antecubital vein and inflating a blood pressure cuff halfway between the systolic and the diastolic pressure. One to one and one-half units of blood may be safely withdrawn slowly, provided that the patient has a normal hemoglobin level.

Placement of an intra-aortic balloon pump is indicated in severe mitral regurgitation that is refractory to maximal pharmacologic therapy. Appreciable augmentation of cardiac output can be achieved with balloon counterpulsation, but the clinician must be cognizant of its potential complications (femoral artery laceration or occlusion, thromboemboli and cholesterol emboli, renal failure, femoral neuropathies, etc.). Nevertheless, insertion of this device may be lifesaving if immediate surgery cannot be performed. Intra-aortic balloon counterpulsation is contraindicated in aortic regurgitation because aortic regurgitation will worsen with inflation of the balloon in diastole.

Considerations in Infective Endocarditis

As emphasized previously, the definitive surgical treatment in severe acute aortic or mitral insufficiency must be undertaken as expeditiously as possible. In bacteremic patients with endocarditis and valvular regurgitation who are otherwise hemodynamically stable, it is prudent to attempt to sterilize the blood with an adequate regimen (7 to 14 days) of appropriate antibiotics before surgical replacement of the valve is performed. Bacteria remaining in the blood may seed the newly implanted prosthetic valve, possibly resulting in prosthetic valve endocarditis or valve ring abscess. Sterilization of an infected prosthetic valve is difficult, and it is not unlikely that implantation of a second prosthetic valve would soon be required. Therefore, surveillance blood cultures should be obtained routinely. Normalization of a previously elevated white blood cell count and body temperature is also a reasonable index of the adequacy of control of the infectious process, especially in culture-negative endocarditis or in instances in which there is coexisting pneumonia or septic emboli. It is advisable to continue antibiotics for several days after the valve is replaced.

CHRONIC VALVULAR REGURGITATION

Pathophysiology, Features, Operative Intervention

Chronic Mitral Regurgitation. There are numerous primary and secondary causes of chronic regurgitation. Primary forms of regurgitation are those that result from structural or functional abnormalities of the mitral valve apparatus, e.g., rheumatic mitral disease, connective tissue disorders, or papillary muscle dysfunction. Secondary forms result from progressive dilatation of the left ventricular cavity, which ultimately distorts the mitral valve annulus, leading to mitral insufficiency. This commonly occurs in dilated cardiomyopathy, for example.

The hemodynamic picture in chronic mitral regurgitation differs from that in acute regurgitation. With longstanding regurgitation that develops over several months to years, there is remodeling and dilation of the left ventricle and atrium so that the increased volumes may be accommodated without a large increase in chamber pressures, i.e., there is an increase in compliance. In this regard, even in severe mitral regurgitation, the PCWP tracing may not demonstrate a prominent "v" wave. Furthermore, with a dilated, compliant left atrium, the left ventricle can unload into a low-pressure, low-impedance chamber through the incompetent mitral valve. Curiously, the increased ventricular volume and low impedance leak actually optimize loading conditions for left ventricular ejection. As such, the left ventricular ejection fraction in compensated chronic mitral regurgitation is frequently normal or even slightly elevated at rest. This state of affairs may be tolerated well for several years to decades, until the left ventricle eventually fails and the ejection fraction begins to drop.

Although many patients with severe chronic valvular regurgitation benefit from valve replacement, other patients with longstanding regurgitation and a dilated, hypocontractile left ventricle may not benefit from valve replacement. Indeed, valve replacement in some patients may be even deleterious because with elimination of the low-impedance leak, the left ventricle will now have to pump against an increased afterload. Mitral valve replacement ideally should be performed before there is significant functional impairment of the left ventricle. A mitral valve or mitral annuloplasty is preferred over valve replacement if the anatomy of the mitral apparatus is conducive to this procedure.

Recommendations for valve replacement are still evolving and must be weighed against the immediate operative mortality and the long-term risks of chronic anticoagulation and thrombotic events from a prosthetic valve. Patients with severe regurgitation and New York Heart Association function class II or class III failure who remain symptomatic despite intensive medical therapy should be considered for operation, provided that the ejection fraction is normal or slightly depressed. Good left ventricular function is seen postoperatively in these patients if the preoperative left ventricular end systolic index is 30 ml per m^2 or greater. Prudence should be exercised in recommending valve replacement in patients with class IV heart failure and significantly reduced ejection fraction, since further deterioration in ventricular function can occur postoperatively. A higher perioperative mortality and depression of left ventricular function is seen postoperatively, especially in patients with a left ventricular end systolic index of 90 ml per m^2 or less; between 30 and 90 ml per m^2 there is intermediate risk.

Occasionally a patient who comes to the attention of a physician for other reasons is found to have severe mitral regurgitation but is asymptomatic or minimally symptomatic. If there is evidence for reduced left ventricular function (ejection fraction, 50 percent), we usually initiate treatment with an angiotensin-converting enzyme inhibitor for afterload reduction in hopes of forestalling further deterioration of myocardial contractile function.

Chronic Aortic Regurgitation. Chronic aortic regurgitation may be caused by abnormalities in the aortic cusps, aortic root distortion or dilatation, or loss of commissural support. In contrast to acute regurgitation, the left ventricle is usually markedly dilated and eccentrically hypertrophied from longstanding volume overload. As with chronic mitral regurgitation, the left ventricle develops increased compliance with time to accommodate the regurgitant volume. Comparing chronic aortic regurgitation with mitral regurgitation, patients with chronic aortic regurgitation ordinarily present with symptoms earlier in the course of the disease than do patients with mitral regurgitation because there is no low impedance chamber analogous to the left atrium into which the left ventricle can unload.

The cardiac examination in chronic regurgitation is similar to that in acute regurgitation, but the peripheral signs indicative of a hyperdynamic circulation are more prominent. These signs include a water-hammer pulse with abrupt distention and quick collapse (Corrigan's pulse), a widened pulse pressure, bifid carotid pulse, Quincke's sign, Duroziez's sign, and head-bobbing (de Musset's sign). The echocardiographic features are also similar to those in acute regurgitation except that the left ventricle is markedly thickened and dilated. The cardiac silhouette on chest film may be greatly enlarged, the so-called cor bovinum.

The same considerations for valve surgery in chronic mitral regurgitation apply to chronic aortic regurgitation. Once left ventricular contractile function becomes moderately impaired (i.e., ejection fraction less than 40 percent), the benefits of valve replacement become marginal and left ventricular function in some instances may even worsen postoperatively.

As an approximate guide, valve operation should be considered in chronic stable regurgitation when the left ventricular end-diastolic diameter on echocardiography approaches 75 mm, the end systolic diameter is 55 mm or greater, and the ejection fraction diminishes to below 40 percent. Echocardiography should be performed routinely at 6- to 12-month intervals in asymptomatic or stabilized patients to track possible deterioration in left ventricular function. When these parameters are borderline in an asymptomatic patient, our approach is to recommend valve replacement at the first sign of symptom development. A fall in ejection fraction with exercise greater than 5 percent as detected by exercise radionuclide angiography may also indicate the need for valve replacement. As with operation for any valve, the benefits of surgery must be weighed against the immediate and long-term risks.

Medical Management

The strategy of pre- and afterload reduction and inotropic intervention utilized for acute valvular regurgitation applies to the medical management of chronic regurgitation (Table 2). If intravenous medications have been used initially to achieve hemodynamic stability, attempts should be made to switch from intravenous medications to oral medications or long-term management, if valve replacement is not contemplated in the near future. Diuretics, digoxin, and oral vasodilators are the mainstay therapy in these patients.

A regimen of loop diuretic (furosemide, 40 to 120 mg per day orally) and digoxin (0.125 to 0.25 mg per day orally) is usually adequate in mild to moderate regurgitation, but in moderate to severe regurgitation, a vasodilator should be added. Our choice for a vasodilator is an angiotensin-converting enzyme (ACE) inhibitor (see the chapter on Congestive Heart Failure: Vasodilator Therapy).

Table 2 Treatment of Decompensated Chronic Valvular Regurgitation

Chronic Mitral Regurgitation
    Hemodynamic stabilization as in Table 1
    Switch to oral medications once hemodynamically stable
- Diuretics, furosemide 40–120 mg daily
- Digoxin, 0.125–0.25 mg daily
- Vasodilators, captopril 50 mg t.i.d, PO
  If angiotensin-converting enzyme inhibitor not tolerated, combination of isosorbide dinitrate (20 mg q.i.d) and hydralazine (75 mg q.i.d.) may be tried.
  Surgical replacement or repair of mitral valve
- Recommended in NYHA functional class II, III, IV patients who remain symptomatic despite maximal medical treatment provided EF > 40%. Patients with depressed EF < 30% and markedly dilated ventricle may not benefit from surgery.

Chronic Aortic Regurgitation
    Hemodynamic stabilization as in Table 1
    Switch to oral medications once hemodynamically stable (as above)
    Surgical replacement of aortic valve
- Recommend in asymptomatic patients or patients who remain symptomatic despite maximal medical treatment when LV end-diastolic diameter approaches 75 mm, end-systolic diameter is 55 mm, and EF diminishes below 40%.

EF = ejection fraction; LV = left ventricle.

Hypotension may result upon administration of ACE inhibitors in patients who are also receiving diuretics, even in patients with a normal to high mean PCWP. Therefore, captopril is the preferred ACE inhibitor to be used initially because of its short half-life. A test dose of 3.125 to 6.25 mg may be given orally; if tolerated, 6.25 mg every 8 hours orally may be continued, or a long-acting agent (enalapril or lisinopril) may be substituted. The dose of captopril may be doubled daily as tolerated to a total of 50 mg every 8 hours. If ACE inhibitors are not tolerated, then the combination of nitrates (20 to 30 mg every 8 to 12 hours) and hydralazine (25 to 100 mg every 6 to 8 hours, as tolerated) may be tried.

SUGGESTED READING

Braunwald E. Valvular heart disease. In: Braunwald E, ed. Heart disease. Philadelphia: WB Saunders, 1988.
Chatterjee K. Vasodilator therapy for mitral regurgitation. In: Duran C, Angell WW, Johnson AD, Oury JH, eds. Recent progress in mitral valve disease. London: Butterworths, 1984.
Dervan J, Goldberg S. Acute aortic regurgitation: pathophysiology and management. In: Frankl WS, Brest AN, eds. Valvular heart disease: comprehensive evaluation and management. Philadelphia: FA Davis, 1986.
Ross J. Left ventricular function and the timing of surgical treatment in valvular heart disease. Am Heart J 1981; 94:498–504.

THE POSTOPERATIVE CARDIAC SURGICAL PATIENT

JOHN PHELAN, M.D.
LLOYD W. KLEIN, M.D.

POSTOPERATIVE CARDIAC CARE

Upon arrival at the intensive care unit (ICU) from the operating room, patients are continuously monitored with an arterial line, balloon-tipped pulmonary artery catheter, Foley catheter for urine output, and a single-lead electrocardiogram (ECG). Chest tube drainage is measured to observe for hemorrhage. In addition, temporary epicardial atrial and ventricular pacing wires are left in place for management of arrhythmias. A 12-lead ECG and chest film are obtained immediately as are serum electrolytes, complete blood count and platelet count, coagulation profile, and arterial blood gases.

Hemodynamic Monitoring

The goals of intensive hemodynamic monitoring are as follows: (1) to provide timely data so that effective interventions can be undertaken prior to the onset of frank clinical decompensation, (2) to aid in the diagnosis and management of various syndromes, and (3) therapeutic decisions to be made objectively. It should be emphasized that all hemodynamic parameters—including cardiac index, pulmonary artery wedge pressure, pulmonary artery pressure and systemic vascular resistance—should be measured on arrival at the ICU to provide a baseline for subsequent reference. These parameters should be followed frequently in patients who require pressor support or who have impaired left ventricular function. In the majority of uncomplicated patients, most invasive apparatus can be removed on the first postoperative day.

Cardiac Function

Concomitant with cross-clamping of the aorta, coronary blood flow ceases and global myocardial ischemia rapidly ensues. To protect the myocardium from acute global subendocardial myocardial infarction, cold cardioplegia is given during cardiopulmonary bypass. Potassium-rich (15 to 35 mEq/L) cold cardioplegia is administered directly in the coronary arteries at 4°C every 20 to 30 minutes, providing excellent myocardial protection and long-term preservation of left ventricular (LV) function. Cross-clamp times of 120 minutes are well tolerated in patients with good preoperative left ventricular function, but shorter times are preferable in the presence of ventricular hypertrophy or functional impairment. Although the ability of the myocardium to recover quickly after cardiopulmonary bypass has markedly improved with the advent of cold cardioplegia, there is still a significant degree of transient myocardial depression that persists for 6 to 12 hours.

Recovery from cardiac surgery is usually uncomplicated when cardiac function in the first 24 to 48 hours provides adequate perfusion of vital organs without the support of inotropic agents or mechanical assistance. The ability of the heart to perform adequately in the early postoperative state is influenced by several factors including preoperative functional classification, type of surgery, and completeness of surgical repair. Patients with severe (class III or IV) functional impairment or markedly diminished global LV ejection fraction (less than 20 percent) are more likely to require pharmacologic assistance or placement of an intra-aortic balloon pump in the early postoperative period. While the majority of these patients survive to leave the hospital, their mortality is greater than average and the first few hours postoperatively are crucial to outcome. In particular, frequent hemodynamic measurements are made in order to maintain adequate filling pressures, mean arterial pressure, and cardiac index. In addition to preoperative left ventricular function, one must also consider the specific type of surgery. The mortality for elective coronary artery bypass grafting is 1 to 2 percent and is usually 5 percent for routine aortic or mitral valve replacement. Undoubtedly, the presence and degree of LV impairment adversely affects outcome in patients who undergo valve replacement for regurgitant lesions. Finally, if for some technical difficulty the surgical repair is incomplete (e.g., incomplete revascularization or repair of a septal defect) and the patient remains hemodynamically unstable, one must utilize the entire scope of diagnostic procedures (e.g., echo, oximetry data) to identify the deficiency and to plan an early definitive surgical approach, if feasible.

Low Cardiac Output States

Perhaps the most crucial challenge in the management of the postoperative patient is the recognition and effective support of reduced cardiac output. A cardiac index of under 2.2 L per minute per m^2 is usually associated with oliguria (less than 25 cc per hour), hypotension, mean arterial pressure (MAP) under 70 mm Hg, and lactic acidosis. The differential diagnosis is presented below in Table 1.

The initial diagnostic approach includes measurement of mean right atrial and pulmonary capillary wedge pressures along with thermodilution cardiac output. From this information, the systemic vascular resistance (SVR) should be derived by the equation:

$$SVR = (MAP-RA)/CO \times 80$$

(normal: 700–1,600 dynes.-sec-cm^{-5}), where MAP = mean arterial pressure, RAP = right atrial pressure, and CO = cardiac output.

There are a number of contributing factors to be taken into account when analyzing low cardiac output in the immediate postoperative period. As previously noted, the effect of cardiopulmonary bypass with cold cardioplegia will transiently depress LV systolic function, which will gradually improve with rewarming. General anesthesia is a significant arteriolar vasodilator, particularly when combined with the physiologic vasodilation accompanying rewarming after hypothermia. Hence, some degree of hypotension and rapid volume status changes are potential consequences. Additionally, one must consider loss of ionized calcium as a cause of impaired pump function. Therefore, if the ionized calcium is reduced, it should be replaced with one ampule of calcium chloride and then monitored frequently in the first 24 hours postoperatively. In addition, preoperative medication, intraoperative infarction, pulmonary status, metabolic acidosis, and anesthetic effects all directly influence cardiac function to variable extents during the immediate postoperative period. Fentanyl and other narcotic analgesics will also inhibit the cardiovascular response to catecholamine loads.

Volume Depletion. If the pulmonary wedge pressure is low with a reduced cardiac index, support should be initiated with both crystalloid and colloid as volume

Table 1 Differential Diagnosis of Low Cardiac Output Following Cardiac Surgery

Preoperative left ventricular dysfunction
Incomplete operative repair
Volume depletion
Incomplete rewarming
Excessive pulmonary vascular resistance
Cardiac tamponade
Perioperative myocardial infarction
Arrhythmia
Sepsis
Drug reaction

replacement. The latter may include albumin, fresh frozen plasma, or packed red blood cells as indicated. In most patients, a wedge pressure of 15 to 18 mm Hg should be adequate. However, there exists a subset of patients with diastolic compliance abnormalities who benefit from slightly higher filling pressures, occasionally as high as 22 mm Hg. These pressures should be tolerated as long as the patient's respiratory status is not compromised. If filling pressures are adequate and a high SVR is found, the use of sodium nitroprusside should be contemplated in doses of 0.5 to 4 μg per kilogram body weight per minute titrated to a MAP greater than or equal to 80 mm Hg. This agent also should be used to maintain MAP below 90 mm Hg in an effort to minimize bleeding at suture lines; it has the advantages of a rapid onset of action and a very short half-life, as the pharmacologic effect disappears within 10 minutes of discontinuation. Additionally, it has direct vasodilating actions on both venous and arterial smooth muscle, leading to marked reductions in both pulmonary and systemic vascular resistances. Alternatively, nitroglycerin can be used in place of nitroprusside. Nitroglycerin is infused intravenously at a rate of 25 to 500 μg per minute and has a more potent effect on venous smooth muscle, thereby reducing preload. While there is a minor direct effect on arterial smooth muscle, the major clinical utility is found in the setting of perioperative myocardial ischemia resulting from coronary vasoconstriction and/or spasm.

Patients with right ventricular dysfunction and/or infarction superficially resemble patients with volume depletion. However, these patients do not tolerate high filling pressures, and elevating the CVP inordinately will frequently result in worse hemodynamics. These patients respond best to catecholamines. In addition, if they can be stabilized, function will almost invariably improve over 24 to 48 hours and they will do well long-term.

Cardiogenic Shock. Once preload and afterload have been optimized, an inotropic agent is selected to ensure peripheral perfusion. Dopamine raises blood pressure by causing peripheral vasoconstriction via alpha-receptor stimulation and by increasing myocardial contractility. This latter effect occurs through a direct effect on beta$_1$-receptors and indirectly through release of norepinephrine in the sympathetic nerves. At low doses (1 to 2 μg per kilogram per minute) dopamine mediates the vasodilation of renal, mesenteric, coronary, and cerebral vascular beds. When infused at 2 to 5 μg per kilogram per minute, dopamine causes enhanced contractility and improvement in cardiac output. At higher doses (5 to 10 μg per kilogram per minute), a chronotropic effect accompanies an increase in SVR and MAP. By contrast, dobutamine stimulates primarily beta$_1$-receptors, and to a lesser degree, beta$_2$- and alpha-receptors, resulting in augmented myocardial contractility without much change in SVR or heart rate. This results in a relatively small elevation of blood pressure despite improved cardiac output with minimally increased cardiac oxygen consumption. Dobutamine typically is administered at doses of 2 to 10 mg per kilogram per minute intravenously. Amrinone has also been administered to enhance myocardial contractility, as well as to cause dose-dependent decreases in filling pressures and SVR. It is usually given as an initial bolus of 0.75 mg per kilogram and then as a continuous infusion of 5 to 10 μg per kilogram per minute. The major disadvantage of this agent is its high incidence of reversible thrombocytopenia when used for lengthy periods. Levophed (norepinephrine) has two principal hemodynamic effects. It acts to increase SVR by alpha-receptor activation and also stimulates cardiac contractility by acting on beta$_1$-receptors. Infusion rates of 1 to 15 μg per minute are used. Epinephrine stimulates beta$_1$, beta$_2$- and alpha-receptors and has found utility for support of both blood pressure and cardiac output. It may be infused at rates of 1 to 10 μg per minute. Isoproterenol is the most potent and pure beta-agonist and therefore will greatly increase both the heart rate and contractility. This yields a decline in both pulmonary and systemic vascular resistances, and therefore its greatest utility may be in the patient who has marked elevation in pulmonary vascular resistance associated with a low cardiac output. Isoproterenol can be infused at rates of 1 to 12 μg per minute. For further discussion of these agents see chapters regarding Distributive Shock and Cardiogenic Shock.

The appropriate selection of an inotropic agent varies with the clinical circumstance. In the presence of left ventricular impairment and ongoing ischemia, dobutamine in combination with nitroglycerin or amrinone appears to offer the most inotropic support with the least cost in terms of increased myocardial oxygen demand and improved oxygen delivery. If renal perfusion and LV function are impaired, dopamine may be the agent of choice and may be particularly beneficial to preserve renal blood flow when used at low doses (2 μg per kilogram per minute) in combination with other pressor agents. Dopamine is probably the treatment of choice for acute heart failure after cardiac surgery, having been shown to be superior to isoproterenol and phenylephrine, and may provide the optimal combination of effects as an aid to discontinuation of cardiopulmonary bypass.

Finally, the use of the intra-aortic balloon pump has increased dramatically in recent years. When inserted either surgically or percutaneously from the femoral artery, this device reduces afterload by lowering aortic impedance and also increases coronary blood flow by elevating diastolic driving pressure; the actual increment produced in cardiac index is surprisingly small (it may increase up to 0.8 L per minute per m^2). One must continuously monitor patients for limb ischemia and infection at the insertion site, especially in small, elderly women or in patients with pre-existing peripheral vascular disease. Every effort should be made to wean the patient from the ventilator prior to discontinuing the balloon pump because in many circumstances the work of independent breathing consumes approximately 25 percent of the cardiac output. Once the patient has been extubated, weaning the balloon proceeds in a gradual reduction from 1:1 to 1:4. If at 1:4 the patient has optimal hemodynamic parameters, the balloon should be removed. Several weaning attempts may be needed and the patient should be observed for several hours at lower levels of support prior to removal. Other mechanical assist devices such as the total artificial heart and left ventricular assist device are used in desperate situations in which patients are not able to be weaned from cardiopulmonary bypass. These patients must be candidates for subsequent cardiac transplantation.

Congestive Heart Failure. Postcardiac surgical patients characteristically have 2 to 4 L of excess fluid in their extravascular space, which begins to be reabsorbed into the intravascular space 24 to 72 hours after surgery. Patients with normal left ventricular function will diurese without difficulty. However, patients with postoperative abnormalities in left ventricular function require vasodilator and diuretic therapy, or clinical congestive failure and supraventricular and ventricular arrhythmias will result with an alarmingly high frequency. An indication of impending problems is frequently the absence of the normally rapid weight reduction experienced by these patients when they leave the ICU.

Cardiac Tamponade. Apart from pump failure and hypovolemia, the presence of cardiac tamponade must always be considered in the differential diagnosis of a low cardiac output syndrome. Typically, tamponade occurs in the setting of a patient who has had brisk output through the chest tubes which abruptly ceases. Hemodynamically, one observes a rise in mean right atrial and pulmonary capillary wedge pressures. These pressures frequently equalize and cardiac index falls; however, posterior accumulation of thrombus causing clinical tamponade may fail to produce diastolic equalization. The mediastinum widens on chest film, and an echocardiogram should confirm (but occasionally may not, in this setting) the presence of a large pericardial effusion with evidence of right ventricular diastolic collapse. Initially, treatment consists of volume infusion to maintain blood pressure. Cardiac tamponade may be temporarily relieved emergently by sterile irrigation of the chest tubes or by pericardiocentesis done at the bedside using a 14-gauge needle. These procedures may fail or succeed only transiently, as the effusion is frequently loculated and consists primarily of blood clot. Consequently, in most circumstances, open surgical drainage must be performed either at the bedside or preferably in the operating room.

Ischemia and Infarction

The presence of myocardial ischemia must always be considered in patients with a low cardiac output. In such cases, a decision to return to the operating room is always in the forefront. On arrival to the ICU, an ECG should be obtained and scrutinized critically for evidence of ST-segment changes diagnostic for ischemia. While transient conduction abnormalities and T-wave changes are frequently observed immediately after surgery, localized ST-segment changes are not. In this setting, a nitroglycerin infusion is initiated and titrated upward as hemodynamically tolerated. The ECG is repeated and if evidence of ischemia or low cardiac output persists, reoperation should be considered and/or an intra-aortic balloon pump inserted.

Patients returning to the ICU with intraoperative Q-waves usually have patent grafts and if the hemodynamic consequences are not severe, they do well. Late-onset ischemia with new Q-wave formation after return to the ICU is usually associated with vessel closure.

Enzymatic evidence for myocardial infarction (MI) should be sought in all patients. Absolute CPK-MB isoenzyme elevations of over 40 to 80 mg per dl or persistently elevated MB fractions (over 8 percent) are highly suggestive of MI, as is evidence of new Q waves or loss of precordial R-wave forces. Moreover, after the early postoperative period, an assessment of left ventricular function should be obtained by either echocardiography or radionuclide ejection fraction. Patients who have sustained a postoperative MI may benefit from the long-term use of beta-blockers to reduce mortality and the incidence of sudden death, provided that there is no evidence of congestive heart failure or other contraindications.

Pericarditis

The occurrence of pericarditis in the first 3 to 5 days postoperatively occurs in up to 40 percent of cases. A pericardial friction rub without symptoms of pericarditis is a very common observation 1 to 5 days postoperatively. This may or may not be associated with ECG evidence of pericarditis (diffuse ST elevation and PR depression). In the asymptomatic patient, no therapy is indicated. However, in the individual who becomes symptomatic with pericarditis, a trial of indomethacin or aspirin is warranted. If this regimen is unsuccessful, the use of oral prednisone or a single dose of 7 mg of dexamethasone intravenously should be contemplated.

Cardiac Arrhythmias

Postoperative cardiac arrhythmias may also occur, and successful management relies on timely and accurate recognition. The occurrence of arrhythmias should trigger a search for an underlying precipitant such as hypokalemia, acidosis, hypoxemia, bleeding, volume shifts, or pulmonary embolus. The arrhythmogenic potential of the increased catecholamine load, especially those catecholamines intravenously or nasally administered, should not be overlooked. The tachyarrhythmias may be separated into ventricular and supraventricular mechanisms for purposes of discussion.

Premature atrial contractions (PACs) are usually benign but can be compromising in patients who are particularly dependent on atrial synchrony for stroke volume—i.e., severe left ventricular hypertrophy with decreased diastolic compliance, aortic stenosis, among others. In these patients, digoxin therapy should be started at the first sign of ectopy unless contraindicated. Whether or not PACs should be treated routinely with digoxin or propranolol is somewhat controversial.

Many patients who have had chronic atrial fibrillation preoperatively will return from surgery with either junctional rhythms, which allows atrial pacing, or sinus activity. These patients usually revert to atrial fibrillation without significant hemodynamic consequence. Under these circumstances, cardioversion is not usually indicated and the use of medication should be limited to appropriate drugs that control rate. These patients are frequently on preoperative digoxin or propranolol and exhibit a relatively slow ventricular response after reconversion to atrial fibrillation.

Supraventricular arrhythmias, particularly atrial fibrillation, occur commonly in postoperative patients, frequently accompanying clinical evident pericarditis. Additionally, volume overload, hypoxia, and other metabolic precipitants must be treated aggressively. PACs are frequent precursors to these arrhythmias. The onset of supraventricular arrhythmia necessitates a search for an underlying cause, as noted above, particularly pericarditis. If oral or intravenous digoxin does not successfully control the rate, intravenous verapamil may be used in 5-mg increments, as long as the patient remains hemodynamically stable. Once rate control is achieved with digoxin or verapamil, a type-Ia antiarrhythmic drug (quinidine or procainamide) may be initiated for chemical conversion to sinus rhythm. Patients who develop transient paroxysmal atrial fibrillation postoperatively but who were in sinus rhythm preoperatively will almost invariably revert spontaneously to sinus rhythm after several hours. Electrical cardioversion is rarely necessary in these patients, and its use should be limited to those with acute decompensation because of the tendency toward recurrence over the first postoperative month. Once the rhythm is controlled, irregularities tend not to recur after the initial 30- to 60-day period and medications can be discontinued. A relatively common precipitating factor is aerosol therapy with Ventolin or Alupent, which should be discontinued in those patients in whom arrhythmias develop. If despite the above measures atrial fibrillation persists, synchronized cardioversion beginning at 50 joules can be performed following intravenous sedation with midazolam or diazepam. The appropriate timing for elective cardioversion depends on the patient's clinical stability, but probably should be attempted before discharge from the hospital.

Transient second- and third-degree atrioventricular (AV) block are common occurrences, especially after valve surgery. These disturbances may be treated rapidly using the atrial and ventricular epicardial pacing wires placed during surgery. In most circumstances, AV sequential pacing yields the optimal hemodynamic effect because of the significant contribution of atrial systole to cardiac output. Rates of 80 to 100 beats per minute usually suffice to maintain normal hemodynamic parameters.

Sustained, monomorphic ventricular tachycardia is actually rare after bypass surgery except in the setting of prior occurrence. Hemodynamically unstable ventricular tachycardia or ventricular fibrillation requires immediate unsynchronized defibrillation with 200 J. If unsuccessful, 300 J should be delivered immediately (see chapter on arrhythmias for full ACLS protocol). Lidocaine (1 to 2 mg per kilogram body weight delivered intravenously as a bolus) should be given and an additional 0.5 mg per kilogram or a 50-mg intravenous dose given 15 to 20 minutes later. A continuous infusion of lidocaine (1 to 4 mg per minute) is started simultaneously. The dose of lidocaine should be attenuated in patients with heart or liver failure. Lidocaine frequently is administered for the first 24 to 48 hours postoperatively in patients with frequent or multifocal PVCs. If lidocaine does not successfully suppress complex ventricular ectopy, one should use procainamide (6 to 12 mg per kilogram) given no faster than 50 mg per minute intravenously until clinical effect is observed or prolongation of the QRS by more than 50 percent occurs. A constant infusion of 2 to 6 mg per minute should then be maintained, and drug levels may be monitored. In some circumstances, patients are refractory to both lidocaine and/or procainamide, and bretylium tosylate should be initiated. Bretylium is administered as a bolus of 5 to 10 mg per kilogram given slowly over 10 to 20 minutes; then a maintenance infusion of 0.5 to 2.0 mg per minute is begun. Rarely, sustained ventricular tachycardia will respond only to overdrive pacing. This may easily be accomplished using the epicardial pacing wires that are left in place following surgery.

When a complex arrhythmia becomes a diagnostic dilemma, the atrial and/or ventricular pacing wire may be attached using an alligator clip to the V lead of the electrocardiographic recorder. This facilitates the recognition of P waves and therefore assists in the diagnosis of atrial arrhythmias. Moreover, these pacing wires can be used therapeutically to overdrive pace and to suppress ventricular tachycardia or atrial flutter.

RESPIRATORY CARE

A chest film should be obtained immediately upon presentation to the ICU to check for endotracheal tube positioning, pneumothorax or hemothorax, and line positioning. Not infrequently, a tube in the right mainstem bronchus may still be associated with bilateral respiratory sounds. Chest films should be repeated to look for changes in tube position or lung status and should be obtained immediately if any significant problems with oxygenation or CO_2 retention occur.

Oxygenation and Acid-base

Immediately after surgery, all patients are intubated and initially managed with the following ventilator settings: tidal volume, 10 to 15 cc per kg; FiO_2, 70 percent; expiratory rate, 10 to 12 per minute; and intermittent mandatory ventilation (SIMV) mode. Some institutions use 5 cm H_2O of positive end-expiratory pressure (PEEP) routinely in all patients, but this has no proven benefit. A tidal volume of 10 cc per kg may be preferable to avoid excessive tension on suture lines when an internal mammary graft has been used. Arterial blood gases should be obtained early after arrival to the ICU and appropriate ventilator adjustments made. The PaO₂ should be maintained at greater than 70 mm Hg, and the PaCO₂ at less than 45 mm Hg. As rewarming occurs, CO₂ production increases and may cause a metabolic acidosis. This situation may be complicated by shivering, which not only further increases oxygen demand and the acidosis, but which may also result in less effective ventilation. If sedation, blankets, and ascertaining the position of the endotracheal tube do not substantially correct the acidosis, treatment with bicarbonate to maintain a pH of over 7.30 may be required. Appropriate bicarbonate replacement can be calculated using the following formula:

$$HCO_3 \text{ replacement} = (\text{weight/kg}) \times (0.3) \times (\text{base deficit})$$

It usually is prudent to give approximately half the calculated amount and repeat the pH measurement before administering the remainder.

Weaning

Once the effects of sedation have receded and the patient breathes spontaneously, the SIMV rate is progressively reduced and continuous positive airway pressure (CPAP) is begun. Successful weaning may be predicted using the following guidelines: peak negative inspiratory force, less than −25 mm Hg; respiration rate, less than 30 per minute: vital capacity, greater than or equal to 10 cc per kilogram; FiO₂ less than 50 percent. Following extubation, an FiO₂ of 50 percent is administered and arterial blood gases are frequently obtained to monitor and ensure adequate ventilation and oxygenation. Incentive spirometry and chest physiotherapy are initiated soon after extubation in order to avoid atelectasis and pneumonia. It must be reiterated that the nebulized bronchodilators are arrhythmogenic and may precipitate atrial fibrillation.

The chest film should be reviewed daily for at least the first 3 days to exclude pneumothorax, pulmonary infiltrates or edema, and pleural effusion. If a large pneumothorax or compromising effusion occurs, a chest tube should be promptly inserted. When evidence for pulmonary edema exists, appropriate therapy is initiated after confirmation with wedge pressures and other clinical parameters. One must also consider noncardiogenic pulmonary edema in the presence of diffuse bilateral interstitial infiltrates and a normal pulmonary capillary wedge pressure. This phenomenon probably occurs to a variable extent in most patients recovering from cardiopulmonary bypass and usually causes a transient decline in lung compliance. The vast majority of patients recover without difficulty, but a few will develop adult respiratory distress syndrome (ARDS) with evidence of increased capillary permeability and leakage of plasma into pleural, peritoneal, and interstitial spaces.

Prolonged intubation may be required in patients with chronic obstructive pulmonary disease (COPD) or asthma following open heart surgery. For patients with COPD it is important to recognize that they may have a chronic compensatory metabolic alkalosis, and thus the goal of ventilation should be to maintain a normal pH. Frequently, the PCO₂ will be greater than 45 mm Hg in these circumstances and a bicarbonate diuresis may be initiated by using potassium chloride or acetazolamide. The use of nebulized bronchodilator therapy often facilitates the weaning process. Inhaled bronchodilators include Bronkosol (isoetharine), 0.5 cc in 2.5 cc of saline every 4 to 6 hours; or Alupent (metaproterenol), 0.2 cc in 2.5 cc of saline every 4 to 6 hours. If additional bronchodilator therapy is required, aminophylline at 5 to 7 mg per kilogram is infused over 30 minutes followed by a continuous infusion of 0.5 mg per kilogram per hour. For refractory patients, a course of systemic steroids may be indicated. With prolonged intubation (longer than 2 weeks), tracheostomy should be performed.

HEMATOLOGIC EFFECTS

Effects of Cardiopulmonary Bypass

Cardiopulmonary bypass evokes a diffuse inflammatory response with increased capillary permeability mediated at least in part by activation of complement and kinins and by exposure to nonendothelial surfaces. As a result, platelet clumping and embolization may occur, in addition to activation and consumption of the coagulation system (factor XII). Polymorphonuclear leukocytes are likewise aggregated, leading to intrapulmonary sequestration of leukocytes and transient postoperative pulmonary dysfunction.

Bleeding

The platelet count, prothrombin time (PT), and partial thromboplastin time (PTT) are routinely measured immediately after surgery. Usually, patients are given 2 U of fresh frozen plasma as they are weaned from cardiopulmonary bypass. If the PT and PTT remain abnormal, additional units of fresh frozen plasma are given. If the fibrinogen level is less than 100 mg per deciliter, one should administer cryoprecipitate, usually 8 U at a time (2 U per 10-kg body weight elevates fibrinogen by 50 mg per dl). If evidence of the fibrinogenolysis is present, with high levels of fibrin degradation products, epsilon-aminocaproic acid (Amicar) may be given at a dose of 5 to 10 gm intravenously over 1 hour and then followed by an infusion of 1 g per hour for 3 to 5 hours. Platelet transfusions are reserved for patients whose postoperative platelet count drops below 80,000 per ml or in those patients who have a prolonged bleeding time.

Of critical importance during the postoperative period is careful monitoring of bleeding through the chest tubes. When drainage exceeds 1,500 cc over the first 12 hours or if a sudden increase (over 300 cc per hour) occurs, exploration should be considered. Occasionally, bleeding of up to 400 cc in the first hour may occur, which, if all other clotting parameters are reasonable, may not require specific therapy if bleeding diminishes subsequently. Recently, bloody drainage from the chest tubes has been collected, filtered, and reinfused. This technique of autologous transfusion significantly reduces the need for multiple transfusions and could be employed routinely. If drainage ceases entirely, consideration that the tube has thrombosed, kinked, or become entrapped must be seriously entertained and immediately corrected.

Anticoagulation and Antiplatelet Agents

Anticoagulation is often employed in the early postoperative recovery period, particularly following valve surgery or aneurysmectomy. For the first 48 hours, patients are maintained without anticoagulants and then heparinization is initiated to maintain the PTT at 1.5 to 2 times control. Most patients with mechanical prostheses who remain in sinus rhythm and have no evidence of emboli may safely be orally anticoagulated without heparinization when extubated. On the second postoperative day, Coumadin therapy may be initiated using 10 mg orally for 3 consecutive days. The PT is then adjusted to 1.5 times control. Recent data have demonstrated that more aggressive anticoagulation therapy does not reduce the incidence of thromboembolic complications but does increase the rate of hemorrhagic complications. Lifetime anticoagulation is required with mechanical prostheses, whereas patients who receive bioprosthetic values may be anticoagulated for only the first 6 months, unless there is evidence of chronic atrial fibrillation with left atrial thrombosis or a prior embolic event. When aortic homografts are used, anticoagulation may be unnecessary unless evidence of embolic phenomena exists.

Following coronary artery bypass grafting, the efficacy of aspirin to maintain graft patency has now been demonstrated. Therefore, 325 mg of enteric-coated aspirin is given once daily, beginning the second postoperative day. More aggressive therapy with preoperative aspirin and Persantine may be more effective and is better studied, but bleeding rates and complications may be increased in some centers.

NEUROLOGIC FUNCTION

Neurologic complications of cardiopulmonary bypass are rare (less than 2 percent) but when present are associated with a high mortality (25 to 30 percent). The causes include inadequate pump perfusion pressure or embolism, either due to air or atherosclerotic debris. Occasionally, intracranial hemorrhage occurs, resulting from the anticoagulation necessary for bypass. Risk factors that predict a neurologic event include advanced age or prior neurologic deficit.

Carotid stenosis is also a well-known risk factor for an acute neurologic event during cardiopulmonary bypass. When asymptomatic bruits are heard, no increased risk exists; therefore, simultaneous carotid endarterectomy should not be pursued. In symptomatic patients, substantial evidence exists to support the practice of simultaneous endarterectomy. Another possibility, if the clinical situation allows, is first to operate on the carotid stenosis. Nevertheless, in some nonelective situations, neither of these options may be a reasonable approach, and the decision to proceed with knowledge of an increased risk is made. Manifestations may include seizure, hemiparesis or persistent unresponsiveness. These findings should prompt a neurologic evaluation including CT scan of the head, electroencephalogram, and consultation by a neurologist. While some institutions routinely give intravenous Decadron (4 mg every 6 hours for several days) in an effort to reduce cerebral edema, no data exist to support such a practice. When seizures occur, diazepam (5 to 10 mg intravenously) should be given; lorazepam (2 mg intravenously) may be substituted. Additionally, dilantin should be given slowly (15 to 18 mg per kilogram intravenously), not exceeding a rate of 50 mg per minute. If these measures fail, prompt neurologic consultation must be obtained. Moreover, one should ensure that all possible metabolic precipitants, including hypoxemia, acidosis, or hypocalcemia are eliminated.

Brachial plexus and peripheral mononeuropathies have also been observed following cardiac surgery. These generally are due to compression and are transient, usually lasting 4 to 8 weeks. They do not require therapy.

Some elderly patients may experience ICU psychosis. This may occur as a result of microemboli from cardiopulmonary bypass, or simply as a result of multiple sedatives and the disruptive ICU environment. If agitation is manifest in the early postoperative phase, this may necessitate heavy sedation. It is crucial that the patient remain without agitation while intubated with chest tubes or while on the intra-aortic balloon pump. Resolution of ICU-induced psychosis frequently occurs as many of the medicines and devices are weaned. Moreover, it is useful for staff and family to restore environmental cues. Persistent agitation may be treated with Haldol, 1 to 5 mg intravenously every 2 to 4 hours.

METABOLIC EFFECTS

An impaired response to insulin, leading to hyperglycemia, may be observed in the immediate postoperative period. This may result in transiently increased insulin requirements in diabetic patients or the need for small doses of insulin in borderline diabetic patients. Other hormonal alterations include elevated circulating epinephrine, norepinephrine, antidiuretic hormone, and aldosterone levels. Consequently, increased total body water with diffuse interstitial edema is a frequent observation. Hence, sodium administration should be closely monitored. The use of 0.25 percent sodium chloride with or without 5 percent dextrose in small amounts (20 to 30 units per hour) is usually sufficient. Alternatively, one can substitute lactated Ringer's solution.

RENAL FAILURE

The incidence of acute renal failure following open heart surgery is very small (less than 0.1 percent). Optimal renal function may be defined by adequate urine output (more than 25 cc per hour), and a normal serum BUN and creatinine. In circumstances where preexisting renal insufficiency is present, postoperative renal function may be adequately determined by changes from the baseline BUN and creatinine. The most effective way to ensure adequate recovery of renal function is to maintain adequate filling pressures and cardiac index. In the presence of normal hemodynamics and oliguria, some have given Lasix or mannitol (up to 25 g) in order to convert oliguric to nonoliguric renal failure. However, because there is no published trial establishing a clear long-term benefit from therapy with Lasix or mannitol, most institutions do not employ this method.

Once acute renal failure has been diagnosed, one should obtain serum and urine sodium, creatinine, and osmolarity. The specimens should be obtained in the diuretic-free state or at least 12 hours after the last diuretic dose. The fractional excretion of sodium (FeNa) may then be calculated using the formula:

$$FeNa = (UNa/UCr) \times (PCr/PNa) \times 100$$

where UNa = urinary sodium, UCr - urinary creatinine, PCr = plasma creatinine, and PNa = plasma sodium. If FeNa is less than 1, the cause of oliguria is prerenal (i.e., poor perfusion). Other findings that are seen in this circumstance include UNa of less than 20, and a U:P ratio of greater than 1.2. When FeNa is greater than 1 and UNa is greater than 20 and isosthenuria is present, then acute renal failure is diagnosed. Among the causes of renal failure that need to be carefully evaluated are drugs (e.g., aminoglycoside) and pigments (usually hemolysis). However, most commonly, acute renal failure in this setting is due to hypotension from poor perfusion during cardiopulmonary bypass (acute tubular necrosis). A nephrology consultation should be obtained and emergent dialysis considered when hypervolemia, hyperkalemia, or acidosis exists.

For hyperkalemia (potassium level greater than 5.6 mEq per deciliter), an ECG should be scrutinized for changes including peaked T waves and QRS widening. If these are present, 10 cc of a 10 percent solution of calcium gluconate may be given and repeated in 5 minutes. Other measures to consider include one ampule of 50 percent dextrose along with 10 U of insulin intravenously. Kayexalate should be initiated simultaneously and administered orally, 30 g in 50 to 100 ml of 20 percent sorbitol every 4 hours. Alternately, a Kayexalate enema of 50 g in 200 cc of 20 percent sorbitol may be given every 4 to 6 hours.

Table 2 Common Causes of Postoperative Fevers During the First Week Following Open Heart Surgery

Atelectasis
Pneumonia
Urinary tract infection
Pericarditis
Drug fever
Thrombophlebitis
Line infection

INFECTIOUS COMPLICATIONS

Postoperative fever confronts a substantial number of patients following cardiac surgery. Broad-spectrum antibiotics that cover species of staphylococci are used prophylactically by most surgeons. Typically, one selects cefazolin, 2 g intravenously given just prior to surgery and then continued every 8 hours for 2 days postoperatively. In some patients who have allergies to penicillin, 1 g of vancomycin is given intravenously on call, followed by 500 mg every 6 hours for the next 2 days.

Despite treatment with prophylactic antibiotics, many patients develop fevers exceeding 38.5°C in the first week. Causes to be considered are shown in Table 2. Appropriate evaluation should consist of several blood and urine cultures, urinalysis, sputum Gram stain, and review of chest film for atelectasis and pneumonia. Once a focus of infection is identified, antibiotics are selected on the basis of culture results and organism sensitivity.

Early postoperative fevers (days 1 to 5) usually result from atelectasis, pneumonia, pericarditis, indwelling vascular lines, thrombophlebitis, and drugs. Atelectasis is the most common cause of early fever and will usually respond well to aggressive pulmonary care including deep respiratory exercises and aerosol therapy. Beyond this time, wound infection appears to be the most important consideration along with endocarditis in the setting of prosthetic valves.

ACKNOWLEDGMENT The authors are indebted to the review and suggestions made by Dr. Michael Feldman.

SUGGESTED READING

Ellison N. Coagulation evaluations and management. In: Ream AK, Fogdall RD, eds. Acute Cardiovascular Management. Philadelphia: JB Lippincott, 1982.

Hotson JR. Neurological sequence of cardiac surgery. In: Aminoff MJ, ed. Neurology and general medicine. New York: Churchill Livingstone, 1989.

Kirklin JW, Barratt-Boyes BG. Cardiac surgery. New York: John Wiley and Sons, 1986.

Kirklin JW, Blackstone EH, Kirklin JK. Cardiac surgery. In: Braunwald E, ed. Heart disease. Philadelphia: WB Saunders Co., 1988.

Saour JN, et al. Trial of different intensities of anticoagulation in patients with prosthetic heart valves. N Engl J Med 1990; 352:428–432.

HYPERTENSIVE EMERGENCY AND AORTIC DISSECTION

ROBERT J. CODY, M.D.

HYPERTENSIVE EMERGENCIES

A hypertensive emergency does not constitute a specific disease process or specific disorder. Rather, it represents a constellation of severe hypertension, a generalized or specific medical problem, and one or more symptoms that combine to produce a morbid or premorbid situation. In an era when hypertension is at least partially treated by a number of classes of antihypertensive agents, the frequency with which patients present with a true hypertensive emergency has decreased. Typically, patients present to an emergency room or are found with urgent decompensation in a hospital setting. The treatment of hypertensive emergencies requires a careful process of differential diagnosis and a well-executed sequence of management decisions. However, it is unusual to be placed in a situation where corrective matters cannot be instituted in a short period of time and where, at the very least, blood pressure cannot be restored to an acceptable range. Table 1 summarizes some of the more common situations that constitute hypertensive emergencies. It is readily apparent from this list that many of the hypertensive emergencies stem from target organ damage of the brain or heart. Special considerations that will be discussed below are malignant hypertension and eclampsia of pregnancy. The hypertensive emergencies associated with central nervous system (CNS) or cardiac events such as impending stroke and CNS hemorrhage, or acute heart failure and myocardial infarction, constitute serious medical problems in and of themselves. However, it is important that control of blood pressure not be withheld or relegated to an unimportant side event. Both short-term outcome of associated CNS and cardiac events is imminently dependent on satisfactory blood pressure control. The control of blood pressure in the setting of hypertensive emergencies can be divided into immediate, short-term, and long-term goals. For the management of hypertensive emergencies, the physician is generally dealing with immediate and short-term goals.

Immediate Management

Some authors have attempted to distinguish hypertensive "emergencies" from hypertensive "urgencies" according to whether blood pressure should be lowered immediately versus situations where blood pressure can be lowered in 30 to 60 minutes. Such distinctions may not be relevant for an individual patient. The immediate management of a hypertensive emergency requires a sequence of assessment and therapy that generally can be applied almost uniformly in patients. While the temporal sequence of soliciting the patient history, physical examination, and blood pressure reduction are not necessarily the same for each patient, the elements within each of these three groupings is generally the same. Several important historical issues must be clarified and should be obtained from a family member or friend, if the patient cannot provide this information. Perhaps the most important historical issue is the duration of hypertension. If hypertension has been longstanding, then essential hypertension is the likely underlying problem; however, one has to be concerned regarding the events precipitating a rapid and unexplained acceleration of hypertension. This may represent superimposition of a secondary problem, such as renovascular hypertension superimposed on essential hypertension or a primary CNS lesion, such as a posterior fossa tumor, superimposed on longstanding hypertension. If there is no known history of hypertension or if hypertension was recently diagnosed, it is important to consider possibilities such as severe renovascular hypertension, pheochromocytoma, or recent-onset malignant hypertension. It is important to learn such things as whether the patient has been treated for hypertension at any time in the past, the nature of pharmaceutical agents that were used, and the effectiveness of these agents. The history should also include on assessment of target organ changes during the 48 to 72 hours immediately preceding the hypertensive emergency. Of particular concern is the occurrence of CNS such as memory changes, lethargy, focal weakness, visual changes, and nausea or vomiting.

The physical examination is also brief and straightforward and will depend to some degree on the nature of the presenting illness. A brief, efficient neurologic examination should be performed to assess communicative skills, cognition, and memory. It should also include a rapid assessment of motor function. The mandatory component of the physical examination in all hypertensive emergencies is the funduscopic evaluation. The eyegrounds of a

Table 1 General Classes of Hypertensive Emergencies

Central nervous system
  Stroke/stroke in progress
  Cerebral/subarachnoid hemorrhage
  Hypertensive encephalopathy

Cardiovascular system
  Unstable angina/myocardial infarction
  Pulmonary edema/decompensated congestive heart failure
  Aortic dissection

Malignant-phase hypertension

Eclampsia

Hypertension in the perioperative setting
  Head trauma/cranial procedures
  Coronary artery bypass surgery
  Major vascular procedures

Less common situations
  Pheochromocytoma
  Interactions with monoamine-oxidase inhibitors

patient with a hypertensive emergency can provide information regarding the duration of hypertension (arteriolar narrowing, anteriovenous nicking, and sclerosis), the severity of hypertension (hemorrhages and exudates), and the diagnosis of malignant-phase hypertension (presence of papilledema or disc blurring). The pulmonary examination should focus on the presence of, or impending, pulmonary congestion. The cardiovascular examination should include assessment of several key features. Cardiac enlargement, with or without an S_3 gallop, provides information regarding acute or long-term congestive heart failure. While cardiac murmurs provide some information regarding the severity of hypertension or coexistent cardiac disease, the most important murmur to note is that of aortic insufficiency. This may be one of the first clues for aortic dissection or aortic aneurysm. The carotid, brachial, and femoral pulses should be assessed to determine evidence of coexistent atherosclerosis (bruit) or loss of pulses consistent with dissection. In addition to the standard examination of the abdomen, particular attention should be focused on the presence or absence of an abdominal aortic aneurysm.

It is necessary to establish which component of the hypertensive emergency is top priority. For instance, in a patient with a stroke in progress, it is appropriate first to lower blood pressure while awaiting radiologic studies to determine whether anticoagulation should be initiated. By contrast, it is necessary to initiate anticonvulsant therapy for a patient with ongoing seizures prior to a decision regarding the initial antihypertensive therapy. It is important to reiterate, however, that at no time during the management of the patient should adequate blood pressure control be neglected.

Laboratory data obtained at the time of management of hypertensive emergencies often are not definitive but may provide clues to the initial management and can provide insight into concomitant illness and choice of antihypertensive therapy. Standard data such as the chest film, electrocardiogram (ECG), serum electrolytes, and serum BUN/creatinine help identify the extent to which cardiac and renal function are impaired in relation to the current hypertensive crisis. Evidence of chronic congestive heart failure, for instance, would favor the use of a vasodilator rather than aggressive therapy with beta-adrenergic blockage. Hypokalemia would necessitate avoidance of aggressive diuresis until potassium is replaced.

Initial Management of Hypertensive Emergencies and Urgencies

The list of potential medications for the management of hypertensive emergencies can be rather extensive (Table 2). Prior to choosing therapy, it is important to address the following question: How quickly and to what level must the blood pressure be lowered? The unwarranted yet seemingly common clinical practice is to lower blood pressure immediately to normotensive levels. In actuality, this may be totally inappropriate and more experienced physicians now shy away from this approach, particularly with the current wide choice of therapeutic agents. The speed with which blood pressure is lowered is dependent on the overall clinical picture. If a patient has been free of symptoms in the previous 2 to 3 days and is currently free of symptoms, then blood pressure in this individual can be brought down with oral medications in the course of the ensuing few hours and may not require intensive care therapy or an extensive work-up. The patient with active seizures or acute pulmonary edema would certainly benefit from a rapid reduction of blood pressure. On the other hand, a patient with stroke in progress (particularly if severe carotid disease is present) or a patient with an acute myocardial infarction may be better served by a more gradual reduction of blood pressure over the ensuing 1 to 4 hours, rather than radical swings of blood pressure within a few minutes. The decision must also be made as to whether this patient would be stabilized with oral medications, or whether parenteral therapy will be required over the next 48 hours. It is important to reiterate the fact that elevated blood pressure alone, particularly with a diastolic blood pressure of less than 110 mm Hg, does not constitute a hypertensive emergency.

For immediate blood pressure reduction, a parenteral administration of "mini bolus" diazoxide remains a safe and effective means of lowering blood pressure. Repeated bolus adminstration of 50 mg at 5- to 10-minute intervals results in a safe, gradual reduction of blood pressure, avoiding the severe hypotension and complications reported when this drug was first administered as a single bolus of 300 mg. Depending on circumstances such as evidence

Table 2 Pharmacologic Classes for the Treatment of Hypertensive Emergencies

Diuretics
  Generally only an adjunct for the treatment of edema

Central Sympatholytics
  Guanethidine
  Alpha-methyldopa
  Trimethaphan

Peripheral Autonomic Blockade
  Beta-adrenergic blockade
  Alpha-adrenergic blockade
  Combined: labetolol

Direct-acting Vasodilators
  Nitroprusside
  Diazoxide
  Hydralazine
  Minoxidil

Angiotensin-Converting Enzyme Inhibitors*
  Captopril
  Enalapril
  Lisinopril

Calcium-channel Antagonists*
  Verapamil
  Nicardipine

*These compounds can be given intravenously.

of coronary ischemia, sublingual nitroglycerin is sometimes helpful. Parenteral administration of hydralazine or alpha-methyldopa remains effective treatment in the appropriate setting. The reflex tachycardia associated with hydralazine and all vasodilators that rapidly lower blood pressure should be avoided in unstable cardiac conditions such as ongoing coronary ischemia. Calcium-channel antagonists that can be administered parenterally (such as verapamil and nicardipine) are very effective. While calcium-channel antagonists can produce a negative inotropic effect of varying degrees, this typically is not a clinical problem in the hypertensive population in this context, and they would certainly have less of a negative inotropic effect than an intravenous beta-blocker. Furthermore, beta-blockers typically require 1 to 2 hours before their antihypertensive effect is appreciable. With the availability of intravenous enalaprilat, converting enzyme inhibitors can now be considered for parenteral administration. If it is evident that a patient will not be able to take oral medications within the next few hours (e.g., a comatose patient), or if blood pressure control must be carefully titrated, then it is reasonable to make plans to proceed to a continuous infusion of intravenous nitroprusside. Otherwise, most patients can proceed to oral therapy within the first 6 to 12 hours of initiation of therapy. The use of sublingual nifedipine squeezed from its capsule has come into vogue for the use of hypertensive emergencies. *This is a dangerous approach* to reducing blood pressure, as administration of nifedipine in this manner can cause rapid uncontrolled reductions of blood pressure within 5 minutes. There have been anecdotal reports of myocardial infarction, arrhythmias, and congestive heart failure in such circumstances. Nifedipine is a rapidly reacting calcium-channel antagonist. Therefore, giving it in a standard oral fashion will produce appreciable reduction of blood pressure within 30 minutes. Simply stated, there is no need to give it sublingually. Labetalol is an effective parenteral compound for the treatment of hypertensive emergencies. Its combined alpha- and beta-adrenergic blocking characteristics have popularized its use, and parenteral therapy can be followed with the oral formulation.

Malignant-phase Hypertension. The malignant phase of hypertension is a distinct and dangerous hypertensive entity. "Malignant" is not a synonym for accelerated hypertension, hypertensive crisis, or hypertensive emergency. It is a discrete constellation of findings, as summarized in Table 3. The diagnosis of malignant-phase hypertension requires the presence of papilledema on funduscopic examination. Malignant-phase hypertension is associated with arteriolar fibrinoid necrosis, which is a marker for the vasculitic aspect of this disorder, occurring within target organs, particularly the retina, brain, and kidney. Clinically, this disorder is characterized by a rapid increase in blood pressure over a few days and is typically superimposed on one of the other forms of hypertension. The one exception to this rule is the fact that the primary hypersecretion of aldosterone is almost never associated with malignant-phase hypertension. Malignant-phase hypertension can proceed to rapid destruction of renal function in a matter of a few days. Unfortunately, this process sometimes occurs despite adequate blood pressure reduction. Malignant-phase hypertension is almost always associated with an abnormal elevation of renin system activity, even when the underlying hypertension is "essential." Therefore, angiotensin-converting enzyme (ACE) inhibitors are very effective initial therapy for these patients, but typically, two or three drugs are required to achieve reasonable blood pressure control.

Eclampsia of Pregnancy. The management of hypertension during pregnancy requires established clinical experience. The spectrum of hypertension that one can encounter is summarized in Table 4. True eclampsia of pregnancy, by definition, requires the presence of seizure disorders, proteinuria, edema, and hypertension. This is differentiated from pre-eclampsia, where seizures have not yet occurred and prompt control of blood pressure can evert further morbidity. Management of eclampsia consists of anticonvulsive therapy, blood pressure reduction, and delivery of the fetus. This course of action should be initiated promptly to avoid serious complications to the mother and the fetus.

Table 3 Clinical Features of Malignant Hypertension

Blood pressure usually greater than 200/130

Neuroretinopathy (papilledema)

Fluctuating signs and symptoms
  Primary (lethargy, visual changes)
  Secondary (mitral insufficiency, cerebrovascular accident)

Underlying hypertension
  Virtually any form of hypertension except aortic coarctation or primary aldosteronism

Rapid progression to renal destruction

Table 4 Factors for the Management of Hypertension in Pregnancy

Classification of hypertension in pregnancy
  Transient hypertension
  Chronic hypertension
  Chronic hypertension/superimposed pre-eclampsia
  Pre-eclampsia/eclampsia

Treatment of severe hypertension in pregnancy
  Hydralazine
  Diazoxide* (may reduce placental blood flow)
  Nitroprusside* (avoid prolonged or high-dose infusions)
  Labetolol (limited experience in pregnancy)

Treatment of eclampsia
  Clinical stabilization
  Anticonvulsants
  Blood pressure reduction
  Delivery of the fetus

*Calcium channel antagonists may produce uterine muscle relaxation and disruption of the uterine placenta interface; experience in pregnancy is limited.

Table 5 Aortic Dissection

Classification by type
   I: Proximal ascending aorta to the level of the carotid artery
   II: Proximal ascending aorta proceeding distal to the carotid artery
   III: Begins distal to the carotid artery proceeding to any distal region thereafter

Initial management
   Monitoring/stabilization in an intensive care unit
   Reduce systolic blood pressure to 100 mm Hg or lower, if necessary (beta-blockers preferred)
   Minimize aortic shear stress
   Definitive diagnostic procedures when stable

Subsequent definitive management
   Proximal dissection (types I and II)
      Surgery unless complicated by myocardial infarction or CVA
   Distal dissection (type III)
      Medical management unless complicated by impending rupture, target organ compromise

AORTIC DISSECTION

Aortic aneurysm and aortic dissection are not synonymous. Dissection may occur in only a small percentage of patients with a documented aneurysm, while at the same time, a dissection may be present in the absence of a clear-cut discrete aortic aneurysm. The diagnosis of dissection, like pulmonary embolism, requires a high degree of suspicion rather than overt clinical manifestation. Sudden sharp chest pain, the presence of a pulseless artery, a new aortic regurgitation murmur, or widening of the mediastinum on chest film remain the best clinical markers. The DeBakey classification of dissection remains the best pragmatic classification (Table 5). Documentation of the dissection flap has improved considerably in the last 5 years. Previously, angiographic methodologies were able to demonstrate the presence of an aneurysm or dissection but at times had difficulty locating the dissection flap in order to permit surgical repair. Newer approaches such as computerized tomography or transesophageal echocardiography have improved the localization of dissection flaps. The medical aspect of the therapy of aortic dissection focus on stabilization of patients requiring surgical repair (types I and II) or on chronic medical management of patients with type III dissection, who typically are not recommended for surgery except under the conditions listed in Table 5.

Medical therapy of aortic dissection follows principles similar to the treatment of hypertensive emergencies, with a few notable exceptions. When hypertension is present, it is necessary to lower blood pressure promptly. Unlike other hypertensive emergencies, however, this is one situation where lowering blood pressure well within the normal range is the primary goal, and systolic blood pressures as low as 100 mm Hg are preferable. Second, the choice of agents is somewhat different. With this disorder, beta-adrenergic blockade is a treatment of choice, not only because of its ability to lower blood pressure, but also for its ability to decrease contractility and shear force within the aorta, thereby minimizing further dissection. Ideally, beta-adrenergic blockage should involve a selective beta-blocker such as metroprolol and must be combined with a parenteral vasodilator such as nitroprusside. These patients should all be treated parenterally so that close titration of blood pressure is possible. If necessary, to maximize the reduction of blood pressure, ganglionic blockade with guanethidine is still recommended as adjunctive therapy for these patients, and if nitroprusside is insufficient to reduce systolic blood pressure, it should be replaced by trimethaphan. Newer approaches to the medical management of aortic dissection have been considered. Generally, calcium-channel antagonists are not recommended. Some individuals have advocated the use of verapamil because of its afterload-reducing properties and its negative inotropic effects. However, when calcium-channel antagonists (including verapamil!) are administered acutely as a bolus, the rapid reduction of blood pressure they produce can stimulate an increase of sympathetic nervous system activity manifested by tachycardia. More promising, however, is the use of parenteral labetalol because of its alpha- and beta-adrenergic blocking properties.

HEART AND GREAT VESSEL TRAUMA

ALFRED S. CASALE, M.D.
WILLIAM A. BAUMGARTNER, M.D.

INITIAL MANAGEMENT

The initial evaluation and resuscitation of victims with thoracic cardiovascular wounds is identical to that of other seriously traumatized patients.

The first priority is evaluation of the airway and, if inadequate, expeditious provision of one, usually by orotracheal intubation. Oxygen should be administered to all patients. Adequate gas exchange may require controlled ventilation and/or relief of a tension or open pneumothorax. Circulatory status is assessed by palpation of pulses, observation of cutaneous signs of perfusion, and measurement of blood pressure. Electrocardiographic monitoring and pulse oximetry is established as large-bore peripheral intravenous lines are placed. Blood is submitted for typing and cross-matching, and chemical, hematologic, and toxicologic analysis.

Many factors may suggest the presence of a serious chest injury, and a high "index of suspicion" is required. Any penetrating wound of the chest or upper abdomen can be associated with cardiovascular injury. In addition, the presence of bruising or hematomas, as well as the history and mechanism of injury may warn of important intrathoracic problems.

Patients may present either in shock or adequately perfused.

Shock

These unstable, hypotensive patients demonstrate classic signs of hypoperfusion and are suffering from one of four syndromes: (1) severe dysrhythmia with cardiac arrest, (2) severe myocardial contusion with cardiogenic shock, (3) pericardial tamponade, or (4) exsanguination.

Dysrhythmia

Dysrhythmia with associated shock should immediately be managed with closed-chest massage and appropriate chemical and electrical interventions as guided by the American Heart Association's Advanced Cardiac Life Support standards. If, however, life-sustaining rhythm and perfusion are not immediately achieved, open-chest resuscitation should be performed. The decision to proceed in these desperate situations must be tempered by the knowledge that the mortality of patients presenting without electrical activity approaches 100 percent.

Myocardial Contusion

Myocardial contusion severe enough to lead to acute cardiogenic shock is rare but lethal. This diagnosis should be made only after all possible mechanical causes of circulatory embarrassment have been excluded. Treatment involves optimization of cardiac function with ionotropes and vasodilators and possibly intra-aortic balloon counterpulsation.

Pericardial Tamponade

A far more common cause of shock in patients with chest injury is pericardial tamponade. The sudden introduction of small amounts of blood into the nondistensible pericardial sac from a penetrating cardiovascular wound or from rupture of a contused cardiac chamber leads to restriction of ventricular filling and compromised coronary perfusion. In addition to hypotension, characteristics of hemodynamically compromising tamponade include an increased central venous pressure (especially when increasing to more than 20 mm of water with fluid administration), distended neck veins, muffled heart sounds, and a 15-mm Hg drop in blood pressure with inspiration (pulsus paradoxus). The last three signs constitute Beck's triad and, although suggestive of tamponade, are rarely all present.

These patients with hemodynamically compromising hemopericardium should receive a rapid infusion of 2 L of crystalloid solution, with further management dictated by their response. If blood pressure increases satisfactorily, the patient should be transferred to an operating room at once for definitive management of the presumptive cardiac wound. Any unavoidable delay can be used to obtain a chest film and to insert pleural tubes, but these procedures should not in themselves delay transfer. If deterioration during transit occurs, therapeutic subxiphoid aspiration of the hemopericardium should be rapidly accomplished. We feel strongly that victims with pericardial tamponade who respond to volume must not be managed expectantly, but should undergo subxiphoid pericardial exploration. Pericardiocentesis should not be considered adequate definitive treatment.

Patients with tamponade who do not improve with a rapid fluid bolus will not survive for definitive repair unless the tension hemopericardium is relieved. Initially, this may be attempted with pericardial aspiration. If hemodynamics improve, immediate transfer to an operating room with a pericardial drainage catheter in place is accomplished. However, should pericardiocentesis fail, immediate open-chest resuscitation is mandated.

Exsanguination

The fourth syndrome leading to shock following cardiovascular injury is exsanguination with consequent hypovolemia. The classic signs of hemorrhagic shock occur in this syndrome, along with either massive hemothorax or external blood loss. Exsanguination most commonly follows gunshot wounds to the heart or great vessels that also cause large pericardial and pleural or chest wall defects, or rupture of the descending thoracic aorta.

Hypotensive exsanguinated patients should receive a rapid infusion of fluid and blood. The few who improve should be rushed to an operating room as volume repletion continues. There is no place for nonoperative management or pericardiocentesis in these patients. Exsanguinated patients who do not improve with rapid fluid administration should undergo immediate open-chest resuscitation. These patients are desperately wounded, and prompt control of ongoing bleeding and volume repletion is emergently required.

Adequate Perfusion

Patients with either penetrating chest wounds or significant blunt thoracic injuries whose blood pressure and perfusion are not depressed at presentation offer a slightly less emergent but often more difficult diagnostic and therapeutic challenge. Here, four classes of patients exist: (1) those with a hemopericardium not causing tamponade, (2) those with limited bleeding, (3) those with cardiac contusion without hemodynamic effects, and (4) those without cardiovascular injury.

Because patients in the first three groups can deteriorate with frightening rapidity, all stable patients with high-risk chest wounds should have chest films, and studies to identify the often subtle signs of cardiac injury. We institute central venous pressure (CVP) monitoring and place chest tubes as appropriate, guided by radiographic and physical findings. The incidence of false-negative pericardiocentesis minimizes its value as a diagnostic test.

Echocardiography can confirm suspected hemopericardium but in our experience is not a reliable technique to exclude injury.

In patients with a pericardial wound and any sign, however subtle, of cardiac injury or in patients who require operation for other injuries, the surgeon should explore the pericardium by a limited subxiphoid incision without delay. The occasional patient with a less suspicious chest wound or a history of blunt injury alone, who has never been hypotensive, has no murmur and no bleeding, and has a normal EKG and CVP can be expectantly managed in an intensive care setting.

OPEN-CHEST RESUSCITATION

We identify three indications for open-chest resuscitation of patients with acute cardiovascular injuries: (1) lethal dysrhythmia not responding to initial therapy, (2) hypotension with tamponade not improved by fluid and/or therapeutic pericardial aspiration, and (3) hypotension with bleeding not responsive to rapid fluid infusion. Thoracotomy in the emergency department is not an initial step in the management of patients with thoracic wounds but should be used as an extension of resuscitation in selected situations. It should be preceded by endotracheal intubation, ventilation, volume infusion, appropriate drug and electrical therapy, and nasogastric intubation. Suction with autotransfusion capability, careful attention to sterility, and suitable operating facilities are desirable.

The patient is placed in a supine position with hands tucked under his head. An incision in the left anterolateral chest is positioned several centimeters below the left nipple (in the inframammary fold in women) and carried from the medial edge of the sternum laterally to the anterior axillary line and then obliquely toward the axilla. The sixth rib usually lies just below this incision and the hemithorax is entered above it, in the fifth intercostal space. Rib spreaders are placed and clots rapidly evacuated. The hemithorax is rapidly evaluated for parenchymal, hilar, or great vessel injury. Any bleeding sites are controlled by direct pressure or packing. Wide longitudinal pericardiotomy, anterior to the phrenic nerve, is performed with rapid manual and suction evacuation of blood and clots. Digital control of cardiac wounds and, if necessary, manual cardiac compression are carried out. If adequate control can be obtained, the patient should be taken to an operating room for definitive repair. Adjuvant clamping of the descending thoracic aorta is possible but should be utilized only if absolutely necessary to restore cardiac and cerebral perfusion.

DEFINITIVE OPERATIVE REPAIR

Those wounded patients who either are stable at presentation or can be rendered stable with fluid administration, therapeutic pericardial aspiration, or open-chest resuscitation are best managed definitively in the operating room. Although full cardiac surgical facilities are desirable, cardiopulmonary bypass is seldom needed. Any wounding missile, blade, or fragment that remains in place should not be removed in the emergency department but should be included in the operative field for controlled, intraoperative removal. Wide skin preparation and draping of the neck, chest, abdomen, both groins, and legs should precede administration of anesthetic agents since sudden deterioration upon induction could mandate emergency incision and open-chest resuscitation.

Positioning the patient with the head dependent helps avoid cerebral air embolism if the left side of the heart has been disrupted. Tube thoracostomy eliminates the risk of tension pneumothorax upon initiation of positive-pressure ventilation.

Most cardiac and intrapericardial great vessel wounds are best approached through median sternotomy, as are injuries to the innominate and right subclavian arteries. If, however, serious pulmonary or posterior mediastinal injuries are suspected, a posterolateral thoracotomy offers better exposure. The descending thoracic aorta, distal aortic arch, and left subclavian artery are best exposed through a left posterolateral thoracostomy.

We explore all stable patients with suspected but not documented intrapericardial bleeding through a subxiphoid incision under light general or local anesthesia.

An 8- to 10-cm incision is located two-thirds below the xiphoid and carried through the linea alba. The xiphoid is excised and retractors are placed superiorly. The pleurae are displaced laterally, the peritoneum inferiorly, and the anteroinferior pericardium is grasped with two long clamps. A small nick is made between the clamps and, if blood is found, the midline incision is extended and full sternotomy carried out, as described below.

If blood is not noted upon entering the pericardium, the pericardial incision is extended and a wider exploration through the same exposure undertaken. Only when this somewhat wider exploration reveals no intrapericardial blood is the exploration considered negative and the wound closed.

When blood is found during subxiphoid exploration, or in patients who are, or have been, unstable, a complete median sternotomy is performed immediately. The anterior pericardium is exposed and opened widely with an inverted "Y" incision. The pericardial space is evacuated, and any bleeding wounds are controlled. Adherent clots over non-bleeding wounds are not removed at this point. In the rare event that release of the hemostatic effect of the tamponade leads to uncontrollable bleeding, Sauerbruch's grip can be helpful. The third finger of the left hand is placed in the transverse sinus under the ascending aorta and pulmonary artery, while the fourth and fifth fingers are placed in the posterior pericardial cavity. Compression with all fingers can partially control cardiac inflow and outflow.

Having located and controlled all gross bleeding, pericardial stay sutures are placed and attached to the sternal retractors, creating a pericardial cradle. The heart is thoroughly explored and the presumptive path of the wounding object is recreated. Any entrance wound without a corresponding exit wound raises the possibility of an intramyocardial or intracavitary foreign body or of an intravascular foreign body embolus.

Many wounds of the ventricles seal spontaneously and can be repaired without displacing adherent clot until suture control is insured. Freely bleeding ventricular wounds can be controlled most directly by digital pressure. Placing a Foley catheter through the wound, inflating the balloon, and gently pulling it against the injured site can also control bleeding. Stay sutures deeply placed on either side of a ventricular wound can be crossed and thus approximate wound edges, temporarily slowing bleeding enough to allow repair. Definitive repair of ventricular wounds requires the placement of 2-0 or 3-0 nonabsorbable sutures buttressed with pericardial pledgets in a horizontal mattress configuration. Wounds in proximity to coronary arteries are sutured with substantial bites placed in mattress fashion under the vessel with buttressing pledgets on both sides. Large defects in the ventricular mass may require placement of a prosthetic patch during cardiopulmonary bypass. Management of all left ventricular wounds requires constant attention to the danger of systemic air embolization.

Injuries to the thin-walled atria seal less often than do ventricular wounds, but they bleed under much less pressure. Digital pressure is the most direct way to control these injuries. A carefully placed curved vascular clamp can isolate the disruption and allow meticulous repair with running layers of nonabsorbable, monofilament suture.

Management of coronary artery injuries requires considerable judgment to avoid meddlesome attempts to repair insignificant vessels, yet minimize ultimate myocardial loss from ischemia. Distal coronary arteries of less than 1-mm diameter can be ligated safely. Larger vessels, more proximally placed, should be repaired or bypassed at the time of initial exploration. This usually requires cardiopulmonary bypass and cardioplegic arrest.

Wounds of the posterior surfaces of the heart are difficult to manage. Elevation of the heart's apex to visualize these injuries usually causes a profound decrease in cardiac output. The risk of air embolization through the wounded, posteriorly located left atrium is high. Temporary cessation of cardiac output by inflow occlusion (occlusion of both venae cavae intrapericardially) or by induced ventricular fibrillation can be utilized for short periods to allow repair, but cardiopulmonary bypass is often needed.

Foreign bodies that enter the heart can be intramyocardial, intracavitary, or embolic to the pulmonary or systemic circulation. If easily accessible, intramural objects should be removed and the wound reinforced. Prolonged attempts to dislodge these foreign bodies are, however, not warranted. Ingenious methods to remove intracavitary foreign bodies without recourse to cardiopulmonary bypass have been described, but we have preferred to remove these on bypass either initially or at a later time. Embolized missiles are removed as soon as they are noted.

Valvular and septal injuries usually do not require acute operative intervention but can initially be managed medically. In the first days following injury, the anatomic extent of the lesion, its hemodynamic consequence, and the need for operative repair should be determined.

AORTIC DISRUPTION

Sudden deceleration of the thorax or the extreme stresses placed on the aorta in crush injuries can cause full- or partial-thickness disruption of the thoracic aorta. Traumatic rupture of the thoracic aorta usually occurs just distal to the left subclavian artery at the site of the ligamentum arteriosum. However, aortic disruption may also occur just above the aortic valve in the proximal ascending aorta. Ninety percent of patients with thoracic aortic disruption die at the scene of the rapid deceleration injury. Of the small percentage who live to present for medical evaluation, 50 percent die within the first 24 hours and survival continues to fall as diagnosis is delayed.

Many radiographic signs of aortic injury have been described. A high index of suspicion is important when a suggestive mechanism of injury has been identified. A low threshold for further investigation must be maintained if these patients are to be saved.

Computed tomographic or magnetic resonance imaging scans can provide valuable information in evaluating the thoracic aorta. However, we continue to rely on aortography as the optimal method of establishing the presence of aortic disruption.

Although primary repair of the disrupted descending aorta has been reported, we favor Dacron graft interposition repair of these injuries. Four operative strategies have been described to provide perfusion to the lower body during the period of aortic cross-clamping required for graft insertion: (1) "clamp and sew," rapid repair without provision of distal perfusion, (2) placement of a heparin-bonded Gott shunt from proximal aorta or left ventricle to distal aorta, (3) left atrial-to-femoral artery bypass with minimal heparinzations, or (4) femoral vein-to-femoral artery partial cardiopulmonary bypass.

When head injury is not serious we prefer left atrial-to-femoral artery bypass with a centrifugal pump. However, if head injury makes even the minimal heparinization required for this method dangerous, we have utilized the Gott shunt. Nevertheless, despite all of these operative strategies, a worrisome incidence of paraplegia persists.

SUGGESTED READING

Casale AS, Borkon AM, Penetrating cardiac trauma. Trauma Q 1988; 4(2): 34–41.
Hood RM, Boyd AD, Culliford AT, eds. Thoracic trauma. Philadelphia: WB Saunders Co., 1989.
Symbas PN. Cardiothoracic trauma. Philadelphia: WB Saunders Co., 1989.

PULMONARY THERAPEUTICS

ACUTE RESPIRATORY FAILURE

ROGER C. BONE, M.D.
RANDALL L. BUSCH, M.D., D.D.S.

Acute respiratory failure (ARF) develops in patients of all age groups, so thorough, organized approaches to the etiologies and laboratory presentations of this condition are mandatory. Prior to and during the 1950s, the primary causes of respiratory failure were barbiturate overdose and poliomyelitis. With improvements in the maintenance of effective airways, mechanical ventilation, and the advent of naloxone for reversal of narcotic respiratory depression, overdose became a less frequent precursor to ARF. Also, the Salk and Sabin vaccines essentially eliminated poliomyelitis as a cause of respiratory failure.

In the early 1960s, arterial blood gas evaluation was an unrefined research tool. For this reason, acute respiratory depression, as it is known today, was seldom recognized. With the advent of clinical arterial blood gas analysis, the true incidence of ARF came to be recognized. ARF was found to result from a myriad of causes: burns, myocardial infarction, pulmonary emboli, shock (of all types), as well as primary pulmonary disorders (Fig. 1).

Today a wide variety of conditions are encompassed under the term "acute respiratory failure." Some authors have used ARF to mean only those circumstances that cause a primary disorder of gas exchange. Others use the term to describe any disruption in the function of the respiratory system. This broader definition of ARF will be used here.

Most clinicians now agree that in the absence of an intracardiac shunt, acute respiratory failure is present if the PaO_2 is greater than 50 mm Hg and/or the $PaCO_2$ is greater than 50 mm Hg, the patient is acutely dyspneic, or the arterial pH shows significant respiratory acidemia. However, it should be noted that these values are somewhat arbitrary. Many patients with ARF do not fulfill all criteria of this definition, but the majority have at least two of the above elements.

Employing this definition, ARF can be subdivided into two types. Type 1 failure (also known as hypocapnic or normocapnic ARF) is manifested by abnormally low PaO_2 with $PaCO_2$ that is either low or normal. Type 2 failure (also termed ventilatory or hypercapnic ARF) is manifested as hypercapnia as well as hypoxemia. Arterial blood gas determinations remain the gold standard for measurement of gas tensions. Today, we have other devices—e.g., pulse oximeters and end-tidal CO_2 monitors—to evaluate oxygenation and ventilation noninvasively.

OXYGEN THERAPY

The fundamental focus in the treatment of respiratory failure caused by chronic obstructive pulmonary disease (COPD) is the judicious use of oxygen. Prudent use of oxygen and the dangers of indiscriminate use have added new perspectives to the management of respiratory failure. The primary danger of high oxygen concentration in the patient with advanced COPD is development of progressive hypercapnia, decreased hypoxic stimulus to breathe, and consequent acidosis. The proper use of oxygen in respiratory failure satisfies tissue needs for oxygen but does not produce narcosis or oxygen toxicity. The proper dose of oxygen is the lowest concentration that produces adequate but not excessive PaO_2. A PaO_2 concentration of 60 mm Hg usually results in greater than 90 percent saturation of arterial oxyhemoglobin (contingent on pH). Once hemoglobin is nearly saturated with oxygen, further increases in the PaO_2 have relatively little effect in increasing arterial oxygen content.

Patients with COPD who develop ARF often have reversible disorders, such as bronchospasm, congestive heart failure, secretions, or other conditions that result in decreased alveolar ventilation and ARF. Bronchodilators, diuretics, antibiotics, and other measures are employed to treat these primary causes. Asynchronous breathing may be an early indicator of diaphragmatic fatigue. The majority of patients with COPD respond favorably to controlled oxygen delivery, and adequate oxygenation is usually obtained without precipitation of severe hypercapnia. If demanding hypercapnia occurs, supplemental oxygen should be decreased in an incremental fashion. Failure to hyperventilate on abrupt withdrawal of oxygen will suddenly drop the PaO_2 to dangerously low levels. Because of the enormous number of poorly ventilating spaces in the lungs of a patient with COPD, increased hypoxia and even cyanosis may not be evident for several minutes after removal of the oxygen supply. Nevertheless, increasing hypoxia will ensue. The use of central nervous system

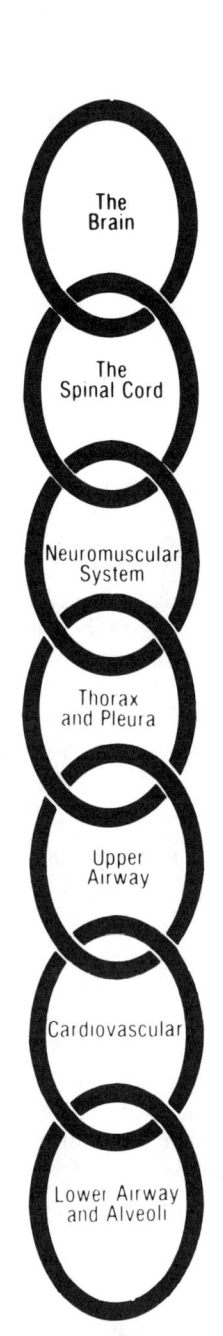

Figure 1 Causes of acute respiratory failure. (Republished with permission from Balk R, Bone RC. Classification of acute respiratory failure. Med Clin North Am 1989; 67:553.)

(CNS) depressants, benzodiazepines, narcotics, barbiturates, and even antihistamines may pose significant hazards to patients with COPD and ARF. These agents uniformly depress respiratory drive and can be responsible for failure of controlled oxygen therapy. If the patient requires endotracheal intubation and mechanical ventilation, however, sedatives may be given.

DELIVERY SYSTEMS

Regulated oxygen delivery can be administered either by nasal cannula or by air-entrainment oxygen masks. A Venturi mask employs the Bernoulli principle, passing a jet of oxygen through a restricted orifice entraining room air to provide known oxygen concentrations (of 24 to 40 percent). The foremost advantage of the Venturi mask is maintenance of known percentages of inspired oxygen. The advantage of a nasal cannula is that it is often better tolerated by patients and remains in place when patients expectorate or eat. With either of these delivery systems, arterial blood gases should be monitored to ensure appropriate results.

Clinical decisions for endotracheal intubation are based on the patient's mental status, ability to clear secretions effectively, fatigue, and impending ventilatory arrest or apnea. Patients should not be intubated because they have modest increases in $PaCO_2$ when supplemented with oxygen; these expected increases in $PaCO_2$ are considered an adaptive response to oxygen administration. When controlled oxygen is judiciously used, only a small proportion of patients will still require intubation.

MECHANICAL VENTILATION

A primary therapeutic goal for patients with COPD in hypercapnic respiratory failure is avoidance of endotracheal intubation and mechanical ventilation, if possible. Potential complications inherent to intubation include reduction in the patient's ability to clear secretions by coughing and the more prolonged requirement for ventilatory support once it is instituted. Also, the weaning process may be more difficult for these patients than it is for patients with most other causes of respiratory failure. These potential disadvantages are much less germane in patients with hypercapnic respiratory failure due to neuromuscular disease or drug overdose.

If mechanical ventilation is required, tidal volumes of 10 to 12 ml per kilogram are usually sufficient. To avoid the problem of air trapping, flow rates should be adjusted to allow adequate time for full expiration. In most instances, inspiratory-to-expiratory time ratios of 1:2 to 1:3 are sufficient, although adjustments in respiratory rate may be needed to accomplish this.

The goal of ventilator therapy is not to achieve normal blood gas values. If chronic carbon dioxide retention was present before the current illness, decreasing $PaCO_2$ to normal levels (i.e., 40 mm Hg) will cause alkalosis and may make it difficult to wean the patient from the ventilator. The desired $PaCO_2$ level—and goal for initial treatment—is one that results in return to the patient's usual pH. Abrupt changes in $PaCO_2$ and pH should be avoided, since rapid alterations may induce seizures, cardiac arrhythmias, or both.

Although tracheostomy may facilitate oral feeding, it does result in greater complications than low-pressure, cuffed endotracheal tubes, so premature tracheostomy should be avoided.

OTHER TREATMENTS

Pneumothorax

Pneumothorax should be considered when abrupt deterioration in respiratory or cardiovascular status occurs, especially in patients with histories of asthma, bullae, or adult respiratory distress syndrome (ARDS). Detection of unilateral tympany upon percussion and/or tracheal deviation on palpation should raise one's index of suspicion of this complication. In the past, unilaterally diminished breath sounds were considered a good diagnostic indicator; however, even the best clinicians can be misled if the patient is intubated and mechanically ventilated, since sound is often transmitted bilaterally. A radiograph usually clinches the diagnosis. Proper placement of a chest tube is the appropriate treatment. If severe hemodynamic compromise occurs, one may place a 16-gauge needle or intravenous catheter in the second intercostal space at the level of the midclavicular line of the appropriate hemithorax.

Pulmonary Embolus

Pulmonary embolus should be thought of early if a patient develops acute onset of tachypnea, dyspnea, and tachycardia, with or without pleuritic chest pain. Pulmonary emboli most commonly occur in patients confined to bed (i.e., those under intensive care or after hip surgery). Normal ventilation-perfusion scans virtually preclude pulmonary emboli. Pulmonary angiograms may be required to confirm a diagnosis in patients with respiratory failure, especially in patients who are at risk for anticoagulation. Therapy should be initiated with 5,000 U of heparin administered intravenously as a bolus, then 1,000 U per hour and adjusted as needed to maintain the partial thromboplastin time at approximately double its control value. A massive embolus producing significant hypotension may require streptokinase.

Aspiration Pneumonia

Aspiration pneumonia should be suspected if a patient with an unprotected airway is obtunded or exhibits an altered level of consciousness. Both the volume and gastric pH determine the extent of the injury. If particulate matter was aspirated, it should be promptly suctioned. There is no evidence that lavage with saline or the administration of corticosteroids or antibiotics reduces acute lung injury. Treatment is primarily supportive.

Obstructive Lung Disease

Sympathomimetic

Treatment of reversible components such as bronchospasm is important. Nebulized bronchodilator solutions such as albuterol (2.5 mg in 3 ml, total volume), metaproterenol (15 mg in 3 ml, total volume), or isoetharine hydrochloride (5 mg in 2 ml, total volume) can be used. Intermittent positive pressure breathing (IPPB) is generally not necessary to deliver bronchodilators.

Treatment of ARF that is secondary to upper airway edema can be managed with high FIO_2 and administration of racemic epinephrine (0.25 ml in 3 ml of saline, via a nebulizer every hour) for the acute episode. Administration of an aerosolized corticosteroid such as dexamethasone (4 mg intravenously every 6 hours) is also used, to decrease edema caused by the acute and chronic inflammatory response.

NUTRITIONAL SUPPORT

Methylxanthines

Theophylline, a xanthine derivative, is an important bronchodilator. Because of its low solubility, it is administered intravenously as aminophylline, a complex of theophylline and ethylenediamine. The usual loading dose of aminophylline is 5 to 6 mg per kilogram body weight. Since this group of compounds gives rise to many toxic side effects, safe maintenance dosage levels have recently been challenged. Theophylline clearance depends on many factors: circulatory and hepatic function, patient variation, drug interactions, and smoking status. The recommended maintenance dosage for nonsmokers without unusual host factors is 0.5 mg per kilogram per hour, which provides mean serum levels of about 10.0 μg per milliliter in most patients. For smokers without unusual factors 0.8 mg per kilogram per hour is given. If a nonsmoker has underlying congestive heart failure or hepatic dysfunction, further reductions in dosage to 0.2 mg per kilogram per hour are indicated. Because safe levels are so variable from patient to patient, drug level monitoring is crucial. Monitoring should begin 12 to 24 hours after theophylline is first administered. Since some patients metabolize the drug slowly, theophylline levels may continue to rise; adjustments may need to be made before levels reach the toxic range.

Steroids

Corticosteroids are indicated for severe bronchospasm that is unresponsive to intravenous or inhaled bronchodilators. Corticosteroids potentiate bronchodilatory effects of the xanthines and sympathomimetic agents. Methylprednisolone (0.5 mg per kg every 6 hours) has been shown to be of benefit to patients with ARF from COPD.

Antibiotics

Antibiotics should be administered at the first sign of infection. Since infection is one of the most frequent factors precipitating ARF in patients with chronic pulmonary disease, a high index of suspicion should be present. Common organisms such as *Streptococcus pneumoniae* or *Haemophilus influenzae* should be treated with a cephalosporin or ampicillin.

Nutritional support is essential for patients in respiratory failure. Since the hypoxic drive to breathe is decreased even in normal volunteers after only a few days of intravenously administered dextrose, adequate and appropriate caloric intake is important. Inadequate nutrition may also make it more difficult to wean some patients. Hypophosphatemia may occur after just a few days of intravenous glucose therapy, impairing oxygen delivery to tissues through its effect on the oxyhemoglobin curve and increasing the likelihood of infection due to altered phagocytosis, chemotaxis of polymorphonuclear leukocytes, and bacterial killing. Enteral alimentation should, therefore, be used early in patients who cannot eat. To reduce the likelihood of aspiration, small-caliber feeding tubes should be selected.

SUGGESTED READING

Bone RC. Treatment of respiratory failure due to advanced chronic obstructive lung disease. Arch Intern Med 1980; 140:1018–1021.

Bone RC. Treatment of severe hypoxemia due to the adult respiratory distress syndrome. Arch Intern Med 1980; 140:85–89.

Bone RC, George RB, Hudson LD. Acute respiratory failure. New York: Churchill Livingstone, 1987.

Bone RC, Pierce AK, Johnson RL. Controlled oxygen administration in acute respiratory failure in chronic obstructive pulmonary disease: a reappraisal. Am J Med 1978; 65:896–902.

Weinberger SE, Schwartzstein RM, Weiss JW. Hypercapnia. N Engl J Med 1989; 321:1223–1231.

ADULT RESPIRATORY DISTRESS SYNDROME

ROGER C. BONE, M.D.

The adult respiratory distress syndrome (ARDS) represents a sequence of pathophysiologic events that develop secondary to a variety of insults. Bacterial sepsis, aspiration, fat embolism, shock, drug injury, and other injuries are known to precipitate this syndrome. Irrespective of etiology, damage is associated with diffuse pulmonary cell injury, and interstitial and alveolar edema and inflammation. ARDS is characterized by pulmonary infiltrates, hypoxemia, and decreased lung compliance.

ARDS affects an estimated 150,000 persons per year in the United States, and despite sophisticated methods of respiratory support, mortality remains greater than 60 percent. Those patients who survive the initial period of injury, however, can regain lung function that is essentially normal, so protective therapies in the early phases of acute lung dysfunction are clearly needed.

Efforts to better define the complex series of pathophysiologic events based on numerous experimental animal models for lung injury have enhanced our understanding of ARDS, but the exact mechanism of acute lung injury remains speculative. ARDS is thought to represent a late stage of a pathophysiologic process; supportive therapy given late in the treatment of ARDS makes survival less likely. Research efforts have focused on identifying clinical entities that precede ARDS, since a better understanding of the injury reaction, the events that precipitate the condition, and the inflammatory sequelae that lead to ARDS will furnish a basis for controlled clinical trials and provide specific pharmacologic therapies to supplement current supportive therapy. Early treatment with blockers of the inflammatory reaction may improve survival.

ETIOLOGY

It is the prevailing view that ARDS is but a complication of another disease process (Table 1); major risk factors predispose individuals to the development of ARDS, and the incidence increases with the number of risk factors present. The sepsis syndrome is the major preexisting disease with which ARDS is clinically associated. It has been useful to group diseases that cause ARDS, since increased quantities of water in the lung is a recurrent pathophysiologic theme, and consequently, basic treatment modalities are similar. A technique has been described by which ARDS can be predicted in hospitalized patients (with varying degrees of accuracy), based on identification of risk factors (Table 2). Correction of underlying disease(s) is generally associated with recovery, except, perhaps, when ARDS contributes to nosocomial complications that protract the clinical course or lead to multiple organ systems failure.

In prospective studies, the percentage of at-risk patients who actually developed ARDS has varied from 21 percent to 36 percent. Even higher rates are associated with the presence of more than one risk factor. Since no

Table 1 Causes of Adult Respiratory Distress Syndrome

Aspiration	Physicochemical
Gastric contents	Inhaled toxin (nitrogen
Near-drowning	dioxide, ammonia,
	chlorine, cadmium,
Drug	phosgene, smoke, oxygen)
Chlordiazepoxide	Pancreatitis
Colchicine	Smoke inhalation
Dextra 40	
Ethchlorvynol	Trauma
Fluorescein	Burns
Heroin	Fat embolism
Leukagglutinin reaction	Fractures
Methadone	Head trauma
Propoxyphene	Lung contusion
Salicylates	Nonthoracic trauma
Thiazides	Shock of any etiology
Infectious	Miscellaneous
Bacterial pneumonia	Amniotic fluid embolism
Fungal and *Pneumocystis*	Bowel infarction
carinii pneumonia (rare)	Carcinomatosis
Gram-negative sepsis	Dead fetus
Tuberculosis	Eclampsia
Viral pneumonia	High altitude
	Pulmonary edema
Metabolic Disorders	
Diabetic ketoacidosis	
Uremia	

Republished with permission from Bone RC. The adult respiratory distress syndrome: new trends. Resident & Staff Physician 1989; 35:25–34; © July 1989 by Romaine Pierson Publishers, Inc.

Table 2 Incidence of ARDS Occurring with Single and Multiple Risk Factors

Condition	Alone	With One Other Condition	With Two Other Conditions	Total
Sepsis syndrome	5/13(13)	2/4	2/2	0/19(47)
Aspiration of gastric contents	7/23(30)	3/9(33)	0/0	10/32(31)
Multiple emergency transfusions	4/17(24)	3/11(27)	12/14(86)	19/42(45)
Pulmonary contusion	5/29(17)	7/12(58)	7/9(78)	19/50(38)
Multiple major fractures	1/12(8)	4/10(40)	10/12(83)	15/34(44)
Near-drowning	2/3	1/1	0/0	3/4
Pancreatitis	1/1	0/0	0/0	1/1
Prolonged hypotension	0/1	0/1	2/2	2/4

Republished with permission from Bone RC. The adult respiratory distress syndrome: new trends. Resident & Staff Physician 1989, 35:25–34; © July 1989 by Romaine Pierson Publishers, Inc.

specified biochemical marker has been found that allows identification of ARDS in its milder stages, any clinical definition must emphasize criteria that would intuitively indicate severe disease (Table 3). It is therefore possible that criteria used in prospective studies to confirm the diagnosis of ARDS might not have identified milder and self-limited cases (cases in which strict radiographic criteria of edema may be difficult to ascertain). This is particularly true for those patients in whom positive end-expiratory pressure (PEEP) was concurrently utilized. Criteria currently used in clinical studies to define ARDS exclude patients who demonstrate pulmonary capillary wedge pressures (PCWP) greater than 15 to 19 mm Hg. Such exclusionary criteria should accurately identify patients with cardiac pulmonary edema (CPE), but at the same time may fail to identify ARDS patients with concurrent hydrostatic contributions to the development of radiologic noncardiac pulmonary edema (NCPE).

CLINICAL COURSE AND OUTCOME

The clinical course of progressive respiratory insufficiency can be characterized by four stages: injury, apparent stability, respiratory insufficiency, and the terminal stage. Clinical signs are usually not evident, and chest

Table 3 Criteria Frequently Used in the Diagnosis of ARDS

Severe defect in oxygenation: PaO_2 < 50 mm Hg on room air
OR
$PaO_2 \leq 50$ mm Hg on an F_IO_2 of $\geq 40\%$ and PEEP of > 5 cm H_2O
New bilateral and changing infiltrates on x-ray examination
PLUS
Pulmonary capillary wedge pressure < 18 mm Hg
PLUS
No other explanation for above findings
PLUS
Identification of a disease process with which ARDS has been described

Republished with permission from Bone RC. The adult respiratory distress syndrome : new trends. Resident & Staff Physician 1989, 35:25–34; © July 1989 by Romaine Pierson Publishers, Inc.

roentgenograms may be clear during the initial stage. This phase may last as long as 6 hours. During the phase of apparent stability, hyperventilation and abnormalities on chest films and physical examination appear. During the next 12 to 24 hours (respiratory insufficiency phase), chest films usually show diffuse, five-lobe alveolar and interstitial infiltrates. Pulmonary findings are generally bilateral and symmetric, and tachypnea and rales are evident on physical examination. The terminal stage is characterized by persistent severe hypoxemia (despite administration of 100 percent oxygen) as well as carbon dioxide retention.

Intrapulmonary shunting is the major cause of hypoxemia in patients with ARDS. It develops because the lung is perfused but not completely ventilated. In addition, many alveoli are ventilated but not perfused, resulting in increased physiologic dead space. Thus, both increased physiologic dead space and increased right-to-left shunting occur; in severe cases, shunting may exceed 50 percent. Of therapeutic importance is the fact that the functional residual capacity, the quantity of air remaining in the lungs at the end of a normal expiration, is decreased; this decreased capacity is a consequence of microatelectasis and edema. Lung compliance is also decreased.

Recent studies of immediate outcomes have shown that patients with ARDS are relatively unlikely to die as a consequence of initial pulmonary damage. Pathophysiologic changes occur with acute injury to the lung's gas-exchanging membrane, but patients with ARDS tend not to succumb from any direct sequelae of respiratory failure (e.g., hypoxemia). Early deaths are more frequently the result of complications of underlying illness. Late deaths appear to be a consequence of the sepsis syndrome, which develops in patients with ARDS with six times the frequency of control populations of critically ill patients without ARDS.

According to one study, patients with ARDS are at increased risk for development of nosocomial sepsis. In such patients, the use of antibiotics apparently does not significantly alter mortality. The sepsis syndrome is, therefore, perhaps the leading risk factor for development of ARDS and is also a major complication of ARDS once the syndrome is established.

Another study emphasized nonrespiratory causes of death in patients with ARDS. So-called systemic aberrations were thought to contribute to both the severity and the high mortality rate of ARDS. High pulmonary vascular resistance and low pulmonary compliance are more common in nonsurvivors of ARDS, compared with survivors. In the context of immediate outcome, these studies would seem to redirect the focus toward more direct respiratory sequelae of ARDS, rather than the systemic sequelae previously inferred. However, pulmonary versus systemic indicators of immediate prognosis may not be mutually exclusive. Pulmonary risk factors of death with ARDS may result from protracted depression of systemic oxygen transport.

The need to understand further the pathophysiology of the systemic sequelae of ARDS is obvious. However, there is as yet no singular examination that can be used to predict the onset of this syndrome. A thorough history, careful physical examination, and demonstration that radiographically defined pulmonary edema coexists with normal PCWP remains the basis for determining the diagnosis of ARDS.

MECHANISMS OF LUNG DAMAGE

Although the exact mechanisms and mediators of lung inflammation that results in permeability pulmonary edema and its consequence, ARDS, have not been identified in detail, there are a number of possibilities. Acute injury may involve agents that are capable of inciting inflammatory responses in the lung. Blood-borne substances may initiate or sustain the intense inflammatory reaction that is characteristic of ARDS. Various agents have been implicated—complement, fatty acids, fibrin split products, histamine, kinins, lysosomes, platelet-active factor, platelets, prostaglandins, proteolytic enzymes, serotonin, and leukotrienes—each of which is capable of producing vascular damage, vasoconstriction, or bronchoconstriction.

Considerable evidence has accumulated that implicates neutrophils as one of the key cellular elements in initiating the inflammatory response that results in capillary permeability, but it has not yet been proved that the initial injury in ARDS is to the capillary endothelium. The importance of enzymes released by leukocytes and mediators such as serotonin (released by platelets) and histamine (released by damaged lung tissue) is unclear, but these agents have been implicated in the pathogenesis of ARDS. An understanding of pathogenesis will come only when the various implicated mechanisms can be separated into "initiators," "perpetrators," and "bystanders." Only then will we be able to successfully block the inflammatory reaction in experimental and clinical studies and increase survival in ARDS.

TREATMENT OF ACUTE RESPIRATORY FAILURE

Treatment of acute respiratory failure of any cause includes provision of adequate tissue oxygenation by respiratory and circulatory support. Since the clinical problems are similar no matter what inciting agent leads to ARDS, the therapeutic goal is to support patients until alveolocapillary membrane integrity is reestablished. Critical factors in ARDS treatment include optimal distention of alveoli to increase functional residual capacity, maintenance of tissue perfusion, and control of the primary problem.

Because alveolar collapse leads to a basic pathophysiologic defect, major efforts are directed toward obtaining optimal distention of alveoli. PEEP is used to increase functional residual capacity (FRC) and to correct the tendency toward progressive atelectasis. Ventilatory assistance is frequently required. Indications for supplemental oxygen include arterial oxygen tension lower than 60 mm Hg (room air; patient with previously normal lungs). If arterial oxygen tension does not increase satisfactorily with high concentrations of oxygen, ventilatory assistance may be necessary.

PEEP is indicated if an FiO_2 above 50 percent is required to maintain satisfactory arterial oxygen tension in a mechanically ventilated patient. Continuous positive airway pressure (CPAP) is a technique whereby PEEP can be given to a patient by mask. This method of PEEP administration is to be condemned in obtunded or stuporous patients but may be useful in alert patients. The PaO_2/FiO_2 ratio and its response to therapy can be used as an index of survival (Fig. 1).

Further treatment includes correction of factors that led to decreased red blood cell oxygen transport, provision of appropriate nutritional support, and avoidance of complications.

POSITIVE END-EXPIRATORY PRESSURE

Since its introduction for use in the management of adult patients with diffuse lung injury more than 20 years ago, PEEP has become an integral component in the treat-

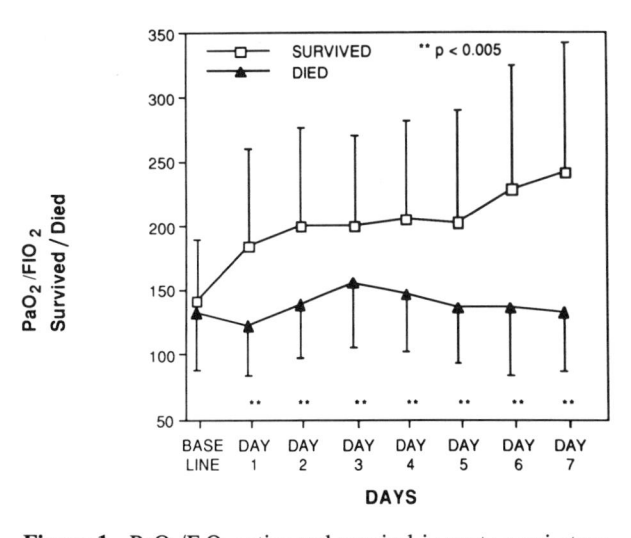

Figure 1 PaO_2/F_IO_2 ratios and survival in acute respiratory failure. Republished with permission from Bone RC, Maunder R, Slotman G, et al. An early test of survival in patients with the adult respiratory distress syndrome. Chest 1989, 96:849–851.

Table 4 Beneficial Effects of PEEP

Increased functional residual capacity
Increased compliance
Decreased shunt fraction ($\dot{Q}_S/\dot{Q}_T$)
Increased PaO$_2$
Ability to reduce the F$_I$O$_2$
Conservation of alveolar surfactant and reduction of alveolar surface tension
Possible effectiveness in preventing ARDS in susceptible patients

Republished with permission from Bone RC. Mechanical ventilation. In: Bone RC, George RB, Hudson LD, eds. Acute respiratory failure. New York: Churchill Livingstone, 1987:218.

ment of ARDS. PEEP is still a mainstay in the treatment of diffuse lung processes, since it supports the PaO$_2$ and allows reduction in inspired oxygen concentrations (F$_I$O$_2$). PEEP produces increases in the alveolar and airway pressures at the end of expiration to levels greater than atmospheric pressure. A continuous positive distending pressure is therefore produced across alveolar and airway walls, regenerating (through the process of recruitment) patency in many closed or atelectatic gas exchange units. Areas of shunt and ventilation/perfusion mismatch may be corrected, which would improve oxygenation. Fluid-filled alveoli may be stabilized by allowing fluid to occupy relatively flat layers on alveolar walls; this would also improve gas exchange. It is important to recognize, however, that PEEP does not decrease absolute amounts of extravascular lung water; in fact, lung water may actually increase at high lung volumes.

The beneficial effects of PEEP therapy (Table 4) include its ability to increase FRC; increase pulmonary compliance; decrease shunt fractions ($\dot{Q}s/\dot{Q}t$); increase PaO$_2$ for given F$_I$O$_2$ levels; and possibly, conserve alveolar surfactant, thereby reducing alveolar surface tension. These attributes have made PEEP a standard in the treatment of respiratory failure secondary to diffuse parenchymal lung disease. Intrapulmonary shunting may also decrease in association with the decreased cardiac output produced by high levels of PEEP.

Although PEEP helps to improve several of the physiologic alterations associated with diffuse lung injury, there is no evidence to substantiate that PEEP therapy is anything more than supportive. Further, despite aggressive supportive therapy, there has been no appreciable change in the survival of patients with ARDS over the past two decades. The use of PEEP has been advocated in the treatment of flail chest and mechanical dysfunction of the chest, in infant respiratory distress syndrome, in postoperative patients (to improve oxygenation), and in the treatment of obstructive sleep apnea. Several reports have even suggested that early use of PEEP might protect susceptible patients from developing ARDS, but investigations of possible benefit of prophylactic PEEP in patients at high risk for the development of ARDS have proved inconclusive. This has been a controversial topic, and the issue will prove difficult to resolve because of the heterogeneity of ARDS.

Another controversial issue in PEEP therapy has been appropriate levels of PEEP to administer. Most would agree that PEEP should be increased or decreased in small increments and that each patient's cardiac output and tissue oxygen delivery need to be carefully monitored. If cardiac output decreases, it must be supported with volume infusions and inotropic agents. The literature contains numerous attempts to specify "optimal" or "best" levels of PEEP. The common theme among these efforts appears to define some "ideal" level of PEEP as that level that allows inspired oxygen concentrations to be reduced to less toxic ranges while maintaining adequate tissue oxygen delivery.

Unfortunately, PEEP therapy has some undesirable effects— intra-alveolar pressures may exceed intracapillary pressures (leading to increased dead space ventilation [V$_D$/V$_T$]) and cardiac output and organ perfusion may decrease. While the use of PEEP is usually associated with increases in PaO$_2$, this parameter may actually decline as a result of decreased cardiac output, alveolar overdistention, or increased pulmonary arterial resistance and decreased pulmonary capillary size. With administration of PEEP, blood may be diverted from well-preserved and ventilated lung units to more poorly ventilated ones, exacerbating pulmonary shunting. PEEP may even elevate cerebral venous and intracranial pressures, potentiating cerebral dysfunction.

It is important to reiterate that PEEP does not decrease extravascular lung water but can significantly decrease intravascular pulmonary fluid volume as a consequence of reduced cardiac output. This PEEP-related decrease in cardiac output is primarily based on diminished venous return caused by elevated intrathoracic pressure. In addition, PEEP is capable of increasing pulmonary vascular resistance, decreasing left ventricular afterload, decreasing myocardial blood flow, and altering the geometry and compliance of the right and left ventricles. PEEP-induced decreases in cardiac output lead to declining hepatic, adrenal, bronchial, fundal mucosal, renal, coronary, and subendocardial arterial blood flow. These changes appear to return to baseline levels when PEEP is discontinued. PEEP may also predispose patients to pulmonary barotrauma (Tables 5 and 6), especially when large tidal volumes are used. Physicians need to be aware of this potential complication and realize that tension pneumothorax may develop rapidly in patients ventilated with PEEP.

Despite its potential detrimental effects, PEEP therapy has a beneficial role in the management of respiratory

Table 5 Pulmonary Barotrauma

Pneumomediastinum
Subcutaneous emphysema
Pneumothorax
Pneumopericardium
Pneumoperitoneum
Air embolus
Bronchopleural fistulas
Perforation of stomach and cecum

Republished with permission from Bone RC. Mechanical ventilation. In: Bone RC, George RB, Hudson LD, eds. Acute respiratory failure. New York: Churchill Livingstone, 1987:218.

Table 6 Conditions Associated with an Increased Incidence of Pulmonary Barotrauma

Gram-negative sepsis, emphysema, necrotizing pneumonia, acid aspiration
Use of volume ventilators
High inflation pressures secondary to low compliance
High levels of PEEP
High tidal volumes (>15 ml/kg)
Complication of intravenous catheter insertion

Republished with permission from Bone RC. Mechanical ventilation. In: Bone RC, George RB, Hudson LD, eds. Acute respiratory failure. New York: Churchill Livingstone, 1987:218.

failure secondary to diffuse parenchymal lung disease. When using PEEP, however, attention must be directed toward maintaining organ perfusion and function. At present, there is no evidence that PEEP decreases extravascular lung water or prevents the development of ARDS in susceptible patients. The primary goal of PEEP therapy, therefore, is to obtain adequate arterial oxygen saturation (on nontoxic FIO_2 levels) while maintaining cardiac output and tissue oxygen delivery.

FUTURE DIRECTIONS

Future treatments for ARDS will involve pharmacologic manipulation of the inflammatory process. Many agents show promise, but final results regarding their efficacy will depend on randomized, placebo-controlled clinical trials. Several drugs have been tested in animal models of septic shock and acute lung injury that might eventually prove useful. However, models in which such drugs have so far been tested were somewhat removed from their clinical correlates. These drugs were often administered prior to, or concurrent with, injurious agents, rather than after development of the full-blown syndrome, as in the clinical situation.

Since sepsis is the major cause of ARDS, the majority of animal studies evaluating pharmacologic modification of disease progression have used an endotoxin model. Even though this type of model may not perfectly reproduce the clinical syndrome, it has helped define the pathophysiology of acute lung injury and has led to an evaluation of drug intervention studies.

It is worthwhile to examine the possibility that manipulation of the arachidonic acid pathway might positively influence the outcome of ARDS. Prostaglandins (PGs) are unsaturated hydroxy-fatty acids that are synthesized in most mammalian nucleated cells. PGs are released in response to a variety of stimuli, including mechanical manipulation. Since the lung has been identified as a site where significant metabolism of PG precursors occurs, biologically active PGs released from other organs are, under certain conditions, prevented from reaching the arterial circulation. Following endotoxin infusion, inhibition of vasoconstrictor PG synthesis with meclofenamate and ibuprofen has been found to prevent increases in airway resistance and decreases in dynamic pulmonary compliance.

Prostaglandins of the "E" series have many anti-inflammatory properties. PG_{E1} and PG_{E2} decrease lymphokine production, depress lymphocyte mitogen response, induce T-lymphocyte suppressor activity, and decrease oxygen radical production by macrophages. In patients with ARDS, PG_{E1} has been reported to reduce pulmonary artery pressure and increase atrial oxygen content and cardiac output. More significantly, administration of PG_{E1} to surgical patients with ARDS has been shown to improve survival. Unfortunately, these data were not confirmed in a recent multicenter clinical trial.

Figure 2 Conventional and proposed treatment of septic shock and multi-organ failure. Conventional therapy is represented by solid lines, proposed therapy by dashed lines.

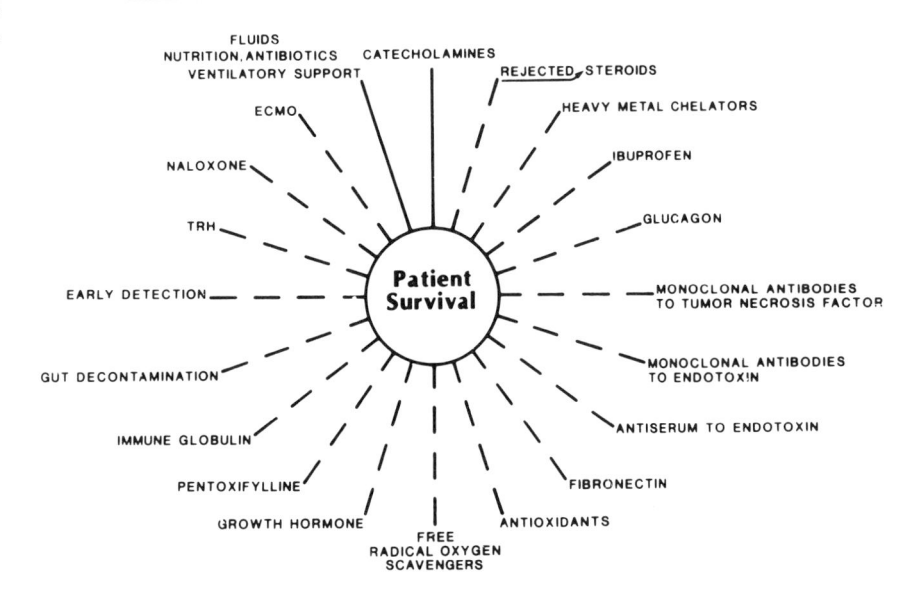

Data from investigations in animal models of the efficacy of steroids in septic shock are impressive. Corticosteroid treatment of sheep given endotoxin inhibits platelet aggregation and release of arachidonic acid products. In humans, however, results have been less clear. Initial investigations found compelling evidence in favor of corticosteroid administration to patients with septic shock, but subsequent studies suggested that corticosteroids do not increase overall survival. At present, it must be concluded that clinical trials would not support the use of corticosteroids in septic shock or ARDS.

Natural antioxidants, iron and heavy metal chelators, oxygen radical scavengers, niacin, endotoxin immunization, endorphins (in endotoxin shock), and surfactant replacement (in neonatal respiratory distress) have all been evaluated for use in the treatment of ARDS, but results have been inconclusive. Treatment modalities currently being tested in either animals or clinical trials are shown in Fig. 2.

SUGGESTED READING

Bone RC. The adult respiratory distress syndrome: new trends. Resident Staff Physician 1989; 35(8):25–34.
Bone RC, Fisher CJ, Jr, Clemmer TP, et al. A controlled clinical trial of high-dose methylprednisolone in the treatment of severe sepsis and septic shock. N Engl J Med 1987; 317:653–658.
Bone RC, Fisher CJ, Jr, Clemmer TP, et al. Early methylprednisolone treatment for septic syndrome and the adult respiratory distress syndrome. Chest 1987; 92:1032–1036.
Bone RC, Slotman G, Maunder R, et al. Randomized double-blind, multicenter study of prostaglandin E1 in patients with the adult respiratory distress syndrome. Prostaglandin E1 Study Group. Chest 1989; 96:114–119.

PNEUMONITIS

ROBERT A. KAPLAN, M.D.
CYRUS C. HOPKINS, M.D.
ROBERT H. RUBIN, M.D.

Pneumonitis, inflammation of the lung parenchyma, is the most common form of life-threatening infection observed in hospitalized patients. Although pneumonitis may result from such noninfectious processes as leukoagglutinin reactions, allergic reactions to organic antigens, and drug hypersensitivity reactions, the focus in this chapter will be on the critically ill patient with pulmonary infection, and the terms pneumonitis and pneumonia will be used interchangeably.

Critically ill patients with pneumonia who will be cared for in an intensive care unit (ICU) can be divided into two major categories: those with severe community-acquired pneumonia that results in respiratory failure sufficient to require admission to the ICU, and those already in the ICU who acquire nosocomial pneumonia. The differential diagnostic considerations and the clinical management of these two groups of patients are very different.

COMMUNITY-ACQUIRED PNEUMONIA

Although clinical manifestations may overlap, it is helpful to divide patients with community-acquired pneumonia into two groups: those with "typical" and those with "atypical" pneumonia. *Typical pneumonia* refers to disease characterized by an acute onset over a time period of less than 24 hours, fever, chills, and systemic toxicity, localized pulmonary findings on physical examination and chest film, a cough productive of purulent sputum which on microscopic examination is shown to contain many neutrophils and one predominant form of bacteria, and an elevated white blood cell count (WBC) that contains an increased number of immature granulocytes ("a shift to the left"). *Atypical pneumonia* refers to disease characterized by a subacute onset over several days, a predominance of constitutional symptoms, a paucity of focal findings on physical examination, diffuse or patchy infiltrates on chest films, variable sputum production, and only minor changes in the WBC.

There are two important variations of this categorization of community-acquired pneumonia as typical or atypical. The first of these is the occurrence of acute bacterial pneumonia in a patient with preceding viral respiratory infection. Some 35 to 50 percent of individuals with acute bacterial pneumonia have a preceding respiratory infection. Typically, these patients have had a viral prodrome (myalgias, malaise, fever, nonproductive cough) for 5 to 7 days, and then have a sudden clinical deterioration (e.g., rigors, high fevers, productive cough, increasing shortness of breath). Often, this is in the setting of widespread respiratory illness in the community. This biphasic course is very different from that of patients who have a progressive decline over several days and are more likely to have viral or *Mycoplasma pneumoniae* pneumonia without bacterial superinfection.

The second variation to be considered is community-acquired Legionella pneumonia. The clinical presentation of this form of pulmonary infection combines elements of both typical and atypical pneumonia: on the one hand, "viral type" symptoms of malaise, myalgias, headaches, nonproductive cough, abdominal discomfort, and diarrhea are common, sputum production is usually scant, and the roentgenographic picture may reveal only interstitial abnormalities similar to those produced by *Mycoplasma pneumoniae*; on the other hand, the rate of progression of the pulmonary process is that of a bacterial infection, bilateral pulmonary involvement is the rule, and the clinical course is suggestive of a virulent bacterial process.

For all forms of community-acquired pneumonia, a careful epidemiologic history can be of great help in arriving at an etiologic diagnosis. Every patient with community-acquired pneumonia should be asked about travel and occupational exposures, contacts with animals and other ill individuals, and other unusual exposures. Thus, primary fungal pneumonia might be considered in individuals with recent geographic exposures to *Histoplasma capsulatum* or *Coccidioides immitis*, psittacosis in an individual who cares for parrots, or tuberculosis in a patient with an appropriate exposure history. The presence of community outbreaks of respiratory infection (particularly influenza) should be ascertained. Particular emphasis should be placed on obtaining information on possible risk factors for human immunodeficiency virus (HIV) infection, remembering that the incubation period between acquisition of HIV and the onset of the acquired immunodeficiency syndrome (AIDS) is not infrequently greater than 7 years. Thus, we have seen several patients who presented with community-acquired atypical pneumonia, which subsequently was shown to be due to *Pneumocystis carinii*, in whom the critical piece of information was the history of blood transfusions 7 to 10 years before.

The most common cause of typical community-acquired pneumonia is *Streptococcus pneumoniae*, which accounts for 25 to 60 percent of such cases. *Haemophilus influenzae* accounts for another 4 to 15 percent; *Staphylococcus aureus*, 2 to 10 percent; and group-A streptococci *(Streptococcus pyogenes)*, 1 to 5 percent. *S. aureus* and *H. influenzae* are particularly prominent as a cause of postinfluenza pneumonia, and group-A streptococci cause pneumonia in the setting of community-wide outbreaks of streptococcal pharyngitis. Aerobic gram-negative bacilli other than *H. influenzae* and mixed aerobic and anaerobic infections account for the remainder of the cases of diagnosed bacterial pneumonia. In elderly patients, particularly those with chronic obstructive pulmonary disease and other debilitating illnesses, there is an increased incidence of infection with *H. influenzae*, enteric gram-negative bacilli, and *S. aureus*. In addition, it has become apparent that *Branhamella catarrhalis*, long thought of as a commensal inhabitant of the upper respiratory tract, can be an important cause of pneumonia in elderly, debilitated individuals.

When there is a history compatible with an aspirational episode (neurologic disease, exposure to sedating drugs, poor oral hygiene, episodes of vomiting, etc.), other diagnostic considerations pertain. Following a major aspirational episode, there are three clinical sequelae that need to be considered: a chemical pneumonitis, bronchial obstruction, and bacterial pneumonia. The first two of these present acutely; the last is often more insidious, presenting several days to weeks after the episode with symptoms of fever, weight loss, and productive cough. Putrid sputum is noted in approximately half of these patients. The chest film usually reveals involvement of dependent portions of the lung, with frequent involvement of the pleural space. In younger patients, particularly those without other diseases or contact with medical institutions, the bacterial etiology is that of the normal upper respiratory flora: such anaerobes as *Bacteroides melaninogenicus*, *Fusobacterium* species, and anaerobic gram-positive cocci (alone in approximately 50 percent of cases) and such aerobes as oral streptococci (together with the anaerobes in the remainder of the cases). In elderly, debilitated patients, whose oropharyngeal flora has been replaced by enteric gram-negative bacilli or *S. aureus*, aspirational episodes will result in a more virulent process in which these organisms will play an important role. Therefore, the treatment of aspiration-related pneumonia should be based, in part, on the clinical status of the patient prior to the aspirational episode.

The diagnostic and therapeutic approach to patients with presumed bacterial pneumonia acquired in the community is based on the appropriate examination of deep pulmonary secretions. Although blood cultures should be drawn in all patients with pneumonia severe enough to merit admission to the ICU (in part to rule out the possibility that the pulmonary process is secondary to hematogenous spread or is an ARDS picture secondary to systemic sepsis), these will reveal the etiology of the process in less than 25 percent of cases. In the majority of patients with typical, community-acquired pneumonia the expectorated sputum provides the necessary diagnostic information. However, rigid criteria based upon microscopic examination of a Gram-stained sputum specimen should be applied to ensure the adequacy of the sample: Under low power (100×), the number of neutrophils and the number of epithelial cells present should be assessed. If more than 25 neutrophils and fewer than 10 epithelial cells are present, the specimen being evaluated has been contaminated minimally by the resident oropharyngeal flora. Such specimens provide clinically useful information and can be utilized both for microscopic and cultural diagnosis. Sputum specimens that do not fulfill these criteria necessitate either an empiric choice of therapy (Table 1) or a more invasive approach to specimen collection. In this circumstance, either transtracheal aspiration or bronchoscopy may be carried out. Our preference, in the patient ill enough from pneumonia to require intensive care, is to proceed directly to bronchoscopy, reserving empiric therapy for patients in whom this cannot be done (practically, this is usually the patient with an unstable cardiac status). Choice of antimicrobial regimen in such individuals is then based upon the clinical characteristics (see Table 1).

The most common causes of atypical community-acquired pneumonia are *M. pneumoniae*, viruses such as influenza and the adenoviruses, *Legionella* species, and *Chlamydia pneumoniae* (TWAR). In certain geographic areas, acute histoplasmosis, coccidioidomycosis, blastomycosis, and Q fever (*Coxiella burnetii*) need to be considered as well. The patient with atypical, community-acquired pneumonia severe enough to require admission to the ICU should be treated with high doses of intravenous erythromycin aimed at the therapy of the most treatable forms of atypical infection: Legionella, Mycoplasma, and Chlamydia. In patients whose clinical presentation does not fit clearly into either the typical or atypical category, then the erythromycin therapy should be combined with

Table 1 Initial Therapy of Patients with Pneumonia*

Category of Pneumonia	Usual Pathogens	Options for Initial Therapy
Community-acquired Typical, in otherwise healthy patient	*Streptococcus pneumoniae*	Penicillin (cefazolin or erythromycin if penicillin-allergic)
Typical, in patient with antecedent influenza	*S. pneumoniae* *Haemophilus influenzae* *Staphylococcus aureus*	Cefuroxime, ampicillin-sulbactam, trimethoprim-sulfamethoxazole
Typical, in patient with "chronic disease"†	*S. pneumoniae* *H. influenzae* *S. aureus* *Branhamella catarrhalis* Enteric Gram-negative bacilli	Cefuroxime, ampicillin-sulbactam, trimethoprim-sulfamethaxazole
Atypical	Viral *Mycoplasma pneumoniae* *Legionella* species *Chlamydia pneumoniae* (TWAR) *Pneumocystis carinii*‡	Erythromycin +/− trimethoprim-sulfamethaxazole
Aspiration, in otherwise healthy patient	Oral anaerobes and streptococci	Penicillin + metronidazole, ampicillin-sulbactam, clindamycin
Aspiration, in patient with "chronic disease"	Oral anaerobes and streptococci *S. pneumoniae* *H. influenzae* *S. aureus* *B. catarrhalis* Enteric gram-negative bacilli	Cefazolin + gentamicin, cefuroxime + metronidazole, ampicillin-sulbactam, clindamycin + gentamicin, clindamycin + aztreonam
Nosocomial§ Sputum with predominant gram-negative rods on smear	*Klebsiella pneumoniae* *Escherichia coli* *Pseudomonas aeruginosa* *Enterobacter* spp. *Serratia marcescens*#	Aminoglycoside# or aztreonam + ceftazidime, tircarcillin, or imipenem-cilastatin
Sputum with mixed flora or gram-positive cocci	*S. aureus* + above	Cefazolin, nafcillin or vancomycin + aminoglycoside or aztreonam

* The listed antibiotics constitute regimens active against the most common respiratory pathogens in each patient category and are appropriate for initial therapy except in the following cases: when the history suggests exposure to an uncommon pathogen, sputum smear reveals a predominance of an unusual organism, or distinctive antibiotic resistance patterns prevail in a hospital or community

† "Chronic disease" = Chronic obstructive lung disease, alcoholism, diabetes, advanced age, nursing home residence, or other debilitating illness (not including specific immunodeficiency states)

‡ In HIV-positive patients

§ Knowledge of the usual indigenous flora and sensitivity patterns is essential to treatment of nosocomial pneumonia, especially in the ICU.

Two drugs should be used for the initial treatment of severe nosocomial pneumonia caused by gram-negative rods. When renal function is a significant concern, aminoglycoside therapy may be limited to one or two doses.

Table 2 Etiology of Nosocomial Pneumonia*

Microorganism	Incidence (%)
Pseudomonas aeruginosa	16.9
Staphylococcus aureus	12.9
Klebsiella spp.	11.6
Enterobacteriaceae spp.	9.4
Escherichia coli	6.4
Serratia marcescens	5.8
Proteus spp.	4.2

*As reported in the National Nosocomial Infections Study Report Annual Summary 1984: MMWR 1986; 35:1755–2955. It should be noted that this reflects the reporting from a number of institutions of varying size and type across the United States. Thus, at some institutions the different Enterobacteriaceae are individually reported, while at others, they are grouped together. Also, such data may not adequately reflect the situation at a particular institution. Thus, at our institution Acinetobacter is an important cause of nosocomial pneumonia, although this is not necessarily true nationally.

more conventional antibacterial therapy as previously outlined. Particularly in such patients, more invasive evaluation by means of fiberoptic bronchoscopy with bronchoalveolar lavage and transbronchial biopsy should be considered. Open lung biopsy is recommended in such individuals who have focal, as opposed to diffuse, lung disease or in those whose clinical course has deteriorated and whose initial bronchoscopic studies have been non-revealing.

NOSOCOMIAL PNEUMONIA

Pneumonia accounts for 15 percent of all nosocomial infections, with approximately 15 percent of all hospital-associated deaths being ascribable to nosocomial pneumonia. Although the incidence of bacteremia in patients with nosocomial pneumonia is less than 10 percent, the mortality has been reported to be as high as 25 to 50 percent, at least three times that of community-acquired pneumonias. In part, this is due to the general debility of the patient population developing nosocomial pneumonia, but in part this is due to the microbial agents causing such pneumonia (Table 2). Mortality from gram-negative pneumonia exceeds 50 percent; for gram-positive nosocomial pneumonia they are less than 25 percent, with nosocomial Legionella infection being somewhere in the middle. Such data emphasize the importance of early and aggressive therapy of gram-negative pulmonary infection in ICU patients.

Impaired airway clearance mechanisms, altered pharyngeal flora, and endotracheal intubation all put the hospitalized patient at increased risk for pneumonia. The ICU patient is at highest risk and is exposed to pathogens that may have acquired significant drug resistance under the selective pressure of prophylactic and therapeutic antibiotics. The usual clinical criteria for the diagnosis of pneumonia lose their sensitivity and specificity in the patient who is critically ill. Infiltrates may be obscured by the presence of pulmonary edema. Fever and leukocytosis may be due to a multiplicity of other causes. Neutrophils seen on Gram's stain and sputum samples may reflect endotracheal tube-related airway irritation. Sputum bacteria may reflect only airway colonization. The diagnosis of nosocomial pneumonia is most definite when there is a clear-cut change in these parameters, usually associated with worsening hypoxemia and a predominant sputum organism. However, treatment must often be initiated on the basis of less clear information, particularly in patients with abnormal chest films due to preceding pneumonia or congestive heart failure. Our own approach to such patients, based upon the need for early therapeutic intervention, is to initiate therapy when two or more of the following events is noted: an unexplained deterioration in gas exchange; an increase in sputum volume, color, and thickness, especially when accompanied by an increase in the number of neutrophils in the sputum; the appearance of a single bacterial species as the predominant organism in the sputum, particularly when this organism is *Pseudomonas aeruginosa*, one of the Enterobacteriaceae, *S. aureus, Acinetobacter,* or *Branhamella catarrhalis*; an otherwise unexplained increase in WBC or fever; or a worsening of the chest film. It should be emphasized that the chest film in such patients, once abnormal, is a rather insensitive indicator of either improvement or deterioration.

Once the decision has been made to initiate antimicrobial therapy, the initial choice of antibiotics is dictated by four major factors: the results of a microscopic examination of a Gram-stained sputum and, when available, cultural information on the previously colonizing flora; the patient's exposure to antibiotics in the 2 to 3 weeks preceding the current episode; a knowledge of the predominant nosocomial flora of the particular ICU and its usual antimicrobial sensitivity pattern; and an assessment of the potential risk of side effects from a given class of antimicrobial agent (e.g., the risk of aminoglycoside toxicity in the patient with unstable renal function). If gram-positive cocci predominate on the microscopic examination, then initial therapy with nafcillin or cefazolin is instituted (reserving vancomycin for patients with beta-lactam allergy or in ICUs with a known risk of methicillin-resistant *S. aureus* infection).

When gram-negative pneumonia is the concern, our practice is to initiate therapy with a beta-lactam drug to which the organism is likely to be sensitive, based on the resident nosocomial flora and previous antibiotic selective pressure (such drugs as ampicillin-sulbactam, cefuroxime, ceftazidime, an antipseudomonal penicillin, and imipenem-cilastatin) plus an aminoglycoside (which aminoglycose is chosen is again based upon the prediction of possible drug resistance). Once the gram-negative organism is identified on culture and its antibiotic susceptibility pattern determined, the antimicrobial regimen should often be modified. If *Pseudomonas aeruginosa* is identified as the causative organism, a two-drug regimen of an antipseudomonal beta-lactam drug plus an aminoglycoside is obligatory to provide synergistic killing and to minimize the development of resistance. Whether this principle should apply to all gram-negative pneumonias is controversial; some organisms have more readily inducible beta-lactamases, such as Enterobacter species, but this problem may apply to many gram-negative organisms. Our practice is to use such a two-drug regimen whenever there is clearcut evidence of pneumonia due to a gram-negative organism, reserving single-agent therapy for patients who are only moderately ill and in whom the evidence of infection is less compelling. In patients for whom aminoglycoside therapy is believed to constitute a significant risk, aztreonam may be safely substituted. When mixed gram-positive and gram-negative infections are suspected, then initial therapy should cover both classes of organisms, with initial use of either a combination such as cefazolin and an aminoglycoside or such drugs as ampicillin-sulbactam, ticarcillin-clavulanic acid, or imipenem-cilastatin. It should be emphasized that the antistaphylococcal activity of third-generation cephalosporins is too limited to support their use as initial single-drug therapy if *S. aureus* infection is a serious concern.

SPECIAL PATIENT CATEGORIES

Some chronic lung diseases are associated with distinctive causes of pulmonary infection. Patients with cystic fibrosis are at particular risk for recurrent infection with mucoid strains of *Pseudomonas aeruginosa*; initial therapy of pneumonia in these patients should include tobramycin plus an antipseudomonal penicillin or ceftazidime. Drug-resistance patterns may modify these recommendations. Once the patient's condition stabilizes, oral ciprofloxacin therapy has been extremely useful in making earlier cessation of intravenous therapy and discharge from the hospital possible. Patients with chronic obstructive pulmonary disease, including those with recurrent bronchitis or bronchiectasis, are much more likely to be colonized with *Haemophilus influenzae*, and initial therapy of pneumonia in these patients should include coverage for this species as well (e.g., cefuroxime, ampicillin, or ampicillin-sulbactam). Patients with pulmonary alveolar proteinosis, perhaps because of impaired alveolar macrophage function, are at increased risk for nocardial infection; in these patients initial therapy should include trimethoprim-sulfamethoxazole (or sulfisoxazole alone). Minocycline is the initial drug of choice in patients with sulfonamide allergy.

Immunocompromised patients are at risk for severe infection with routine pathogens and for infection with opportunistic agents that would be unlikely to produce disease in the intact host. The specific nature of the immune defect may allow prediction of the likely pathogens. However, because specific diagnosis and early initiation of therapy is critical in determining the prognosis in these patients, and because routine examination of expectorated sputum from these patients is often misleading, invasive diagnostic techniques are often required. The choice of procedure is based on the status of the patient and the location of the pulmonary lesions. Transtracheal aspiration has been largely supplanted by bronchoscopy in these patients but may help clarify the diagnosis of bacterial pneumonia. Transthoracic needle aspiration is particularly useful in the evaluation of focal, pleural-based lesions, especially when cavitation is present. In general, the two most useful diagnostic procedures are bronchoscopy and open lung biopsy. Bronchoscopy with protected brush, lavage, and/or transbronchial biopsy is most appropriate in the patient whose chest film reveals a diffuse rather than a focal process, and whose illness is more of a diagnostic dilemma than a therapeutic emergency. Open lung biopsy, the definitive diagnostic procedure, is most appropriate in patients in whom previous diagnostic procedures have been nondiagnostic, and when deteriorating patient status mandates the emergent initiation of appropriate therapy. The use of such invasive procedures is, of course, modified by the clinical status of a patient. Patients terminally ill with acute leukemia, advanced cancer, or AIDS are poor candidates for invasive diagnostic procedures; by contrast, transplant patients, whose long-term prognosis is excellent if they recover from their pneumonia, merit an extremely aggressive approach.

ONGOING CARE OF THE ICU PATIENT WITH PNEUMONIA

Along with the initiation of antimicrobial therapy, management of the critically ill patient with pneumonia has several other components. The clinician must be aware of the potential effects of pneumonia both locally and systemically. These effects include fever and the metabolic consequences of fever (e.g., for each degree of temperature elevation above 100°F., there is an increase in cardiorespiratory workload of approximately 10 percent, which can be clinically important in patients with severe cardiorespiratory disease), and abnormalities in gas exchange, which can occur in all forms of pneumonia. In addition, there are three other potential adverse events that can develop in the course of pneumonia, which occur to varying degrees depending on the particular etiologic cause of the pneumonia: the occurrence of bacteremia and the resulting potential for metastatic seeding of microorganisms, lung necrosis, and contiguous spread to the pleural and pericardial spaces (Table 3). Part of the clinical management of patients with pneumonia includes an assessment and approach to these potential problems. For example, because bacteremia and a risk of meningitis is common in pneumococcal pneumonia, a lumbar puncture is part of the initial assessment in patients with pneumococcal pneumonia who have headaches or even slight changes in mental status. By contrast, patients with Klebsiella pneumonia, who are usually at least as toxic as patients with pneumococcal infection, with similar chest films and abnormalities in gas exchange, uncommonly have bacteremia or metastatic infection. Therefore, the index of suspicion for meningitis is very low, and a lumbar puncture is rarely a part of the diagnostic approach in these patients. Conversely, patients with pneumococcal pneumonia rarely cavitate portions of the lung, and when they do, an alternative explanation should be sought; patients with Klebsiella and staphylococcal pneumonia commonly do so. This difference in lung pathology will affect other aspects of these patients' care as well: with a necrotizing

Table 3 Likelihood of Potential Complications With Different Forms of Pneumonia

Etiology of Pneumonia	Bacteremia	Contiguous Spread: Pleural and/or Pericardial	Necrotizing Pneumonia
Streptococcus pneumoniae	20–50%	1+	0
Klebsiella pneumoniae	<10%	3+	4+
Staphylococcus aureus	<10%	4+	4+
Streptococcus pyogenes	<10%	almost invariable	1–2+
Aspiration (anaerobic or mixed aerobic/anaerobic)	<10%	3+	4+
Haemophilus influenzae			
Nontypable	<10%	—	0
Type B	15–35%	2+	0
Escherichia coli	<10%	2+	2+
Pseudomonas aeruginosa	10%	2+	4+

pneumonia, high airway pressures can be associated with the sudden development of a pneumothorax; this is rarely a problem with pneumococcal disease. Therefore, the clinician should attempt to define the etiology of the process not only for the selection of antimicrobial therapy, but also to guide in the identification and management of possible complications from a particular form of pneumonia.

In the ambulatory patient, mucociliary clearance and cough are usually sufficient to provide drainage of infected secretions. In the critically ill patient, particularly when intubated, mechanical assistance is mandatory to facilitate the drainage of secretions and thus help prevent spread of the pneumonia, necrosis of lung tissue, abscess, and empyema. Postural drainage, percussion, vibration, assisted cough, and suctioning all play a role; in the patient with obstructive airway disease, bronchodilatory therapy may be a useful adjunct to vigorous pulmonary toilet. Although controlled trials of the efficacy of therapeutic bronchoscopy are lacking, suctioning under direct visualization through the fiberoptic bronchoscope should be considered to facilitate drainage when routine chest physical therapy and sunctioning are inadequate.

A variety of significant adverse drug reactions may occur during therapy for severe pneumonia. Cutaneous hypersensitivity reactions and *Clostridium difficile*-associated colitis are well recognized. Of particular concern in the critically ill patient are nephrotoxicity and ototoxicity associated with vancomycin and aminoglycoside therapy. Serum creatinine and antibiotic levels should be monitored and doses adjusted accordingly, especially in patients with underlying renal disease and other conditions that appear to predispose to toxicity (i.e., diabetes, diuretic therapy, etc.). In these high-risk patients, alternative nontoxic drug regimens should be employed whenever possible.

In most cases of pneumonia a decrease in the magnitude of fever, leukocytosis, and sputum purulence and an improvement in gas exchange should begin within 48 to 72 hours of initiation of effective therapy, though chest films will respond much more slowly. Recrudescence or failure of clinical improvement should trigger a search for an undiagnosed infectious agent, a noninfectious cause of pneumonitis, the development of antibiotic resistance, superinfection, or the presence of one of the complications outlined in Table 3. In patients who manifest a clinical response, the last issue to be addressed is the duration of therapy, which depends on the type and severity of infection and the clinical course. For example, severe, necrotizing gram-negative, staphylococcal, or mixed aerobic-anaerobic pneumonia often requires 4 to 6 weeks of parenteral therapy; less severe infection, treated early, with a prompt response, may require only 10 to 14 days of therapy. Many gram-negative pneumonias will fall in the middle, requiring 2 to 3 weeks of therapy. This clinical decision should be individualized for each patient on the basis of the following: nature of the invading organism (in general, such organisms as *Pseudomonas aeruginosa, Klebsiella pneumoniae, Legionella pneumophila, S. aureus*, and anaerobic infection require prolonged therapy); amount of lung necrosis present; presence of extrapulmonary infection; and rapidity of response to therapy. If this is done, cure of such life-threatening processes can be accomplished, although exquisite attention to detail is essential throughout the sometimes extended courses of therapy that may be required.

SUGGESTED READING

Donowitz GR, Mandell GL. Acute pneumonia. In: Mandell GL, Douglas RG Jr, Bennett JE, eds. Principles and practice of infectious diseases. 3rd ed. New York: John Wiley & Sons, 1989.

Fraser RG, Paré JA. Infectious diseases of the lungs. In: Fraser RG, Paré JA, eds. Diagnosis of diseases of the chest. 2nd ed. Vol. 2. Philadelphia: WB Saunders Company, 1978.

Glanville AR, Martin GE. Pneumonia. In: Wilson JD, ed. Drug use in respiratory disease. Sydney: Williams & Wilkins, 1987.

Kovacs JA, Masur H. Opportunistic infections. In: DeVita VT. AIDS: etiology, diagnosis, treatment, and prevention. 2nd ed. Philadelphia: JB Lippincott, 1988.

Neu HC. Principles governing use of antibiotics in pulmonary infections. In: Fishman AP, eds. Pulmonary diseases and disorders. 2nd ed. New York: McGraw-Hill, 1988.

Rubin RH, Young LS, eds. Clinical approach to infection in the compromised host. 2nd ed. New York: Plenum, 1988.

OBSTRUCTIVE LUNG DISEASE

ROBERT A. BALK, M.D.

The obstructive lung diseases encompass a wise range of disorders, including asthma, cystic fibrosis, bronchiectasis, bronchiolitis obliterans, and chronic obstructive pulmonary disease (COPD). The term "COPD" is used to describe patients with chronic bronchitis, emphysema, or a combination of the two disorders. These patients characteristically manifest airflow obstruction and have frequent episodes of acute and chronic respiratory failure, and so are commonly evaluated and treated by critical care specialists.

Patients with COPD may manifest chronic respiratory failure, evidenced by hypoxemia and/or hypercapnia. This is particularly true in the chronic bronchitic ("blue bloater" or type-B patient), whose clinical course is marked by recurrent episodes of acute decompensation. The extra stress placed upon the heart in this circumstance may result in right-sided cardiac failure secondary to the lung disease, cor pulmonale. Several decades ago the mortality for acute respiratory failure in COPD was 10 to 40 percent; however, with the advances in technology and medical therapeutics the acute mortality is now less than 10 percent. Unfortunately this population of patients continues to have a high late mortality, with the vast majority of patients not surviving 5 years. Approximately one half of the patients requiring mechanical ventilation will not be alive in 2 years.

The patient with COPD and acute respiratory failure (ARF) usually presents with breathlessness, cyanosis, and tachypnea. There is utilization of the accessory muscles of respiration, and often there is a change in the quantity and color of daily sputum production. The arterial blood gases will usually reflect a decrease in the partial pressure of oxygen (PaO_2) and an increase in the partial pressure of carbon dioxide ($PaCO_2$) in the arterial blood. The abnormal blood gas dictates the initial goals of management: to correct the hypoxemia and improve the elimination of CO_2.

CAUSES OF ACUTE RESPIRATORY FAILURE IN COPD

A number of different clinical situations have been associated with the exacerbation of COPD (Table 1). The deterioration in pulmonary function may be a manifestation of the progression of the underlying lung disease. Infection of the tracheobronchial tree or the lung parenchyma is the most common precipitating factor for the development of ARF in patients with COPD. The infectious agents are frequently viral, with the most common pathogens being rhinovirus, influenza virus, parainfluenza virus, and coronavirus. The common bacterial pathogens include *Haemophilus influenzae*, *Streptococcus pneumoniae*, *Mycoplasma pneumoniae*, and *Branhamella catarrhalis*. Previously published autopsy studies have reported a relatively high (20 to 51 percent) incidence of pulmonary thromboembolism associated with the exacerbation of COPD. These results are probably not truly representative of the majority of patients with COPD. Left ventricular failure may be very difficult to appreciate in the setting of an acute exacerbation of COPD, and diagnosis may require the use of balloon-tipped pulmonary artery catheters. In the past, respiratory failure related to oversedation with or without the use of injudicious oxygen therapy was frequently encountered. Fortunately, there has been an appreciation of the potential for respiratory center depression associated with the combination of sedation and too high a concentration of inspired oxygen (FIO_2).

Table 1 Common Precipitating Causes of an Acute Exacerbation of COPD

Progression of the underlying lung disease
Tracheobronchial or parenchymal lung infection
Left ventricular failure
Pulmonary embolus
Pneumothorax
Acute bronchospasm
Thoracoabdominal surgery or trauma
Uncontrolled oxygen administration
Oversedation
Increased atmospheric pollution
Medication noncompliance

TREATMENT

The treatment of ARF in patients with COPD can either be conservative or invasive (Table 2). The conservative approach describes the initial attempt to manage the patient without the use of assisted ventilation. When confronted with a COPD patient with ARF, the clinician needs to concentrate first on ensuring adequate oxygenation and preventing the deleterious effects of hypoxemia.

Table 2 Treatment of Acute Respiratory Failure in COPD

Controlled oxygen therapy
Bronchodilators
  Beta-agonists
  Anticholinergic agents
  Corticosteroids
  Theophylline
Antibiotics
Diuretics in patients with evidence of heart failure
Digitalis in patients with evidence of left ventricular failure or biventricular failure
Chest physiotherapy when appropriate
Mechanical ventilation when conservative management fails
Prevention of complications and multi-organ system dysfunction
  Prophylaxis of deep vein thrombosis
  Stress ulcer prevention
  Avoid metabolic/contraction alkalosis
  Correct electrolyte imbalance
  Ensure adequate nutrition

Conservative Approach

Oxygen Therapy

Oxygen should be administered in sufficient quantity to raise the oxygen saturation of hemoglobin (SaO_2) to approximately 90 percent. At this saturation, 90 percent of the hemoglobin oxygen-binding sites contain oxygen and there is little additional benefit associated with increasing the PaO_2 above this level. In fact, if the PaO_2 increases far beyond this level of saturation, there may be depression of the hypoxic drive and subsequent increase in CO_2 retention with worsening of the respiratory acidosis. Low-flow oxygen can be administered either via nasal cannula or using a Venturi mask. The advantage of the Venturi mask is that a precise FIO_2 can be delivered to the patient, while the exact FIO_2 delivered by nasal-cannula oxygen varies, depending on the flow rate and breathing characteristics of the patient. Mouth breathing and the patient's inspiratory flow pattern can alter the delivered FIO_2.

Oxygen is essential to reverse the hypoxic pulmonary vasoconstriction and to ensure adequate delivery of oxygen to tissues. The administration of adequate amounts of oxygen therapy will reduce the pulmonary artery pressure, decrease pulmonary vascular resistance, increase right ventricular ejection fraction, and with time return the hematocrit back toward normal in polycythemic patients. In those patients who manifest chronic hypoxemia or who desaturate with exercise, the use of supplemental oxygen has been shown to improve survival significantly.

Bronchodilator Therapy

Despite the fact that the majority of patients with COPD have irreversible obstruction, bronchodilators are routinely employed in the treatment. The beta-adrenergic agonists stimulate adenyl-cyclase and increase levels of cyclic adenosine monophosphate (cAMP), a bronchial smooth muscle dilator. Because of their ease of use, rapid onset of action, and relatively low toxicity-to-benefit ratio, they are the initial agents employed in the treatment of acute exacerbations of COPD. Recent innovations have resulted in new $beta_2$ selective agents which cause less cardiac toxicity and have a longer duration of action (Table 3). This is particularly important in the COPD population since the majority of patients are older and may be at risk for concomitant coronary artery disease. The preferred route of administration is topical, either by metered-dose inhaler or by nebulizer. This form of administration has less systemic toxicity yet still produces the beneficial bronchodilatory effect with a rapid onset of action. In the intensive care unit, I prefer to use either metaproterenol or albuterol given by nebulizer every 2 to 6 hours, depending on the patient's response and severity of illness.

Anticholinergic blockade will decrease levels of cyclic guanosine monophosphate (cGMP), which is a bronchoconstrictor. Atropine has traditionally been used to promote bronchodilation in this manner. Unfortunately, atropine has a variety of untoward side effects (arrhythmias, bladder outlet obstruction, dry mouth, and dry

Table 3 Commonly Used Beta-Adrenergic Agonists

Drug	Metered-Dose Inhaler	Nebulization	Oral Route	Subcutaneous Route
Epinephrine	—	—	—	0.3 mg q 20 min. up to 3 doses†
Isoproterenol	2 puffs q 1–2 hr	0.25 ml 1% solution in 1.75 ml saline q 4–6 hr	—	—
Isoetharine	2 puffs q 4 hr	0.5 ml 1% solution in 1.5 ml saline q 4–6 hr	—	—
Terbutaline	2 puffs q 4–6 hr	5 ml 0.1% solution q 4 hr	2.5–5.0 mg q 8 hr	0.25 mg may repeat in 15-30 min.
Metaproterenol	2 puffs q 4–6 hr	0.3 ml 5% solution in 2.5 ml saline q 4–6 hr	10–20 mg qid	—
Albuterol	2 puffs q 4–6 hr	1 ml 0.5% solution in 1.5 ml saline q 4–6 hr	2–8 mg qid	—
Fenoterol‡	—	1 ml 0.5% solution q 4–6 hr	—	—

*Adapted and modified from Dorinsky PM, Gadek JE. Obstructive lung disease. In: Parrillo JE, ed. Current therapy in critical care. Toronto: BC Decker Inc.
†Not recommended for patients with COPD
‡Currently not available for general use in the US

secretions) that have limited its use in some patients with COPD. Ipratropium bromide is a quaternary congener of atropine and has been shown to promote bronchodilation as effectively as the beta-2 agonists in patients with COPD. Ipratropium bromide has a somewhat delayed onset of action yet appears to last longer than the beta-2 agonists. Ipratropium bromide does not cause the arrhythmia and drying of secretions seen with atropine. The most common side effects are dry mouth and a bitter metallic taste. Theoretically, there is an advantage to using ipratropium bromide in the early treatment of bronchospasm because it does not dilate the pulmonary arteries like the beta-agonists and theophyllines do. Therefore, there is no increase in the ventilation/perfusion ($\dot{V}/\dot{Q}$) abnormality related to loss of hypoxic vasoconstriction. This $\dot{V}/\dot{Q}$ abnormality can lead to early worsening of the arterial blood gases during the initial treatment of bronchospasm.

Currently, a solution of ipratropium bromide is not available for use in a nebulizer. There are special adapters to allow the use of ipratropium through an endotracheal tube, and a spacer device can be used in a nonintubated patient with ARF. Since the effectiveness of metered-dose inhalers is dependent on the technique used, the clinician may elect to use atropine given by nebulizer if the special adapter or the spacer device is not available or ineffective.

Corticosteroids have been shown to help improve airflow and increase the forced expiratory volume (FEV_1) in patients with obstructive lung disease. Up to 30 percent of patients with irreversible airway obstruction were found to have an improvement in FEV_1. The mechanism of action is unknown but may involve decreasing circulating lymphocytes, monocytes, eosinophils, and basophils; increasing neutrophils; stabilization of the lysosomal membranes of the neutrophils and monocytes; enhanced action of catecholamines through decreased uptake and deactivation and increased receptor sites; inhibition of phospholipase A_2 with a decrease in arachidonic acid metabolism; decreased inflammation; and improved integrity of the vascular endothelium. Corticosteroids are associated with a variety of side effects when used either acutely or chronically. However, their ability to produce improved airflow has led to their frequent use in COPD patients with ARF. The usual dose is 0.5 to 1.0 mg of methylprednisolone or its equivalent per kg body weight, administered intravenously every 6 hours. With response there is a gradual tapering over 2 to 4 weeks.

Aminophylline and other theophylline derivatives are phosphodiesterase inhibitors. This inhibition results in an increase in cyclic AMP levels and the resultant bronchodilation. Theophylline was once the mainstay of therapy for airflow obstruction, but it has recently been downgraded to a third- or fourth-line drug because of its narrow therapeutic index. There are a number of side effects associated with its use, and the disturbing feature is that the onset of side effects corresponds to the recommended therapeutic levels. The frequent arrhythmias including multifocal atrial tachycardia (MAT) in patients with COPD are now thought to be related to theophylline rather than a manifestation of the severe lung disease or hypoxemia.

In addition to its ability to relax airway smooth muscle, theophylline is also a mild diuretic and a positive inotrope, can augment diaphragmatic contractility, and is a central respiratory stimulant. Theophylline is still used in the treatment of ARF in COPD patients but is no longer a first-line agent. Care must be taken to avoid producing side effects, especially arrhythmias and seizures.

When using theophylline in a patient who has not previously been receiving the medication or who has not been receiving treatment for several doses, it is necessary to give an intravenous loading dose of 5.6 mg per kg body weight over 20 minutes. This is followed by a constant intravenous infusion, with the rate of administration dependent on the patient's age, liver function, and additional factors that may disturb theophylline pharmacokinetics (Table 4). A young healthy individual would receive an infusion of 0.9 mg per kilogram per hour, whereas an elderly patient with liver failure or congestive heart failure would receive an infusion of 0.2 to 0.3 mg per kilogram per hour. In those individuals who are not as acutely ill, the decision to use theophylline should be weighed against the risks associated with its narrow therapeutic index. In this circumstance, if theophylline therapy is chosen, oral dosing may be substituted for the intravenous infusion, in

Table 4 Factors Affecting Theophylline Clearance

Decreased Clearance	Increased Clearance
Severe liver disease	Tobacco use
Congestive heart failure	Marijuana use
Acute illness in critical care unit	Phenytoin
Cimetidine	High-protein, low-carbohydrate diet
Troleandomycin	Charcoal-broiled meat
Erythromycin	
Propranolol	
Allopurinol	
Phenobarbital	
Oral contraceptives	
Viral infections	
Fever	
Age, over 60 years	

which case it is important to remember that the bioavailability of the drug may be altered by food intake. The most important rule to remember when using theophylline is to follow drug levels closely in an attempt to avoid problems with toxicity. A goal of 10 to 15 μg per milliliter should be satisfactory.

Antibiotics

As previously mentioned, infection is the most common precipitating cause of ARF in patients with COPD. A broad-spectrum antibiotic that is effective against *H. influenzae* and *S. pneumoniae* should be administered. There is evidence that patients with acute infectious symptoms (i.e., cough, purulent sputum, and dyspnea) improve more rapidly when antibiotics are given.

Diuretics and Digitalis

In those patients with cor pulmonale who are having difficulty with diuresis after adequate oxygen therapy, a brisk diuresis can be promoted with the use of diuretics. It is important to closely monitor fluid and electrolyte losses to avoid producing a severe contraction alkalosis, which can exacerbate retention of carbon dioxide and aggravate weaning. Alkalosis can also predispose the patient to arrhythmias.

The use of digitalis in the setting of ARF and cor pulmonale is still controversial. Most would favor the addition of digitalis to the regimen of those patients who manifest left-sided cardiac failure or biventricular failure. On the other hand, digitalis is not recommended for those patients with only right-sided cardiac failure. The controversy continues to rage, however. Digoxin may benefit respiratory muscle function, as evidenced by improved electromyograms of the diaphragm in mechanically ventilated COPD patients with ARF.

Chest Physiotherapy

Chest physiotherapy is frequently employed in the routine treatment of patients with COPD, but data supporting its routine use remain controversial. It has been demonstrated that there may be deleterious effects on gas exchange when chest physiotherapy is performed on patients who have less than 30 ml of sputum production per day. In addition to this consequence, the procedures are time-consuming and require special training.

Vasodilators and Respiratory Stimulants

Current evidence does not support the use of vasodilators in the treatment of ARF with COPD. Even in the population of patients who have pulmonary hypertension, this therapy may have deleterious effects upon the cardiac output and oxygen delivery to tissues.

Respiratory stimulants such as doxapram are also to be avoided in the usual treatment of ARF. While the ventilation of an occasional patient may increase and improve after this therapy, the majority of patients already are maximally working and are using accessory muscles of respiration. These patients literally have no further effort to give, and "whipping" them with a stimulant will have no beneficial effect.

Mechanical Ventilation

Despite initial efforts aimed at quickly improving the ARF, a number of patients will continue to deteriorate and will require assisted ventilation. Such patients tire easily and are more likely to fail; the clinician can directly observe the patient for signs of paradoxical respiration. The abdomen will sink in during inspiration, instead of protrude. This finding is seen with diaphragmatic dysfunction from a variety of causes and is usually taken as a sign of respiratory muscle fatigue. Paradoxical respirations coupled with worsening arterial blood gases are usually signs that the patient will fail conservative management; therefore, elective intubation is a wise choice so that the respiratory muscles can relax.

Oral or nasal intubation is preferred. Early tracheostomy is associated with a greater number of early complications and can always be performed at a later time if weaning is difficult. It is important to use a tube with a large enough diameter, as the airway resistance is inversely proportional to the radius.[4] When initiating mechanical ventilation, I recommend using a volume-cycled ventilator with an initial tidal volume of 10 to 12 ml per kg. The initial FIO_2 should be 100 percent to ensure proper oxygenation during the transition to mechanical ventilation. The minute volume should be chosen to achieve a normal pH for the given condition being treated and not to obtain a normal level of carbon dioxide if that results in a respiratory alkalosis. Acid-base equilibrium, electrolyte balance, and weaning management will be much easier to address if this rule is followed. The mode of mechanical ventilation is left to the discretion of the clinician. My bias is to rest the patient and use the assist-control mode; however, there is controversy regarding the merits of this maneuver.

PREVENTION OF COMPLICATIONS AND MULTIPLE ORGAN SYSTEM DYSFUNCTION

The COPD patient with ARF, like other critically ill patients, is more prone to the development of complications and multi-organ failure, such as deep vein thrombosis and pulmonary thromboembolism. Unless there are specific contraindications such as bleeding diathesis, heparin allergy, uncontrolled hypertension, or thrombocytopenia, minidose heparin (5,000 U subcutaneously every 12 hours) is recommended. Patients with ARF are also at risk for bleeding and stress ulceration of the gastrointestinal tract. The use of histamine-2 receptor blockers has been shown to be adequate prophylaxis; these agents may decrease the clearance of theophylline and care must be taken to avoid toxicity. Fluid and electrolyte abnormalities must be avoided, and particular attention should be directed toward preventing the development of a contraction alkalosis from over-diuresis and/or inadequate potassium replacement.

Critically ill patients also benefit from adequate nutritional replacement. In patients with COPD who have limited ability to excrete CO_2 it is important to avoid large carbohydrate loads, which may not be adequately eliminated and may promote further retention of CO_2. Specialized enteral and parenteral formulae currently exist to assist with this problem.

The final point to remember in caring for these acutely ill patients is to anticipate and prevent nosocomial infections and additional organ system dysfunction. Both complications adversely effect survival and are two of the most common causes of death in today's intensive care unit.

SUGGESTED READING

Derenne JP, Fleury B, Pariente R. Acute respiratory failure of chronic obstructive pulmonary disease. Am Rev Respir Dis 1988; 138:1006–1033.
Rice KL, Leatherman JW, Duane PG, et al. Aminophylline for acute exacerbations of chronic obstructive pulmonary disease. Ann Intern Med 1987; 107:305–309.
Timms RM, Khaja FU, Williams GW, et al. Hemodynamic response to oxygen therapy in chronic obstructive pulmonary disease. Ann Intern Med 1985; 102:29–36.

AIRFLOW OBSTRUCTION CAUSED BY BRONCHOSPASM

REYNOLD A. PANETTIERI, Jr., M.D.
MARK A. KELLEY, M.D.

Increasing mortality from asthma in the United States and other countries has focused recent attention on the management of severe bronchospasm in the critical care unit. Although most deaths from asthma and other chronic obstructive lung diseases occur while the patients are outside the hospital, there is evidence that inadequate assessment and treatment of severe bronchospasm may contribute to increasing mortality in these patients. Fortunately, advances in the use of more selective bronchodilators, the early initiation of corticosteroids, and improved mechanical ventilation for patients with life-threatening obstructive airways diseases has led to an in-hospital mortality of less than 1 percent.

Airway smooth muscle contraction, production of tenacious mucoid secretions, and bronchial mucosal inflammation and edema are the three mechanisms that induce severe reversible bronchospasm. Although all three mechanisms are operative in causing airway luminal narrowing, the onset of airway smooth muscle contraction and bronchial mucosal edema can occur within minutes after exposure to specific allergens. By contrast, the late-phase reaction to allergen exposure, which provokes bronchospasm within 2 to 8 hours and persists for 1 to 2 days, is the result of marked bronchial wall inflammation with infiltration of mononuclear cells and epithelial desquamation. Therapeutic strategies to reduce bronchospastic airflow obstruction are aimed at promoting airway smooth muscle relaxation and reducing airway inflammation.

APPROACH TO THE PATIENT

Although the initial assessment of the dyspneic patient with a history of asthma or chronic obstructive airways disease should alert the physician to the likely probability of an acute exacerbation of the patient's underlying disease, it is important to consider the differential diagnosis of other treatable conditions manifested by dyspnea and wheezing (Table 1). Abnormal phonation and/or an inability to clear upper airway secretions suggests upper airway obstruction, laryngospasm (allergic or functional), or anaphylaxis. The presence of profound orthostatic hypotension especially when accompanied by urticaria or angioedema likely indicates an anaphylactic or an anaphylactoid reaction. The older patient who presents with wheezing and a history of smoking, or other risk factors for coronary artery disease, but without a history of asthma or significant atopy raises the clinical suspicion of congestive heart disease. Unfortunately, clinical response to inhaled bronchodilators may not discriminate laryngospasm, anaphylaxis, or congestive heart failure from asthma, given the nonspecific increase in airway hyperreactivity induced by these disorders. Nonetheless, dyspnea and wheezing unresponsive to conventional bronchodilator therapy should suggest an alternative etiology for the bronchospasm.

During severe episodes of bronchospastic airflow obstruction, air trapping and ventilation-perfusion imbalance cause marked hypoxemia. This hypoxemia coupled with expiratory and inspiratory respiratory muscle fatigue in-

Table 1 Differential Diagnosis of Respiratory Distress and Wheezing

---
Central Airway Obstruction
  Goiter
  Tumor
  Epiglottis
  Foreign body
  (Rarely, sarcoidosis and amyloidosis)

Anaphylaxis and Anaphylactoid Reactions
  Laryngeal edema and laryngospasm

Congestive Heart Failure

Table 2 Risk Factors for Respiratory Failure Caused by Severe Bronchospasm

History
  Long history of asthma
  Poorly controlled and labile bronchospasm
  Bronchospasm refractory to inhaled sympathomimetics
  Previous ICU admissions with/without requiring mechanical ventilation
Physical Examination
  Patient sitting erect often unable to lie flat
  Diaphoresis and/or accessory muscle use
  Pulsus paradoxus of greater than 20 mm Hg
  Markedly decreased breath sounds and lack of wheezing
Laboratory Tests
  Repeated measurements of FEV_1 (<1 L/sec) or PEFR (80 L/min) despite therapy
  Hypercapnia
  Severe hypoxemia (PaO_2 <60 mm Hg) despite supplemental oxygen

duces a lactic acidosis that further compromises muscle function and can ultimately lead to hypercapnic respiratory failure. Early identification of patients with severe airway obstruction requires a focused history and attention to physical findings predictive of impending respiratory failure (Table 2). Because no one finding predicts respiratory failure in patients with severe airway obstruction, frequent physician reassessments, serial measurements of airflow (peak expiratory flow (PEFR) or forced expiratory volume over one second (FEV_1)), and repeated arterial blood gas measurements are mandatory. Patients with a previous history of respiratory failure requiring mechanical ventilation and/or evidence of respiratory muscle fatigue, mental confusion/obtundation, or hypercarbia should be admitted to an intensive care unit (ICU) for careful monitoring. Fortunately, the majority of these patients improve progressively and uneventfully with appropriate therapy.

TREATMENT

Therapeutic goals in the treatment of life-threatening bronchospasm are to promote airway smooth muscle relaxation and to decrease bronchial wall inflammation. Because patients with severe airflow obstruction universally have hypoxemia and experience marked increase in the work of breathing, the use of supplemental oxygen may temporarily improve oxygen delivery and respiratory muscle function. Often the marked increases in minute ventilation in these patients will require the administration of high-flow supplemental oxygen by nasal cannula (4 to 6 L per minute) or preferably by nonaerosolized face mask in order to raise arterial PO_2 significantly. Although oxygen saturation monitoring and telemetry are essential in the initial assessment of patients with severe airflow obstruction, these monitors are insensitive for predicting impending hypercapnic respiratory failure. Close supervision and reassessment of the patient by the physician is necessary.

Few randomized controlled studies exist to address efficacy, dosage, and frequency of various therapeutic modalities in the treatment of severe bronchospasm. The most common therapy includes a combination of aerosolized and/or subcutaneous beta-adrenergic agonists, aminophylline, and systemic corticosteroids.

Beta-Adrenergic Agonists

Aerosolized beta-agonists—with ease of administration, rapid onset of bronchodilation, and fewer side effects than the same agents delivered orally or parenterally—are the first agents of choice in the treatment of acute bronchospasm. These agents presumably cause relaxation of bronchial smooth muscle by reversibly binding to smooth muscle beta-2-adrenoreceptors and increasing cytosolic cyclic adenosine monophosphate (cAMP) levels that inhibit smooth muscle contraction. Other possible mechanisms of action may include alteration of bronchial mucous gland secretion, enhanced mucociliary clearance, and decreased release of mediators from inflammatory cells.

The most frequently administered beta-adrenergic agents are listed in Table 3. Although isoproterenol is the drug of choice in the treatment of pediatric patients with severe bronchospasm, more selective beta-adrenergic agents are used in adults. The majority of beta-adrenergic agents can be administered orally, parenterally, or aerosolized. However, there is no evidence that orally or parenterally delivered beta-adrenergic agents are more

Table 3 Aerosolized Beta-Adrenergic Agents

Drug	Beta$_2$-Specific	Onset of Action (min)	Peak Effect (min)	Duration (hr)	Aerosol Dose by Nebulizer	Aerosol Dose by Metered Dose Inhaler
Isoproterenol	no	5	15	1	2.5–5 mg	250 μg/2 puffs
Isoetharine	yes	10	30	2–3	5 mg	680 μg/2 puffs
Metaproterenol	yes	10	45	3–6	15 mg	1,300 μg/2 puffs
Terbutaline	yes	10	60	4–6	—	400 μg/2 puffs
Albuterol	yes	10	60	4–6	2.5–5 mg	180 μg/2 puffs
Bitolterol†	yes	10	60	3–8	—	1,050 μg/3 puffs
Fenoterol†	yes	10	60	4–8	—	400 μg/2 puffs

*Aerosol dose by nebulizer diluted in 3 ml of saline
†Not available in US

efficacious than the aerosolized preparations (see Table 3). Furthermore, the subcutaneous use of beta-adrenergic agents including epinephrine in combination with aerosolized isoproterenol has shown no benefit in improvement in airflow when compared with aerosolized isoproterenol alone. Moreover, increased systemic side effects of nausea, vomiting, tachyarrhythmias, and palpitations occur with the parenteral and oral preparations as compared with the aerosolized agents. Similar improvement in bronchospasm is attained whether the beta-adrenergic agent is aerosolized by metered-dose inhalers with spacer devices or by nebulization. However, given the inability of the critically ill patient to coordinate use of the metered-dose inhaler, most physicians treat severe life-threatening bronchospasm with nebulized beta-agonist agents.

Optimal frequency of administration of beta-adrenergic agents is controversial. More frequent use of aerosolized albuterol or isoproterenol (2.5 to 5.0 mg every 20 minutes) has been suggested to be superior in improving bronchospasm with no increase in adverse effects when compared with conventional dosing. One mechanism by which more frequent dosing could improve bronchospasm may relate to the more distal deposition of inhaled particles in smaller airways. Repeated peak expiratory flow rate (PEFR) or forced expiratory volume over one second (FEV_1) measurements in patients receiving aerosolized beta-adrenergic agents every 20 minutes allows the titration of further treatments to attainment of maximum bronchodilation (Table 4). When no further benefit from frequent treatments is obtained, more conventional dosing (every 4 to 6 hours) is indicated. It is unclear whether more frequent administration of aerosolized beta-adrenergic agents should be the rule for all patients with airflow obstruction; however, the severely bronchospastic patient may benefit from this therapy. In pediatric patients, intravenous isoproterenol has been efficacious in treatment of severe, life-threatening bronchospasm. By contrast, current evidence does not support intravenous beta-agonist therapy in adults.

Adverse effects of beta-adrenergic agents are dose-dependent. The more selective $beta_2$-adrenergic agents (terbutaline, albuterol, metaproterenol, or isoetharine) have the same side effects at high doses as more potent but less specific agents (epinephrine or isoproterenol). Beta-agonists induce tachycardia, premature ventricular contractions, and atrial and ventricular tachyarrhythmias. Patients with chronic obstructive lung disease who are receiving steroids and/or diuretics can develop hypokalemia that may be exacerbated by the use of beta-adrenergic agents that promote shifts of potassium from the extracellular to intracellular space. As a result of this hypokalemia, the threshold for life-threatening arrhythmias is lowered. Apart from the cardiovascular effects of these agents, beta-agonists rarely can induce bronchospasm and may worsen hypoxemia by dilating pulmonary arteries and increasing ventilation-perfusion mismatch. The majority of these adverse effects are enhanced in combination with theophylline.

Aminophylline

Theophylline preparations are one of the most frequently prescribed bronchodilators worldwide. Despite the frequent use of this drug, the mechanism of theophylline-induced smooth muscle relaxation is unknown. Phosphodiesterase inhibition of both cAMP and cyclic guanosine monophosphate (cGMP) pathways, antagonism of adenosine-mediated bronchoconstriction, or alterations in phosphatidylinositol breakdown are only a few of the proposed cellular mechanisms by which theophylline may induce bronchodilation. Other systemic effects of theophylline include cardiac inotropy and chronotropy, central nervous system (CNS) stimulation, increased gastric acid production, relaxation of the gastroesophageal sphincter, diaphragmatic inotropy, and induction of a mild diuresis.

Aminophylline, the intravenous theophylline preparation complexed with ethylenediamine, is the most commonly used intravenous methylxanthine for the treatment of airway obstruction. Unfortunately, the numerous extrapulmonary effects, the complicated pharmacokinetics, and the narrow therapeutic index of aminophylline result in difficulty predicting dosing and serum levels. Table 5 summarizes physiologic factors and drug interactions that alter theophylline metabolism, and Table 6 reviews an adult dosing schedule for use of intravenous aminophylline therapy. The elimination half-life of theophylline in normal subjects varies widely from 3 to 10 hours. Bronchodilator effects of theophylline in asthmatics are proportional to the log of the plasma concentration over a range of 5 to 30 mg per liter. The optimal concentration is 10 to 20 mg per liter. To minimize adverse effects, physicians must individualize theophylline dosages and frequently obtain serum levels.

Table 4 Management Severe Bronchospasm

1. Initiate maximal beta-adrenergic therapy
   Inhaled beta-agonists administered by aerosol:
   Albuterol 2.5–5.0 mg diluted in 3 ml saline over 20 min
   Isoetharine mesylate, 5.0 mg diluted in 3 ml saline over 20 min
   Nebulized treatments should be administered every 20 min until there is no further improvement in bronchospasm as measured by PEFR or FEV_1, or adverse side effects occur.
   If no response after 2 nebulized treatments, then 0.15 ml of epinephrine (1:1000) may be given subcutaneously; dose may be repeated once if no objective improvement is observed within 10 min.

2. Initiate steroid therapy
   Unless patient's bronchospasm has resolved corticosteroids are begun within 1 hour of the patient's presentation to medical attention (methylprednisolone, 0.5–1.0 mg/kg every 6 hr).

3. If there is no improvement in 30–60 min of aggressive beta-adrenergic therapy, then aminophylline infusion is begun.

4. Persistent bronchospasm with worsening of the patient's condition as evidenced by severely diminished PEFR or FEV_1 measurements or hypercapnia, and severe hypoxemia on arterial blood gas determinations necessitates intubation and ventilatory support.

Table 5 Physiologic Factors and Drug Interactions Altering Theophylline Metabolism

Increases Serum Levels	Decreases Serum Levels
Advanced age	Carbamazepine
Obesity	Dilantin
Erythromycin	Rifampin
Cimetidine	Cigarette smoking
Oral contraceptives	Phenobarbital
Propranolol	
Allopurinol	
Hepatic disease/congestion	
Congestive heart disease	

Although theophylline has been proved effective in the management of chronic airway obstruction, theophylline in the management of acute bronchospasm is less well established. Comparison of patients receiving high-dose aerosolized beta-agonists with patients receiving aminophylline alone or aerosolized beta-agonists and aminophylline together showed no additive benefit from aminophylline. Moreover, the addition of methylxanthines significantly increased symptoms of tremor, nausea, anxiety, and palpitations in patients receiving aminophylline. Some studies have demonstrated an additive effect of aminophylline when used in conjunction with aerosolized beta-agonist in the treatment of severe bronchospasm; other studies that used maximum doses of aerosolized beta-agonist have shown no additive benefits of theophylline. This suggests that aminophylline therapy should only be considered for acute bronchospasm if the patient does not respond to maximal doses of aerosolized beta-agonists or is intolerant of high-dose beta-agonists. Further studies are needed regarding theophylline's efficacy in preventing or shortening hospitalizations from exacerbations of acute airway obstruction. Until such studies are performed, aminophylline should be administered to patients who require hospitalization but not as first-line therapy (see Table 4).

Life-threatening adverse effects of theophylline include seizures, supraventricular and ventricular tachyarrhythmias, and hypokalemia. Less serious side effects of nausea, tremulousness, and headache are common. Although theophylline toxicity is dose-dependent and associated with serum levels above 50 μg per milliliter, seizures and ventricular arrhythmias can occur in patients with therapeutic levels especially if patients have preexisting CNS or cardiac diseases. Theophylline-induced seizures are life-threatening and require immediate discontinuation of the drug. Diazepam, phenytoin, and phenobarbital are recommended for treating theophylline-induced seizures. Lidocaine is the treatment of choice for theophylline-induced ventricular arrhythmias.

Corticosteroids

Because airway luminal narrowing is the result of both bronchial smooth muscle contraction and bronchial mucosal edema with inflammation, corticosteroid administration is essential in the management of severe airway obstruction. Often patients with airflow limitation can obtain transient improvement in bronchospasm after treatment with aerosolized bronchodilators. However, the inflammatory agents that mediate bronchoconstriction during the late-phase reaction induced by allergens are unresponsive to aminophylline or aerosolized beta-agonists. By contrast, corticosteroids are effective in decreasing this late-phase response. Although the onset of bronchodilation induced by corticosteroids is reported to occur 3 to 6 hours after initial administration (with peak effects occurring 12 to 24 hours later), alterations in beta-adrenergic receptor function may occur more quickly. The precise mechanism of corticosteroid-induced bronchodilation is not known. Corticosteroids, however, have been shown to increase beta-adrenergic receptors on lymphocytes; decrease circulating eosinophils, basophils, and neutrophils; reduce IgE synthesis; inhibit eicosanoate release and secretion of mucus; and induce vasoconstriction.

Although controversy exists regarding maximal dose, frequency, and mode of administration, effects of corticosteroids on airway function appear to be dose-dependent. Maximal improvements in airflow in patients with severe airway obstruction can be obtained with use of intravenous high-dose, methylprednisolone therapy (60 mg every 6 hours). Since methylprednisolone is the active metabolite of prednisone and has a longer half-life than hydrocortisone, there may be a theoretical advantage in using this preparation. Adverse effects from short courses of corticosteroids are minimal. Hyperkalemia, hyperglycemia, and altered mental status can occur in patients treated with short courses of high-dose steroid therapy (prednisone, 1 to 2 mg per kg) but resolve after discontinuation of these agents. Exacerbations in airway obstruction that result from rapid tapering of corticosteroid therapy are likely the major complication of corticosteroid treatment. Few studies have prospectively studied the

Table 6 Theophylline Dosing* in Adults with Acute Bronchospasm

Dosing	Intravenous aminophylline
Loading Dose†	
History of theophylline use:	
None	6 mg/kg over 20 min
Oral Theophylline Use	0–3 mg/kg over 20 min
Maintenance Dose‡	
Patient category	
Nonsmoker	0.5 mg/kg/hr
Smoker	0.3 mg/kg/hr
Critically ill	0.5 mg/kg/hr
Congestive heart failure	0.2 mg/kg/hr
Severe pneumonia	0.2 mg/kg/hr

*Dosing expressed in aminophylline equivalents (theophylline dose = 0.8 × aminophylline dose).
†If possible, serum theophylline levels should be obtained prior to administration. Initial target serum concentration for theophylline is 10 μg/ml.
‡Theophylline levels should be measured 12–24 hr after loading and more frequently if symptoms or signs of theophylline toxicity are evident.

optimal tapering regimen for corticosteroid use. Most physicians continue intravenous corticosteroids until there is objective evidence of airflow improvement and decrease the dosing frequency of methylprednisolone over 36 hours. The patient is then maintained on prednisone (0.5 to 1 mg per kg daily).

Anticholinergic Agents

Ipratropium bromide, a synthetic congener of atropine without systemic side effects, is the only anticholinergic agent approved for the treatment of acute bronchospasm. Other agents such as glycopyrrolate and atropine methionate are quaternary ammonium anticholinergic agents that have been extensively studied in Canada and Europe but are unavailable in the United States. Recent evidence suggests that the addition of a single 0.5-mg dose of nebulized ipratropium to an aerosolized beta-adrenergic agonist is more effective in the treatment of severe bronchospasm than either drug alone. As a single agent, ipratropium bromide is less effective than beta-adrenergic agents. At present, ipratropium is supplied in a metered-dose inhaler (36 μg every 6 hours). The lack of serious adverse effects in conjunction with the potential for augmenting beta-agonist–induced bronchodilation may suggest a role for ipratropium bromide in the treatment of severe, refractory bronchospasm. Although studies have demonstrated the efficacy of ipratropium bromide in the treatment of chronic obstructive lung disease caused by chronic bronchitis or emphysema, its routine use in acute bronchospastic airway obstruction needs further study. Given the adverse systemic side effects and short half-life of atropine in addition to the availability of more effective agents that reduce bronchospasm, atropine is not recommended in the treatment of severe bronchospasm.

Antibiotics and Hydration

There is well-established evidence that respiratory viruses induce exacerbations of acute bronchospasm. However, the role of bacterial infections in inducing exacerbations of asthma has not been well established. The routine use of antibiotics in the treatment of acute airway obstruction may not be indicated, and significant adverse effects from antibiotics can include severe hypersensitivity reactions and adverse drug interactions. Studies in children with acute exacerbations of severe asthma show no apparent clinical benefit from the routine use of antibiotics. Alternatively, the association between purulent sinusitis and asthma is well established. Since purulent sinusitis appears to exacerbate bronchospasm in susceptible patients, uncontrolled studies have suggested a beneficial role for antibiotic therapy in the treatment of purulent sinusitis with a resultant decrease in the severity in the patient's bronchospasm.

Parenteral fluids should be administered judiciously. The goal of replenishing increased respiratory and insensible losses is prudent. No studies have demonstrated the efficacy of aggressive fluid repletion in augmenting the expectoration of mucus. Studies in animal models suggest that overhydration had no effect on mucociliary clearance.

Table 7 Life-Threatening Complications of Mechanical Ventilation in Patients with Severe Airflow Obstruction

Hypotension
  Increased end-expiratory pressures (auto-PEEP)
  Tension Pneumothorax
  Drug-related (postintubation)

Alveolar Hypoventilation
  Severe respiratory acidosis
  Mild hypoxemia

Pulmonary Barotrauma
  Tension pneumothorax
  Pneumomediastinum
  Bronchopulmonary fistula development

Self-Extubation
  Oropharyngeal bleeding
  Loss of airway

Mechanical Ventilation

Only 2 percent of asthmatic patients who present to the hospital with dyspnea require intubation and mechanical ventilation. However, a mortality of 5 to 38 percent is reported in these patients, and a threefold increase in ventilator-related complications occurs in severely bronchospastic patients when compared with patients receiving mechanical ventilation for all other causes. For the critical care physician, patients with severe airflow limitation present particular challenges in management.

Indications for intubation of patients with severe airflow limitation include severe deterioration in mental status, progressive hypercapnia with evidence of respiratory muscle fatigue, and/or progressive metabolic acidosis despite maximal bronchodilator therapy. Table 7 reviews the most frequent complications of mechanical ventilation and their associated causes in patients with severe airflow obstruction.

The majority of severely bronchospastic patients who require intubation will need sedation and paralysis with intravenous diazepam (5 to 20 mg) and pancuronium (0.04 to 0.1 mg per kilogram) prior to orotracheal intubation. Since severely bronchospastic patients may have edematous nasal mucosa and chronic sinusitis, orotracheal intubation is preferred. To facilitate the clearance of thick secretions and to decrease airflow resistance, an endotracheal tube of the largest diameter possible should be placed.

Ventilator management of the severely bronchospastic patients requires prolonged expiratory times to minimize pulmonary hyperinflation and end-expiratory pressures that may result in hypotension. High inspiratory flow rates (80 to 100 L per minute) with relatively low tidal volumes (0.7 to 1.0 cc per kilogram) and reduced respiratory rates can decrease the likelihood of ventilator-related complications while increasing expiratory time necessary to decrease pulmonary hyperinflation. Unfortunately, the arterial Pco_2 will increase and may require administration of sodium bicarbonate to compensate for the respiratory acidosis. In order to avoid high peak pressures, which are associated with pulmonary barotrauma, patients require sedation and paralysis. The majority of severely asthmatic patients who are mechanically ventilated improve dramatically within 12 to 24 hours after intubation.

Severe Refractory Bronchospasm

It is the rare patient with severe refractory bronchospasm who does not improve despite maximal bronchodilator therapy, corticosteroids, and mechanical ventilation. In such patients, uncontrolled case-report studies have suggested the use of alternative modes of therapy.

General anesthesia (0.5 to 1.0 percent halothane or enflurane) has been effective in reducing life-threatening bronchospasm. This therapy requires an anesthesiologist and careful cardiac monitoring since these drugs are arrhythmogenic.

Bronchial lavage may improve severe airway obstruction by removal of bronchial mucus plugs. Patients who appear to benefit from this therapy have evidence of atelectasis and hyperinflation on chest films. Bronchial lavage by bronchoscopy may markedly increase peak airway pressures and may lead to significant pulmonary barotrauma.

Extracorporeal membrane oxygenation may be the only alternative for the severely bronchospastic patients refractory to all other modes of therapy. In two reports, this treatment appears to have been successful. Physicians must recognize that these alternative modes of treatment should not supersede maximal conventional therapies of beta-adrenergic agonists, aminophylline, corticosteroids, and mechanical ventilation (see Table 4).

SUGGESTED READING

Daroli R, Parret C. Mechanical controlled hypoventilation in status asthmaticus. Am Rev Respir Dis 1984; 129:385-387.
Fanta CH, Rossing TH, McFadden FR. Treatment of acute asthma: is combination therapy with sympathomimetics and methyl xanthines indicated? Am J Med 1986; 80:5-10.
Jenne JW, Murphy S. Drug therapy for asthma. In: Lenfant C, ed. Drug therapy for asthma: research and clinical practice. Vol. 31. New York: Marcel Dekker, 1987.
Nelson HS. Adrenergic therapy of bronchial asthma. J Allergy Clin Immunol 1986; 77:771-790.
Scoggins CH. Acute life threatening asthma. In: Lenfant C, ed. Drug therapy for asthma: research and clinical practice. Vol. 31. New York: Marcel Dekker 1987.
Scoggins CH, Sahn SA, Petty TL. Status asthmaticus, a nine-year experience. JAMA 1977; 238:1158-1162.
Siegel D, Sheppard D, Gelb A, Weinberg PF. Aminophylline increases the toxicity but not the efficacy of inhaled beta-adrenergic agonists in the treatment of acute exacerbations of asthma. Am Rev Respir Dis 1985; 132:283-286.

SYNDROMES CAUSED BY ASPIRATION OF STOMACH CONTENTS

PETER SZIDON, M.D.

The aspiration of gastric contents causes acute hypoxemic respiratory insufficiency. The predominant pattern of pathological response to injury and its duration depend on the nature and volume of the material aspirated. When the aspirate is acidic (with a pH less than 2.5), or when it is hypertonic (such as enteral feeding solutions), or toxic (as with the aspiration of regurgitated hydrocarbons ingested accidentally), the inflammatory response will be severe and prolonged. Nonparticulate fluids having a pH approaching 7 can produce severe respiratory insufficiency, provided that sufficient volume is aspirated, but the duration of the syndrome will be shorter. Large food particles cause impaction of the airways, localized inflammatory exudate, and infection but do not elicit diffuse damage.

By contrast, aspirate containing very small, nonobstructing food particles will behave as hypertonic solution.

The pulmonary consequences of aspiration of gastric contents are sometimes designated as "aspiration pneumonia." This term is more appropriate for the pulmonary infections resulting from the aspiration of oropharyngeal bacterial pathogens, which is discussed elsewhere in this text.

MANAGEMENT

Prevention

The aspiration of gastric contents can be avoided in many cases. Thus prevention is the most effective therapy. It is important to recognize groups of patients with predisposing factors in order to be able to adopt measures that may anticipate or reduce their risk (Table 1).

Patients requiring emergency surgery, especially if they are obese, and pregnant patients undergoing cesarean section are perhaps among those with the highest risk. The effects of pregnancy on gastric emptying and esophageal sphincter tone can continue for some time after delivery. Patients who have early postpartum procedures under anesthesia (e.g., tubal ligation) may still be predisposed.

Table 1 Predisposing Factors to Aspiration of Gastric Contents

Depressed Level of Consciousness
(e.g., seizures, alcoholic intoxication, general anesthesia)

Laryngeal Incompetence
   Neurologic disorders (e.g., myasthenia gravis, Guillain Barré)
   Trauma to the larynx
   Oropharyngeal surgery

Disorders of the Digestive Tract
   Esophageal (e.g., achalasia, scleroderma)
   Gastric (e.g., outlet obstruction, nasogastric feeding, effects of pregnancy)
   Intestinal (e.g., ileus)

We prefer to reduce the risk of aspiration in these patients by selecting regional rather than general anesthesia, but no controlled studies are available to support or refute this choice. When regional anesthesia is not appropriate we recommend, whenever possible, endotracheal intubation with the patient awake before the induction of general anesthesia. We recommend rapid-sequence induction coupled with the Sellick maneuver when awake intubation is impractical. The Sellick maneuver consists of applying pressure with the thumb and index fingers over the cricoid cartilage during endotracheal intubation and maintaining the pressure until the endotracheal cuff is inflated. We do not recommend evacuation of the stomach contents prior to intubation by either the use of induced emesis or gastric tubes. Aspiration can result from these maneuvers and, by and large, they are not well tolerated by patients who are about to have emergency surgery. Lavage of the stomach after ingestion of hydrocarbons should be postponed until a cuffed endotracheal tube is in place. The use of esophageal balloon devices to block reflux is strongly discouraged.

Gastric acidity can be reduced acutely by the ingestion of soluble antacids. We prefer to use either 30 ml of a solution of sodium citrate (0.3 mol per L) or two tablets of Alka-Seltzer dissolved in half a glass of water. It is important to avoid using particulate antacids. Experimental evidence has shown that aspiration of antacid particles causes severe and sustained lung damage. When consideration for surgery is not immediate we use H_2-receptor antagonists (cimetidine or ranitidine) for their ability to reduce the volume and acidity of gastric fluid. The recommended parenteral dose for cimetidine is 300 mg intramuscularly and that of ranitidine, 50 mg. However, H_2-receptor antagonists will not reduce the acidity of gastric fluid that has already been secreted. The rationale for using oral antacids is superior when acute reductions in gastric acidity are desired. A number of significant drug interactions can be encountered between the short-term use of H_2-receptor antagonists and drugs commonly used in critical care settings, the most important being warfarin, phenytoin, lidocaine, and theophylline. The use of antacids and H_2-receptor antagonists can promote, in a relatively short time, the colonization of gastric and oropharyngeal secretions with enteric flora, thereby increasing the risk of nosocomial pneumonia. At present there is insufficient data on the competing risks of acute gastrointestinal bleeding and nosocomial pneumonia to allow the expression of a preference on the routine use of these agents, based on scientific evidence.

Nasogastric tubes used for decompression of the stomach or for feeding are another common factor predisposing to aspiration. Nasogastric tubes interfere with the function of the gastroesophageal sphincter and promote bacterial colonization of the stomach. We prefer percutaneous transpyloric feeding tubes, which deliver solutions beyond the duodenum to minimize the risk of aspiration of feeding solutions. However, since the stomach continues to secrete gastric juice, the risk of aspiration of gastric contents is not eliminated.

Endotracheal or tracheostomy tubes are sometimes used prophylactically in patients who are considered to be risks for chronic, recurrent aspiration. The use of these devices is associated with hypersecretion of mucus, impaired mucociliary clearance, decreased effectiveness of cough, and colonization of the trachea with oropharyngeal flora. The incidence of nosocomial pneumonia is increased several times in patients with endotracheal tubes, and the evidence for aspiration of oropharyngeal secretions is greater in these patients than in comparable ones without tubes. We do not recommend this type of prophylaxis.

Selected patients, mostly those with neurologic disorders, can have disabling pharyngeal or laryngeal dysfunction but are otherwise capable of sustaining a good quality of life. These patients can be considered as candidates for surgical procedures designed to eliminate the continuous entry of aspirated material into the larynx and trachea.

Initial Approach

Our initial concerns in the management of patients who aspirate gastric contents include an attempt to determine, whenever possible, the characteristics of the aspirate—i.e., to estimate its volume, acidity, and the extent to which it contains particles of food. It is also important to establish the baseline appearance of the chest film and the composition of arterial blood gases. The most significant initial goals are to protect the airway, to administer oxygen and to monitor subsequent oxygenation using pulse oximeters or, if these are not available, by repeating arterial blood gas samples.

It is estimated that approximately half of the episodes of aspiration occurring in hospitalized patients are witnessed. The pH of the remaining regurgitate should be determined promptly. If the pH of the fluid is less than 2.5, the inflammatory response is certain to be severe and protracted even if the volume aspirated is not large. However, the finding of a pH over 2.5 is not an assurance that the recovery will be rapid.

Intubation and Suctioning

We recommend intubation of the trachea using high-volume, low-pressure cuffed tubes for suctioning regurgitate and preventing recurrence of acute aspiration in patients who have decreased level of consciousness (e.g., in alcoholic intoxication) or in those who have dysfunction of pharyngeal motility and are at risk of repeated acute episodes of aspiration (e.g., those with Guillain Barré). We do not recommend endotracheal intubation for conscious patients who are able to cough and cooperate with care and whose oxygenation can be provided with an FIO_2 of less than 0.50. Nasotracheal suctioning is usually sufficient to establish airway patency in many of these patients. However, suctioning should not be expected to play a major role in therapy. Acidic or hypertonic aspirates are dispersed very rapidly and cause immediate tissue damage. We do not recommend lavage of the airways with saline or with alkaline solutions, as this practice is probably harmful.

Bronchoscopy

We consider bronchoscopy when there is evidence of aspiration of particulate matter. Clinically, these patients may present initially with choking, dysphonia, stridor, or wheezing; inspection of the regurgitate may reveal fragments of food. Radiographically there may be atelectasis. However, localized hyperinflation can be present if a check-valve phenomenon leads to air trapping. Films of expiration vs. inspiration may reveal a shift of the mediastinum. Fiberoptic bronchoscopy can be a hazardous procedure in patients who develop severe respiratory failure following gastric aspiration. We believe that the risk is considerably lessened if the procedure is performed through an endotracheal tube, with ventilatory support, while monitoring airway opening pressure (for barotrauma) and arterial oxygenation with a pulse oximeter. Fiberoptic bronchoscopy is an excellent method for identifying and locating the presence of impaction in the tracheobronchial tree. However, its ability to remove particles is limited to those that are small. Rigid bronchoscopy should be used to remove large particulate matter.

Ventilatory Support

Ventilatory support—using endotracheal intubation, positive pressure ventilation, and positive end-expiratory pressure (PEEP)—is indicated when the arterial PO_2 cannot be maintained above 60 mm Hg without using an FIO_2 greater than 0.50. Many authorities favor the use of continuous positive airway pressure (CPAP) through a tightly fitting mask in selected patients who are alert and can cooperate. This maneuver often can reduce inspired oxygen requirements. We do not advocate this approach for two reasons: (1) CPAP masks can induce gastric distention in some patients and thereby increase their risk of vomiting; (2) patients can aspirate more than once. Vomiting into a tight-fitting mask can result in catastrophic consequences. Instead of using CPAP masks we prefer early intubation and mechanical ventilatory support when faced with progressively worsening hypoxemia or increasing oxygen requirements.

The rapidly forming and sometimes extensive pulmonary edema associated with aspiration of acid or hypertonic gastric contents can lead to acute depletion of intravascular volume. With the application of PEEP or CPAP there may be significant reductions in cardiac output resulting from decreases in preload. If mixed venous oxygen tension decreases, there can be marked worsening of hypoxemia. We recommend using fluid replacement with crystalloid solutions. Monitoring of fluid status can be accomplished satisfactorily by following urinary output and vital signs. Pulmonary artery catheters should not be used routinely. Some authors recommend them in selected patients who have concurrent primary cardiovascular or fluid balance disorders. We have difficulties with the interpretation of wedge pressure data and have not used them frequently.

Bronchodilators and Corticosteroids

Bronchoconstriction and wheezing are commonly seen in patients with aspiration of gastric contents. We recommend the routine use of beta-agonist aerosols delivered using hand-held nebulizers or into the inspiratory line of respirators: metaproterenol sulfate 5 percent solution, 0.3 ml diluted in 2.5 ml of saline every 4 hours. Several experimental studies have shown that the use of corticosteroids is associated with no benefit with respect to outcome or to attenuation of severity, in the various aspiration syndromes. Their routine use is not recommended. The use of steroids may be harmful by interfering with lung healing or by predisposing to infection. When patients with asthma sustain aspiration of gastric contents they tend to sustain major bronchoconstrictive, often fatal responses. The use of steroids is appropriate in this setting, the suggested dose being 1 mg of methylprednisolone per kilogram body weight per day, intravenously, in four divided doses.

Antibiotics

We do not recommend the prophylactic use of antibiotics in patients who aspirate gastric contents. However, we recognize that it is often very difficult to identify the onset of infection since excess sputum, fever, elevation of the white count, or pulmonary infiltrates are all expected to occur nonspecifically in sterile, chemical lung damage. Approximately 25 to 50 percent of patients with acid aspiration develop a bacterial pulmonary infection within 1 week of the aspiration episode. Patients who get infections tend to have a higher mortality and worse oxygenation than those who do not get this complication. Radiographic extension of lung infiltrates after the second day of illness, a change in character of the sputum, and new onset of fever can be used as clinical clues for the beginning of infection. The predominant organisms are aerobic bacteria such as gram-negative enteric bacilli, *Pseudomonas* and

Staphylococcus species. Antibiotic coverage should be active against *Pseudomonas* and *Staphylococcus aureus*. Initial broad-spectrum coverage for nosocomial pneumonias depends, to some extent, on patterns of institutional bacterial flora. At our institution we select a third-generation cephalosporin, e.g., ceftazidime and vancomycin. In other institutional settings an antipseudomonas aminoglycoside, imipenem or ciprofloxacin may be appropriate alternatives. We use cultures of protected brushings obtained by bronchoscopy to refine the initial antibiotic coverage. This is especially so when we suspect that food particles have been aspirated, resulting in obstructive pneumonia; in this case, the pathogenic bacteria can be derived from oropharyngeal flora and may be more appropriately treated with clindamycin.

SUGGESTED READING

Bynum LJ, Pierce AK. Pulmonary aspiration of gastric contents. Am Rev Respir Dis 1976; 114:1129–1136.
Gibbs CP, Modell JH. Aspiration pneumonitis. In: Miller RD, ed. Anesthesia 2nd ed. New York: Churchill Livingstone, 1986.
Wynne JW, Modell JH. Respiratory aspiration of stomach contents. Ann Intern Med 1977; 87:466–474.

ALVEOLAR HYPOVENTILATION AND RESPIRATORY MUSCLE FATIGUE

BENNETT P. DeBOISBLANC, M.D.
WARREN R. SUMMER, M.D.

Ventilatory failure is observed in up to 30 percent of critically ill patients. Alveolar hypoventilation may result from either excessive ventilatory loads or ineffective operation of the ventilatory pump. Since proper function of the ventilatory pump requires the integrated activity of neural, muscular, and skeletal systems, dysfunction at any level can precipitate alveolar hypoventilation. In critically ill patients, fatigue of the respiratory muscles, particularly the diaphragm, is a common cause of ventilatory failure.

INITIAL APPROACH

Alveolar hypoventilation may occur acutely or chronically and may be observed in patients with normal or abnormal lungs. The first step in the approach to a patient with hypercapnia is to evaluate the entire respiratory system (Table 1). Alveolar hypoventilation may result from failure at any level; often several levels are impaired.

Initially we try to decide if hypoventilation is due to an abnormality of the lungs. Regardless of the functional integrity of the musculoskeletal parts of the ventilatory pump, excessive ventilatory loads due to lung disease or to increased carbon dioxide production can precipitate or aggravate alveolar hypoventilation (Table 2). Thus the initial therapeutic goal is to identify and treat existing airflow obstruction, pneumonia, pulmonary edema, sepsis, shock, hyperthermia, and hypoxemia to reduce the load on the ventilatory pump.

TREATMENT

Alveolar Hypoventilation Associated with Depressed Ventilatory Drive

Characteristically patients with inadequate central respiratory drive have hypercapnia and hypoxemia without significant dyspnea or respiratory distress. Respiratory excursions are usually infrequent and shallow, and the $P(A-a)O_2$ is usually preserved. Rapid and shallow respirations, use of accessory muscles, or thoracoabdominal dyssychrony should suggest an alternative diagnosis, such as neuromuscular disease or respiratory muscle fatigue. The etiologies of central hypoventilation are varied. Patients with blunted respiratory drives may have established neurologic disease—e.g., encephalitis or stroke, sedative-

Table 1 Malfunction of Any Component of the Respiratory System May Lead to Alveolar Hypoventilation

Anatomic Component	Insults That May Precipitate Alveolar Hypoventilation
Chemoreceptors	Trauma, carotid surgery
Upper respiratory motor neurons	Stroke, encephalitis, drug overdose, hypothyroidism, obesity
Spinal cord	Trauma, tumors
Peripheral motor neurons	Polio, ALS, Guillain-Barré, phrenic nerve injury
Neuromuscular junction	Aminoglycoside toxicity, myasthenia gravis
Muscle	Malnutrition, electrolyte disturbances, fatigue, deconditioning
Chest wall	Obesity, kyphoscoliosis, flail
Pleura	Pneumothorax, large effusions
Lung parenchyma	Severe fibrosis, pulmonary edema, pneumonia, hemorrhage
Airways	Asthma, COPD, tracheal stenosis

Table 2 Physiologic Determinants of Ventilatory Compensation

Ventilatory Load	Ventilatory Drive
Airways resistance	Reduced with
Bronchospasm	Depressed mental status
Airway edema and secretions	Chronic loading
Upper airway obstruction	Sleep deprivation
Lung compliance	Metabolic alkalosis
Intrinsic PEEP	Sedative drugs
Interstitial edema and inflammation	High PaO_2
Atelectasis	Muscle Function
Chest wall compliance	Integrity of chest wall and pleural space
Kyphoscoliosis	Flail
Massive ascites	Pneumothorax
Ileus or abdominal surgery	Neuromuscular transmission
Obesity	Spinal cord
Chest wall pain	Motor neuron
Pregnancy	Neuromuscular junction
Minute ventilation requirement	Muscle power
Dead space	Mass: age, sex, nutrition
Metabolic acidosis	Coordination
Anemia	Fiber length (hyperinflation)
Hypermetabolism: fever, infection, trauma, burns, carbohydrate load	Nutrient supply
	Extracellular electrolyte milieu
	Muscle endurance
	Duty cycle (T_I/T_{TOT})
	Load ($P_{pleural}/P_{pleural}$ max)
	Blood flow
	Arterial O_2 content

hypnotic drug overdosage, hypothyroidism, extreme obesity, primary metabolic alkalosis, disease of the peripheral chemoreceptors, or idiopathic central hypoventilation.

The initial treatment of acute or severe alveolar hypoventilation in patients with depressed ventilatory drive is mechanical ventilation. Support usually requires the insertion of an endotracheal tube, although in rare cases assisted ventilation by face mask or negative pressure ventilation is possible if the patient is awake and alert. Because many patients with central hypoventilation have normal lungs, required minute ventilations and developed pressures on the ventilator are frequently low. Initial tidal volumes are set at 5 to 10 ml per kilogram, based on ideal body weight, and respiratory frequencies are set at 8 to 10 breaths per minute in the assist-control mode. Often respiratory alkalosis develops even with these low minute ventilations. In these patients, when the tidal volume remains fixed, alveolar ventilation is constant. Because carbon dioxide partial pressure (PCO_2) is inversely proportional to alveolar ventilation under steady-state metabolic conditions, one can estimate the required change in respiratory rate (RR) to correct overventilation by the following equation:

$$\text{desired RR} = \text{present RR} \times (\text{present } PaCO_2/\text{desired } PaCO_2).$$

Because this is only an estimation, results should be verified by an arterial blood gas in 20 to 30 minutes. Such formulas are less helpful in patients with large ventilation-perfusion imbalance and dynamic airways or parenchymal lung disease.

Three methods of *long-term* artificial ventilation are used in patients with blunted respiratory drive: negative-pressure ventilation, positive-pressure ventilation, and phrenic nerve pacing.

Negative-pressure Ventilation. Negative-pressure ventilation has found utility primarily as a nocturnal assist device in stable patients with central alveolar hypoventilation or chronic neuromuscular disease and reasonably good lung function. Patients who require continuous mechanical ventilation are better treated with volume-cycled positive-pressure ventilator. Although alveolar ventilation normally decreases during sleep, this response may be exaggerated in primary hypoventilators. A vicious circle is set up in which nocturnal hypoventilation leads to microatelectasis; pulmonary hypertension; and sodium, water and bicarbonate retention, further impairing lung function and blunting respiratory drive. Nocturnal-assisted ventilation can break this cycle. The hemodynamic and ventilatory improvement can be carried over to a lower mean daytime $PaCO_2$, improved oxygenation, and reversal of existing polycythemia and cor pulmonale.

Candidates for nocturnal negative-pressure ventilation are generally those with moderate to severe daytime hypercapnia and hypoxemia. These patients have the most pronounced sleep-associated hypoventilation. It is recommended that patients with central hypoventilation undergo a modified sleep study prior to and during the first night of negative-pressure ventilation. This screening sleep study should include at least inductance plethysmography and oximetry. Patients with untreated obstructive sleep apnea are generally excluded from negative-pressure ventilation, since occlusive apneas may be aggravated by this therapy.

If frequent severe arterial desaturations occur with negative-pressure ventilation, the addition of nasal continuous positive airway pressure (CPAP) or tracheostomy is often helpful. Institution of negative-pressure ventilation is an empiric exercise. The level of negative pressure and the respiratory rate are adjusted to maintain arterial blood gases or oximetry in an acceptable range. Noninvasive studies such as oximetry, capnometry, and inductance plethysmography can be used to monitor respiratory support. Negative-pressure ventilators can be used with a metal or plastic tank, a cuirass, or an airtight suit, depending upon setting, patient comfort, and monitoring needs.

Positive-Pressure Ventilation. Positive-pressure ventilation may be delivered through a tracheostomy, an endotracheal tube, a face mask, or a nasal mask. Ventilation by face or nasal mask has been satisfactory in patients needing only periodic assisted ventilation, usually during sleep. The obvious advantage to mask ventilation is that an endotracheal or tracheostomy tube is not required. The primary complications of face or nasal mask ventilation are patient discomfort, aerophagia with abdominal bloating and vomiting, and inadequate alveolar ventilation. Nasal positive-pressure ventilation (NPPV) produces fewer of these side effects than does mask ventilation and may be tolerated for longer periods of time. Ventilation can be started using the assist-control mode. Adequacy of ventilation is assessed by blood gases, capnometry, and oximetry. A face or nasal mask should not be used for patients who require more than 15 cm H_2O of positive pressure.

The obesity-hypoventilation syndrome (OHS) usually occurs in massively obese individuals. Relatively small changes in weight can dramatically improve alveolar ventilation in these patients. Caloric intakes 500 kcal below predicted requirements (Harris-Benedict equation) will usually provide a weekly weight loss of approximately 0.5 kg. In massively obese individuals, this rate of weight loss may be too slow, requiring restriction of calories to 1,000 kcal below requirements. Fluid, protein, and electrolyte requirements must be supplemented during such severe caloric restriction.

Obese patients with persistent hypercapnia often have evidence of cor pulmonale. Treatment of right-sided cardiac failure can improve ventilation, oxygenation, and respiratory muscle blood flow. Supplemental oxygen is the most important drug in treating cor pulmonale, although the patient with OHS may develop severe CO_2 narcosis with minor elevations in FIO_2. Oxygen induces a spontaneous diuresis by lowering pulmonary vascular resistance, which increases cardiac output and renal blood flow. Oxygen administration has been demonstrated to enhance CO_2 responsiveness in chronically hypoxemic hypoventilators. Oxygen therapy usually reverses secondary polycythemia, if present, which obviates the need for repeated phlebotomies. In the acute setting, phlebotomy to reduce the hematocrit below 55 percent can dramatically lower pulmonary vascular resistance and improve cardiac output. Therapy with thiazide or loop diuretics is reserved for patients who are unresponsive to oxygen or who have marked edema. Cardiac glycosides are useful only in patients with concomitant left ventricular failure. Obstructive sleep apnea is exceedingly common in patients with OHS. Occasionally a nasopharyngeal airway will correct the occlusive apneas, but sinusitis and patient intolerance are common complications of this treatment. Nasal CPAP may be effective in improving hypoxemia but in our experience rarely obviates the need for intubation. NPPV is usually ineffective acutely in the obese patient with obstructive sleep apnea. Tracheostomy is curative for obstructive sleep apnea but is reserved for patients with life-threatening arrhythmias or severe cor pulmonale who cannot be maintained on nasal CPAP. Uvulopalatopharyngoplasty (UPPP) improves the apnea index in only 50 percent of patients thus treated. UPPP is therefore reserved for patients with severe upper airway narrowing and as an adjuvant to nasal CPAP.

The pharmacotherapy of central alveolar hypoventilation or OHS has been disappointing but, because other therapies are often invasive, a drug trial is usually attempted. Medroxyprogesterone acetate, a progestational agent, is occasionally effective in increasing respiratory drive in obese men and postmenopausal women without significant obstructive sleep apnea. We usually begin with a dose of 40 mg three times per day. Responders usually demonstrate improved alveolar ventilation within 2 to 4 weeks. The ability of a patient to hyperventilate voluntarily and to lower the $PaCO_2$ is predictive of a beneficial response to medroxyprogesterone. Acetazolamide, a carbonic anhydrase inhibitor, is indicated in the treatment of significant metabolic alkalosis complicating or causing alveolar hypoventilation. Its role in OHS is questionable and its side effects, principally paresthesias, are common. Acetazolamide induces a mild metabolic acidosis, which functions to stimulate ventilation. The usual starting dose is 250 mg per day; the dose may then be titrated until effective. Acetazolamide is not indicated as a treatment for pure respiratory acidosis or for metabolic alkalosis secondary to hypokalemia. Nonsedating tricyclic antidepressants, analeptics, and narcotic antagonists are only anecdotally effective for treating patients with depressed respiratory drive, OHS, or obstructive sleep apnea and are not recommended. Theophylline is a weak respiratory stimulant, but it has not proved to be effective in management of primary alveolar hypoventilation in the adult. Because of its potential toxicity it should be reserved for patients with coexisting reversible airways obstruction. Hypothyroidism must be considered in all patients with blunted respiratory drive. There is currently no role for the use of thyroxine in the treatment of euthyroid patients with central alveolar ventilation.

Phrenic Nerve Pacing. Electrophrenic pacing has been used to support ventilation on a permanent basis in two patient populations: those with primary alveolar hypoventilation and those with high cervical cord transections. Phrenic nerve pacing should not be employed in patients with abnormal lungs as diaphragmatic fatigue and phrenic nerve fibrosis occur if high stimulation frequencies are required. For this reason patients with alveolar hypoventilation due to chronic lung disease are not candidates for electrophrenic pacing. Morbidly obese patients, patients with kyphoscoliosis, and those with phrenic nerve or neuromuscular junction disease also do not benefit. Patients adequately ventilated by electrophrenic pacing often require alternative modes of ventilation if the work of breathing is increased owing to intercurrent illness. Because the pacing electrodes are usually applied to the phrenic nerves in the chest through bilateral thoracotomies to insure that all phrenic nerve roots are being paced, this further limits the applicability of electrophrenic pacing to patients who can tolerate the surgery.

Alveolar Hypoventilation Due to Neuromuscular Disease or Kyphoscoliosis

Many neuromuscular diseases may precipitate alveolar hypoventilation. Among the most notable are spinal cord injury, poliomyelitis, amyotrophic lateral sclerosis (ALS), Guillain-Barré syndrome, myasthenia gravis, and phrenic nerve injury. Alveolar hypoventilation is usually a late observation in patients with progressive neuromuscular disease such as Guillain-Barré syndrome, although early, unexpected decompensation can occur. Use of the accessory muscles or dyspnea aggravated by the supine position suggests that the respiratory muscles are affected. Evidence of decreased inspiratory muscle forces often precedes the onset of ventilatory failure and permits the institution of mechanical ventilation in a timely fashion prior to sudden respiratory arrest. Maximum static inspiratory pressure at the mouth is the most practical indicator of respiratory muscle involvement. This pressure may be reduced to as low as 50 percent of baseline before the vital capacity begins to fall. Although the vital capacity and the maximum static inspiratory pressure at the mouth are effort-dependent and therefore lack specificity, both are useful in following the progression of respiratory muscle involvement.

Newly diagnosed neuromuscular patients should undergo serial bedside spirometry and static mouth pressures at least daily. Maximum static inspiratory pressures of less than -20 cm H_2O and vital capacities of less than 40 percent of predicted value suggest impending need for mechanical ventilation. It is important to note, however, that intercurrent systemic or respiratory illness may suddenly precipitate ventilatory failure when muscle forces exceed this level. A rapidly falling vital capacity and inspiratory force are indications for earlier intubation than would normally be the case, although the ultimate decision to intubate depends on close observation and clinical judgment. Once the $PaCO_2$ begins to rise, respiratory arrest is imminent. There is no proven value in "exercising" the respiratory muscles of patients with motor neuron or neuromuscular disease in an attempt to maintain muscle strength. This practice will actually aggravate muscle failure in myasthenia gravis. Intubation and assist-control mode of ventilation are therefore preferable once respiratory failure occurs. Early institution of negative-pressure ventilation or NPPV may noninvasively provide ventilatory support and reduce inspiratory muscle energy expenditure. Prevention of respiratory muscle fatigue by this method may improve patient comfort and delay or obviate the need for mechanical ventilation in borderline cases. Patients with more fulminant disease will require translaryngeal intubation or tracheostomy. Mechanical ventilation should be continued unless the disease is in remission and the muscle forces and vital capacity exceed 30 percent of the predicted values.

Intermittent positive-pressure breathing (IPPB) has been demonstrated to improve lung compliance in patients with hypoventilation whose vital capacities are reduced because of severe kyphoscoliosis or neuromuscular disease. Additional benefits noted have been improved alveolar ventilation and oxygenation. Because this therapy is well tolerated and has no common significant side effects, it should be routinely employed in these populations. Incentive spirometry and inspiratory muscle training may be of some benefit in kyphoscoliosis, but overzealous training may lead to fatigue of weak muscles as can occur in neuromuscular patients. Patients with kyphoscoliosis are among the most difficult to wean from assisted ventilation. Periodic sigh breaths, 1.5 times the normal tidal volume, may improve weaning in ventilator-dependent patients. Negative-pressure ventilation and NPPV have been used chronically.

Respiratory Muscle Dysfunction

Dysfunctional respiratory muscles may be deconditioned and therefore may benefit from training; they may be fatigued and therefore in need of rest; or they may be functionally impaired because of derangements of blood flow, disturbances of extracellular electrolytes, or malnutrition.

By definition a muscle that is fatigued will be functionally improved after a period of rest. This is in contrast to respiratory muscle dysfunction related to disuse atrophy, electrolyte disturbances, or malnutrition. In these conditions even rested muscles fail to generate adequate force. Often the pathophysiology of respiratory muscle dysfunction is multifactorial. Weak muscles are more prone to fatigue than are strong muscles, since weak muscles must work at a higher percentage of maximum workload (high tension-time index).

In critical illness inspiratory muscles (principally the diaphragm) perform most of the work of breathing and are therefore more prone to fatigue than expiratory muscles. In patients subjected to a fatiguing ventilatory load, the sequence of clinical events preceding alveolar hypoventilation is predictable. Rapid, shallow breathing occurs within the first few breaths. A tidal volume/respiratory rate ratio of less than 10 is usually indicative of an unsustainable ventilatory state. Rapid, shallow breathing is usually followed by progressively dyssynchronous thoracoabdominal movements. At this point the patient's muscular apparatus is unable to sustain the current load. Hypercapnia is a relatively late finding in these patients.

The treatment of choice for severe respiratory muscle fatigue associated with alveolar hypoventilation is rest by assisted ventilation. Both positive- and negative-pressure ventilation have a role in treating respiratory muscle fatigue. Unlike the case for central hypoventilation, most patients with acute respiratory muscle fatigue and alveolar hypoventilation have severe lung disease. Required minute ventilations and inflation pressures are much higher than for patients with normal lungs. This usually mandates endotracheal intubation and positive-pressure ventilation, but we have on numerous occasions reversed inspiratory muscle fatigue with the use of an iron lung. Clinical stabilization of the patients obviated the need for intubation. If negative-pressure ventilation is to be used in this fashion, it must be accomplished before CO_2 narcosis develops, as the risk of aspiration in the iron lung is high. NPPV may also be used in this fashion if overnight ventilation allows for significant improvement of fatigue.

Treatment of mild-to-moderate degrees of diaphragmatic fatigue in patients with chronic hypoventilation is less labile. Several clinical trials have demonstrated that in ambulatory patients with severe chronic obstructive pulmonary disease, inspiratory muscle strength and endurance are improved by rest periods. Because nocturnal negative-pressure ventilation by body wrap or suit is usually well tolerated in this population, it is being more frequently employed in the ambulatory setting. NPPV may also play a role in this group.

Recently several drugs have been demonstrated to improve inspiratory muscle function in critically ill patients with ventilatory failure complicated by diaphragmatic fatigue. Theophylline has been shown to increase transdiaphragmatic pressure in patients with chronic obstructive pulmonary disease and may also prevent or delay the onset of fatigue. The drug does not, however, seem to reverse existing fatigue. Because it is arrhythmogenic and has variable effects on inspiratory muscle fatigue, the use of theophylline should be restricted to patients with concomitant airflow obstruction. Therapeutic doses of digoxin have also been shown to increase transdiaphragmatic pressure development. Again, because of potential cardiac toxicity, digoxin should be used only in patients with coexisting left ventricular failure.

Because hypoxemia decreases diaphragmatic endurance time during loaded breathing, and because oxygen administration decreases minute ventilation requirements during exercise, oxygen administration should play a major role in the treatment of respiratory muscle fatigue.

True disuse atrophy of the diaphragm occurs rarely in the ICU, being confined primarily to patients with high spinal cord transections. When one considers that the majority of critically ill patients perform significant work of breathing even while mechanically ventilated, other mechanisms of respiratory muscle dysfunction must be operational. The majority of ventilated patients who fail to be weaned have a combination of excessive ventilatory demands and chronic respiratory muscle fatigue. Patients with catabolic illnesses lose diaphragmatic muscle mass in proportion to the loss of lean body weight. The resultant diaphragmatic weakness may be mistaken for deconditioning. Training such a patient is of little utility unless adequate calories and nitrogen are given to support positive nitrogen balance. Even if adequate nutrition is supplied, new protein may not be assimilated in the presence of ongoing sepsis, trauma, or burns. Enteral or parenteral nutritional support should be started soon after a critically ill patient is admitted to the ICU. Postponing treatment until laboratory evidence of malnutrition exists will likely prolong the period of required mechanical ventilation.

Several extracellular electrolytes are important in normal excitation-contraction coupling of respiratory muscles. During nutritional repletion special attention should be given to replenishing phosphate, calcium, magnesium, and potassium. Even modest depletion of phosphate may lead to inspiratory muscle weakness in critical illness.

Though seldom thought of as an electrolyte, hydrogen ion also may affect diaphragmatic function. Both metabolic and respiratory acidoses decrease diaphragmatic tension generation in animal models and humans. Correction of any underlying acid-base disturbance should be a high priority in a patient with respiratory muscle dysfunction, although the administration of bicarbonate has not been shown to improve patient outcome.

Finally, it has been demonstrated that endurance of the diaphragm in hypotensive patients is improved by restoring the blood pressure to normal. During periods of high work loads, blood flow through the maximally dilated phrenic vascular bed is proportional to mean aortic pressure. Spontaneously breathing patients who are hypotensive are at great risk of developing acute respiratory muscle fatigue. Respiratory arrest may occur suddenly in these individuals. Institution of mechanical ventilation is indicated as a specific therapy for refractory shock and as a preventive measure to avoid respiratory failure. Although administration of parenteral cardiac inotropes may improve respiratory muscle mechanics in shocked patients, these drugs should not be used to wean hemodynamically unstable patients. However, it seems reasonable that sympathomimetic drugs could be used to support ventilation in shocked patients until intubation can be accomplished.

SUGGESTED READING

Celli B. Respiratory muscle function. Clin Chest Med 1986; 7:567–584.
Grassino A. Determinants of respiratory muscle failure. Am Rev Respir Dis 1986; 134:1091–1093.
Luce JM. Respiratory complications of obesity. Chest 1980; 78:626–631.
Rochester DF, Esau SA. Critical illness, infection, and the respiratory muscles. Am Rev Respir Dis 1988; 138:258–259.

UPPER AIRWAY OBSTRUCTION

ROBERT S. LEBOVICS, M.D.

Few diseases are potentially as rapidly fatal or are as likely to lead to serious morbidity as mismanaged obstruction of the upper airway. Because time is critical in effecting proper therapy, recognition of the problem in its early phases is as important as its subsequent management. Irreversible cerebral damage classically occurs after 4 minutes of anoxia. The time period of desaturation of hemoglobin varies according to many factors—i.e., metabolic, ventilatory, respiratory, hemodynamic, as well as hematologic. The shortest time in which arterial oxygen saturation may decrease to near zero is as little as 2 minutes. For practical purposes, therefore, the clinician has 6 minutes from the onset of upper airway obstruction to irreversible brain damage. Occasionally, a few more minutes might be available; however, this is a luxury one should not rely upon.

ANATOMY OF THE UPPER AIRWAY

The upper airway begins in the nasal vestibule, proceeds through the nasal cavity and, certainly from a histologic point of view, includes the paranasal sinuses, middle ear, and mastoid. It continues inferiorly to the pharynx, where it joins the oral cavity, which is a second conduit to join the upper airway in a region called the oropharynx. The oropharynx begins at the level of the soft palate and continues distally, subsequently dividing at the level of the cricopharyngeal muscle, which acts as the introitus to the esophagus and continues down the alimentary tract. The larynx, which is the continuation of the upper airway, is a unique structure found in humans that is involved in deglutition, speech production, and protection of the airway. The subglottic space below the vocal cords is the narrowest portion of the upper airway and hence is the most frequent site of clinically significant obstructions. The upper airway continues down the trachea and ends at the bifurcation of the mainstem bronchi. The subsequent subdivisions down to the alveoli constitute the lower airways. From a clinical point of view, therefore, disease from the nasal vault and the oral cavity down to and including the carina can directly affect a patient's ability to breathe or a physician's ability to assist a patient's ventilation.

ETIOLOGY

The causes of airway obstruction can be acute or chronic; specific causes include infection, trauma, neoplasm, foreign body, and autoimmune and allergic disorders. Acute obstruction of the upper airway presents with a variety of signs and symptoms. Generally, the previously normal patient becomes agitated and begins to progress from a stage of restlessness to one of panic. Occasionally, the patient's ability to phonate is compromised, as in the case of a foreign body aspirated into the larynx. Patients will universally attempt to sit up and lean forward, open the jaw, protrude the tongue, and often will be unable to manage oral secretions. Inspiratory stridor is nearly universal. One must realize, however, that in order for stridor to be present at least some air must be moving through the obstructed airway. When symptoms do not resolve and the stridor disappears, one must assume the worst and be prepared immediately to secure the airway through either nasal intubation, insertion of a nasal airway, oral intubation, and occasionally emergent tracheotomy (cricothyrotomy being the preferred mode in most emergent settings).

Chronic obstruction presents more insidiously, with symptoms including shortness of breath, stridor, and vocal changes. The minute ventilation is a direct function of the amount of air that has been inspired and expired from the lungs per unit time. A given minute ventilation may comfortably support a patient at rest but not while exercised. This flow of air is contingent upon a patent airway and it should be stressed that airflow is a function of the fourth power of the radius. Basic calculus shows, therefore, that the airflow will decrease very rapidly over a given period of time once a critical airway size is reached at constant pressure. This leverage in terms of airway works for the patient by providing significant leeway at diameters greater than 4 mm. However, once the critical point is reached, insufficient ventilation will occur and exponentially continue to decrease as airway size is further compromised.

Infections

There are many pathogens that can cause laryngeal infections. The most common symptom, regardless of the etiology, is hoarseness or vocal changes. Dysphagia, odynophagia, and weight loss are symptoms that need to be detailed in a history. Actual laryngeal pathology is usually apparent on indirect (mirror) laryngoscopy, although cultures for organisms or biopsies may be required to render a correct diagnosis and effect proper therapy.

Epiglottitis. Epiglottitis is a subcategory of a more general disorder that is categorized as supraglottitis. This disease is primarily one of children from ages 4 to 10; adults, however, are certainly susceptible to infection. Acute epiglottitis is an infectious bacterial process that primarily involves the epiglottis. The aryepiglottic folds, the arytenoid cartilages, and the hypopharyngeal mucosa may be grossly swollen and inflamed. The causative bacterial agent is usually *Haemophilus influenzae*, type B, and bacteremia is frequently concomitant. The typical history is one of a healthy child who rapidly develops throat pain with subsequent odynophagia after an upper respiratory infection. The child often becomes restless quickly and develops a "hot potato voice." In order to satisfy air hunger, the child will often lean forward with mouth open, frequently drooling and gasping for air. A child afebrile

6 hours earlier now may have a temperature of 105°F with a significant leukocytosis. If any patient is near death at the time of presentation, attempts at physical manipulation and examination of the airway are contraindicated. If the patient is not in acute distress, a limited examination can be done in the emergency room or intensive care setting, but it should be done by a senior staff physician. With a stable patient, the safest way of confirming the diagnosis is a well-penetrated lateral neck film, which shows the classic features of an enlarged epiglottis.

Treatment of epiglottitis over recent years has evolved, with most hospitals initiating their own specific protocols. In general, pediatric epiglottitis is a surgical emergency to be treated with emergency laryngoscopy and intubation in the operating room. Special techniques for anesthetic induction and for handling the compromised airway are required by the surgeon. At the time of surgery, nasotracheal intubation is the preferred method for securing an airway. Orotracheal intubation and tracheotomy can be performed as the specific situation warrants; this will usually be decided by the operating surgeon and the anesthesiologist. The diagnosis is confirmed endoscopically with direct visualization of a cherry-red swollen epiglottis, which usually has white fibrinous material and pus overlying its mucosa. Direct cultures are not so useful in obtaining bacterial identification as are blood cultures taken at this time.

In an adult with acute epiglottitis, the clinical presentation is frequently more subdued. The patient will complain of dysphagia, odynophagia, and fever that has been progressing over 1 to 2 days. Stridor may not be a sign, although the patient may have some features of the "hot potato voice." Because the caliber of the airway is larger in the adult, intubation and tracheotomy may not be necessary. The diagnosis is confirmed with the same radiographic studies or with a carefully performed flexible fiberoptic examination through the nasopharynx. The adult patient must be admitted to an intensive care unit, where adequate clinical monitoring is available. After blood and sputum cultures are obtained, the patient is best started on a combination of ampicillin and chloramphenicol to avoid the problem of antibiotic-resistant organisms. Other third-generation cephalosporins may be considered after consultation with the infectious disease service. At all times it is necessary to have an emergency tracheotomy set-up available by the patient's bedside. For an adult patient, it is also advisable to keep an endotracheal intubation set-up at the bedside since there are some cases in which oral intubation may be accomplished by a skilled physician.

High humidity with increased oxygen saturation by face-tent is advisable for adult patients in an intensive care unit for whom management by observation has been chosen. Should the patient's condition deteriorate, he should be immediately taken to the operating room to secure the airway. The efficacy of steroids in the face of acute infection has been debated in the past and there has been no consensus on this issue. In both the child and the adult, rapid resolution of clinical findings and subjective symptomatology occurs. However, a child should not be extubated and an adult should not be removed from an intensive care setting unless there is endoscopic confirmation for resolution of the infectious disease process. It must be stressed that while an adult may be managed without endotracheal intubation in an intensive care setting, this is not a suitable approach for the treatment of acute epiglottitis in children. Because of their size, children must be taken to an operating room to have the airway secured early in the treatment process even though general anesthesia would be necessary.

Acute Laryngotracheobronchitis. Acute laryngotracheobronchitis (croup) is an acute infection of the lower air passages and is most commonly seen in young children up to 3 years of age. The most common pathogen is the parainfluenza virus. However, bacterial organisms such as *Staphylococcus aureus* and *Streptococcus* have been found. The pathophysiology of croup is primarily one of circumferential mucosal inflammation in the subglottic larynx and trachea. Because children have a much smaller anatomic airway, the potential for rapid and fatal complications should always be foremost in the clinician's mind. Usually the child will present with the symptomatology of an upper respiratory tract infection, including nasal discharge, cough, and coryza. Hoarseness may develop, and as inflammation of the mucosa proceeds inspiratory stridor may occur. As the disease progresses, use of the accessory muscles of respiration will produce retraction of the chest. Pallor and cyanosis are ominous signs and should lead the clinician to do an emergency endotracheal intubation. Restlessness, dehydration, and exhaustion as well as progressive agitation and tachycardia may be signs of advanced croup. Blood gas analysis may reveal hypercarbia in such cases. Anteroposterior neck films often show a classic "steeple sign" in the subglottic larynx that is highly suggestive of the diagnosis. Treatment of laryngotracheobronchitis often requires hospitalization and close observation. Ultrasonic humidification and racemic epinephrine should be given in a pediatric intensive care setting. Hydration of the patient is necessary. Although the efficacy of steroids has been debated, they are more effective against croup than against epiglottitis.

Tuberculous Laryngitis. Tuberculous laryngitis is almost associated with active pulmonary tuberculosis. It will classically present with hoarseness, cough, and blood-tinged sputum. The most common site of disease in the larynx is in the interarytenoid fold, in the posterior portion of the larynx. Because granulomas tend to be subepithelial, deep biopsies may be essential for diagnosis. Appropriate antituberculous therapy needs to be instituted in addition to symptomatic measures, such as voice rest and analgesics. Occasionally tracheotomy to protect the airway and later reconstruction to open secondary stenosis are required.

Syphilis. Syphilis of the larynx is generally a painless disease with hoarseness as its predominant symptom. Lesions may be noted on endoscopic examination. While the diagnosis may be suspected based on serologic testing and other systemic manifestations of the disease, confirmatory biopsy is required. Generally, laryngeal involvement occurs in the tertiary stage of syphilis. Treatment involves appropriate antibiotics (i.e., penicillin) and other supportive measures as required for any airway problem. Should there be airway complications, tracheotomy may be required for breathing and laryngotracheoplasty performed to correct scarring and secondary stenosis.

Sarcoid. Sarcoid can present as a granulomatous disorder of the upper airway. While it is a rare manifestation of sarcoidosis in this location, it is characterized histopathologically by its noncaseating granulomata. Appropriate systemic evaluation is required for confirmation. Hoarseness and airway compromise are presenting symptoms. Treatment consists of steroids for the systemic disorder and occasionally intralesional injections of steroids. It is thought that these injections may relieve only local obstruction within the airway and lessen the need for tracheotomy. Leprosy in the larynx is caused by *Mycobacterium leprae* and can be found in 10 percent of the cases of systemic leprosy. Treatment includes long-term diaminodiphenylosulfone (dapsone) and possibly also steroids. Glanders is an infectious disease caused by the bacterium *Pseudomonas mallei*. It is a fairly invasive infection and often causes a local inflammatory response within the cartilage of the larynx. Treatment is primarily with antibiotics.

Perichondritis. Perichondritis of the larynx can be caused by an infectious or inflammatory process. It is often difficult to distinguish among bacterial, traumatic, neoplastic, or post-therapeutic irradiation changes. Perichondritis often leads to an abscess in the spaces beneath the mucoperichondrium. The thyroid cartilage is the most common cartilage affected by perichondritis. The symptomatology is generally slow and progressive, although sudden acute forms have been noted in association with pain, tenderness, and swelling. Hoarseness and airway compromise with symptoms of dysphagia and odynophagia imply surgical emergencies. In an emergency situation, radiographic studies should be performed, if possible, to rule out a foreign body; the airway should then be secured in the operating room. Treatment for perichondritis is directed at the underlying cause and may require long-term antibiotics, conservative debridements of laryngeal granulations in the operating room, and possibly steroids.

Diphtheria. While less common today in the United States because of immunization, diphtheria can present insidiously in the larynx. Generally, hoarseness followed by a progressive croupy cough is a first symptom. Physical examination will reveal a grayish white membrane on the laryngeal structures. Airway obstruction and permanent tracheotomy were common at the turn of the century because of progressive destruction of the laryngeal framework by the infection. Current treatment consists of penicillin and antitoxin. Tracheotomy is clinically indicated to protect the airway.

Fungal Infections. The most commonly found mycotic infections of the larynx are histoplasmosis candidiasis, and blastomycosis. Probably the most serious mycotic infection is blastomycosis. The signs are fairly nonspecific: hoarseness, dyspnea, dysphagia, and odynophagia. Physical examination may reveal small nodules on the vocal cords, but vocal cord fixation in the absence of neoplastic disease should alert one to the possibility of blastomycosis. Diagnosis is confirmed by biopsy showing microabscesses in an epithelium that is infiltrated with giant cells and mononuclear cells. Often the hyphae of the fungus can be seen on special stains. Treatment for blastomycosis is intravenous amphotericin B and tracheotomy to secure the airway, should a significant obstruction be present. Actinomycosis is caused by *Actinomyces bovis* and results in a yellowish granulomatous infiltration of the pharynx and larynx. Infection may involve the mandible from adjacent mucosal ulcerations within the oral cavity. Occasionally the organisms can be found within the tonsillar crypts. Diagnosis is established by culture or histology. Treatment involves a course of penicillin for several weeks.

Tumors

Benign Tumors. The most common type of benign laryngeal tumor is the papilloma. Other less common tumors include hemangioma, angiofibroma, chemodectoma, neurofibroma, chondroma, and granular cell myoblastoma. As with most infectious causes of laryngeal dysfunction, benign tumors will usually present with hoarseness. Dyspnea, dysphagia and pain usually reflect late findings. Fiberoptic endoscopy can be done in an outpatient setting to evaluate hoarseness. If a laryngeal tumor is seen, formal endoscopic evaluation and biopsy are necessary. The histopathology is generally diagnostic and will predicate subsequent treatment. The papilloma, a benign tumor of the larynx that requires special attention, is believed to be caused by the human papilloma virus and has six predominant serotypes involved in laryngeal disease. At present there is some debate as to whether there are two clinical forms: an adult form and a juvenile form. Generally, the adult form tends to be unifocal and is easier to treat. Juvenile laryngeal papillomatosis occurs in younger children and can be a devastating infection that is often multifocal. Such children usually present with stridor, but routine examination can be difficult, especially if the child is uncooperative and will not tolerate mirror or fiberoptic examination. Endoscopic evaluation in the operating room is mandatory. While direct examination is highly suggestive, actual pathologic diagnosis is required. It is also essential that the surgeon manipulating the airway of a child suspected of having laryngeal papillomatosis does not inadvertently seed the tracheobronchial tree as this may compromise subsequent therapy.

At present, the treatment of laryngeal papillomatosis in either adults or children is controversial. Currently the mainstay of therapy is the carbon dioxide laser. Since there is a significant chance of recurrence, most patients require several operative procedures to extirpate the disease process. Histopathology is mandatory for all patients, and especially in adults, in order to rule out a malignant lesion. Other surgical therapies that have been used to treat papillomas include mechanical debridement with cupped forceps, cryotherapy, and wide surgical excision, which is more commonly performed in the oropharynx and the oral cavity. Children with laryngotracheal papillomatosis will often require long-term tracheostomies as part of their medical and surgical management. Interferon, often used to treat papilloma virus infections, has been shown to result in significant improvement and decreased morbidity. However, few long-term remissions have been obtained with interferon alone. Whether the duration of medical therapy, the dosing amount, or other factors are involved is not clear at present. There is now some evidence that photosensitization with subsequent obliteration of the tumor with an argon laser may be a promising new modality of treatment. Finally, patients with papilloma-virus infections of the larynx and trachea often have low serum magnesium levels, although the significance of this is unclear.

Malignant Tumors. The most common cancer of the upper aerodigestive tract is the squamous cell carcinoma. Risk factors include excessive alcohol intake and smoking. Other less common tumors include salivary gland tumors, neuroendocrine tumors, and metastatic cancer. Airway obstruction presents in a manner similar to that associated with other causes; however, there is often a prior history available to the clinician. Obstruction at the level of the base of tongue, the supraglottic larynx, and the upper trachea all have a similar presentation, depending on the degree of obstruction. If a history cannot be obtained, a careful physical examination will establish the diagnosis. In addition, the feasibility of endotracheal intubation through either the nose or the mouth can be assessed at this time by means of flexible fiberoptic endoscope. If the examining surgeon believes that it is not safe to secure the airway from above, emergency tracheotomy should be performed under local anesthesia.

Foreign Bodies

Choking on food and other foreign bodies causes over 2,000 deaths per year in the United States. It is the sixth most common cause of accidental death. The majority of episodes of foreign body aspirations into the respiratory tract occur in children under 4 years of age. In such cases, they are *infrequently observed and may not be suspected initially.* Peanuts seem to be the most common foreign body aspirated in children, followed by other foodstuffs and metallic objects. Most of the foreign bodies lodge within the bronchial tree, whereas only 5 percent will get stuck in the larynx. In adults, aspiration of poorly chewed foods is often associated with inebriation, poor dentition, and swallowing disorders, the most common causes of foreign body obstruction. Symptoms can include a sticking pain localized in the larynx, spasm of the larynx, and changes in voice quality up to and including complete aphonia, stridor, or dyspnea, or a complete lack of air movement despite repeated respiratory excursions. For acute obstruction with aphonia and no air movement, a sharp blow to the back followed by necessary forced pressure to the epigastrium, the Heimlich maneuver, is indicated to dislodge the material. Foreign bodies retained in the tracheobronchial tree require prompt endoscopic removal in the operating room.

Traumatic Causes

Generally, facial fractures secondary to maxillofacial trauma are not life-threatening and have a relatively low priority in the management of the patient with multiple injuries. Certain of these fractures, however, may be the source of airway obstruction and hemorrhage, which makes their immediate management more urgent. In addition to bony fractures, mucosal lesions and penetrating trauma affecting large arteries and veins in the neck may also contribute to obstruction of the upper airways. Hematoma in the neck from bleeding vessels may significantly displace the pharyngeal structures and decrease one's ability to breathe. Initial therapy for victims of trauma includes a complete systemic evaluation of the patient in addition to an evaluation of facial fractures. The airway may be compromised by blood, secretions, or the tongue. The mandible provides support for the tongue, and for example, a bilateral parasymphyseal fracture of the mandible may permit the tongue to fall back into the oropharynx, obstructing the airway. This can be quickly managed by grasping the tongue with a towel clip and pulling it forward. Nasoethmoidal fractures, LeFort fractures, and mandibular fractures all can sometimes produce obstruction of the upper airway. An experienced surgeon should be called to evaluate the airway and to effect any management necessary.

Trauma to the larynx and the trachea is occurring with increasing frequency. Penetrating trauma causes the most obvious injuries to the trachea and larynx. Blunt trauma, however, may also cause severe injuries. Some patients may not survive the initial injury and will die before reaching the hospital. However, there are some patients with significant injuries who may have minimal symptoms at initial presentation. Early treatment of laryngeal and tracheal injuries is essential for a successful outcome.

The signs and symptoms of upper airway trauma are varied and include pain over the larynx with either dysphonia or aphonia. Obstruction, while not initially present, may slowly develop with progressive stridor, hoarseness, and dyspnea. Hematomas may be present as well as ecchymosis over the area of injury. Loss of the laryngeal framework may manifest itself by diminution of the landmarks, e.g., the thyroid and cricoid cartilages. Subcutaneous emphysema may be present, and in more severe cases either saliva or air may leak from penetrating wound. Roentgenographic examination is helpful, although a portable flexible fiberoptic examination of the upper airway will usually facilitate emergency diagnosis and direct initial treatment.

Treatment is always directed first at maintaining the airway. Severe mucosal lacerations and swelling may make endotracheal intubation difficult and dangerous, as passage of the endotracheal tube into a false lumen may further compromise the patient's condition. When in doubt, emergency surgical exploration of the larynx and trachea is recommended. Surgical approaches and techniques may vary, however, but generally the trachea, larynx, and carotid sheath should be explored and evaluated. When technically possible, tracheal injuries should be repaired if the wound is not severely contaminated. Closure of simple lacerations may suffice, or resection of a severely injured area with primary anastomosis and appropriate tracheal and laryngeal immobilization may be indicated. If a patient's condition is not stable, a tracheostomy tube can be placed through the injury and definitive repair deferred to a later time. Complications of facial and airway trauma include stenosis of the larynx or trachea due to inadequate treatment at the time of injury, hoarseness secondary to vocal cord paralysis, or chronic aspiration due to an incompetent glottis.

Allergic and Immunologic Causes

Severe allergic reactions may cause mucosal inflammation within the oropharynx and hypopharynx. In severe cases this will effectively shut down the abilities of the upper airway to conduct air. Other diseases such as hereditary angioedema, the cause of which is unknown, may invoke choking or gasping for air. Emergency tracheotomy is required, as endotracheal intubation will be impossible.

MANAGEMENT

Tracheotomy

For all causes of airway obstruction, be they acute or chronic, a tracheotomy is often necessary to save a life. An emergency bedside tracheotomy is indicated only when a delay required to transport a patient to an operating room may be life-threatening. Experience has shown that complication rates are much higher in an emergency setting than in procedures that are planned for the operating room. Even in the hospital, morbidity and mortality dramatically increase when tracheotomy is attempted on struggling, panic-stricken patients who are hungry for air by physicians who are not experienced and do not have adequate assistance, lighting, equipment, or suction. *Threatened* airway compromise by extension of hematoma, edema, or abscess should be recognized and the airway secured. Patients with upper airway obstruction will expend their last energy reserve to maintain adequate alveolar ventilation. Tracheotomy should be performed *prior to exhaustion* and *prior to unfavorable arterial blood gas analysis*. Tracheotomy should be considered in patients not only as a last resort but for palliative support and also as a prophylactic measure to avoid serious potential complications. Tracheotomy will facilitate a patient's subsequent respiratory support and pulmonary hygiene and will decrease the amount of ventilatory dead space.

Cricothyrotomy

Cricothyrotomy has been advocated when emergency intubation or ordinary tracheotomy is not possible. In less experienced hands or in patients with thick necks or who are obese, standard tracheotomy in an emergency setting is hazardous. Cricothyrotomy is indicated for emergent establishment of an airway when time and circumstances prevent transportation to the operating suite. The procedure is technically simple because the cricothyroid membrane is directly under the skin and subcutaneous tissue. The cricothyroid cartilage is easily palpated, and the membrane between the cricoid and thyroid cartilage can easily be determined. The cricothyroid membrane is relatively devoid of blood vessels, so this should be a relatively bloodless procedure. There are physicians who condemn cricothyrotomy because of subsequent complications, including laryngeal stenosis. It is, however, my opinion that in emergency situations, when no other means of establishing an airway are available, it is certainly indicated and appropriate. Conversion to a standard tracheotomy should be undertaken at the first reasonable opportunity.

The technique of cricothyrotomy is relatively simple, and commercially prepared kits are available in many hospitals. After the neck has been extended with a roll under the shoulders and the cricothyroid membrane is visualized, a knife or cannula is used to puncture the membrane and a standard tracheostomy tube is inserted directly through the puncture site into the airway. Air sounds will be heard immediately, and it is critical that this tube be suctioned immediately. If the suction catheter *does not* easily pass down the tube, one should immediately suspect having entered a false lumen and therefore should remove the cannula and repeat the procedure. Once the airway is established and the patient is ventilated and oxygenated, appropriate surgical revision may be undertaken.

SUGGESTED READING

English G, ed. Otolaryngology. Philadelphia: WB Saunders, 1990.
Johnson J, et al. Tracheotomy: self-instructional package (#84100). American Academy of Otolaryngology, Head and Neck Surgery, 1984.
Mayo Smith MF, Hirsch PJ, Wodzinski, et al. Acute epiglottitis in adults: an eight-year experience in the state of Rhode Island. N Engl J Med 1986; 314:1133–1139.
Myer CM III, Orobello P, Cotton RT, et al. Blunt laryngeal trauma in children. Laryngoscope 1987; 97:1043–1048.
Ward RF, Arnold JE, Healy GB. Flexible minibronchoscopy in children. Ann Otol Rhinol Laryngol 1987; 96:645–649.

OXYGEN TOXICITY

ERIC R. PACHT, M.D.
PAUL M. DORINSKY, M.D.

Supplemental oxygen, with or without mechanical ventilation, is frequently required by critically ill patients who are admitted to intensive care units. In general, the potential untoward effects of supplemental oxygen are of minimal clinical concern in the first 12 to 24 hours. That is, initial efforts in the management of critically ill patients are focused on reversal of the underlying illness and maintenance of an arterial Po_2 that is sufficient to meet the metabolic demands of individual tissues. This latter point, in particular, is important since the demands of individual organs for oxygen are instantaneous and dependent upon "adequate" levels of arterial oxygen, which are generally believed to be met when the arterial partial pressure of oxygen (Po_2) exceeds 55 mm Hg and/or oxygen saturation is at least 90 percent. At these levels, the patient will generally be on the flat portion of the oxyhemoglobin dissociation curve and have less risk of developing dangerous levels of tissue hypoxia.

In practice, the level of inspired oxygen (e.g., FiO_2) is adjusted to the lowest level necessary in order to maintain an arterial Po_2 between 55 and 60 mm Hg and/or an oxygen saturation of 90 percent. This therapeutic strategy will minimize the risk imposed by high levels of supplemental oxygen in most patients. However, many critically ill patients will require excessive levels of inspired oxygen to maintain adequate arterial oxygenation. In this regard, exposure to high levels of inspired oxygen for a prolonged period of time (i.e., in excess of 12 to 14 hours) results in a number of pathologic, physiologic, and clinical changes (Table 1). Specifically, the toxicity attendant to high levels of inspired oxygen may include irreversible lung damage, which is similar pathologically to adult respiratory distress syndrome (ARDS). Finally, although specific treatment strategies for these toxic effects of high levels of supplemental oxygen do not exist, a number of supportive measures can be employed in order to reduce the level of inspired oxygen and therefore minimize the toxic effects of oxygen.

PATHOPHYSIOLOGY OF OXYGEN TOXICITY

During normal cellular respiration, molecular oxygen is metabolized by mitochondrial cytochrome oxidase in a four-electron reduction in which water is the end product ($O_2 + 4 H^+ + 4 e^- \rightarrow 2 H_2O$). During this series of reactions, highly reactive oxygen species such as superoxide anion (O_2-), hydrogen peroxide (H_2O_2), hydroxyl radical ($\cdot OH$), perhydroxyl radical ($\cdot HO_2$), and singlet oxygen ($^1O_2$) are produced. These oxygen radicals are toxic and can cause lipid peroxidation, depolymerization of mucopolysaccharides, oxidation of sulfhydryl groups and subsequent inactivation of proteins and enzymes, and nucleic acid damage. If extensive, peroxidation of membrane lipids leads to loss of cellular integrity, cell lysis, and death. Natural defense mechanisms to protect the lung from oxygen-centered radicals include superoxide dismutase, catalase, glutathione peroxidase, as well as radical quenchers such as tocopherol (vitamin E) and ascorbate (vitamin C). At normoxia, these enzymes and radical quenchers are able to protect the lung from damage by detoxifying any oxygen radicals that are produced during normal metabolism. However, during hyperoxia, when the lung is directly exposed to high partial pressures of oxygen, the cellular and extracellular defense mechanisms are overwhelmed and the lung is injured by the excess of oxygen-centered radicals. In addition, inflammatory cells such as neutrophils are attracted to the lower respiratory tract by specific chemotactic factors released by alveolar macrophages during hyperoxia. Although inflammatory cells are not required for the characteristic injury of hyperoxia, potentially they can release large quantities of reactive species, which can cause further lung damage.

In humans, the clinical manifestations of hyperoxia have predominantly been studied in normal volunteers. Exposure to high concentrations of oxygen causes a characteristic substernal chest pain after 12 to 16 hours, which is due to a tracheitis and damage to the tracheal epithelium. Other symptoms include cough, dyspnea, paresthesia, conjunctivitis, nausea, vomiting, and general malaise (see Table 1). Numerous investigators have documented the physiologic consequences of exposure of normal subjects to high concentrations of oxygen, which include a reduction of tracheal mucociliary transport, a decreased vital capacity, a decrease in the diffusing capacity, a

Table 1 Pathologic, Physiologic, and Clinical Sequelae of Oxygen Toxicity

Pathologic Sequelae	*Physiologic Sequelae*	*Clinical Manifestations*
Atelectasis	Reduced vital capacity	Substernal chest pain
Interstitial edema/inflammation	Reduced total lung capacity	Paresthesias
Alveolar hemorrhage/inflammation	Reduced diffusing capacity	General malaise
Hyaline membranes		
Endothelial cell damage		
Tracheobronchitis		

decrease in pulmonary compliance, and a widening of the alveolar-arterial oxygen gradient (see Table 1). These physiologic changes may in part be due to oxygen-induced damage to the alveolar capillary membrane and subsequent fluid and protein "leak" across the damaged membrane. In fact, it has been demonstrated that normal subjects exposed to high concentrations of oxygen for only 16 to 17 hours develop a reversible increase in albumin and transferrin concentrations in bronchoalveolar lavage fluid. This implies that even short exposures to hyperoxia damage the integrity of the alveolar capillary membrane and cause a leak of protein-rich fluid into the alveolar spaces.

Although comprehensive pathologic studies have been performed in animals, very few studies have been done in humans. Most of these studies have involved patients who died after prolonged and complicated illnesses who were exposed to high concentrations of oxygen. Grossly, the lungs of patients who died after prolonged exposure to oxygen are hemorrhagic, congested, and edematous. Microscopically, the prominent features include fibrin thrombi, hyaline membrane formation, alveolar septal edema, capillary endothelial cell damage, loss of type-I pneumocytes, and fibrosis (see Table 1). The lung pathology seen in oxygen toxicity parallels the pathologic picture in acute lung injury such as ARDS. Since most of the human studies have been done on patients with diffuse lung injury, it is difficult to distinguish damage from ARDS versus damage from hyperoxia. In fact, oxygen toxicity is regarded as one of the many factors that can predispose toward the development of ARDS.

MANAGEMENT

Two general principles underlie the use of oxygen in the management of critically ill patients (Table 2). First, and perhaps most important, is the maintenance of an adequate level of arterial oxygen tension. Although uncertainties remain, there is a general consensus that an arterial oxygen tension in the range of 55 to 60 mm Hg (which corresponds to an oxygen saturation of 90 percent) is the minimum level of oxygen tension necessary to meet the metabolic demands of individual organs. Clearly, variations intrinsic to pathophysiologic alterations that occur in individual patients, as well as conditions that may affect the oxyhemoglobin dissociation curve (e.g., pH, temperature, carbon dioxide partial pressure [PCO_2]) can affect the minimum "acceptable" level of arterial oxygen pressure (PaO_2). Nonetheless, in most situations, a PaO_2 of at least 55 to 60 mm Hg will be adequate. Moreover, since oxygen availability to individual tissues is affected not only by PaO_2, but also by hemoglobin concentration and cardiac output, it stands to reason that these factors should be optimized as well. In this context, hemoglobin concentration should be maintained at a level of 10 to 12 g per deciliter in females and 12 to 14 g per deciliter in males. Likewise, cardiac output can be augmented in order to provide "adequate" tissue oxygen delivery. Unfortunately, an adequate level of tissue oxygen delivery is difficult

Table 2 Management of Patients Who Require High Levels of Supplemental Oxygen

General Measures
  Maintain PaO_2 at 55-60 mm Hg
  Monitor PaO_2 and/or SaO_2 frequently
  Maintain adequate cardiac output
  Correct anemia (i.e., target Hgb at 10-12 in female, 12-14 in males)
  Maintain normal body temperature
  Evaluate thyroid function

Specific Measures
  Diffuse Lung Injury
    PEEP ventilation
    Diuresis
    Extracorporeal membrane oxygenation (?)

  Unilateral Lung Injury
    Independent lung ventilation

to define except in general terms. Nonetheless, tissue oxygen delivery can be presumed to be adequate in those situations in which clinical evidence of end-organ dysfunction is absent (e.g., adequate urine output, stable BUN and creatinine, normal liver function tests, normal mental status) and there is no evidence of anaerobic metabolism (e.g., normal lactic acid levels).

The second general principle of oxygen therapy in the management of critically ill patients relates to the prevention of oxygen toxicity. Namely, every effort should be made to use the lowest level of FIO_2 necessary to maintain a PaO_2 in the range of 55 to 60 mm Hg. In this regard, it is important to maintain the FIO_2 below 0.5, when possible, since an FIO_2 in excess of approximately 0.5 will result in pulmonary oxygen toxicity. Furthermore, these toxic effects of oxygen will increase in severity as both the FIO_2 and the duration of exposure to the high FIO_2 increase. Nonetheless, this therapeutic principle is impossible to achieve in some patients and may not be valid in patients with diffuse lung injury. That is, most studies related to the pathogenesis of oxygen toxicity have been performed in normal study subjects. In addition, there is some evidence to indicate that lung injury and/or previous exposure to high levels of inspired oxygen may confer some degree of protection against the toxic effects of inspired oxygen. Consequently, the upper limit of inspired oxygen that is considered safe for long-term administration is unknown. Nonetheless, it is reasonable to postulate that an FIO_2 at or below 0.5 can be administered for prolonged periods with a minimum of untoward side effects.

Although it is undesirable, many patients require an FIO_2 in excess of 0.5 for maintenance of adequate arterial oxygen tension. Generally, these patients have either acute, diffuse lung injury (e.g., ARDS) or extensive unilateral lung disease (e.g., pneumonia), and they require mechanical ventilatory support. Moreover, measures employed to reverse the underlying disease and/or correct factors known to potentiate oxygen toxicity (e.g., hyperthyroidism, hyperpyrexia) too often have few short-term effects on inspired oxygen tension levels. Nonetheless, certain supportive measures may be beneficial in lowering very high levels of inspired oxygen. In addition, although some degree of overlap exists, these supportive measures are different for patients with diffuse lung injury and patients with extensive unilateral lung disease.

Acute Lung Injury

For patients with acute diffuse lung injury (e.g., ARDS), the use of positive end-expiratory pressure (PEEP) ventilation may markedly improve gas exchange. PEEP is thought to work by reexpanding collapsed or partially collapsed alveoli, thereby increasing functional residual capacity (FRC) and decreasing the number of lung units that are perfused but not ventilated (e.g., intrapulmonary shunt). The therapeutic endpoint for PEEP in ARDS is the lowest level of PEEP necessary to maintain an adequate PaO_2 (e.g., 55 to 60 mm Hg) using an inspired FIO_2 of 0.5 or less. This approach takes advantage of the salutary effects of PEEP while minimizing cardiopulmonary barotrauma attendant to its use. Likewise, a number of new modes of mechanical ventilatory support for patients with ARDS have recently been developed. These include pressure-controlled inverse ratio ventilation and high-frequency ventilation. However, at the present time, these techniques either have not been shown to be superior to conventional mechanical ventilation with PEEP and/or have not been subjected to controlled prospective trials. For these reasons, their use in the management of severe gas-exchange abnormalities attendant to ARDS remains largely investigational.

Diuretic therapy may also be a useful adjunct in the management of the refractory hypoxemia attendant to ARDS. In particular, ARDS results in a marked increase in pulmonary capillary permeability. As a consequence, hydrostatic forces play a major role in the movement of fluid from the intravascular to the interstitial and alveolar spaces of the lung. Through the judicious use of diuretics in these patients, fluid flux across the alveolar capillary membrane can be diminished. To the extent that this occurs, gas exchange will improve and the need for excessively high levels of inspired oxygen can be reduced.

Finally, extracorporeal membrane oxygenation (ECMO) has been used as a means of respiratory support for patients with severe gas exchange abnormalities due to ARDS. The putative advantage of ECMO is its potential to support gas exchange (e.g., oxygenation of mixed venous blood and removal of carbon dioxide) without exposing the alveoli to high levels of inspired oxygen. Although it is theoretically appealing, initial studies using ECMO failed to demonstrate an improved survival compared with conventional treatment in patients with end-stage respiratory failure. In addition, there is the theoretic concern that ECMO, while reducing pulmonary barotrauma and the risks of oxygen toxicity, may, in fact, increase the incidence of nonpulmonary organ failure. Despite these limitations, ECMO has received a recent resurgence of clinical interest. Although the data from ongoing clinical trials are incomplete, survival appears much better than that reported in the original ECMO trials. In this future, ECMO may play a much more important role in the management of acute respiratory failure due to ARDS.

Extensive Unilateral Lung Injury

Patients with extensive unilateral lung injury (e.g., pneumonia) may develop respiratory failure and severe gas-exchange abnormalities similar to those observed in patients with ARDS. However, unlike ARDS, refractory hypoxemia (e.g., intrapulmonary shunting) is due almost entirely to an extensive alveolar filling process. In this regard, many of the therapeutic modalities used in the treatment of ARDS (e.g., PEEP) will worsen gas exchange in these patients. For example, the use of PEEP in these patients has the effect of increasing pulmonary capillary resistance in the unaffected alveolar units. As a consequence, blood flow to the involved lung may increase and result in a worsening of gas exchange.

Despite these limitations, it is still reasonable to institute PEEP cautiously in these individuals in an attempt to improve gas exchange and thus reduce the requirements for high levels of inspired oxygen. If this is unsuccessful, which is often the case, independent lung ventilation should be considered. This requires placement of a Carlon tube and the use of two separate mechanical ventilators. Each ventilator is used for independent ventilation of one lung. The advantage of this approach is that PEEP can be applied only to the involved lung. Disadvantages of this approach involve some degree of patient discomfort and tube malplacement. Nonetheless, most patients will tolerate asynchronous, independent lung ventilation with the concomitant use of sedatives. However, tube malplacement is a serious potential problem that needs to be monitored closely. Clearly, the use of independent lung ventilation represents a heroic endeavor in the management of the gas-exchange abnormalities attendant to extensive unilateral lung injury. However, if patients are selected carefully, it can be beneficial.

FUTURE DIRECTIONS

The treatment of oxygen toxicity outlined above essentially involves a vigorous attempt to limit the duration of exposure to high concentrations of oxygen to as brief a period of time as possible. However, more specific forms of therapy may be available in the future to benefit patients who require high concentrations of oxygen for prolonged periods of time. As previously mentioned, the toxicity of oxygen is due to the overproduction of reactive oxygen species. In this context, efforts to increase the antioxidant defense systems of the lung may be beneficial in preventing some of the toxic effects of hyperoxia. In support of this postulate, it has been established that both endotoxin and prior exposure to oxygen enable animals to survive for extended periods of time in environments of

100 percent oxygen. This protective effect of both endotoxin and oxygen is linked to their ability to stimulate the production of intracellular antioxidant enzymes such as superoxide dismutase and catalase. This may also have clinical relevance, as some critically ill patients, presumably those with prior exposure to endotoxin and/or low-flow oxygen, survive for long periods of time on extremely high concentrations of oxygen. In this regard, if an attenuated endotoxin-like compound could be developed to stimulate the in vivo production of antioxidant substances, it could potentially have significant therapeutic benefit.

An alternative approach to the management of oxygen toxicity involves the administration of antioxidant compounds in an effort to bolster the lung's defenses and ameliorate some of the toxic effects of high partial pressures of oxygen. Vitamin E appeared to be the most promising agent, as initial reports indicated that it could decrease the incidence of bronchopulmonary dysplasia in premature infants subjected to high concentrations of oxygen. Unfortunately, that study has since been refuted and it appears that vitamin E, as well as vitamin C, while necessary for protection against the toxic effects of oxygen, do not afford additional protection when given in high supplemental doses. Finally, catalase and/or superoxide dismutase, encapsulated in liposomes and administered intratracheally have been shown to increase the pulmonary levels of these enzymes as well as prolong survival and decrease lung injury, when compared with animals that do not receive the supplemental antioxidant enzymes.

Though still experimental, this appears to be a promising approach to human oxygen toxicity.

It has also been demonstrated that hypothyroid, adrenalectomized, or hypothermic animals are protected from the toxic effects of oxygen. The probable mechanism involves decreases in the level of cellular respiration and thus decreases in the production of reactive oxygen species. Therefore, another possible approach would be to induce either a hypothermic, hypothyroid, or hypoadrenal state transiently until oxygen requirements are reduced to acceptable levels.

Despite all the possible future interventions, the focus on the treatment of oxygen toxicity must be on prevention, because once established, the pathologic damage due to oxygen toxicity cannot be reversed.

SUGGESTED READING

Carlon GC, Ray C, Klein R, et al. Criteria for selective positive end-expiratory pressure and independent synchronized ventilation of each lung. Chest 1978; 74:501–507.
Davis WB, Rennard SI, Bitterman PB, Crystal RG. Pulmonary oxygen toxicity: early reversible changes in human alveolar structures induced by hyperoxia. N Engl J Med 1983; 309:878–883.
Deneke SM, Fanburg BL. Normobaric oxygen toxicity of the lung. N Engl J Med 1980; 303:76–86.
Frank L, Massaro D. Oxygen toxicity. Am J Med 1980; 69:117–126.
Matthay MA. New modes of mechanical ventilation for ARDS. How should they be evaluated? Chest 1989; 95:1175–1177.

RADIATION PNEUMONITIS AND FIBROSIS

R. DWAINE RIEVES, M.D.
JAMES H. SHELHAMER, M.D.

Radiation-induced lung damage is the most common serious complication of thoracic radiotherapy. The clinical characteristics of radiation-induced pulmonary damage were recognized shortly following the introduction of radiotherapy for malignancy. Recent refinements in radiotherapy, including limitation of dose rate, precise portal field adjustment and dosimetry, have resulted in a much lower incidence of clinically significant pulmonary toxicity. However, more penetrating radiation energies combined with aggressive chemotherapy regimens utilizing drugs with pulmonary toxicity and radiosensitizing properties, continue to produce the occasional case of life-threatening pulmonary toxicity.

Pulmonary toxicity rarely appears during the initial administration of radiotherapy. Radiation pneumonitis, the acute sequela of lung radiation injury is manifested following a latency of several weeks. Radiation fibrosis, the chronic consequence of radiation damage, develops 4 to 12 months following radiotherapy. Pulmonary toxicity following radiation is related to the radiation regimen, as well as to individual patient characteristics (Table 1). Most radiation lung damage results from exposure in excess of 20 Gy (1 Gy is equivalent to 100 rad). Fractionation of the total radiation dose and a reduction in the individual dose administration rate has been shown to lessen the likelihood of pulmonary injury. Rarely does symptomatic lung damage result when less than 25 percent of the lung volume is radiated. Likewise, radiation to the apices is usually less consequential than radiation of the lung bases. Exposure to certain chemotherapeutic agents may result in significant lung damage at lower radiation doses. Prior treatment with actinomycin D, adriamycin, or bleomycin has been associated with "radiation recall," the more severe and acute onset of radiation pneumonitis. The development of radiation pneumonitis has been well described following the abrupt termination of steroid therapy in cancer patients receiving combined chemotherapy and radiation. The pathology of radiation pneumonitis is nonspecific, consisting of alveolar septal edema with a mononuclear cell infiltrate, fibrin membrane lining of alveoli, and desquamation of atypical alveolar lining cells.

Table 1 Risk Factors for Radiation-Induced Lung Disease

Radiotherapy Administration
  Increasing
    Total radiation dose
    Fractionation administration schedule
    Dose delivery rate
    Volume of radiated lung

Concomitant Therapy
  Chemotherapeutic agents
    Actinomycin D, adriamycin, bleomycin, methotrexate, cyclophosphamide
  Prednisone, especially abrupt termination of steroid therapy
  High concentrations of supplemental oxygen

Patient Factors
  Underlying lung disease
  Prior radiotherapy
  Prior therapy with actinomycin D, adriamycin, or bleomycin

Pathologically, radiation fibrosis is indistinguishable from other causes of fibrosis, with septal fibrosis and alveolar obliteration.

RADIATION PNEUMONITIS

Recognition and Management

Radiation pneumonitis manifests clinically 6 to 16 weeks following radiation. Symptoms develop insidiously, most commonly with nonproductive cough and exertional dyspnea. Dyspnea may worsen and a low-grade fever may be noted. Chest tightness, although uncommon, has been described. A productive cough, hemoptysis, or night sweats is unusual and suggests another pulmonary process. Most patients will have radiographic findings at the time of initial symptoms. Usually, a pulmonary infiltrate is noted within the area of the radiation port. Unlike an infectious process, the infiltrate commonly crosses anatomic boundaries, corresponding appropriately to the radiation port. Should the chest radiograph be inconclusive, computerized tomography (CT) may be necessary to localize more accurately the infiltrate. Chest CT scanning has been shown to be more sensitive than radiography in the detection of radiation pneumonitis. Occasionally, radiation pneumonitis will present with pulmonary infiltrates extending beyond the field of radiation. This may be due to tangential radiation, but other etiologies for lung infiltrates should be considered. Diagnostically, pulmonary function tests are of little value, although radiation pneumonitis has been associated with decreased lung volumes and diffusing capacity. Sequential pulmonary function tests are useful in monitoring the course of lung impairment. The combination of symptoms with chest radiographic findings are usually adequate for diagnosis and initiation of therapy. However, atypical symptoms or unusual radiographic patterns, especially in immunocompromised patients, may require more extensive evaluation. The clinical approach to the diagnosis of pulmonary infiltrates in patients following radiotherapy does not differ from that of other patients with infiltrates. Usually, the history, physical examination and sputum examination are adequate for diagnosis. Especially in immunocompromised patients or patients with rapidly progressing symptoms and radiographic abnormalities, expeditious diagnostic efforts are indicated. An abrupt onset of symptoms or extensive progression of pulmonary infiltrates over several hours is uncharacteristic of radiation pneumonitis. In these patients, bronchoscopic lavage and biopsy may be crucial to the diagnosis of an infection or recurrent malignancy.

Unlike the focal infiltrates commonly seen with radiation pneumonitis, a form of diffuse interstitial pneumonitis may develop in patients following total body radiation. The interstitial pneumonitis is usually seen in bone marrow transplant patients and uncommonly can be solely attributed to radiation therapy. Cytomegalovirus and other opportunistic infections, as well as cytotoxic chemotherapy and graft-versus-host diseases are confounding diagnostic considerations. Invasive diagnostic procedures are usually required to exclude infectious agents. The role of radiation in the pathogenesis of the interstitial pneumonitis is unsettled, but therapy with combination methotrexate chemotherapy and radiation has been most clearly associated. In the absence of infection, the prognosis is poor, as no effective therapy has been described.

Manifestations of radiation pneumonitis range from the more common asymptomatic chest radiographic findings to progressive respiratory failure. Consequently, therapy must be tailored to the clinical setting and moderated by the patient's symptoms. Patients who present with minimal symptoms and lack risk factors for severe pulmonary damage can be treated symptomatically, with cough suppressants, antipyretics, and rest. Although no consistent indicators of incipient severe pulmonary toxicity have been described, more aggressive therapy is indicated in patients at higher risk for radiation damage. A larger dose of radiation or larger volume of radiated lung especially prompt more intense therapy. Although no randomized, prospective clinical trial has verified the utility of glucocorticosteroids in the treatment of radiation pneumonitis, a wealth of clinical data supports their use. Prompt initiation of prednisone is recommended in patients at high risk for radiation pneumonitis and intractable cough, limiting dyspnea or hypoxemia. The recommended dose is 60 to 100 mg per day, to be continued at this level for a week or more, until symptoms improve. Usually, symptomatic improvement is noted within 48 hours. Once improvement has been noted, the steroid therapy is very slowly tapered, usually over a 6- to 12-week period. Many examples of rebound pneumonitis, following abrupt cessation of steroids, have been described. Occasionally, hospitalization for observation and supplemental oxygen is required, although most patients can be managed as outpatients with close follow-up. Rarely, radiation pneumonitis will progress to respiratory failure and require mechanical ventilation. Acceleration of symptoms despite steroid therapy has been described, but progressive deterioration should prompt an evaluation for complicating factors, such as infectious pneumonia, thromboembolic disease, or cardiac failure. The action of steroid therapy in radiation pneumonitis is unknown, but a few studies have suggested an immunologic basis for radiation injury. Conceivably, steroid therapy may modulate the immune response to the lung injury. Few other drugs have been utilized as therapy for radiation pneumonitis. Anticoagulants and nonsteroidal anti-inflammatory drugs have been used in a limited number of patients with no success.

Complications of Radiation Pneumonitis

Although uncommon, a number of complications have been associated with radiation pneumonitis. Many case reports of spontaneous pneumothorax have been described, usually in the setting of acute radiation pneumonitis. No predisposing factor for pneumothorax was evident in these patients. The possibility of spontaneous pneumothorax should be considered in patients with radiation pneumonitis and chest pain. Another cause for chest pain during radiation pneumonitis is rib fracture. Rib fracture is believed to be due to direct radiation-induced bone damage. Exudative pleural effusions have been described in association with radiation pneumonitis, although symptoms of pleural irritation are uncommon. The development of a tracheoesophageal fistula may coincide with radiation pneumonitis, as suggested by concurrent bacterial pneumonitis and radiation pneumonitis. A striking clinical presentation is the occlusion of a proximal airway by tumor edema, following radiation. Unlike in radiation pneumonitis, the chest radiograph demonstrates lobar or total lung atelectasis. Profound hypoxemia may progress to ventilatory failure. The diagnosis is confirmed by bronchoscopy. Steroids, supplemental oxygen, and bronchodilators are recommended as initial therapy.

RADIATION FIBROSIS

Radiation fibrosis is the chronic manifestation of radiation-induced lung injury. Chest radiographic evidence of fibrosis is usually fully developed by 12 months following radiation. Fibrosis is most commonly asymptomatic, the major clinical challenge being the distinction of fibrosis from recurrent malignancy. Symptomatically, radiation fibrosis rarely results in more than exertional dyspnea. Other symptoms such as persistent or productive cough, hemoptysis, or fever are not characteristic of fibrosis and suggest an alternate diagnosis. Although most cases of symptomatic radiation pneumonitis culminate in fibrosis, more commonly the development of fibrosis is clinically silent. The role of steroids in the prevention of fibrosis has not been evaluated. Radiation fibrosis is radiographically manifest as dense consolidation or interstitial thickening, in the area of the radiation port. Contraction of the radiated lung tissue is evident, and tracheal or bronchial deviation is common. Cavitation within an area of fibrosis is unusual and suggests another process. Chest CT scanning is valuable in the distinction of fibrosis from recurrent neoplasm. Clinically, the development of a recurrent laryngeal nerve palsy, Horner's syndrome, or superior venal caval syndrome is most suggestive of malignancy. As most cases of radiation fibrosis are asymptomatic, no treatment is necessary. For patients with exertional dyspnea, supplemental oxygen therapy may be of benefit. Steroid therapy is not indicated for treatment of fibrosis. Pulmonary function tests should be obtained in symptomatic patients, especially to evaluate for the possibility of underlying obstructive lung disease. If obstruction is demonstrated, bronchodilator therapy may result in symptomatic improvement.

SUGGESTED READING

Coggle J, Lambert B, Moores S. Radiation effects in the lung. Environ Health Perspect 1986; 70:261–291.

Gibson P, Bryant D, Morgan G, et al. Radiation-induced lung injury: a hypersensitivity pneumonitis? Ann Intern Med 1988; 109:288–291.

Watchie J, Coleman C, Raffin T, et al. Minimal long-term cardiopulmonary dysfunction following treatment for Hodgkin's disease. Int J Radiat Oncol Biol Phys 1987; 13:517–524.

Weiner R, Bortin M, Gale R, et al. Interstitial pneumonitis after bone marrow transplantation. Ann Intern Med 1986; 104:168–175.

WEANING FROM MECHANICAL VENTILATION

MICHAEL R. SILVER, M.D.
ROBERT A. BALK, M.D.

For most patients, termination of mechanical ventilation is relatively straightforward. The simplest approach is abrupt termination of mechanical ventilation with concurrent extubation and is most appropriate for patients that have been electively intubated and mechanically ventilated for some reason other than respiratory failure. Patients successfully weaned using this approach are those with little or no preexisting lung disease, such as patients undergoing elective surgery or patients intubated for airway protection. In this setting, termination of mechanical ventilation, or "weaning," occurs when four basic criteria are satisfied: (1) The patient must be awake and alert enough to breathe spontaneously and protect himself from aspiration. (2) The condition necessitating mechanical ventilation has resolved to the extent that the patient no longer requires ventilatory assistance. (3) The main airways are freed of secretions, either by suctioning or spontaneous

Table 1 Parameters for Weaning Patients from Mechanical Ventilators

Routine Weaning Parameters
  PEEP $\leq$ 5 cm H_2O
  $F_IO_2 \leq 0.5$
  Spontaneous tidal volume $\geq$ 5 ml/kg ideal body weight
  Vital capacity $\geq$ 10 ml/kg ideal body weight
  Maximum inspiratory force more negative than -20 cm H_2O
  Resting minute ventilation < 10 L/min
  Maximum voluntary ventilation > 2 × resting minute ventilation
  Spontaneous respiratory rate $\leq$ 25 breaths/min
  Static compliance $\geq$ 30 ml/cm H_2O

Potential Weaning Parameters
  Reduced tracheal occlusion pressures ($P_{0.1}$)
  Dead space/tidal volume $\leq$ 0.6
  $T_I/T_{TOT} \leq 0.4$

coughing. (4) There must be personnel available to deliver respiratory support (humidified oxygen, medication nebulizer treatments, and reintubation and reinstitution of mechanical ventilation) as required. Weaning parameters (Table 1) or alternative modes of ventilation are usually not required in weaning these patients from mechanical ventilation. Weaning parameters may help to confirm the clinical impression that the patient has adequate respiratory function to permit a return to spontaneous ventilation.

Mechanically ventilated patients with underlying lung disease, chronic debilitating diseases, or slowly resolving disease processes are usually not candidates for abrupt termination of mechanical ventilation and concurrent extubation. These patients benefit from one of the other two approaches to weaning: increasing time periods during which the patient receives no mechanical ventilation (T-piece trials) or reducing over time the patient's respiratory support [intermittent mandatory ventilation (IMV) or pressure-support wean]. Studies to date have not clearly shown that weaning by increasing durations of T-piece trials is superior to weaning by reducing the amount of mechanical ventilation the patient receives each minute. Clinicians are thus left to choose the method of weaning with which they are most comfortable and which satisfies the individual patient's needs. When a previously healthy patient has recovered completely from the disease process that necessitated ventilation, weaning from mechanical ventilation occurs readily regardless of the method used.

A small percentage of intubated patients require weeks of mechanical ventilation. The majority of this chapter will be devoted to a discussion of weaning these "difficult" patients from mechanical ventilation. Weaning should not begin until the disease process that precipitated respiratory failure has significantly resolved, regardless of a patient's previous medical health. While this improvement may be clinically apparent, functional pulmonary improvements include an improvement in the alveolar-arterial oxygen tension gradient, an increase in pulmonary compliance, and a reduction in ventilatory requirements. In general, while we may reduce ventilatory support for patients requiring positive end-expiratory pressure (PEEP), we do not actively wean patients from mechanical ventilation until the required level of PEEP is less than or equal to 5 cm H_2O.

GENERAL CONSIDERATIONS IN WEANING

Prior to weaning the patient with prolonged ventilator requirements, we find several parameters useful in our assessment. Most of these parameters are described by the mnemonic "weans now" (Table 2). In patients requiring long-term mechanical ventilation, weaning parameters are used to *support* a clinical decision, rather than to serve as the basis for the decision. Weaning patients with an ongoing metabolic acidosis requires consideration of respiratory compensation required for acid-base balance, which can significantly increase the work of breathing. Patients with a metabolic alkalosis, usually from excessive diuresis, should have their metabolic derangement corrected before weaning is attempted.

Nutritional support should begin soon after the patient is intubated. Adequate nutrition is important to maintain respiratory muscle function and immunologic competence. Nutritional and electrolyte deficiencies such as kwashiorkor, hypophosphatemia, and hypomagnesemia can lead to difficulties in weaning. Because of the increased respiratory demands of patients fed high-carbohydrate diets, nonfat calories should be limited while one is weaning patients with pre-existing lung disease. In addition, patients with significant medical illnesses tend to be catabolic, resulting in additional loss of respiratory muscle mass and even more difficulty in weaning. Adequate protein intake, coupled with an anabolic hormone such as growth hormone, may help maintain muscle mass and facilitate weaning from mechanical ventilation. If significant retention of carbon dioxide occurs during periods of spontaneous ventilation, carbohydrate and caloric intake should be reduced by increasing fat intake. Twenty-four-hour urinary nitrogen excretion levels (nitrogen balance determination) are measured in patients to ensure that dietary protein needs are met.

Table 2 Optimizing Weaning Potential

"Weans Now"
  W Check *W*eaning parameters
  E Use the largest possible *E*ndotracheal tube to minimize airway resistance
  A Optimize *A*rterial blood gases
  N Resume an appropriate *N*utrition program
  S Clear any *S*ecretions before weaning

  N Optimize *N*euromuscular status
  O Institute therapy to minimize airway *O*bstruction
  W *W*ean when patient is *W*akeful

Other Considerations
  Minimize volume overload
  Assess patient's motivation to wean
  Aggressively treat low-grade infections

Adapted from Beaton N, Bone R. Criteria for weaning your patients from respirators. J Respir Dis 1985; 6:80–83.

Both bronchial secretions and bronchospasm increase airway resistance, increase the work of breathing, and decrease the likelihood of successful weaning. Increasing airway resistance is detected by an increase in the patient's peak airway pressures without a change in the plateau pressure. Aggressive bronchodilator therapy coupled with bronchial hygiene reduces airway resistance, thereby minimizing the work of breathing and facilitating weaning.

Additional considerations in weaning patients are level of wakefulness and neuromuscular status. Although some patients may require narcotics or sedatives, the process of weaning may be facilitated by discontinuing long-acting sedatives and reducing narcotic doses. It is also important to ensure that the patient has had adequate rest and is not fatigued prior to initiation of weaning trials.

Two other considerations not directly addressed by the mnemonic "weans now" are the physician's subjective impression of the patient's ability, interest, and motivation in weaning from mechanical ventilation and the patient's fluid-volume status. While this factor is not easily quantified, we find that patients who appear highly motivated generally wean more quickly than patients who are despondent and uninterested in weaning. Many patients develop significant increases in extravascular fluid. Both pleural effusions and pulmonary interstitial edema (congestive heart failure) decrease pulmonary compliance and increase the work of breathing. Unrecognized volume overload is one of the most easily correctable and commonly overlooked reasons for why patients are unable to wean.

WEANING PREVIOUSLY HEALTHY PATIENTS WITH ACUTE LUNG INJURY

Patients who require prolonged mechanical ventilation are of two distinct types: previously healthy patients with acute lung injury and patients with permanent or preexisting lung disease. The first type of patient is typified by the young, previously healthy victim of trauma with adult respiratory distress syndrome (ARDS). This patient has an acute pulmonary process that necessitated intubation and mechanical ventilatory support. Weaning from mechanical ventilation will occur when the underlying disease has been resolved.

Weaning parameters are useful in assessing the pulmonary status of this type of patient (see Table 1). These parameters indicate inspiratory muscle strength [negative inspiratory force, and tidal volume (V_T)], static and dynamic ventilatory reserve (vital capacity and maximum voluntary ventilation), and respiratory needs [minute ventilation and fraction of inspired oxygen (FIO_2)]. In patients with no pre-existing lung disease, the respiratory rate during a trial of spontaneous breathing is a good indicator of how well the patient will do without mechanical ventilation. Respiratory rates significantly and consistently above 25 breaths per minute usually indicate the need for continued ventilatory support, and/or a different weaning modality than simple T-piece trials.

Another parameter indicative of the inspiratory muscle work is the lung and chest wall compliance. The plateau pressure ($P_{plateau}$) is proportional to pulmonary compliance. If the V_T remains constant and there are no chest wall binders or variable air leaks from dysfunctional endotracheal tube cuffs or bronchopleural fistulae, changes in $P_{plateau}$ correlate well with changes in lung static compliance. Reducing ventilatory support in patients recovering from ARDS is usually unsuccessful in patients with a static compliance below 30 cc per centimeter H_2O. The patient's main difficulty is the extremely high work of breathing imposed by the stiff, noncompliant lung.

Patients recovering from ARDS frequently show marked improvement in arterial oxygen partial pressure (PaO_2), allowing a reduction of their FIO_2. In our experience, reducing PEEP before the $P_{plateau}$ falls can result in a deterioration of oxygenation over the next several hours. To restore oxygenation to its previous level may require increasing PEEP above the initially prescribed level. One problem with $P_{plateau}$ measurements is that volume overload, atelectasis, pneumonia, dwelling peritoneal dialysis fluid or ascites, and changes in position can all increase $P_{plateau}$. Despite these limitations, an unexplained fall in $P_{plateau}$ in patients recovering from ARDS is one of the best indicators of their ability to tolerate weaning from PEEP.

When the patient requires PEEP at a level of less than or equal to 5 cm H_2O and then FIO_2 is less than or equal to 0.5, weaning parameters are useful in predicting ability to wean. Our approach to weaning these patients is to allow them short periods (15 to 30 minutes) of spontaneous ventilation, usually through a Briggs T-piece. We often increase the FIO_2 by 5 to 10 percent before beginning a T-piece trial and monitor the patient with continuous pulse oximetry. Using patient discomfort and a respiratory rate of more than 25 breaths per minute as endpoints, the duration of these periods of spontaneous ventilation is gradually increased. Survivors of ARDS without preexisting lung disease often wean by increasing T-piece trials alone.

For those patients who are unable to wean by progressive T-piece trials, the addition of 5 to 10 cm H_2O of pressure support ventilation (PSV) to the T-piece trials is often helpful. With the introduction of PSV, there is little difficulty in weaning patients through a small-bore endotracheal tube and few problems in overcoming the inherent resistance in the ventilator circuits. Patients with tracheostomies do not usually have significant problems with airflow resistance through the tracheostomy tube unless it is a very small tube. Shorter tube lengths help patients tolerate smaller radius tubing. We empirically use 5 cm H_2O of PSV for patients with large endotracheal or tracheostomy tubes, low respiratory rates, and low inspiratory flows. For patients with small endotracheal or tracheostomy tubes with high inspiratory flow rates, 10 cm H_2O of PSV is used. For patients unable to wean by T-piece trials with PSV, the algorithm of Figure 1 is useful.

When the patient has successfully tolerated 4 to 8 hours of spontaneous breathing or a therapeutic intervention has markedly improved weaning parameters (e.g., plasmapheresis in patients with myasthenia gravis), the tube is removed. Extubation should occur in the morning after the patient has been rested with ventilatory support.

WEANING PATIENTS WITH PRE-EXISTENT OR PERMANENT LUNG DISEASE

The most difficult type of patient to wean from mechanical ventilation is the patient with chronic hypercapnic respiratory failure (CRF). Causes of CRF include emphysema, chronic bronchitis, kyphoscoliosis, previous thoracoplasty, surgical resection of lung tissue, and neuromuscular disease. Mechanical ventilation is required in these patients when an additional medical illness (e.g., superimposed infection, congestive heart failure, pulmonary embolism, or pneumothorax) further compromises ventilation or oxygenation status and exacerbates CRF.

Our general approach to weaning these patients is to review the items in Table 2, with special attention to blood gases, airway obstruction, and nutrition. Weaning parameters are not always useful when weaning patients with CRF, in that baseline weaning parameters may have already been marginal or poor, and may still be "unacceptable" at the time of successful weaning.

Many patients with CRF have had a chronic respiratory acidosis with a compensatory metabolic alkalosis prior to the institution of mechanical ventilation. During a prolonged hospital course, and prior to active weaning, the patient's acid-base status may have been altered by relative hyperventilation with normalization of the arterial carbon dioxide partial pressure ($PaCO_2$) and resultant alkalemia. Weaning these patients requires hypoventilating them and allowing them to retain carbon dioxide back to their normally compensated CRF level. With time, the level of bicarbonate (HCO_3^-) will also rise to buffer chronically elevated carbon dioxide partial pressure (PCO_2). When PCO_2 and bicarbonate level are restored to the patient's baseline level (pH between 7.33 and 7.37), active weaning can begin. Oxygen therapy during this period is important; we maintain oxygen saturation at or near 90 percent. Higher oxygen saturations can decrease respiratory drive during periods of spontaneous breathing and may result in marked and acute retention of carbon dioxide acute respiratory acidosis, and carbon-dioxide narcosis. Maintaining levels significantly above 90 percent saturation is therefore not recommended. Airway obstruction secondary to increased secretions or narrowed airways increases the patient's work of breathing and must be avoided. In addition to frequent suctioning, aggressive treatment with inhaled beta-2 agonists and anticholinergic agents, intravenous theophylline, corticosteroids, and occasional antibiotics is appropriate. In patients requiring chronic steroid therapy for obstructive airway disease, therapy is continued until mechanical ventilation is discontinued. The beneficial effect of steroids in reducing airway inflammation is probably greater than their deleterious effects.

Patients with Chronic Respiratory Insufficiency

An algorithm for weaning patients with preexisting lung disease is shown in Figure 1. The first step in weaning is to correct the underlying process that resulted in the institution of mechanical ventilation. The next step involves optimizing factors likely to facilitate weaning (Table 2). The weaning of mechanical ventilation can be achieved with a reduction in the rate of IMV or with T-piece trials.

The physician's response to an elevated respiratory rate during an IMV wean should depend on the patient. Some patients have resting rates of 25 to 30 breaths per minute and are comfortable with low IMV rates despite rapid respiratory rates. In these patients, T-piece trials of increasing durations seem most appropriate. Other patients complain of intense dyspnea and anxiety during an IMV wean. In several extremely anxious patients, adding "flow-by" to the IMV circuit has successfully reduced anxiety. Flow-by delivers a constant airflow to the breathing circuit during the period between end-expiration and the beginning

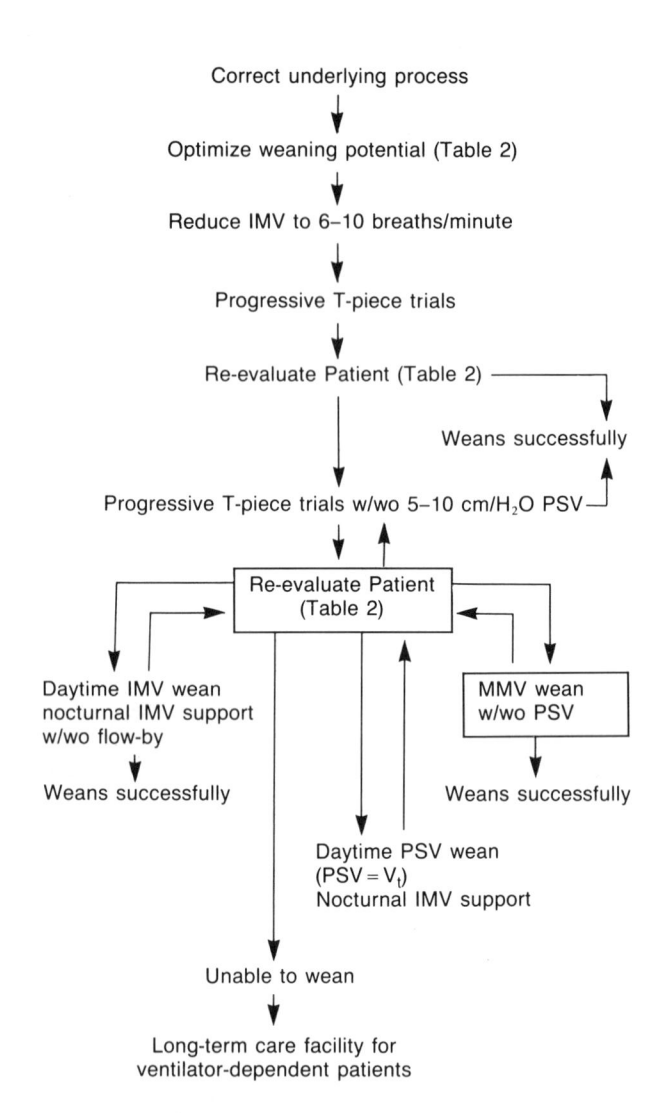

Figure 1 Algorithm for weaning patients from prolonged mechanical ventilation.

of inspiration, resulting in minimal delay in delivery of airflow to the patient at the beginning of a spontaneous breath. Using a baseflow of 10 L per minute and a sensitivity of 3 L per minute, there is no significant pressure support delivered with this flow. Flow-by results in a more rapid response to the patient's spontaneous respiratory efforts and avoids the delays in inspiratory flow that have been reported with circuits using pressure-triggered IMV demand valves. To date, there are no data supporting use of flow-by to improve weaning, so at present we do not use flow-by on all patients on IMV. In patients with a rapid respiratory rate, dyspnea, and significant lung disease (e.g., unresectable lung cancer), we have found that small doses of narcotics (codeine or morphine, but not benzodiazepines) often reduce dyspnea and allow successful weaning.

For patients with CRF, our preference is for T-piece trials rather than IMV weaning. After tailoring the respiratory support to permit restoration of the patient's normal blood gas status, we begin periods of spontaneous breathing with a T-piece apparatus. The patient is allowed several short periods (15 to 30 minutes) of spontaneous ventilation each day; these periods are gradually increased. Crucial to the success of this approach are periods of increased respiratory support between T-piece trials to allow appropriate rest of the respiratory muscles. In some cases, this may require increasing the IMV rate by 1 to 2 breaths per minute, especially at night. Resting patients between T-piece trials and at night minimizes the respiratory muscle fatigue that patients experience when they begin successive T-piece trials. Weaning patients by using intermittent T-piece trials and reducing the IMV between the T-piece trials is strongly discouraged. Rather than monitor arterial blood gases during T-piece trials, we use clinical acumen, pulse oximetry, and occasionally capnometry to monitor patients. Patients who fatigue after short periods (less than 1 hour) of spontaneous ventilation are allowed to breathe spontaneously on the ventilator with the addition of small amounts of PSV. If the patient becomes intensely dyspneic, fatigues, or retains carbon dioxide to an unacceptable degree during low level PSV, an IMV wean is resumed. Weaning then proceeds by lowering the IMV rate toward zero during the day and reinstituting ventilatory support at night. Some patients tolerate this reduction well, but others require short periods of partial reduction in the IMV and a gradual increase in the duration of these periods. Patients ventilated with an IMV rate of 4 to 6 breaths per minute who do not tolerate T-piece trials rarely successfully complete an IMV wean.

Several patients have been successfully weaned using levels of PSV sufficient to deliver the patient's tidal volume when on IMV. These were patients unable to wean with low levels of PSV or gradual reduction of IMV. Patients are ventilated with PSV during the day and IMV support at night. The initial level of PSV is sufficient to maintain the patient's spontaneous tidal volume and is gradually decreased by 5 cm H_2O per day until a PSV of 0 cm H_2O is reached. At this point, the nocturnal IMV is reduced and supplemented with low levels of PSV. Many of these patients are not able to wean completely from mechanical ventilation, but with full nocturnal support they are not ventilator-dependent during the day.

Our philosophy has been to use PSV weaning only after the patient has failed a T-piece and IMV wean. Teleologically, PSV involves converting a volume-cycled ventilator to a pressure-cycled ventilator. In unmonitored patients receiving PSV, atelectasis, bronchospasm, or increased secretions can all result in decreased tidal volumes with disastrous effects. We do not routinely add PSV to the regimen of all patients who are beginning to wean for two reasons: low levels of PSV still provide significant respiratory support, and adding ventilator support during the weaning process is counterproductive.

Two other weaning modalities are gradual reduction in the tidal volumes with a constant IMV rate and mandatory minute ventilation (MMV). Reduction of tidal volumes with a constant rate attempts to mimic the patient's smaller tidal volumes. Although superficially appealing, reducing ventilatory support in this fashion probably is associated with a high rate of atelectasis unless sighs are added. MMV is an excellent support mode that guarantees the patient a desired minute ventilation. In addition to setting the minimum minute ventilation tolerated, the "back-up" respiratory rate and minimum tidal volume can be designated. During spontaneous ventilation, if the patient's respiratory rate exceeds a predetermined value or if the minute ventilation falls below a preset value, mechanical ventilation using the back-up rate and tidal volume is initiated. After a period of time, the respiratory support is reduced to the initial level. Because MMV "rescues" the patient during periods of inadequate patient ventilation, monitoring the weaning trials may be difficult. In situations in which supervision of the patient is not optimal, MMV is an excellent way of ensuring adequate ventilatory support during weaning trials even in absence of a caregiver. Weaning by reducing MMV does not seem to offer any significant advantages to IMV or T-piece weaning in a well-supervised patient-care setting.

SUGGESTED READING

MacIntyre NR. Weaning from mechanical ventilatory support: volume-assisting intermittent breaths versus pressure-assisting every breath. Respir Care 1988; 33:121–125.

Morganroth ML, Morganroth JL, Nett LM, Petty TL. Criteria for weaning from prolonged mechanical ventilation. Arch Intern Med 1984; 144:1012–1016.

Perel A. Newer ventilation modes—temptations and pitfalls. Crit Care Med 1987; 15:707–709.

Sahn SA, Lakshminarayan S, Petty TL. Weaning from mechanical ventilation. JAMA 1976; 235:2208–2212.

Schachter EN, Tucker D, Beck GJ. Does intermittent mandatory ventilation accelerate weaning? JAMA 1981; 1210–1214.

THERAPEUTICS FOR INFECTIOUS DISEASE

NOSOCOMIAL INFECTION

DENNIS G. MAKI, M.D.

Hospital-acquired (nosocomial) infections are among the most common and serious complications encountered in the intensive care unit (ICU) and usually result from monitoring or life support therapies. It is therefore appropriate that measures to prevent nosocomial infections be addressed.

Critical care units have contributed greatly to the care of patients with life-threatening conditions and trauma, but they are associated with a greatly increased risk of nosocomial infection: rates of nosocomial infection in patients requiring more than 1 week of advanced life support in an ICU are three to five times higher than in hospitalized patients who do not require ICU care. Infection is the most common cause of death—directly or indirectly—of patients who survive major trauma or full-thickness burns and is the most frequent precipitating event in multiple system organ failure.

During the past decade, much has been learned of the pathogenesis and, especially, the epidemiology of nosocomial infections—the hospital reservoirs of nosocomial pathogens and their modes of transmission. Published guidelines for the prevention of these infections are now available, based increasingly on controlled studies that have established the efficacy of specific preventive measures, especially within the ICU. Knowledge and technology of asepsis with regard to surgery and high-risk medical devices are now advanced enough that, if they are applied consistently, they can greatly reduce the risk of nosocomial infection.

PROFILE AND EPIDEMIOLOGY

Profile of Nosocomial Infection in the Intensive Care Unit

The rates of nosocomial infection are highest in burn units, surgical ICUs, and ICUs for low–birth weight neonates (15 to 30 percent), with intermediate risk in medical and pediatric ICUs (5 to 10 percent), and with the lowest rates in coronary care units (1 to 2 percent). Approximately one-third of ICU infections are catheter-related urinary tract infections, and one-fourth are pneumonias associated with endotracheal intubation and mechanical ventilatory support; postoperative surgical wound and intra-abdominal infections, nosocomial bacteremias, and antibiotic-associated colitis account for the remainder. More than 10 percent of patients hospitalized in a surgical ICU for more than 72 hours acquire a nosocomial bacteremia, most commonly from an intravascular device. The microbial profile of these infections at individual sites and their major associated risk factors are shown in Table 1.

In the ICU, as contrasted with non-ICU patient care units within the same institutions, rates of primary bacteremia—most of which originate from the use of intravascular devices—and of ventilator-associated pneumonia are ten times higher. Moreover, a far higher proportion of nosocomial infections are caused by antibiotic-resistant bacteria; the intensive antimicrobial therapy characteristic of ICUs grossly distorts the patient's microflora and fosters colonization and, ultimately, nosocomial infection with methicillin-resistant *Staphylococcus aureus* and coagulase-negative staphylococci, enterococci, aminoglycoside- and third-generation cephalosporin-resistant Enterobacteriaceae, *Pseudomonas*, and yeasts such as *Candida*.

Epidemiology

It is no surprise that the ICU is a milieu uniquely conducive to the occurrence of epidemic nosocomial infection, especially infections caused by antibiotic-resistant pathogens. During the past decade, two-thirds of reported outbreaks of nosocomial infection have occurred in ICUs, even though less than 10 percent of all hospitalized patients require ICU care.

In the ICU, the major reservoir of nosocomial organisms is the infected or colonized patient (Fig. 1). Most bacteria, many viruses (e.g., hepatitis A, herpes simplex virus, respiratory syncytial virus), and possibly even *Candida* are spread primarily on the hands of medical personnel, who themselves are rarely permanently colonized or infected. The exanthems of childhood—Varicella-Zoster and measles particularly—*Legionella*, *Mycobacterium tuberculosis*, and, in granulocytopenic patients, *Aspergillus*, are transmitted by the airborne route. Aspiration (often around cuffed endotracheal tubes), surgery, and exposure to invasive devices of all types greatly amplify transmission, colonization, and vulnerability to nosocomial infection by all routes (see Fig. 1). Resistant nosocomial

Table 1 Profile of Nosocomial Infection in the Intensive Care Unit

Infections	Major Pathogen	Risk Factors
Urinary tract	*Klebsiella* and *Enterobacter* spp. *Pseudomonas aeruginosa* Enterococci *Staphylococcus epidermidis* *Candida* spp.	Urinary catheter Monitoring of urine output Other urologic manipulation or bladder irrigations Renal transplantation Diabetes Female gender
Pneumonia	*Klebsiella* and *Enterobacter* spp. *Serratia marcescens* *P. aeruginosa* *Acinetobacter* spp. *Staphylococcus aureus* Oral anaerobes	Tracheostomy Endotracheal tube Nasogastric tube Intracranial pressure monitoring Stress ulcer prophylaxis with H_2-blocker or antacids Immunosuppression Granulocytopenia
Postsurgical wound or intraabdominal	*S. aureus* *Escherichia coli* and other gram-negative bacilli Enterococci *Bacteroides fragilis*, and other bowel anaerobes	Trauma, especially penetrating abdominal injury Postgastrointestinal or radical gynecologic surgery Immunosuppressive therapy Granulocytopenia Hepatic transplantation
Bacteremia from Intravascular devices Catheter-related	Coagulase-negative staphylococci *S. aureus* *Candida* spp.	Central venous catheter in place >5 days Heavy colonization of insertion site skin Hemodynamic monitoring Exposure of catheter to remote source bacteremia
Contaminated infusate	*Enterobacter* spp. *S. marcescens* *Citrobacter* spp. *Pseudomonas cepacia* or *Pseudomonas maltophilia*	
Antibiotic-associated diarrhea or colitis	*Clostridium difficile*	Prolonged antibiotic therapy, especially with clindamycin or broad-spectrum beta-lactams Enteral tube feeding

organisms from colonized and infected patients can also be perpetuated and spread in contaminated mechanical apparatus, such as urine collection receptacles, respiratory therapy equipment, chamber domes of transducers used for hemodynamic monitoring, dialysis machines, or fiberoptic bronchoscopes or endoscopes.

Critical care medicine is synonymous with cutting-edge, high-tech medicine: mechanical ventilatory support, hemodynamic monitoring, total parenteral nutrition, hemodialysis, intracranial pressure monitoring, innovative forms of surgery, and a huge arsenal of drugs, especially anti-infectives of every genre. Notably, technology more than anything else has forced critical care medicine to confront the necessity of nosocomial infection control; prospective studies have shown that various invasive devices (Table 2) play a far more important role in determining susceptibility to nosocomial infection than underlying disease. But this should be viewed as good news. There is far greater hope that nosocomial infections can be reduced by more attention to aseptic technique and advances in technology with respect to devices than that the ravages of chronic organ failure and debilitating systemic diseases (e.g., Type 1 diabetes) can be reversed through medical breakthroughs.

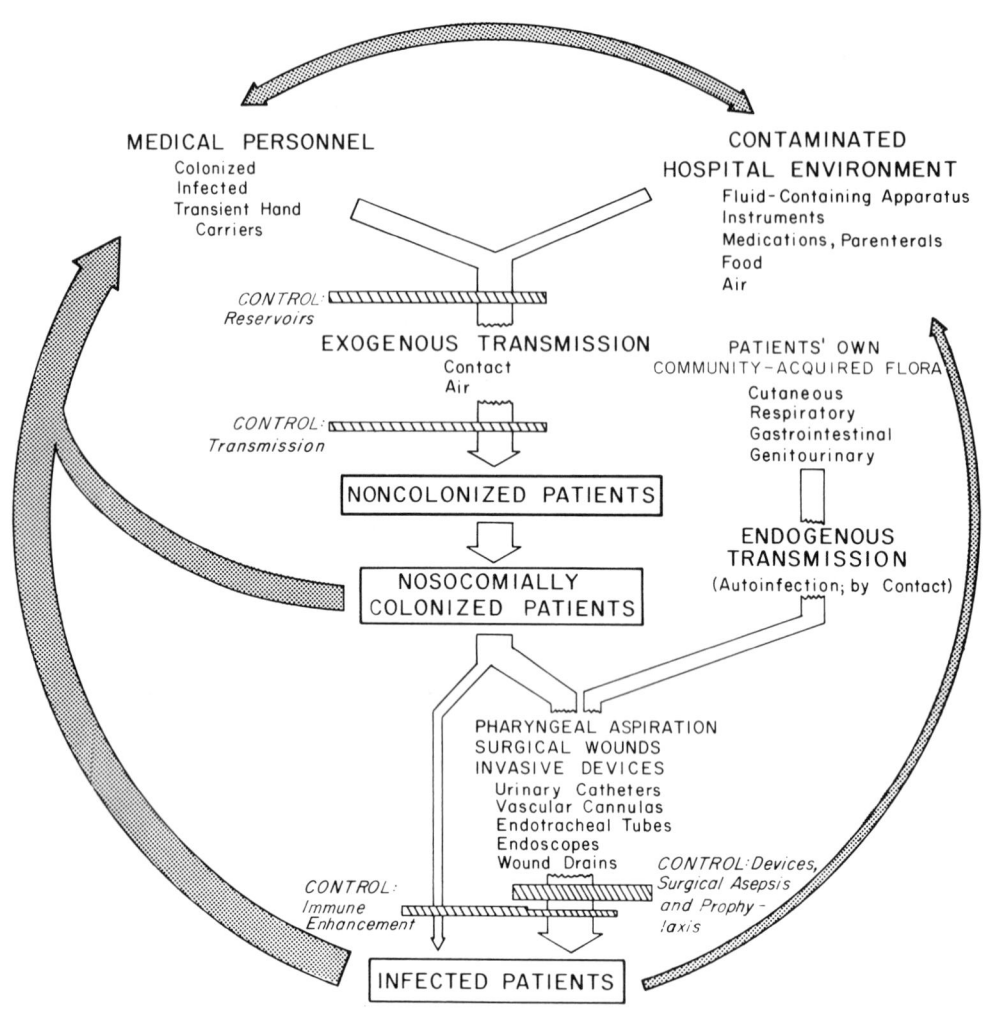

Figure 1 The epidemiology of nosocomial infection. Transmission occurs mainly by contact spread, to a much lesser extent by the airborne route. Antimicrobial therapy greatly modulates the profile of colonizing microorganisms. Aspiration, surgical wounds, and especially exposure to invasive devices amplify transmission, colonization, and susceptibility to infection by all routes. Republished with permission from Maki DG. Control of colonization and transmission of nosocomial bacteria in the hospital. Ann Intern Med 1978; 89:77.

CONTROL OF NOSOCOMIAL INFECTION

The Basic Hospital Infection Control Program

As explicitly mandated by the Joint Commission on Accreditation of Hospitals, every hospital is required to have an active Infection Control Committee, with representation from the major clinical services and hospital departments, including staff physicians, nurses, or respiratory therapists working in the institution's ICUs. The key members of the hospital's infection control program are the infection control nurse or nurses and the physician hospital epidemiologist, who implement policies developed by the committee, investigate suspected epidemics, and are responsible for assuring that hospital personnel are informed about nosocomial infection control (Table 3).

It is essential that individuals working in an ICU receive training in the epidemiology of nosocomial infection and especially in essential control measures. This is particularly important for houseofficers in teaching hospitals, who turn over rapidly and frequently come into the ICU with only the most rudimentary knowledge of asepsis. ICU physicians and nurses must be familiar with their hospital's protocols for the management of invasive devices, especially intravascular lines, urinary catheters, endotracheal tubes, and tracheostomies. Moreover, ICU physicians need to be sensitive to the hazards of broad-spectrum antimicrobial therapy, which greatly increases the risk of superinfection by antibiotic-resistant bacteria and *Candida*, and antibiotic-associated colitis caused by *Clostridium difficile*.

Table 2 Significant Risk Factors for Nosocomial Infection in the Intensive Care Unit as Determined by Multivariate Analysis of Prospectively-Collected Data Bases

Type of ICU (Investigators)	Risk Factors	Approximate Magnitude of Increased Risk*
Pediatric ICU (Goldmann et al)	Patent ductus arteriosus	28.2
	Low birth weight	—†
	Endotracheal tube	7.0
	Hyperalimentation	5.9
	Surgery	—
	High FIO_2	—
	Umbilical catheter	—
	Blood product therapy	—
Adult medical or surgical ICU (Craven et al)	Urinary catheter >10 days	3.2
	ICU confinement >3 days	2.5
	Intracranial pressure monitor	2.5
	Arterial line	1.5
	Shock	2.5

*Relative risk or odds ratio; values >1.0 denote significantly increased risk of infection, and ratios <1.0 denote decreased risk, vis-a-vis, a protective effect.
†Not reported or indeterminant (e.g., zero denominator).
Adapted from Maki DG. Risk factors for nosocomial infection in intensive care. Arch Intern Med 1989; 149:30–35.

Handwashing

Given the evidence that the major mode of spread of nosocomial organisms from patient to patient in the hospital is via the hands of hospital personnel, handwashing is imperative *before* a health care employee has manual contact with a vulnerable ICU patient, especially before examining an open wound, performing an invasive procedure, or even handling the patient's invasive devices; it is equally important *after* contact with a long-term patient, during which microbial contamination of the hands is likely to have occurred. More than 40 percent of ICU personnel randomly sampled can be shown to be carrying gram-negative bacilli, and approximately 10 percent can be shown to be carrying *S. aureus*, at any time. Yet, inexplicably, handwashing is performed inconsistently by many ICU personnel, especially physicians.

Three controlled trials have now demonstrated that the use of a chlorhexidine-containing solution, rather than a nonmedicated soap, for routine handwashing in an ICU significantly lowers the incidence of endemic nosocomial infection.

Reliable Chemical Disinfectants and Antiseptics

Reliable sterilization and disinfection embrace virtually all measures aimed at the prevention of nosocomial infection. Numerous epidemics of gram-negative infection have stemmed from the failure of a chemical germicide to disinfect critical reusable medical apparatus, such as respiratory therapy equipment, or to disinfect the skin before insertion of invasive devices. Remarkably, in many

Table 3 Facets of an Effective Hospital Nosocomial Infection Control Program

Active Infection Control Committee, with representation from most major departments and services, including the ICUs

Surveillance of nosocomial infections, especially in the ICUs

Comprehensive and regularly updated institutional policies and procedures for prevention of nosocomial infection

    Surveillance of nosocomial infections
    Isolation and universal precautions
    Sterilization and disinfection
    Indications for the use and management of invasive procedures and devices
        All types of intravascular catheters
        Hemodynamic monitoring
        Tracheostomies and endotracheal tubes
        Mechanical ventilation and other respiratory therapy
        Bronchoscopy and gastrointestinal endoscopy
        Hemodialysis
        Intracranial pressure monitoring
        Anesthesia and the operating room
        Intra-aortic balloon pumps
        Cardiopulmonary bypass
    Guidelines for use of antibiotics and utilization review
    Epidemic investigation

Educational programs for new employees and regular in-service updates dealing with nosocomial infection control

Active Employee Health Department:
    Free immunizations (hepatitis B, measles, rubella, influenza A)
    Post-exposure protocols

Quality assurance review of infection control practices

outbreaks, the epidemic organisms were actually cultured from an in-use solution of the germicide. Most of these outbreaks were traced to the use of unreliable chemical disinfectants or antiseptics, such as quaternary ammonium compounds or phenolic germicides. But alarmingly, iodophors such as povidone-iodine, which are the most widely used antiseptics for cutaneous disinfection in U.S. hospitals, have been implicated in four outbreaks of nosocomial infection over the past decade: *Pseudomonas* organisms were found to have contaminated the products in the manufacturers' plants.

Simple tincture of iodine (1 percent iodine in 70 percent alcohol), 70 percent alcohol alone, or an iodophor is currently recommended for skin disinfection. However, in a recent prospective trial in which ICU patients receiving central venous or arterial catheters were randomized to have 70 percent alcohol, 10 percent povidone-iodine, or a 2 percent chlorhexidine solution used for disinfection of the catheter insertion site, 70 percent alcohol was shown to be equivalent to povidone-iodine for the prevention of catheter-related infection, whereas the use of 2 percent chlorhexidine was associated with a threefold lower incidence of infection.

It is extremely important that the agent used be applied with vigorous rubbing for a minimum of 30 seconds, to allow adequate time for germicidal activity. Defatting the skin with acetone does not improve cutaneous antisepsis or reduce the risk of infection but has been shown to produce excessive inflammation.

Isolation Precautions

Isolation or special precautions for infected patients are the only means of curtailing the spread of contagious organisms and preventing epidemics, especially in ICUs, where the risk of cross-infection is very high. Although requiring all persons entering a patient's room to wear gloves and a gown, even a mask, may seem ritualistic, each aspect of the isolation procedure is directed at interrupting a potential mode of spread and is based on the known epidemiology of the infecting organism. To be maximally effective, however, isolation procedures require compliance by every individual coming into contact with the patient, including physicians. Isolation is indicated, usually for the entirety of hospitalization, for all patients infected (or even only colonized) by antibiotic-resistant nosocomial pathogens, such as methicillin-resistant *S. aureus* or gram-negative bacilli resistant to aminoglycosides or third-generation cephalosporins.

The world epidemic of acquired immunodeficiency syndrome (AIDS) and information indicating that in the U.S. more than one million persons are silent carriers of the human immunodeficiency virus (HIV) have engendered great concern among health care professionals regarding the risk of exposure to HIV in the hospital or clinic. In 1987, the Centers for Disease Control and the Department of Labor issued detailed guidelines for "Universal Precautions"—barrier precautions to prevent exposure of health care workers to potentially hazardous blood or body fluids which must be used with *all* patients:

1. It is recommended that gloves be worn when one is performing any venipunctures or insertions of intravascular devices, and whenever it can be anticipated that there could be potential for contamination of hands by blood or body fluids.
2. If there is potential for spatter of blood or body fluids or contamination of clothing, a gown should be worn.
3. Where there is potential for aerosolization of body fluids, such as during surgery, intubation, endoscopy, or insertion of an arterial catheter, a mask and eye shielding are included.
4. Since most occupation-related acquisitions of HIV have involved needle sticks or other "sharp" injuries, resulting in percutaneous inoculation of HIV or other bloodborne viruses, intense efforts must be made to avert accidental "sharp" injuries.

It has also been stated in the guidelines for "Universal Precautions" that it is important for ICU personnel not to wear gloves for prolonged periods. Unfortunately, this practice is quite common, resulting in heavy contamination of gloves and, ironically, in an increased risk of nosocomial cross-infection between patients.

Precautions for Use of Invasive Devices

As previously noted, the vast majority of nosocomial infections, especially in immunologically competent patients and in ICUs, are causally related to surgical operations or exposure to invasive devices of various types (see Tables 1 and 2 and Fig. 1). Comprehensive guidelines for the prevention of infection with those procedures or devices that pose the greatest risk (urinary catheters, endotracheal intubation and mechanical ventilatory support, intravascular catheters and infusion therapy, surgery, and hemodialysis) have been published and should form the basis for institutional policies and procedures (see Suggested Reading at the end of this chapter). Although discussion of specific control measures is beyond the scope of this chapter, all health care professionals working in ICUs are obligated to be informed about measures for prevention of infection associated with those devices that they use in their daily activities.

Restricted Use of Antibiotics

Antimicrobial therapy has its greatest ecologic impact in the confines of the ICU; most nosocomial outbreaks caused by antibiotic-resistant microorganisms and even yeasts have occurred in the small fraction of hospitalized patients in an ICU, and antibiotic pressure was usually found to be one of the most important factors predisposing patients to epidemic infection with resistant organisms. Modern-day ICUs are breeding grounds for the multiply resistant bacteria that are now being encountered in hospitals throughout the world—e.g., methicillin-resistant staphylococci, vancomycin-resistant enterococci, *Enterobacter*, *Serratia marcescens*, *Citrobacter*, Proteus-Providencia, and *Pseudomonas aeruginosa*, which are frequently resistant to aminoglycosides or extended-spectrum beta-lactams. Moreover, broad-spectrum antimicrobial therapy is the underlying cause of antibiotic-associated diarrhea and colitis caused by *C. difficile*. It is imperative that physicians and pharmacists direct much more attention to improving the use of systemic antibiotics, especially in ICUs.

Excellent resources, including other chapters in this book, are available to guide the selection and optimal use of anti-infective drugs in critically ill patients. Unnecessary antimicrobial therapy will be implicitly reduced and the drugs employed in this therapy used more effectively when the principles listed below are followed:

1. Fever without other indications of infection does not automatically mandate beginning antimicrobial therapy in an ICU patient.
2. Whenever antimicrobial therapy is begun, the reason should always be documented in the patient's record (e.g., "for treatment of pneumonia," "for prophylaxis in penetrating abdominal trauma").
3. The most narrow-spectrum drug or drugs should be used whenever possible, especially if the infecting organisms or organisms are known at the outset.

4. The need for continued antimicrobial therapy should be reassessed daily, and if cultures identify the infecting organisms, therapy should be modified, aiming for the most narrow-spectrum drugs likely to be effective.
5. Beyond monitoring for efficacy, it is essential that monitoring include surveillance for superinfection by resistant bacteria, *Candida* and *C. difficile.*

Many institutions place very expensive or the most broad-spectrum drugs (e.g., third-generation cephalosporins, imipenem, amikacin, ciprofloxacin, fluconazole, ganciclovir) on a restricted list, requiring that physicians who wish to use these drugs justify their use to a representative of the institutional antibiotic review committee. Such programs implicitly reduce the use of these antibiotics and are gaining increasing acceptance.

Avant Garde Control Measures

Selective Antimicrobial Decontamination

There has been intense interest in Europe and, increasingly, in the United States in the use of "selective antimicrobial decontamination" for prevention of bacterial pneumonia and other nosocomial infections in mechanically ventilated ICU patients. These studies are based on the concept that upper respiratory tract flora is in a continuum with the gastrointestinal flora and that, in concert, microorganisms from these two sources comprise the major reservoir of pathogens causing pneumonia and other nosocomial infections, especially in mechanically-ventilated patients. Most ventilated ICU patients have a nasogastric tube that provides a direct conduit for reflux of microorganisms from the heavily colonized stomach to the oropharynx, from which organisms gain access to the lower respiratory tract.

Selective digestive decontamination consists of scheduled applications of a nonabsorbable antimicrobial combination with activity against aerobic bacteria and yeasts but not anaerobes (such as polymyxin, gentamicin or tobramycin, and amphotericin B or nystatin) in a paste to the oropharynx and instillation into the stomach through a nasogastric tube; a broad-spectrum systemic antibiotic, such as a third-generation cephalosporin, may also be administered intravenously for the first 4 days that the patient is hospitalized in the ICU.

Although studies have demonstrated that selective antimicrobial decontamination results in a significant reduction in the incidence of ventilator-associated nosocomial pneumonia, it is difficult not to have reservations about the use of prophylactic antibiotics in large numbers of ICU patients. In the past, the heavy use of topical antibiotics prophylactically in ICUs has had catastrophic effects on the ecology of the institution, and until selective decontamination has been subjected to further scrutiny, it may be prudent to use it only in selected patients in institutions that have had a prohibitively high incidence of ventilator-associated nosocomial pneumonia.

According to recent reports, the use of a gastric barrier agent for stress ulcer prophylaxis (such as sucralfate) that preserves the natural gastric-acid barrier against bacterial overgrowth, rather than the use of antacids or H_2-blockers (such as cimetidine or ranitidine), significantly reduces the incidence of nosocomial pneumonia. These reports suggest an ecologically more attractive control measure for ventilated ICU patients than prophylactic topical and systemic antibiotics.

Protective Isolation

The use of simple barrier precautions prophylactically to prevent colonization and infection warrants further study. In a recent prospective randomized trial in a pediatric ICU, the use of disposable, nonwoven polypropylene gowns and latex gloves for all patient contacts reduced by 50 percent the incidence of nosocomial infection, fever days, and use of systemic antibiotics, and it did not compromise care in terms of reducing contacts with patients. Whether prophylactic barrier precautions would prove to be of similar benefit in adult ICU patients, however, is unproven, except in patients with major full-thickness burns.

APPROACH TO A NOSOCOMIAL EPIDEMIC

As noted, nosocomial epidemics are most likely to occur in ICUs. The epidemiologic approach to a suspected outbreak must be methodical and thorough, yet expeditious, directed towards establishing the existence of an epidemic, defining the reservoirs and modes of transmission of the epidemic pathogens, and most importantly, controlling the epidemic, quickly and completely (Table 4).

Table 4 Evaluation of a Possible Epidemic of Nosocomial Infections

1. Be prepared administratively

2. Retrieve putative epidemic isolates *immediately,* for subtyping to determine commonality

3. Make preliminary evaluations:
   Identify and characterize individual cases
   Ascertain if situation represents an *epidemic*
   Provisional control measures
   Intensify surveillance
   Review general infection control policies
   Determine need for assistance — especially extramural

4. Conduct epidemiologic investigations:
   Clinical-epidemiologic studies
   Microbiologic studies

5. Definitive control measures

6. Report findings

Adapted from Maki DG. Epidemic nosocomial bacteremias. In: Wenzel RR, ed. Handbook of hospital infection. West Palm Beach: C.R.C. Press, Inc., 1981:371.

It is essential that each hospital, through its Infection Control Committee, be prepared administratively to carry out an investigation and implement needed control measures. Detailed protocols have been published to guide the work-up of a nosocomial epidemic.

If epidemiologic or microbiologic studies suggest or indicate intrinsic contamination of a widely distributed commercial product or device, the local and state health authorities, the Food and Drug Administration, the Centers for Disease Control, and the manufacturer should be informed immediately. Remaining products should be quarantined and retained for evaluation by the public health authorities.

PROTECTION OF HEALTH CARE WORKERS IN THE INTENSIVE CARE UNIT

Persons working in ICUs and those exposed daily to critically ill patients (many of whom have contagious but unrecognized infections) are at risk for developing occupationally related infections—especially tuberculosis and, if the individual is susceptible to these diseases, hepatitis B, rubella, and measles. Although the risk of occupationally acquired HIV infection is very low, it is not zero; to date there have been approximately 30 instances of health care professionals who have acquired HIV infection from contact with an infected patient's blood, with nearly all of these incidents involving accidental needle sticks or other "sharp" injuries. The recent national epidemic of measles has resulted in severe measles in susceptible health care workers, who in turn exposed additional patients to the infection during its incubation phase.

Every effort must be made to assure that health care workers who have contact with patients and ICU personnel or their body fluids are immune to those pathogens for which effective vaccines are available, particularly measles, rubella, and hepatitis B. The vaccines for these viruses are highly effective and extremely safe. It is also recommended that health care workers be immunized against poliomyelitis and that they receive the influenza A vaccine annually.

Furthermore, every hospital should have an employee health service and written protocols for the management of health care workers sustaining biohazardous exposures. Such protocols permit expeditious and comprehensive evaluation and timely administration of postexposure prophylaxis with immune serum globulin or a hyperimmune globulin, or antimicrobial prophylaxis after exposure to virulent bacterial pathogens, such as *Neisseria meningitidis*. Some centers now offer zidovudine (AZT) for personnel sustaining a needle stick or other inoculation exposure to HIV, if the drug can be begun within several hours after the exposure.

The importance of uncompromising compliance with the guidelines for "Universal Precautions" of the Centers for Disease Control and Department of Labor to protect health care workers from exposure to HIV and other blood borne viruses has been discussed. It is most important that the greatest emphasis be placed on precautions to prevent needle sticks and other "sharp" injuries; the prohibition of recapping used needles and making impervious needle disposal containers available at the bedside of every ICU patient are mandatory.

ANTI-INFECTIVE THERAPY

Although it is beyond the scope of this chapter to discuss in detail the management of specific infections, particularly the selection and use of systemic antimicrobial therapy, which are addressed in detail elsewhere in this text, several facets of the management of *nosocomial* infection occurring in the ICU patient should be emphasized:

1. In the individual case, every effort must be made to identify the source of infection and, if possible, to remove that source—for example, through surgical drainage of an abscess, decompression of an obstructed ureter or common bile duct, closing of an intestinal perforation, removal of an infected intravascular catheter, surgical resection of a suppurative peripheral vein segment, discontinuation of an intravenous or intra-arterial infusion that contains huge numbers of gram-negative bacilli, or removal of a heavily contaminated hemodialysis machine. Such measures are crucial to survival and, in the case of nosocomial infection, may supersede antimicrobial therapy in assuring the patient's survival.

2. In most cases, the local infection giving rise to the symptoms of sepsis—especially with septic shock—is apparent clinically. If it is not, however, symptoms of overwhelming sepsis occurring in a patient with one or more risk factors for infection originating from a specific site (see Table 1) should intensify diagnostic efforts to identify infection at that site; in such cases, it is also recommended that all of the patient's intravascular catheters and infusions be replaced.

    Recovery of certain species in blood cultures points strongly towards specific sites of local infection (see Table 1). For example, *Bacteroides fragilis* almost invariably indicates an intraabdominal source; *Enterobacter* species, especially *Enterobacter agglomerans* or *Enterobacter cloacae*, *Pseudomonas cepacia*, *Pseudomonas maltophilia* or *Citrobacter* cultured from the blood of a patient receiving infusion therapy should prompt suspicion of contaminated infusate and may well signal an epidemic; high-grade bacteremia or candidemia, persisting after all of the patient's intravascular lines have been removed, should cause one to have a high index of suspicion for an endovascular focus of infection, and in the ICU, is much more likely to reflect septic thrombosis of one of the great central veins originating from a central venous catheter than it is to reflect endocarditis.

3. Nosocomial infections, in contradistinction to community-acquired infections, are far more likely to be caused by bacteria that are intrinsically

more resistant to antibiotics than community-acquired organisms: methicillin-resistant staphylococci; enterococci; resistant gram-negative bacilli such as *Enterobacter* species, *Serratia*, *Citrobacter*, or *P. aeruginosa*. In the initial antimicrobial regimen, this fact must always be taken into account.

Also, whereas it has been shown that effective prophylaxis for surgery rarely requires the use of more potent antibiotics than first-generation cephalosporins (e.g., cefazolin), in patients who have spent prolonged periods in an ICU and require surgery, the organisms most likely to produce postoperative surgical infection are usually resistant to such drugs, and it may therefore be appropriate to use more broad-spectrum drugs for surgical prophylaxis, such as a third-generation cephalosporin or even an antibiotic combination of a beta-lactam and an aminoglycoside. In general, the results of respiratory tract, skin, and urinary surveillance cultures can guide the selection of drugs most likely to be effective for preventing postoperative infection in a long-term ICU patient who requires surgery.

SUGGESTED READING

Centers for Disease Control. Guidelines for the Prevention and Control of Nosocomial Infections. Atlanta, GA: U.S. Department of Health and Human Services, 1981.
Centers for Disease Control. Recommendations for prevention of HIV transmission in health-care settings. Morbidity and Mortality Weekly Report. 1987; 36:801–816.
Craven DE, Kunches LM, Lichtenberg DA, et al. Nosocomial infection and fatality in medical surgical intensive care unit patients. Arch Intern Med 1988; 148:1161–1168.
Driks MR, Craven DE, Celli BA, et al. Nosocomial pneumonia in intubated patients randomized to sucralfate versus antacids and/or histamine type 2 blockers: the role of gastric colonization. N Engl J Med 1987; 317:1376–1382.
Farber BF, Infection control in intensive care. New York: Churchill Livingstone, 1987:1–214.
Garner JS, Farero MS. Guidelines for handwashing and hospital environmental control. Infect Control 1986; 7:231–243.
Goldmann DA, Durbin WA Jr, Freman J. Nosocomial infections in a neonatal intensive care unit. J Infect Dis 1981; 144:449–459.
Klein BS, Perloff WH, Maki DG. Reduction of nosocomial infection during pediatric intensive care by protective isolation. New Engl J Med 1989; 320:1714–1721.
Leddingham I Mc A, Alcock SR, Eastaway AT, et al. Triple regimen of selective decontamination of the digestive tract, systemic cefotaxime, and microbiological surveillance for preventions of acquired infection in intensive care. Lancet 1988; 1:785–790.
Maki DG. Epidemic nosocomial bacteremias. In: Wenzel RR, ed. Handbook of hospital infection. West Palm Beach: C.R.C. Press Inc., 1981:371.
Maki DG. Pathogenesis, prevention, and management of infections due to intravascular devices used for infusion therapy. In: Bisno A, Waldvogel F, eds. Infections associated with indwelling medical devices. Washington, DC: American Society for Microbiology, 1989:161–177.
Maki DG. Risk factors for nosocomial infection in intensive care. Arch Intern Med 1989; 149:30–35.

THE IMMUNOSUPPRESSED HOST

JOSEPH A. KOVACS, M.D.

For immunosuppressed patients who are infected and seriously ill, the approach to treatment is different from that for critically ill immunocompetent individuals. In either group of patients, an untreated or inadequately treated infection can rapidly cause irreversible damage or death. In immunosuppressed patients, however, the spectrum of causative organisms is different from that in immunocompetent individuals and thus demands different diagnostic and therapeutic approaches. To a large extent, the causative organisms in immunosuppressed patients are predictable, based on knowledge of their immunologic defect (Table 1), but the clinician must recognize that these patients are also exposed to the same pathogens as immunocompetent patients. Much of the therapy for immunosuppressed patients involves drugs or drug combinations that are directed against opportunistic pathogens and are thus different from therapies for immunologically normal patients when either empiric or specific therapy is considered (Table 2).

In a critical care setting, the infectious syndromes most commonly encountered in immunosuppressed patients are fever and neutropenia, septic shock, diffuse pneumonia, and meningitis. The first of these topics is covered elsewhere in this text; the latter three topics are the subject of this chapter.

SEPTIC SHOCK

The general approach to septic shock and other forms of distributive shock (discussed in detail elsewhere in this text) is applicable to immunosuppressed patients. In choosing broad-spectrum antimicrobial agents, however, certain modifications are appropriate. These modifications do not replace the need to evaluate the patient thoroughly so that a likely causative agent can be identified. For the neutropenic patient, the antibacterial regimen should include at least two drugs with activity against likely gram-negative bacilli, including *Pseudomonas aeruginosa*. Acceptable adult regimens are chosen on the basis of microorganism-susceptibility patterns and drug cost in individual hospitals, but in the absence of localizing clues the regimen would include (1) cephalothin, 2 g intravenously every 4 hours; and gentamicin, 1 to 1.5 mg per kilogram intravenously every 6 hours; and ticarcillin, 3 g intravenously every 4 to 6 hours; (2) ceftazidime, 2 g intravenously every

Table 1 Common Causative Organisms for Infectious Disease Syndromes in Immunosuppressed Patients

Inflammatory and Immune Defect	Septic Shock	Pneumonia	CNS Infection
Neutropenia	Gram-negative and gram-positive bacteria, especially *Pseudomonas aeruginosa*, *Klebsiella-Enterobacter* species, *Escherichia coli*, and *Staphylococcus aureus;* after prolonged antibiotics, *Candida* species	Gram-negative and gram-positive bacteria, after prolonged antibiotics, *Aspergillus* species	Gram-negative and gram-positive bacteria, *Aspergillus* species
Complement deficiency	*Neisseria* species	—	*Neisseria meningitides*
Humoral deficiency	*Streptococcus pneumoniae*, *Haemophilus influenzae*	*S. pneumoniae*, *H. influenzae*	*S. pneumoniae*, *H. influenzae*
Cell-mediated deficiency	*Listeria monocytogenes*	*Pneumocystis carinii*, *Legionella* species, herpes simplex virus, herpes zoster virus, cytomegalovirus	*Listeria monocytogenes*, *Cryptococcus neoformans*, *Toxoplasma gondii*

Table 2 Drugs of Choice for Common Causative Organisms in Immunosuppressed Patients

Organism	Drug(s)	Route	Minimum Duration or Dose*
Virus			
Herpes simplex	Acyclovir, 5 mg/kg, q8h	IV	7–14 days
Herpes zoster	Acyclovir, 10 mg/kg, q8h	IV	7–14 days
Cytomegalovirus	Ganciclovir, 5 mg/kg, q12h	IV	14 days
Bacteria			
Staphylococcus aureus	Nafcillin, 2 g, q4h; *or* cefazolin, 2 g, q6h	IV	10–14 days
Staphylococcus epidermidis	Vancomycin, 1.0 g, q12h	IV	10–14 days
Pseudomonas aeruginosa	Tobramycin, 1.5 mg/kg, q6h *plus* ticarcillin, 3.5 g, q6h	IV	10–14 days
Klebsiella-Enterobacter species	Gentamicin, 1.5 mg/kg, q8h	IV	10–14 days
Other enteric gram-negative organisms	Gentamicin, 1.5 mg/kg, q6h; *and* cefazolin, 2 g q6h	IV	10–14 days
Haemophilus influenzae	Cefamandole, 1.5 g, q4h; *or* third-generation cephalosporin (e.g., cefotaxime)	IV	10–14 days
Fungi			
Candida species	Amphotericin B, 0.6 mg/kg/d	IV	1–2 g total dosage
Aspergillus species	Amphotericin B, 0.6 mg/kg/d	IV	1–2 g total dosage
Cryptococcus neoformans	Amphotericin B, 0.3–0.6 mg/kg/d *plus* flucytosine	IV PO	6 weeks
Pneumocystis carinii	Trimethoprim, 5 mg/kg, q6h, *plus* sulfamethoxazole, 25 mg/kg, q6h	IV IV	14 days 14 days
Protozoa			
Toxoplasma gondii	Pyrimethamine, 25 mg/d, *plus* sulfadiazine, 1 g, q6h	PO PO	4–6 weeks 4–6 weeks

*Patients with AIDS will usually require a suppressive regimen following acute therapy because of the high incidence of relapse of virtually all opportunistic infections.

8 hours; and amikacin, 7.5 mg per kilogram intravenously every 12 hours; (3) vancomycin, 1 g intravenously every 12 hours; and tobramycin, 1.0 to 1.5 mg per kilogram intravenously every 6 hours; and piperacillin, 3 to 4 g intravenously every 4 to 6 hours. To achieve optimal levels immediately, the initial dose of tobramycin or gentamicin should probably be 2 mg per kilogram. In certain clinical settings, these regimens must be modified by the addition of other drugs: (1) if the patient is known to be colonized by an organism resistant to the broad-spectrum regimen chosen or if the patient has recently been in a hospital or a unit known to be experiencing an outbreak with a resistant pathogen, a drug with activity against the resistant organism should be added or substituted into the "standard" regimen; (2) if an anaerobic organism is suspected, the addition of clindamycin, 600 mg intravenously every 6 hours, or metronidazole, 750 mg intravenously every 8 hours, would be appropriate; (3) if intravenous line sepsis is a strong possibility, the regimen should include vancomycin, 1 g intravenously every 12 hours; (4) if a respiratory source suggestive of *Haemophilus* is suspected, cefamandole, 2 g intravenously every 6 hours or cefuroxime, 1.5 g intravenously every 8 hours, or a third-generation cephalosporin would be appropriate; or (5) if results of culture or a Gram's stain indicate a causative organism not covered by the initial regimen, another drug might be added, e.g., vancomycin would be added, if gram-positive rods consistent with *Corynebacterium* were seen in a gram-stained sample from a wound. Empiric antifungal therapy for most immunosuppressed hosts who present with septic shock is not generally given initially. Once the results of blood cultures or cultures of other sites reveal a likely causative organism, a broad-spectrum regimen should be adjusted to include appropriate coverage and continued until symptoms resolve and for at least 10 days to 2 weeks.

For patients with defects in humoral immune function, the broad-spectrum regimen for septic shock should include coverage for *Streptococcus pneumoniae* and *Haemophilus influenzae*; chloramphenicol, 1 g intravenously every 4 to 6 hours, or cefamandole, 2 g intravenously every 6 hours, or cefotaxime, 2 g intravenously every 6 hours, would be an appropriate antibiotic to include in the broad-spectrum regimen covering other likely pathogens.

For patients with cellular immune defects, antimicrobial therapy must consider coverage of *Listeria monocytogenes* (ampicillin, 2 g intravenously every 4 hours, and gentamicin, 1.0 to 1.5 mg per kilogram intravenously every 6 hours) and *Cryptococcus neoformans* or *Candida* species (amphotericin B), depending on the specific underlying disease, the clinical presentation, and the results of rapidly available tests such as serum cryptococcal antigen determination.

For patients with certain complement disorders (especially deficiencies in C1a, C3, C5 through C8) coverage of neisserial infections (particularly *Neisseria meningitides*) is important: ampicillin, 2 g intravenously every 4 hours, or chloramphenicol, 1 g intravenously every 6 hours, would be appropriate.

The duration of antimicrobial therapy in any immunosuppressed patient who has been septic should be at least 10 to 14 days. Longer courses may be needed if the patient has a slow response to therapy, an undrained focus of infection, or a persistent immunologic defect, but there are no firm and objective guidelines to delineate what the optimal duration is.

The serum antibiotic concentrations of all patients with septic shock must be carefully monitored, especially for aminoglycosides, which have a low therapeutic-to-toxic index. Dose modification made on objective or empiric grounds are particularly important in immunosuppressed patients whose hepatic and renal functions have often been compromised by the underlying disease, hypotension, or previous therapies. Gentamicin and tobramycin levels should be measured at least three times weekly and maintained at peak concentrations of 4 to 10 μg per milliliter and trough concentrations of 1 to 2 μg per milliliter; amikacin peak and trough levels should be 20 to 35 μg per milliliter and 5 to 10 μg per milliliter, respectively.

Recent randomized studies have documented that bolus administration of corticosteroids at the onset of septic shock is not beneficial and may be harmful in certain subpopulations; therefore, corticosteroids should not be routinely administered to patients with septic shock. Consideration, however, must be given to the need for stress coverage with hydrocortisone acetate, 100 mg intravenously every 8 hours, for any patient who might have adrenal insufficiency due to steroid therapy for the underlying disease during the previous year or due to destruction of the adrenal glands by disease or therapy. Surgical drainage of abscesses is as urgent in septic immunosuppressed patients as in immunocompetent individuals.

Immunoadjuvant therapies such as immunoglobulin infusions, granulocyte transfusions, or administration of complement or transfer factor have uncertain efficacy in most clinical situations, although for certain disorders they may occasionally be useful.

DIFFUSE PNEUMONIA

In immunocompromised patients, multilobed pneumonia can be caused by a wide spectrum of infectious and noninfectious processes, and thus a definitive diagnostic procedure is usually necessary to determine the appropriate therapy. Pending a definitive diagnosis based on evaluation of induced sputum or other pulmonary secretions, bronchoalveolar lavage, or lung tissue it is appropriate to initiate empiric therapy for likely infectious processes.

If infiltrates are bilateral and interstitial, sputum production is scanty or nil, and induced sputum is nondiagnostic, appropriate empiric therapy would include erythromycin, 1 g intravenously every 6 hours, for *Legionella* and *Mycoplasma pneumoniae* and trimethoprim-sulfamethoxazole, 320 mg of trimethoprim and 1,600 mg of sulfamethoxazole intravenously every 8 hours, for *Pneu-*

mocystis. If the history or physical examination or Gram's stain of sputum strongly suggests a bacterial process, one of the regimens suggested in this chapter for septic shock should be added, since gram-positive or gram-negative bacterial processes can occasionally cause diffuse interstitial disease.

If the infiltrates are alveolar on the chest roentgenogram, a broad-spectrum regimen would be appropriate, such as one of those suggested in this chapter for sepsis—i.e., cephalothin-gentamicin-ticarcillin, or ceftazidime-amikacin. Erythromycin and trimethoprim-sulfamethoxazole should be added, since *Legionella* and *Pneumocystis* can cause diffuse alveolar infiltrates, particularly in advanced cases. Fungal pneumonias caused by *Cryptococcus, Aspergillus, Mucor,* or occasionally by *Candida* are also considerations, and these would require therapy with amphotericin B. Aggressive attempts to establish the specific diagnoses are highly recommended. Placement of a pulmonary artery catheter to evaluate the contribution of cardiac dysfunction should also be considered.

If *Pneumocystis* is established as the causative agent, trimethoprim-sulfamethoxazole is usually preferred over pentamidine isethionate (4 mg per kilogram once daily given over 60 to 90 minutes intravenously) because trimethoprim-sulfamethoxazole is usually less toxic than pentamidine, though both are equally effective. Even in patients with acquired immunodeficiency syndrome (AIDS) in whom trimethoprim-sulfamethoxazole is associated with an unusually high frequency of adverse reactions, trimethoprim-sulfamethoxazole is preferred. When trimethoprim-sulfamethoxazole therapy is given, the intravenous route is preferred over the oral route until the patient clearly improves; peak serum levels of sulfamethoxazole 60 to 90 minutes after infusion should be maintained between 100 and 150 μg per milliliter and adjusted for renal dysfunction; leucovorin calcium may be given concurrently (5 to 10 mg intravenously daily) to prevent bone marrow depression. For patients who fail on either pentamidine or trimethoprim-sulfamethoxazole, no useful data are available to support adding the alternative drug as opposed to switching agents. Alternative therapies with trimetrexate, dapsone, clindamycin-primaquine, or alpha-difluoromethyl ornithine (DFMO) have been inadequately evaluated to date. Recent studies suggest that corticosteroids are beneficial as adjunctive therapy in patients with hypoxia (PaO$_2$ $\leq$70 mm Hg) due to *P. carinii* pneumonia. Although the optimal dose, time for intervention, and duration of steroids has not been determined, methyl prednisolone at 40 to 60 mg one to four times per day, administered on a tapering schedule over 21 days appears beneficial.

Antimicrobial therapy should be continued for a minimum of 14 to 21 days. Repeat bronchoscopy at the end of therapy is not clinically necessary. Following successful completion of therapy, a prophylactic regimen for prevention of recurrent *P. carinii* should be initiated in patients with AIDS, in whom there is a high relapse rate. Regimens with documented efficacy include trimethoprim-sulfamethoxazole (one double strength tablet twice a day) or aerosol pentamidine (300 mg administered monthly by the Respirgard II nebulizer).

If legionellosis is established as the etiology, many authorities recommend using a high-dose regimen of erythromycin (1 g intravenously or orally every 6 hours) for at least 4 weeks. There is no convincing evidence that such a regimen is more effective than 500 mg every 6 hours for 14 to 21 days. Rifampin, 600 mg orally daily, should be added to erythromycin regimens in desperately ill patients. Alternative therapies to erythromycin have received limited testing, but tetracycline (500 mg orally every 6 hours), trimethoprim-sulfamethoxazole (320 mg of trimethoprim and 1,600 mg of sulfamethoxazole intravenously every 8 hours), and ciprofloxacin (750 mg orally every 12 hours) are reasonable possibilities.

If a viral process is shown to be the etiologic agent, only herpes simplex, herpes zoster, and cytomegalovirus (CMV) are among commonly identified etiologic agents potentially treatable at this time. Acyclovir—5 mg per kilogram intravenously every 8 hours for herpes simplex, and 10 mg per kilogram every 8 hours for herpes zoster—can be effective if instituted early and continued for at least 14 to 21 days. Urine flow should be maintained to prevent crystalluria, and the dose reduced if renal failure ensues. Both ganciclovir, which has been recently approved, and foscarnet, which is currently available on an experimental basis only, are active in vitro against CMV and will lead to improvement in CMV retinitis in immunosuppressed patients. The experience in patients with CMV pneumonia has been more limited and less promising, but these agents should be considered in patients with documented CMV pneumonia.

CENTRAL NERVOUS SYSTEM INFECTION

Compared with immunocompetent patients, immunosuppressed patients have a relatively higher incidence of intracranial abscess and empyema than meningitis. Even when cerebrospinal fluid (CSF) analysis suggests meningitis, strong consideration should be given to documenting whether abscess or empyema is present so that therapy can be directed appropriately.

For meningitis, the choice of empiric therapy is based on evaluation of the individual patient and knowledge about the underlying immunologic defect. For neutropenic patients in whom gram-negative bacillary meningitis is a major concern, particularly if diagnostic or therapeutic procedures involving their central nervous system (CNS) have been performed, appropriate empiric regimens, when no source is obvious, are as follows: ceftazidime alone, 2 g intravenously every 6 hours; or gentamicin, 1.0 to 1.5 mg per kilogram every 6 hours, and 3 to 6 mg intrathecally every 24 hours (the latter using preservative-free drug); plus piperacillin, 3 to 4 g intravenously every 4 hours. If these patients have intracranial foreign bodies such as Ommaya reservoirs or various types of shunts, or have had recent neurosurgery, vancomycin, 1.0 g intravenously every 12 hours, should be added.

For meningitis in patients with humoral or complement deficiencies, empiric regimens with coverage of *S. pneumoniae* and *H. influenzae* would include chloramphenicol, 1 g intravenously every 6 hours, or cefotaxime, 2.0 g intravenously every 6 hours.

For patients with cellular immune defects, regimens should include adequate coverage for *Listeria monocytogenes*. Such regimens would include ampicillin, 2 g intravenously every 4 hours, and gentamicin, 1.0 to 1.5 mg per kilogram intravenously every 6 hours; or erythromycin, 1.0 g intravenously every 6 hours, and choloramphenicol, 1.0 g intravenously every 6 hours.

Patients with meningitis should be treated for a minimum of 14 days; longer courses are indicated in severely immunosuppressed patients, particularly if the immunosuppression is likely to be transient. The dosage of aminoglycosides needs to be monitored and adjusted, as already discussed. Follow-up assessment with repeat lumbar punctures is useful, but not mandatory.

If India ink or CSF cryptococcal antigen documents cryptococcal meningitis, amphotericin B (0.5 to 1 mg per kilogram per day) alone or combined with flucytosine should be administered. In patients who do not have AIDS, the combination is preferable and therapy can be discontinued after 6 weeks if clinical and laboratory improvement have occurred. In patients with AIDS, no advantage of combination therapy has been documented; after 1 to 2 gm of amphotericin B, a suppressive regimen of either amphotericin B or fluconazole, a recently approved antifungal agent, should be initiated and continued for life.

If a brain abscess is suspected because of focal neurologic signs or increased intracranial pressure, a computed tomography (CT) scan with contrast material should be performed prior to the spinal tap. If an abscess is present, the puncture should not be done from a lumbar approach if the lesion is subtentorial or if there are signs of increased intracranial pressure. If CSF analysis is needed and an abscess if either suspected or known to be present, a cisternal tap is probably safer than a lumbar puncture.

Therapy of a space-occupying CNS mass lesion must often be empiric while awaiting a definitive diagnostic procedure. For patients with cellular immune defects, pyrimethamine, 25 to 75 mg orally daily; and sulfadiazine, 1 to 2 g orally every 6 hours; with leucovorin calcium, 10 mg intravenously daily; plus ampicillin, 2 g intravenously every 4 hours, would be appropriate if the serum and CSF cryptococcal antigen tests are negative. For leukopenic patients, a regimen of vancomycin, 1.0 g intravenously every 12 hours; and ceftazidime, 2 g intravenously every 8 hours; or vancomycin and amikacin, 7.5 mg per kilogram intravenously every 12 hours; and piperacillin, 3 to 4 g intravenously every 4 hours, would be appropriate. The concurrent administration of dexamethasone to prevent cerebral edema prior to surgery is controversial but should probably be avoided unless increased intracranial pressure and herniation are imminent problems.

If *Toxoplasma gondii* is documented to be the cause of the mass lesion, pyrimethamine and sulfadiazine should be continued with leucovorin for at least 6 weeks, and for life, possibly at a lower dose, if the patient has AIDS. If the patient cannot take oral drugs, a sulfa drug can be given intravenously; the pyrimethamine must be administered by nasogastric tube. Trimethoprim-sulfamethoxazole is a less desirable therapeutic alternative. No other drugs have been documented to be effective, although high-dose pyrimethamine (75 mg per day) alone or combined with clindamycin, has anecdotally been reported to be effective. Corticosteroids have no therapeutic role in this disease unless increased intracranial pressure is a life-threatening problem. Bone marrow function should be carefully monitored (by granulocyte and platelet counts) at least twice weekly during therapy.

SUGGESTED READING

Armstrong D, Brown E, eds. Controversies in the management of infectious complications of enoplastic disease. Rev Infect Dis 1989; 11:S1527–S1710.

Hughes WT, Armstrong I, Bodey GP, et al. From the Infectious Disease Society of America: Guidelines for the use of antimicrobial agents in neutropenic patients with unexplained fever. J Infect Dis 1990; 161:381–396.

Pizzo PA. Empiric therapy and prevention of infection in the immunocompromised host. In: Mandell GL, Douglas RG Jr., Bennett JE, eds. Principles and practice of infectious diseases. 3rd ed. New York: Churchill Livingstone, 1990.

Rubin RH, Young LS, eds. Clinical approach to infection in the compromised host. New York: Plenum Publishing Corp, 1981.

Walzer PD, Gentra RM, eds. Parasitic infections in the compromised host. New York: Marcel Dekker, 1989.

ANTIBIOTIC USAGE IN THE INTENSIVE CARE UNIT

HENRY MASUR, M.D.

Infections are frequently the cause for patient admission to intensive care units (ICUs). Infections are also common complications for patients already in the ICU for other life-threatening problems. When there is evidence suggesting that infection is occurring in either of these situations, it should be intuitively obvious that prompt and potent therapy is needed if the patient's chance for survival and optimal recovery is to be maximized.

The administration of antimicrobial therapy for critically ill patients differs from the management approach in other patient populations: (1) antimicrobial therapy must be instituted more promptly, (2) it is more crucial that the offending pathogen be covered by the initial regimen, (3) one drug alone may not suffice for certain organisms, (4) pharmacokinetics are likely to be distorted, and (5) drug interactions and toxicities are more likely to occur.

INITIATION OF ANTIBIOTIC THERAPY

Urgency is an important principle when initiating antimicrobial therapy in the ICU. Initial efforts to stabilize a critically ill patient may require emphasis on airway control, mechanical ventilation, intravascular volume augmentation, pressor administration, and surgical exploration or repair. If there is a reasonable possibility that infection is causing some or all of the life-threatening process, then an expeditious work-up to identify the specific offending pathogen is appropriate. Very quickly, however, either specific antibiotics must be administered, if the offending organism and its likely antimicrobial susceptibility are known, or empiric therapy must be administered. Meningitis is the best example of where several hours' delay can have a major detrimental effect on outcome. It makes sense, similarly, to start therapy for sepsis, extensive pneumonia, or peritonitis as soon as possible. Health care professionals must recognize that writing an order for antibiotics is not the same as administering the antibiotic. Although this concept is intellectually obvious, all too often drugs may not be administered to the patient promptly because the antibiotic order was not written or the drug was not administered expeditiously because the pharmacy, the messenger service, the nurse, or the physician had competing claims on their time and attention. Thus, the intensivist must complete the preliminary evaluation quickly and, if antibiotic therapy is needed, must make certain that the patient receives the indicated drug(s) promptly. This may require providing additional intravenous access sites so that numerous important drugs can be administered simultaneously.

BROAD-SPECTRUM EMPIRIC THERAPY

When a patient has a life-threatening infection that requires intensive care or which develops in the ICU, the antimicrobial therapy chosen must cover all likely pathogens. For non–life-threatening processes treated on general hospital wards or in outpatient settings, failure to treat the offending pathogen may allow the infection to exacerbate, but such failure does not usually lead directly to death or severe morbidity. In the ICU it is always desirable to identify the offending microorganism quickly so that antimicrobial therapy can be directed and specific. Practically, however, the offending organism and its susceptibility are often not known initially. Even if Gram's stain or serology (e.g., cerebrospinal fluid counter-immunoelectrophoresis or serum cryptococcal antigen test) or preliminary culture report (from material submitted previously) identifies a likely cause, there is often uncertainty about several matters: (1) if the identified pathogen is relevant (i.e., could it be unrelated to the life-threatening process?); (2) if the identified pathogen is the only causative agent (i.e., if gram-negative bacilli are seen in ascitic fluid, could anaerobic cocci or *Enterococcus faecalis* also be present?); and (3) if the susceptibility of the pathogen can reliably be predicted (e.g., if 90 percent of the hospital's *Haemophilus influenzae* are sensitive to ampicillin, and 98 percent are sensitive to chloramphenicol, should ampicillin alone be used, or should chloramphenicol alone be used, or should both be used until final susceptibility results are known?). In life-threatening circumstances, most prudent clinicians prefer to cover for all pathogens and all susceptibility patterns that are reasonably likely to occur. Not every conceivable microbial etiology can be treated empirically. Some pathogens almost never cause certain clinical syndromes (e.g., *S. faecalis* virtually never causes pneumonia or meningitis). Also, for most common pathogens, no single drug is universally and invariably active (e.g., penicillin-resistant *Streptococcus pneumoniae* exist, as do vancomycin-resistant *S. faecalis*, nafcillin-resistant *Staphylococcus aureus*, amikacin-resistant *Pseudomonas aeruginosa*, acyclovir-resistant herpes simplex, and ganciclovir-resistant cytomegalovirus), but it is not reasonable or practical to add enough drugs to cover all conceivable possibilities, especially when multiple pathogens may be included in the differential diagnosis. There is a fine margin between providing broad, comprehensive coverage and providing redundant, unnecessary coverage. With each additional drug added, the risks for drug toxicity, undesirable drug interactions, superinfection, and excessive cost increase. Only experience and good judgment can determine what is reasonable for an individual patient.

The choice of empiric antimicrobial regimens for severely ill patients is complicated by the fact that the differential diagnosis is often much more extensive than in other patient populations. The differential diagnosis may be relatively narrow in an immunologically normal patient who is admitted to the ICU with a community-acquired meningitis or pneumonia. For a patient who has acquired an infection while in the ICU, however, the differential diagnosis may include a wide variety of gram-positive cocci, gram-negative bacilli, and fungi, some of which may have very unusual susceptibility patterns because of selective pressures in hospital environments. Thus the physician must recognize how extensive the differential diagnosis is and must treat for all likely pathogens until the etiologic agents are known. This may involve the use of one to three, four, or even five antibiotics, depending on the need to cover fungal, viral, protozoan, bacterial, or mycobacterial pathogens. The choice of empiric regimens requires knowledge of the susceptibility patterns in a specific hospital. Gentamicin, for example, may be a reasonable choice for empiric therapy of gram-negative bacillary infections in hospitals with infrequent gentamicin-resistant pathogens. Amikacin may be a better alternative, however, in hospitals where a substantial fraction of *Serratia*, *Klebsiella*, or *Enterobacter* species, for example, are gentamicin-resistant. Similarly, in hospitals where methicillin-resistant *S. aureus* (MRSA) is common, vancomycin should be used in preference to nafcillin for possible *S. aureus* infections.

SINGLE VERSUS COMBINATION DRUG REGIMENS FOR SPECIFIC PATHOGENS

When a patient has a potentially life-threatening infectious process, many experts believe that certain pathogens are optimally treated with multidrug regimens. Thus, when designing either empiric or specific regimens, physicians may need to choose several drugs for an individual pathogen. With the advent of potent new agents such as imipenem, timentin, and ceftazidime, the need for multiple-drug therapy directed against individual pathogens has become more controversial. Nevertheless, multiple-drug regimens are often advocated for optimal therapy of enteric gram-negative bacilli (such as *Escherichia coli*, *Klebsiella* species, and *Enterobacter* species), *Pseudomonas* species, *Staphylococcus aureus*, enterococci, and *Cryptococcus neoformans*. If the combination can be shown to be synergistic and to produce bactericidal activity in serum, studies suggest better clinical efficacy. In some situations, the need for two-drug therapy has been well documented: *Pseudomonas aeruginosa* infections appear to respond better to synergistic combinations of an aminoglycoside and a penicillin derivative with antipseudomonas activity (e.g., gentamicin and piperacillin) than to an aminoglycoside alone. There are in vitro microbiologic data and animal studies to support these clinical observations. Thus, in any life-threatening situation in which *P. aeruginosa* is suspected, an aminoglycoside alone would never be used, regardless of whether the patient were neutropenic. For suspected or proven infection due to enteric gram-negative bacilli, clinical data from neutropenic patients support the use of multiple-drug regimens, and those data have been extrapolated to life-threatening infections regardless of the neutrophil count. For fungi such as *C. neoformans* or *Candida* species, or for bacteria such as *S. aureus* (nonendocarditis), *Legionella pneumophila*, or enterococci (nonendocarditis), the enhanced efficacy of combination regimens has not been as well established, although many experts believe strongly that combination therapy should be used based on in vitro observations, animal models, or suggestive but uncontrolled clinical observations. When choosing empiric or specific antimicrobial regimens, clinicians must recognize that life-threatening infections may be most effectively treated by combination therapy. When treating specific infections such as cryptococcal meningitis, clinicians also need to be cognizant that combination therapy may offer the benefit of decreased toxicity: When flucytosine is used in combination with amphotericin B, for example, lower doses of amphotericin can be administered without sacrificing efficacy, but this results in decreased amphotericin B toxicity. Thus, combination therapy is an important strategy that can influence efficacy and toxicity.

PHARMACOKINETICS IN CRITICALLY ILL PATIENTS

When administering antimicrobial agents to critically ill patients, clinicians need to recognize that the pharmacokinetics of the drug may be quite abnormal, requiring alterations in dosing regimens. Patients often have renal insufficiency, hepatic insufficiency, altered volumes of distribution, and hypoalbuminemia. They may be receiving other drugs that influence hepatic metabolism or cause hepatic or renal toxicity. Thus, drug doses need to be chosen carefully. In life-threatening situations, loading antibiotic doses must often be given to achieve effective serum levels quickly. The loading dose may have to be increased if a patient's volume of distribution has recently increased owing to, for example, 10 L of fluid resuscitation. If the patient develops acute tubular necrosis due to hypotension, or renal failure due to cisplatin toxicity, then subsequent dosing intervals will have to be adjusted. The use of drugs for which laboratory monitoring of serum levels is readily available greatly enhances the likelihood that effective but nontoxic regimens will be used. Thus, the ability to obtain regular serum aminoglycoside levels may be of sufficient benefit so that aminoglycosides may be very attractive agents in some situations despite their toxicity.

TOXICITIES AND DRUG INTERACTIONS

Antimicrobial agents are associated with adverse effects and toxicities. These adverse effects and toxicities may be additive or synergistic with those associated with other drugs that the patient is receiving. The choice of antimicrobial agents needs to be influenced by the likelihood that a specific patient will develop toxicity and how well that patient is likely to be able to tolerate the toxicity. The use of a drug like ganciclovir to treat cytomegalovirus (CMV) colitis in a patient receiving zidovudine for acquired immunodeficiency syndrome (AIDS) dementia, or trimethoprim-sulfamethoxazole for active pneumocystis pneumonia, may be undesirable because of the high probability that significant neutropenia may occur. Thus, if the trimethoprim-sulfamethoxazole or zidovudine is believed

Table 1 "Standard" Antibiotic Armamentarium for Intensive Care Specialists

Penicillins	Macrolides
Penicillin G	Erythromycin
Nafcillin	Clindamycin
Ampicillin	
Piperacillin	Antifungal Agents
	Amphotericin B
Cephalosporins	Fluconazole
Cefazolin	
Cefuroxime	Antimycobacterial Agents
Ceftriaxone	Isoniazid
Ceftazidime	Rifampin
	Ethambutol
Other Antibacterial Agents	
Vancomycin	Antiviral Agents
Metronidazole	Acyclovir
	Ganciclovir
Aminoglycosides	
Gentamicin	Antiprotozoan Agents
	Pentamidine

to be essential, a nonmarrow suppressive agent for CMV such as phosphonoformate (Foscarnet) may be necessary. Beta-lactam drugs generally have less severe toxicities than aminoglycosides, for instance, and are therefore preferred by some intensivists for the therapy of gram-negative bacillary infections, especially if the patient may already have poor renal function due to hypotension, urinary tract obstruction, previous exposure to nephrotoxins, or diabetes mellitus. If the beta-lactams are equally as effective as aminoglycosides, this may be a reasonable strategy, although many experts prefer aminoglycosides even in such a setting because of their extensively proven efficacy and the availability of serum concentration monitoring.

When choosing antimicrobial regimens, clinicians must recognize that alteration of host microbial flora can adversely affect outcome. Multiple-drug regimens may be necessary to prevent clinical deterioration and death, but reducing the number of administered drugs as soon as possible reduces the number of potential toxicities, the number of potentially deleterious drug interactions, and the alteration of host flora. Antibiotic pressure allows colonization and overgrowth by fungi and by drug-resistant bacteria. Life-threatening superinfections due to *Candida*, *Aspergillus*, resistant *Pseudomonas* species, enterococci, multiple-drug resistant gram-negative bacilli, or *Clostridium difficile* may result. Thus, while broad-spectrum regimens may be desirable as initial therapy, reduction in the number of drugs and extent of antimicrobial coverage as expeditiously as possible has many potential benefits.

MONITORING DRUG LEVELS

Monitoring antibiotic levels is especially important in critically ill patients. Failure to attain therapeutic levels can have life-threatening consequences; thus regular measurement of levels is important for maximizing the likelihood of successful therapy. In addition, monitoring to avoid toxicity is especially important in a patient population in which pharmacokinetics may be difficult to predict. This

Table 2 Empiric Antimicrobial Regimens for Adults With Common Life-Threatening Infections

Clinical Syndrome	Potential Regimens	Usual Initial Adult Dosing Regimen	Comments
Septic Shock			
Community-acquired	Nafcillin and	2 g IV q4h	No coverage for
	Piperacillin and	3 g IV q4h	*Staphylococcus*
	Gentamicin	1.5 mg/kg IV q6h	*epidermidis*, some
	or		anaerobes.
	Ceftriaxone and	2 g IV q12h	No coverage for
	Gentamicin	1.5 mg/kg IV q6h	*Staphylococcus*
			epidermidis, *Streptococcus*
	or		*faecalis*, many anaerobes.
	Vancomycin and	1 g IV q12h	
	Clindamycin and	900 mg IV q8h	
	Cephalothin and	2 g IV q4h	
	Gentamicin	1.5 mg/kg IV q4h	
Hospital-acquired	Vancomycin and	1 g IV q12h	Amikacin or tobramycin
	Ceftazidime and	2 g IV q8h	may be preferable in
	Gentamicin and	1.5 mg/kg IV q6h	some patients
	Clindamycin	900 mg IV q8h	
	or		
	Vancomycin	1.0 g IV q12h	
	Timentin	3.1 g IV q4h	
	Gentamicin	1.5 mg/kg IV q6h	
Meningitis			
Community acquired/ immunologically normal	Ceftriaxone or Chloramphenicol	2 g IV q12h 1 g IV q6h	
Community-acquired/ immunologically abnormal	Ceftazidime and Ampicillin +/−	2 g IV q8h 2 g IV q4h	Ampicillin needed to supplement ceftazidime if *Listeria* is possibility.
	(Amphotericin B) +/−	1.0 mg/kg qd after loading	Amphotericin B indicated if fungus, especially cryptococcus, is suspected.
	(Vancomycin) +/−	1 g IV q12h	Vancomycin indicated if *Staphylococcus* species likely.
	(Amikacin)	7.5 mg/kg IV q12h	Amikacin indicated if gram-negative bacillus suspected.
Hospital-acquired/ immunologically normal or abnormal	Ceftazidime and Vancomycin (and Amikacin)	2 g IV q8h 1 g IV q12h 1.5 g/kg IV q8h	Amikacin indicated if gram-negative bacillus suspected.

Table 2 (*Continued*)

Clinical Syndrome	Potential Regimens	Usual Initial Adult Dosing Regimen	Comments
Line Sepsis	Vancomycin and Piperacillin and Gentamicin	1 g IV q12h 3 g IV q4h 1.5 mg/kg IV q6h	
Pneumonia			
Community-acquired, immunologically normal	Ceftriaxone and erythromycin *or* Cefuroxime and erythromycin	2 g IV q12h 1 g IV q6h 2 g IV q8h 1 g IV q6h	If aspiration suspected, anaerobic coverage must be added; if gram-negative bacillary infection suspected, gentamicin should be added.
HIV with CD4 count <200/mm³	Trimethoprim-sulfamethoxozole and erythromycin	Trimethoprim at 5 mg/kg and Sulfamethoxazole at 20 mg/kg IV q6h 1 g IV q6h	
Immunosuppressed, HIV-negative	Vancomycin and clindamycin and piperacillin and gentamicin and +/−	1 g IV q12h 900 mg IV q12h 3 g IV q4h 1.5 mg/kg IV q6h	Double coverage for gram-negative bacillus pneumonia, especially indicated for neutropenic patients.
	(Trimethoprim-sulfamethoxazole)	5 mg/kg IV 20 mg/kg q6h	Trimethoprim-sulfamethoxazole indicated if *pneumocystis* is a possibility.
	(Erythromycin)	1 g IV q6h	Erythromycin is usually indicated to cover *Legionella* and perhaps TWAR.
Acute Abdomen	Vancomycin and metronidazole and ceftazidime and gentamicin	1 g IV q12h 650 mg IV q8h 2 g IV q8h 1.5 mg/kg IV q6h	

is especially true for patients with changing renal or hepatic function, who are undergoing some form of ultrafiltration or dialysis. At most hospitals, serum levels can be monitored regularly for aminoglycosides and vancomycin. Sulfa levels are available at many reference laboratories. By obtaining peak and trough levels at least two or three times weekly, the likelihood of obtaining adequate levels and minimizing toxicities can be enhanced. Unfortunately, for most beta-lactam, macrolide, antiviral, and antifungal drugs, serum levels cannot readily be obtained at most hospitals.

NEWER ANTIBIOTICS

Many new antibiotics are becoming available for therapy of critically ill patients, especially broad-spectrum agents in the beta-lactam and quinolone families. In recent years, cefotaxime, ceftriaxone, cefoperazone, ceftazidime, imipenem, timentin, sulbactam, aztreonam, and ciprofloxacin have been introduced into clinical practice.

Each of these drugs has unique features regarding its antimicrobial spectrum, toxicity profile, and pharmacokinetics. Each of these drugs is more expensive than many older alternatives. Should critical care physicians introduce these newer agents into their ICU practice? When deciding whether or not to introduce a new agent into clinical practice, physicians must recognize that the more antibiotics that are used in a given ICU, the more potential there is for error. It is difficult to remember the unique features of each drug. Thus, when the physician is choosing a drug, the pharmacist is preparing the unit dose, or the nurse is administering it, there is much more likelihood of error if they are using drugs that are unfamiliar. Whether the drug crosses the blood-brain barrier, whether it should be used in patients with recent seizures, whether it is compatible with cimetidine, whether its dose should be reduced in the presence of hepatic or renal failure, how rapidly the drug should be infused, and whether it should be administered in saline or sterile water are difficult issues to remember and issues that health care professionals often do not have time to search out in reference books. It is thus preferable to limit the number of antibiotics used in the ICU to as small a list as possible. A reasonable antibiotic armamentarium that should be adequate in most situations is presented in Table 1. Additional drugs can be used in unique situations as needed, usually in consultation with the infectious disease service, which can provide specific advice about how to use rarely employed agents. Thus, each ICU can choose one broad-spectrum beta-lactam drug with antipseudomonal activity for general use. Ceftazidime, imipenem, or timentin can be chosen, and the remaining two drugs used only in situations in which they are uniquely appropriate. Among the aminoglycosides, one agent can be chosen for general use among gentamicin, tobramycin, amikacin, and netilmicin. Similarly, among ceftizoxime, cefotaxime, ceftriaxone, and perhaps cefotetan, one agent can be chosen for regular use: the choice depends on each hospital's patient population, pathogen susceptibility pattern, and drug cost, as well as other factors.

THERAPY OF SPECIFIC DISORDERS

Table 2 provides some examples of antibiotic regimens that would be reasonable for the initial treatment of life-threatening infections while the causative agent is being sought. The precise regimen of choice for an individual patient depends on many unique features of the patient and must be selected with local antibiotic resistance patterns in mind. Specific chapters in this book provide more details about each syndrome.

SUGGESTED READING

Abramowicz M, ed. The choice of antimicrobial drugs. Med Lett Drugs Ther 1988; 30:33.
Donowitz GR. Third generation cephalosporins. Infect Dis Clin North Am 1989; 3:595-612.
Moellering RCJ. Principles of antiinfective therapy. In: Mandell GL, Douglas RG, Bennett JE, eds. Principles and practice of infectious diseases. 2nd ed. New York: Churchill Livingstone, 1990:206-218.
Rahal JJ. Choices of new penicillins and cephalosporins in the DRG era. Curr Clin Top Infect Dis 1988; 9:173-184.
Wolfson JS, Hooper DC. Treatment of genitourinary tract infections with fluoroquinolones: activity in vitro, pharmacokinetics, and clinical efficacy in urinary tract infections and prostatitis. Antimicrob Agents Chemother 1989; 33:1655-1661.

ANTIFUNGAL THERAPY

THOMAS J. WALSH, M.D.
PHILIP A. PIZZO, M.D.

Invasive fungal infections are increasingly major causes of morbidity and mortality in critically ill hospitalized patients. The incidence of *Candida* as one of the major nosocomial bloodstream pathogens has continued to rise. Pulmonary aspergillosis continues as a threat to many immunosuppressed patients. Many other less common opportunistic fungi have since emerged as causes of refractory mycoses. The advent of the acquired immunodeficiency syndrome (AIDS) has been associated with a marked increase in the frequency of cryptococcal meningitis and, in endemic areas, disseminated histoplasmosis and coccidioidomycosis.

Although in the past, developments in antifungal therapy did not keep pace with this expanding problem of life-threatening fungal infections, this has been changing during the past five years. While amphotericin B is still the "gold standard," some of these new antifungal compounds may have an impact on the treatment of invasive mycoses in critically ill patients.

ANTIFUNGAL COMPOUNDS

The chemical classes of antifungal compounds that are currently available and undergoing clinical investigation for treatment of fungal infections are listed in Table 1. These compounds consist of polyenes, fluorinated pyrimidines, imidazoles, triazoles, and echinocandins.

Polyenes

The polyene antifungal agents are macrolide rings with a hydrophilic region and conjugated double-bond hydrophobic region of the carbon chain. Amphotericin B, nystatin, and pimaricin (natamycin) are the three medically relevant polyenes. Nystatin is used only as a suspen-

Table 1 Chemical Classes of Antifungal Compounds

Polyenes
  Amphotericin B
  Nystatin
  Pimaricin
  Liposomal formulations of Amphotericin B*

Fluorinated Pyrimidines
  Flucytosine

Imidazoles
  Miconazole
  Ketoconazole
  Clotrimazole

Triazoles
  Fluconazole
  Itraconazole*
  SCH 39304*

Echinocandins
  Cilofungin*

*Investigational in the United States at the time of this writing (June 1990).

sion or cream for mucocutaneous infections. Pimaricin is a shorter chain polyene that is used for fungal keratitis. Amphotericin B is administered parenterally and is the drug of choice for most invasive mycoses.

Mechanism of Action

Amphotericin B and other polyenes bind to fungal cell membranes, resulting in cell membrane injury, increased permeability of intracellular contents, especially potassium, and ultimately cell death. Amphotericin B has higher affinity for ergosterol in fungal cell membranes than for cholesterol in mammalian cell membranes. However, this affinity is not exclusive, and binding of amphotericin B to mammalian cell membranes probably accounts for many of the toxic events.

Pharmacology

Amphotericin B is supplied in 50-mg vials and is currently formulated as a desoxycholate micellar suspension. This suspension is dissolved in 5 percent dextrose in water. Electrolyte solutions should be avoided, as they cause precipitation of the amphotericin B suspension. An in-line filter may trap the colloidal particles and also should be avoided. Intravenously administered amphotericin B binds initially to serum lipoproteins and then redistributes from the blood into tissues. Approximately 5 percent of the amphotericin B is excreted in the urine and bile. An infusion of 0.5 to 1 mg of amphotericin B per kilogram body weight achieves peak serum concentrations of approximately 1 to 3 μg per milliliter with plateau levels of approximately 0.2 to 0.5 μg per milliliter. However, measurement of serum concentrations of amphotericin are not clinically useful. Although amphotericin B desoxycholate is routinely administered on a once-daily basis to seriously ill patients, its long serum half-life also permits alternate-day dosing in clinically stable patients. Amphotericin B penetrates poorly into the cerebrospinal fluid (CSF) but does penetrate relatively well into peritoneal, pleural, and synovial spaces. Pre-existing renal dysfunction, hepatic failure, or hemodialysis has no effect on serum concentrations.

An exciting advance may be the encapsulation of amphotericin B into liposomes. Preclinical data are encouraging, and phase-1 assessments are currently underway.

Toxicity

Acute Toxicity. Virtually all patients have an acute febrile reaction, which may be severe, following infusion of amphotericin B. A small proportion of immunocompromised patients may have an acute bronchospasm and laryngospasm in response to amphotericin B. For these reasons, a 1-mg test dose is administered to monitor the patient for tolerance. If the patient tolerates this test dose, then a dose of 0.5 mg per kilogram may be initiated and infused over 2 to 4 hours. Most critically ill patients require prompt antifungal therapy, and the goal should be to reach therapeutic levels as rapidly as possible. A stepwise increase in dosage over days, therefore, may only delay the initiation of potentially effective treatment.

Fever, chills, and rigor frequently follow administration of amphotericin B, perhaps through the release of tumor necrosing factor (TNF). Hydrocortisone succinate in low doses (25 to 50 mg) may prevent the development of these symptoms in some patients. However, the doses of steroids should not be increased further, as this may exacerbate the infection. Acetaminophen may attenuate the fever. Although aspirin may have a similar effect, its use should be avoided in myelosuppressed patients with thrombocytopenia. Low doses (0.2 to 0.8 mg per kilogram) of intravenous meperidine generally abate the chills, fever, and rigor in patients with cancer receiving amphotericin B. Nausea and vomiting may also occur with the administration of amphotericin B. Although uncommon, an acute respiratory distress syndrome has been described with the simultaneous transfusion of granulocytes and infusion of amphotericin B, probably due to aggregation of polymorphonuclear leukocytes in the pulmonary capillary bed.

Nephrotoxicity. The principal adverse effect of amphotericin B is nephrotoxicity, which includes azotemia, hypokalemia, hypomagnesemia, renal tubular acidosis, and nephrocalcinosis. Amphotericin B–associated azotemia is due to diminished glomerular filtration rate (GFR), which appears to be related to tubuloglomerular feedback.

Tubuloglomerular feedback is a mechanism whereby increased delivery of chloride ions to the macular densa of the distal tubule causes a rapid decrease in GFR, apparently due to increased afferent arteriolar vascular resistance. Tubuloglomerular feedback is amplified by sodium deprivation and suppressed by previous sodium loading. This mechanism of amphotericin B–induced suppression of GFR may be suppressed by prior sodium loading. Consequently, our approach is to saline-load patients receiving amphotericin with the administration of the adult equivalent of 1 L of normal saline solution alternated by half-normal saline, every 8 hours, with potassium supplementation. Patients must be monitored carefully for hypernatremia, hyponatremia, hypokalemia, and pulmonary edema.

Hypokalemia due to amphotericin B may require the administration of several hundred milliequivalents of supplemental potassium per day. Hypomagnesemia may also develop, particularly in patients receiving extended courses of amphotericin B or those who have also received other drugs toxic to renal tubules that cause a divalent cation–losing nephropathy (e.g., cisplatin [dichlorodiamminoplatinum]). Conversely, hyperkalemia and ventricular arrhythmias have been reported in anephric patients receiving too rapid an infusion of amphotericin B (i.e., in less than 1 hour). The mechanism of this potentially fatal reaction appears to be due to increased permeability of mammalian cell membranes by amphotericin B and leakage of intracellular potassium into extracellular fluid, leading to hyperkalemia and potentially fatal arrhythmias. Amphotericin B when used concomitantly with other nephrotoxic agents, such as an aminoglycoside or cyclosporine, may cause acute renal toxicity.

Hematologic Toxicity. Amphotericin B may suppress erythropoiesis when used for chronic periods (over 1 month). There is no apparent effect of amphotericin B in suppressing neutrophils or platelets.

Major Critical Care Uses. Amphotericin B is the drug of choice for treatment of virtually all life-threatening mycoses in critically ill patients. It is utilized in critically and immunocompromised patients for treatment of invasive candidiasis, invasive pulmonary aspergillosis, zygomycosis, cryptococcosis, disseminated histoplasmosis, coccidioidomycosis, and blastomycosis. It is also used as the drug of choice for empirical antifungal therapy in persistently febrile granulocytopenic patients.

Flucytosine

Flucytosine (5-fluorocytosine) is a fluorinated pyrimidine that has been utilized in combination with amphotericin B for treatment of cryptococcal meningitis, other mycoses of the central nervous system (CNS), and disseminated candidiasis.

Mechanism of Action

Flucytosine is taken up by the fungus and is converted by fungal cytosine deaminase to 5-fluorouracil, an antineoplastic compound. The 5-fluorouracil is then converted to 5-fluorodeoxyuridine monophosphate, which inhibits thymidylate synthetase and, consequently, DNA synthesis.

Pharmacology

In contrast to the properties of amphotericin B, flucytosine is cleared approximately 90 percent unchanged in the urine, is minimally protein-bound, has a short plasma half-life of 3 to 5 hours, and penetrates into cerebrospinal fluid by more than 70 percent. Moreover, the compound is cleared by hemodialysis and serum levels are affected by renal insufficiency. Serum concentrations of flucytosine should be followed and dosage adjusted to achieve peak concentrations of 40 to 60 μg per milliliter. Serum levels of 100 μg per milliliter or more are associated with increased frequency of side effects, especially bone marrow suppression.

Major Critical Care Uses

Flucytosine is utilized in combination with amphotericin B in critically ill patients for life-threatening infections due to cryptococcosis, CNS candidiasis, *Candida* endophthalmitis, disseminated candidiasis, renal candidiasis, and possibly invasive mycoses refractory to amphotericin B.

Imidazoles

The class of imidazoles relevant to critically ill patients include clotrimazole, miconazole, and ketoconazole. All imidazoles possess the property of inhibiting fungal cytochrome P450–dependent conversion by C_{14} demethylase of lanosterol to ergosterol, thereby depleting the fungal cell membrane of its major sterol.

Miconazole

Pharmacology. Miconazole is an intravenously administered, water-insoluble, N-substituted imidazole formulated as a colloidal suspension in polyethoxylated castor oil. Miconazole penetrates the CSF poorly. Renal excretion of miconazole is insignificant, and elimination appears to occur principally via slow metabolism.

Toxicology. Local toxicity related to intravenous administration includes thrombophlebitis and irritation at the site of administration following extravasation. Manifestations of systemic toxicity include anorexia, nausea, vomiting, headache, hepatitis, thrombocytopenia, and pruritus, the last of which may persist long after cessation of miconazole. Many of the toxic effects of miconazole may be due to the formulation's colloidal stabilizing oil.

Major Critical Care Uses. The only remaining clinical indication for miconazole in critically ill patients is treatment of deep infection due to *Pseudallescheria boydii*.

Ketoconazole

Pharmacology. Ketoconazole is the first commercially available, orally administered and systemically absorbed N-substituted antifungal imidazole. The plasma alpha half-life of ketoconazole is approximately 2 hours, and the plasma beta half-life approximately 9 hours. Peak serum concentrations following a 200-mg dose of 2 to 4 μg per milliliter are variably attained 2 to 3 hours after ingestion. Ketoconazole penetrates the CSF poorly. Ketoconazole is metabolized by the liver and excreted principally in the bile as an inactive compound. There is minimal urinary excretion. Renal or hepatic insufficiency does not apparently require modification of dosage. Bioavailability of ketoconazole is reduced by achlorhydria, antacids, and H_2-receptor blocking agents (e.g., cimetidine or ranitidine). Serum concentrations of ketoconazole are decreased with concomitant administration of rifampin, apparently by rifampin-induced activation of hepatic microsomal enzymes and acceleration of metabolism of ketoconazole. Another adverse drug interaction with ketoconazole involves prolongation of the serum half-life of cyclosporine A.

Toxicity. Anorexia, nausea, and vomiting are the most frequent dose-limiting side effects of ketoconazole. Hepatotoxicity and endocrinologic abnormalities are less common, albeit important, side effects of ketoconazole. Asymptomatic elevation of serum transaminases develops in 2 to 5 percent of patients receiving ketoconazole. In most cases, elevation of serum transaminases associated with ketoconazole will spontaneously resolve or stabilize during continuation of treatment. Approximately one in 10,000 patients receiving ketoconazole sustains progressive hepatitis, which most frequently develops within the first 3 months of therapy and generally is not dose-related.

The endocrinologic side effects of ketoconazole are related to the inhibition of cytochrome P450–dependent corticosteroid and androgen synthesis. The antiandrogen effects of ketoconazole include gynecomastia and transient dose-dependent suppression of serum testosterone. Ketoconazole also induces a transient dose-dependent decrease in the ACTH-cortisol response by inhibition of cytochrome P450–dependent enzymes involved in adrenal corticosteroid synthesis. The fact that the inhibition of steroid synthesis is transient and dose-dependent probably accounts for the infrequent development of gynecomastia or clinically overt adrenal insufficiency. The antiandrogen properties of ketoconazole have permitted its use in treatment of metastatic adenocarcinoma of the prostate and cortisol-producing tumors of the adrenal gland.

Major Critical Care Uses. Ketoconazole has little role in the initial treatment of invasive mycoses in critically ill patients. Nevertheless, an understanding of this compound is relevant to utilizing other antifungal azoles. Moreover, immunocompromised patients may have been receiving this compound at the time of arrival at a critical care unit.

Triazoles

The triazoles applicable to critically ill patients are fluconazole and itraconazole. This mechanism of action is similar to that of imidazoles—i.e., inhibition of cytochrome P450–dependent conversion of lanosterol to ergosterol.

Fluconazole

Pharmacology. Fluconazole is a water-soluble bistriazol-difluorophenyl-2-propanol antifungal compound. Fluconazole, formulated as a tablet and as a parenteral saline solution, has unique pharmacologic properties in comparison with the previously cited azoles. Fluconazole is principally excreted as the active agent through the kidney. Dosage should be adjusted for renal failure. The rate of serum protein binding is only 11 percent in comparison with over 99 percent for itraconazole and ketoconazole. Unlike the aforementioned azoles, fluconazole penetrates the CSF of inflamed and normal meninges. The drug is well absorbed in human volunteers and not significantly affected by achlorhydria. Its plasma beta half-life is approximately 22 to 30 hours in normal renal function.

Toxicity. Like other antifungal azoles, fluconazole has the potential to cause nausea, vomiting, and elevated transaminase levels. However, these side effects are generally less frequent than those associated with ketoconazole.

Major Critical Care Uses. Although recently approved for treatment of cryptococcosis and candidiasis, there are insufficient available clinical data at this time to support the routine use of fluconazole in the treatment of invasive fungal infections in critically ill patients. It should be used in this setting only after consultation with infectious disease service.

Itraconazole

Pharmacology. Itraconazole is a lipophilic compound of the triazole class of antifungal agents. To date, it has been studied in clinical trials in an oral formulation. Itraconazole is well absorbed in nonimmunocompromised hosts in the fasting state. Depending on the formulation, bioavailability may be impaired in patients receiving cytotoxic chemotherapy, radiation therapy, or antacids. Itraconazole has a high degree of protein-binding and has a serum beta half-life of approximately 17 hours in humans. Less than 1 percent of the active compound is excreted through the urinary tract. No modification of dosage appears to be necessary in cases of hepatic or renal insufficiency. Itraconazole poorly penetrates the CSF. On the other hand, it is widely distributed into various tissues, including the brain, lung, and kidney, and has a large volume of distribution and high tissue-to-plasma concentration ratios.

Toxicology. Current data from early clinical trials indicate that itraconazole has few side effects. The frequency of nausea and elevated serum hepatic transaminase levels appears to be less than for ketoconazole. A few patients have been found to have hypokalemia and pedal edema, suggesting an aldosterone-like effect; however, the mechanism for these effects remains to be elucidated. Unlike in the case of ketoconazole, there have been no apparent adverse effects of itraconazole on adrenal or testicular steroid synthesis.

Major Critical Care Uses. Itraconazole is currently an investigational agent that has been used in the treatment of invasive aspergillosis in granulocytopenic patients and for histoplasmosis in HIV-infected patients. However, its role in treating these infections in critically ill patients awaits further study.

PREVENTION OF FUNGAL INFECTIONS IN CRITICALLY ILL PATIENTS

Nystatin, clotrimazole, and ketoconazole are not effective for significant prevention of deep fungal infections in critically ill patients. Whether newer agents, such as fluconazole or itraconazole, will offer an advantage in preventing fungal infections in critically ill patients is currently being evaluated.

TREATMENT OF FUNGAL INFECTIONS IN CRITICALLY ILL PATIENTS

Mucocutaneous Fungal Infections

Oropharyngeal candidiasis may respond to nystatin, clotrimazole, ketoconazole, or fluconazole. Esophageal candidiasis may be more difficult to treat successfully.

Table 2 Treatment of Systemic Fungal Infections

Organism Causing Infection	Drug of Choice	Dose	Duration of Therapy	Alternative Therapy	Comments
Candida sp.	Amphotericin B	0.5–0.6 mg/kg/day	3–8 wk (1.0–2.5 g or 15–35 mg/kg)	? Fluconazole	See comment under chemotherapy regarding use of concomitant 5-FC.
Aspergillus sp.	Amphotericin B	1.0–1.5 mg/kg/day	8–12 wk (2.5–3.5 g or 35–50 mg/kg)	? Itraconazole	The combination of AmB and 5-FC may be additive/synergistic. Aspergillosis may develop in patients already receiving empirical amphotericin B 0.5 mg/kg/day.
Blastomyces dermatitidis	Amphotericin B	0.4–0.5 mg/kg/day	6–8 wk (1.5–2.5 g or 25–35 mg/kg)	Ketoconazole, 400 mg/d for indolent disease; 6–12 months' duration	Amphotericin B should be used in critically ill patients.
Coccidioides immitis	Amphotericin B	0.5–0.6 mg/kg/day	8–14 wk (2.5–4.0 g or 35–57 mg/kg)	Ketoconazole, 400–800 mg/day for indolent infection;	For patients with meningitis, administration of intrathecal amphotericin B is almost always essential.
Cryptococcus neoformans	Amphotericin B plus Flucytosine	0.3 mg/kg/day plus 150 mg/kg/day	6 wk	Amphotericin B as a single agent (0.5–0.6 mg/kg/day for 6 wk)	Fluconazole, 200–400 mg qd for maintenance of suppression in HIV infection
Histoplasma capsulatum	Amphotericin B	0.4–0.5 mg/kg/day	8 wk (2.5 g or 35 mg/kg)	Ketoconazole, 400–800 mg/day for 6–12 months for indolent, nonmeningeal infection	For HIV-associated histoplasmosis.
Agents of zygomycosis (e.g., Mucor, Absidia, Rhizopus)	Amphotericin B	1.0–1.5 mg/kg/day	8–12 wk (2.5–4.0 g or 35–57 mg/kg)	None	Surgical debridement of infected focus when possible; control of acidosis, when present, is also important; hyperbaric oxygen?
Fusarium sp.	Amphotericin B	1.0–1.5 mg/kg/day	8–? wk (2.5–? g or 35–? mg/kg)	? Triazole	—
Dematiacious fungi (e.g., Cladosporium, Curvularia, Drechslera, Phialophora, Wangiella)	Amphotericin B	0.5–0.6 mg/kg/day	8–? wk (2.5–? g or 35–? mg/kg)	None	Surgical debridement of an infected focus (e.g., sinus or localized pulmonary infection) almost always required.
Paracoccidioides brasiliensis	Ketoconazole	400 mg/day	6–12 months	Amphotericin B 0.4–0.6 mg/kg/day 1.5–2.5 g or 25–35 mg/kg ? Itraconazole	Amphotericin B in critically ill patients
Pseudallescheria boydii	Miconazole	400–1,200 mg q8h	6–12 wk; 1.5–3.5 g or 15–30 4–? wk	? Itraconazole	Surgical debridement helpful in localized infection; some strains are resistant to amphotericin B.
Trichosporon beigelii	Amphotericin B	0.5–1.5 mg/kg/d	8–? wk (2.5–? g or 35–? mg/kg)	? Fluconazole	Some strains are resistant to amphotericin B.

Nonneutropenic patients, including those with human immunodeficiency virus (HIV) initially respond to clotrimazole, ketoconazole, or fluconazole. Granulocytopenic and other heavily immunocompromised patients should receive amphotericin B. Critically ill granulocytopenic patients with esophageal candidiasis require therapy for duration of granulocytopenia, as deep mycosis cannot be excluded.

Deeply Invasive or Systemic Fungal Infections

The approach to treatment of systemic fungal infections are summarized in Table 2. The presence of fungus in any normally sterile body fluid or tissue in a critically ill patient is an indication for initiation of amphotericin B. In addition, in neutropenic patients who remain persistently febrile in spite of broad-spectrum antibiotic therapy, amphotericin should be administered empirically. Amphotericin B is administered in different dosages and durations, depending upon the infection and immune status of the patient.

Therapy with amphotericin B begins with an initial test dose of 1 mg in adults (0.5 mg in children weighing under 30 kg) over 1 hour, followed for 2 to 3 hours, then followed by a dose of 0.5 to 0.6 mg per kilogram given over 2 to 3 hours. This permits the achievement of therapeutic dosages within hours after the decision to initiate antifungal therapy. Empirically administered amphotericin B for persistently febrile granulocytopenic patients is given until recovery from granulocytopenia. Fungemia without another focus is treated usually with a total dose of 15 mg per kilogram (approximately 1 g). Fungemia developing in a nongranulocytopenic patient is treated with approximately 500 mg (7 mg per kilogram) in an adult. Candidemia associated with an indwelling catheter is sufficient criteria for removal of the catheter. Deep visceral infection is treated with a total dose of at least 22 mg per kilogram (approximately 1.5 g). However, certain infections such as hepatosplenic candidiasis may require total doses exceeding 100 mg per kilogram. Granulocytopenic patients with pulmonary aspergillosis should receive early aggressive therapy with amphotericin B at 1 mg to 1.5 mg per kilogram per day.

Preliminary data suggest that liposomal formulations of amphotericin B appear to be less toxic in the host but as effective as amphotericin B desoxycholate in treating invasive mycoses. These formulations are currently being studied in limited clinical trials and offers hope for the future. These agents are not currently approved but may, in some cases, be obtained through protocols.

Combination Antifungal Therapy

Amphotericin B Plus Flucytosine. The combination of flucytosine with amphotericin B may be useful in treatment of systemic mycoses in critically ill immunocompromised patients. Cryptococcal meningitis, however, is the only systemic mycosis for which the combination of amphotericin B with flucytosine has been shown to have superior antifungal activity compared with amphotericin B alone in a prospective, randomized trial. Therapy with the combination of amphotericin B (0.3 mg per kilogram per day) with flucytosine (150 mg per kilogram per day) administered for 6 weeks eliminated the infecting organism from the CSF more rapidly, achieved a higher cure rate, and was associated with a lower rate of nephrotoxicity than therapy with amphotericin B (0.4 mg per kilogram per day) administered alone for 10 weeks. There was, however, no difference in mortality between the two groups. The combination of amphotericin B and flucytosine is also effective against large cryptococcal intracerebral masses (cryptococcomas), obviating the need for surgical intervention.

The dosage of flucytosine often needs to be decreased during the first 2 weeks of therapy, owing to increased blood levels consequent to the decreased GFR caused by amphotericin B. We recommend that peak serum concentrations be maintained between 50 and 75 µg per milliliter in order to avoid flucytosine-associated toxicity. Granulocytopenia due to cytotoxic chemotherapy is not a contraindication to the appropriate use of flucytosine for life-threatening invasive fungal infections.

Given the ability of flucytosine to penetrate the CNS, the combination of amphotericin B plus flucytosine may be indicated in any patient with clinically overt cryptococcosis or other deep mycosis of the CNS. Moreover, flucytosine may be added to amphotericin B for patients with disseminated candidiasis or pulmonary aspergillosis that does not respond to high-dose amphotericin B alone. The combination of flucytosine with amphotericin B may also be of benefit to patients with overt CNS infection, endophthalmitis, hepatosplenic candidiasis, renal candidiasis, persistent fungemia, or refractory invasive pulmonary aspergillosis. However, the routine coadministration of rifampin or imidazoles with amphotericin B is not recommended until more clinical data are available.

Amphotericin B Plus Other Agents. Rifampin, which has no intrinsic antifungal properties, augments the in vitro antifungal activity of amphotericin B against *Candida albicans*, *Candida neoformans*, *Histoplasma capsulatum*, and *Aspergillus* spp., as measured by a reduction in the minimum inhibitory dose of amphotericin B. In vivo studies demonstrate that a combination of rifampin and amphotericin B decreased the amount of amphotericin B necessary to extend survival in experimental murine histoplasmosis and aspergillosis, but not candidiasis. None of these studies demonstrates that the combination of rifampin and amphotericin B confers significantly superior antifungal activity compared with high doses of amphotericin B administered as a single agent. There are no clinical trials demonstrating that rifampin improves antifungal response or patient survival. Therefore, rifampin should not be routinely administered in cases of invasive mycoses.

Combinations of antifungal imidazoles or triazoles with amphotericin B remain controversial. Since amphotericin B binds to ergosterol in the fungal cell membrane and since antifungal imidazoles inhibit synthesis of ergosterol, imidazoles could possibly antagonize the activity of amphotericin B. Such antagonism has been demonstrated experimentally for amphotericin B with miconazole and with ketoconazole. The combination of antifungal azoles and amphotericin B should not be used routinely.

Miconazole

As the first parenterally administered antifungal imidazole, miconazole promised to be an important advance in treatment of invasive mycoses; however, the toxicity of the drug carrier has precluded its routine usage. We therefore suggest that use of miconazole be reserved for treatment of invasive infections due to *Pseudallescheria boydii* (*Scedosporlum apiospermum*).

Ketoconazole

Ketoconazole is a drug that is seldom used in critically ill patients. However, ketoconazole is considered to be a first-line antifungal agent for nonmeningeal paracoccidioidomycosis, chronic cavitary pulmonary histoplasmosis, disseminated histoplasmosis in clinically stable and nonimmunosuppressed patients, and nonmeningeal histoplasmosis. Certain conditions of coccidioidomycosis may be amenable to treatment with ketoconazole such as cutaneous lesions, soft tissue abscesses, draining sinus tracts, synovitis, osteomyelitis and noncavitary pulmonary infiltrates. Since ketoconazole penetrates the CSF poorly, it is not definitively recommended for treatment of any fungal infection of the CNS.

Clinical data so far do not support the use of ketoconazole in treatment of established candidiasis in critically ill and immunocompromised patients. Ketoconazole is available only as an oral formulation and has limited bioavailability in achlorhydric patients and those receiving antacids or H_2-blocker agents. Transaminase elevation, nausea, and vomiting also preclude the use of this agent in critically ill patients.

Fluconazole

Fluconazole may be used for primary treatment or for prevention of recurrence of cryptococcal meningitis in AIDS. Fluconazole is the preferred agent for the prevention of recurrence of cryptococcal meningoencephalitis. Fluconazole is less toxic and reportedly more effective than amphotericin B for preventing recurrent cryptococcal meningoencephalitis in patients with AIDS. Daily dosages used for treatment of cryptococcal meningoencephalitis should range from 200 to 400 mg in patients with normal renal function.

However, amphotericin B remains the drug of choice for critically ill patients with primary cryptococcal meningitis, especially when neurologic deficits are present, such as confusion, obtundation, or focal neurologic deficits.

In our opinion, fluconazole also is not indicated in the treatment of disseminated candidiasis in critically ill patients until more data are forthcoming or unless all other measures have been exhausted and the patient is unable to tolerate amphotericin B therapy. Nonetheless, pending further studies with adequate doses (more than 4 mg per kilogram), fluconazole may become an important agent in the management of systemic fungal infections in critically ill patients.

Itraconazole

Itraconazole is active at doses ranging from 100 mg to 400 mg per day against the following invasive mycoses: disseminated histoplasmosis, paracoccidioidomycosis, blastomycosis, chronic cavitary histoplasmosis, and selected cases of coccidioidomycosis, sporotrichosis, and aspergillosis.

Although itraconazole is active against *Aspergillus* species and has been used in treatment of selected cases of pulmonary aspergillosis, further studies are required to clarify its use in the critical care setting. Amphotericin B remains the drug of choice for treatment of invasive pulmonary aspergillosis in critically ill patients. Factors such as cytotoxic chemotherapy, radiation therapy, intrinsic gastric hypochlorhydria, or gastric antacid therapy may seriously compromise oral bioavailability in severely immunocompromised patients.

Itraconazole may be a less toxic but an equality effective alternative to ketoconazole for treatment of endemic mycoses.

Special Problems

Empirical Amphotericin B in Persistently Febrile Granulocytopenic Patients

Disseminated fungal infections in granulocytopenic patients carry a high mortality. Fungemia or other signs of established systemic fungal infection may not be detected in the granulocytopenic host until the infection is already advanced. Consequently, empirical antifungal therapy in the persistently febrile granulocytopenic patients may provide early treatment for an occult fungal infection and systemic prophylaxis for patients at high risk of invasive mycoses. Empirical antifungal therapy, of course, does not obviate the necessity to diagnose the source of fever and to continually reassess persistently febrile granulocytopenic patients.

Refractory Disseminated Candidiasis

Amphotericin B in doses of 1 to 1.5 mg per kilogram per day may be necessary to manage disseminated candidiasis in critically ill immunocompromised patients, particularly those with *Candida tropicalis* or occasionally *Candida parapsilosis*. These higher dosages should be utilized in conjunction with appropriate saline hydration and particular attention to fluid and electrolyte balances. The combination of amphotericin B and flucytosine may also prove useful in cases of persistent fungemia and progressive deep infection. Removal of vascular catheters is an important adjunct in clearing refractory fungemia.

Pulmonary Aspergillosis

Pulmonary aspergillosis may develop in granulocytopenic patients who are already receiving empirical amphotericin B. In such cases, the dosage of amphotericin B should be initially increased to 1.5 mg per kilogram per day. Whether flucytosine should be added is controversial. Life-threatening hemoptysis is another problem that may complicate the course of critically ill patients with established pulmonary aspergillosis. Hemoptysis due to pulmonary infarction may be one of the first signs of pulmonary aspergillosis in granulocytopenic patients. Alternatively, hemoptysis due to formation of mycotic aneurysms may not become apparent until the time of recovery from granulocytopenia.

Microbiologic Resistance to Amphotericin B

Trichosporon beigelii Fusarium species, *Pseudallescheria boydii* and certain dematiacious hyphomycetes, such as *Exserohilum, Bipolaris,* and *Cladosporium* (Xylohypha) species have been increasingly described as disseminated or locally invasive fungal pathogens occurring especially in critically ill patients. Although *Candida* species and *Aspergillus* species certainly are the most common nosocomial fungal pathogens, these other fungi are presenting increasing challenges to amphotericin B therapy.

Microbiologic resistance to amphotericin B (minimal inhibitory concentration of greater than 2.0 µg per milliliter in *Candida* species) also has been reported in *Candida albicans, Candida tropicalis, Candida krusei, Candida parapsilosis, Candida lusitaniae,* and *Candida guillermondi, Trichosporon belgelii, Pseudallescheria boydii,* and *Fusarium* species. Most polyene-resistant isolates of *Candida* species have caused only colonization or superficial mucosal infection. Polyene-resistant *Candida* species, however, have been an uncommon cause of life-threatening infections in severely immunocompromised patients. *Trichosporon, Fusarium,* and *Pseudallescheria,* however, are increasingly recognized causes of infection in critically ill immunocompromised patients. Initial strategies should include high-dose amphotericin B (1.5 mg per kilogram per day) with flucytosine. If this regimen is not successful, an antifungal triazole, such as fluconazole, perhaps with the addition of flucytosine, may be considered for treatment of systemic fungal infection due to polyene-resistant fungi.

Clinical Resistance to Amphotericin B

Clinical resistance to amphotericin B is defined here as the absence of clinical response to amphotericin B by an infection due to a susceptible fungus. Clinically resistant fungal infections develop especially in patients with infection of foreign bodies, profound immunosuppression, or advanced fungal lesions of the viscera, such as hepatosplenic candidiasis.

Hepatosplenic candidiasis is a clinically resistant infection, which often requires a total dose of several grams of amphotericin B administered over several months in order to achieve cure. The development or persistence of fever, abdominal pain, and/or elevated alkaline phosphatase level after recovery from granulocytopenia, is a common clinical presentation of patients with hepatosplenic candidiasis. Diagnostic imaging of liver and spleen should be pursued with ultrasonography, computerized tomographic scanning, or magnetic resonance imaging to monitor response to therapy. During the scanning of liver and spleen, other sites, such as the kidney, may be found to be infected. In our experience, the combination of amphotericin B and flucytosine administered at the onset of treatment appears to have been more effective than amphotericin B alone in the treatment of hepatosplenic candidiasis. However, therapy may need to be extended over several months to be successful. Splenectomy may also be warranted in the following situations: for massive splenic candidiasis refractory to medical therapy, refractory left upper-quadrant pain attributable to splenic candidiasis, persistent fungemia in the absence of other clearly involved foci, and persistence of splenic lesions and fever after resolution of all sites of infection following medical therapy.

Fungal infection of a foreign body, especially an intravascular device, may result in a systemic mycosis that is clinically refractory to amphotericin B if the infected focus is not removed. Valvular resection is considered essential for cure of fungal endocarditis in most cases. Current findings support removal of infected devices in the following fungal infections: central venous catheters associated with candidemia; umbilical artery catheters in fungemic neonates; dialysis catheters in fungal peritonitis associated with peritoneal dialysis; and infected ventriculoatrial shunts in cryptococcal meningitis. Moreover, both removal of the intravascular catheter and segmental resection of the infected vein may be required for cure of candidal supportive peripheral thrombophlebitis.

Fungemia and pulmonary vasculitis due to the lipophilic fungus *Malassezia furfur* is a newly recognized syndrome in infants and adults receiving parenteral lipid emulsions through central venous catheters. Removal of the central venous catheter and discontinuation of the lipid emulsion generally has been successful in treating this infection. Systemic antifungal therapy does not appear to be required. Infected patients respond well clinically to removal of the catheter and discontinuation of the lipid. Late infectious complications, such as fungal endophthalmitis or pyelonephritis due to *Malassezia furfur*, have not been reported in conservatively treated patients.

Systemic Mycoses in AIDS

Patients with AIDS have an increased frequency and refractoriness of cryptococcal meningoencephalitis. These patients also appear to have an increased risk of disseminated histoplasmosis and coccidioidomycosis. They may present with fulminant deep mycoses due to these endemic pathogens. Such patients should receive amphotericin B until completely stabilized.

Meningoencephalitis due to *Cryptococcus neoformans* in AIDS is a refractory systemic mycosis with frequent relapses. Patients with AIDS, in contrast to patients without AIDS, seldom achieve sustained clinical remission after completion of a course of amphotericin B with or without flucytosine. Such clinical resistance to amphotericin B is most likely attributable to the profound cellular immune deficit associated with AIDS. Outpatient administration of maintenance amphotericin B to patients with AIDS after initial remission of cryptococcal meningoencephalitis has substantially decreased the relapse rate of cryptococcosis.

Disseminated coccidioidomycosis and histoplasmosis have become increasingly prevalent in endemic areas. These infections may cause rapidly fatal pneumonias and hemodynamic deterioration. Amphotericin B remains the drug of choice in initial treatment of these infections.

SUGGESTED READING

Bennett JE. Antifungal agents. In: Mandell GL, Douglas RG, Bennett JE, eds. Principles and practice of infectious diseases. New York: Churchill Livingstone, 1990.

Drutz D, ed. Systemic fungal infections: diagnosis and treatment I and II. Infect Dis Clin North Am 1988; 2:779-969; and 1989; 3:1-133.

Rippon JW. Medical mycology. In: The pathogenic fungi and the pathogenic actinomycetes. Philadelphia: WB Saunders, 1988:119.

Walsh TJ, Pizzo PA. Fungal infections in granulocytopenic patients: current approaches to classification, diagnosis, and treatment. In: Holmberg KJ, Meyer RD, eds. Diagnosis and therapy of systemic mycoses. New York: Raven Press, 1989:47.

Walsh TJ, Rubin M, Pizzo PA. Respiratory disease in patients with malignant neoplasms. In: Shelhamer J, Pizzo PA, Parrillo JE, Masur H, eds. Respiratory diseases in the immunosuppressed host. Philadelphia: JB Lippincott (in press).

NEUROLOGIC THERAPEUTICS

HEAD TRAUMA

ANN MARIE FLANNERY, M.D.

Because damaged brain tissue cannot be repaired, the goal of medical management of head trauma is to avoid circumstances that will impose a secondary injury on the already damaged neural tissue. Cerebral edema is the major cause of secondary injury. Salvage of a maximally functional individual depends on avoiding conditions that may cause or increase cerebral edema: hypoxia, hypercarbia, hypotension, and overhydration.

During the initial evaluation and stabilization of patients with head trauma, attention must be given to adequacy of the airway, ventilatory support as needed, and intravenous vascular access. The cervical spine, which may be fractured or dislocated, should be rigidly immobilized until adequate radiographic evidence of normal bony anatomy is available.

The initial assessment should include the use of the Glasgow Coma Scale (GCS) (Table 1). This standard examination is brief and usually reproducible. Worsening in the GCS can warn of expanding hematomas or increasing intracranial pressure. Patients who score under 8 on the GCS can be classified as having a severe head injury. These patients are likely to require the most intensive care and will be the focus of the remainder of this chapter.

The majority of patients with severe head injury will require endotracheal intubation in order to secure the airway needed for adequate oxygenation, and possible hyperventilation, as discussed below. If there is uncertainty as to whether intubation is necessary, it should be done. Care should be taken to minimize stimuli such as coughing or bucking, which may increase intracranial pressure. The use of short-acting muscle relaxants and barbiturates and the presence of a person experienced in airway management will diminish the risk of those complications. The neurologic examination, especially of the cranial nerves and including the GCS, should be done prior to the administration of agents that make such assessment impossible (Table 2).

Table 1 Glasgow Coma Scale

Eyes open	Spontaneous	4
	To verbal command	3
	To pain	2
	No response	1
Best motor response	To verbal command — Obeys	6
	To painful stimulus	
	Localizes pain	5
	Flexion withdrawal	4
	Flexion abnormal	3
	Extension	2
	No response	1
Best verbal response	Oriented and converses	5
	Disoriented and converses	4
	Inappropriate words	3
	Incomprehensible sounds	2
	No response	1
TOTAL		3–15

Table 2 Initial Management of Head Trauma

Maintain airway
Assess and supplement breathing as needed
Access circulation: insert two large-bore intravenous catheters
Examination:
 Pupils
 Ocular motility
 Corneas
 Gag reflex
 Respiration
 Glasgow Coma Score
Expect, search for, and treat associated injuries of the neck, chest, abdomen, extremities

Avoid hypercarbia, hypoxia, hypotension, overhydration

SURGICALLY CORRECTABLE LESIONS

Early detection and correction of surgical lesions significantly improves outcome in head trauma. Computed tomography (CT) scan, therefore, is mandatory in the initial management of severe head trauma. Medical management of intracranial pressure may be required by most patients after surgery.

Acute Subdural Hematoma. Usually seen on CT as a crescent-shaped collection of fresh blood between the skull and brain, acute subdural hematoma is treated by a craniotomy. Patient outcome is affected by three factors: the time elapsed from injury to surgery, the associated parenchymal brain damage, and the condition of the patient before surgery.

Chronic Subdural Hematoma. Chronic subdural hematomas are found in the same location as acute subdural hematomas but are composed of old hemorrhage, although some fresh blood may be present. These lesions are treated by drainage through a burr hole. Cortical atrophy from age or chronic alcoholism will predispose to chronic subdural hematoma.

Epidural Hematoma. Epidural hematoma is usually a lentiform collection of acute hemorrhage between the dura and the brain, limited by the dural insertion at the

Table 3 Methods of Monitoring Intracranial Pressure

Intraventricular Catheter	Subarachnoid Bolt	Epidural Monitor	Subdural Catheter	Intraparenchymal (fiberoptic)
Risks: Highest rate of infection. Possible hematoma or infarction with insertion or removal. May be technically more difficult to insert.	Risks: Damped by brain swelling: • Less reliable at higher pressure, • Falsely low values. Unable to drain CSF.	Risks: Probably least reliable. Loss of reliability at higher pressure. Unable to drain CSF.	Risks: Unable to drain CSF. Insertion may be more difficult than subarachnoid bolt, or epidural monitor. Will become unreliable at higher pressure.	Risks: Expensive adapter. Cannot be recalibrated after insertion. Fibers may fracture. Cannot drain CSF.
Benefits: "Gold standard" for pressure monitors. Reliable at high pressure. Allows removal of CSF	Benefits: Relative ease of insertions. Intermediate to low infection rate.	Benefits: Easiest and least invasive to insert. Low risk of infection.	Benefits: More reliable than epidural monitor or subarachnoid bolt.	Benefits: Very easy to place. Will work in any brain parenchyma.

cranial sutures. When treated by craniotomy, clot removal, and control of hemorrhage, the outcome of epidural hematoma can be good. Outcome is dependent on the same factors that affect outcome of acute subdural hematoma.

Intraparenchymal Hematoma. The surgical treatment of intraparenchymal hematoma depends on the judgment of the neurosurgeon. Factors that influence the decision to operate include size and location of the lesion and condition of the patient. A single large superficial hematoma in a noneloquent region, associated with deteriorating mental status or rising intracranial pressure may benefit from surgical removal. Multiple or deep hematomas and relatively asymptomatic ones are best managed medically.

Late Complications. Delayed development of extra-axial and intraparenchymal hematomas may occur following serious head trauma. A CT repeated 24 hours after injury may detect the evolution of surgically correctable lesions. In the monitored patient, a trend of increased intracranial pressure may also signal the development of hematomas.

Acute post-traumatic hydrocephalus may also cause increased intracranial pressure. If hydrocephalus is present, placement of an intraventricular catheter will allow drainage of cerebrospinal fluid (CSF) and will control intracranial pressure.

Cerebrospinal Fluid Leaks. Basilar skull fractures are often found to have associated CSF leaks presenting as otorrhea or rhinorrhea. Most of these leaks cease spontaneously. Positioning of the patient and the use of prophylactic antibiotics are controversial and matters of individual preference. A program of bed rest with head elevation of 30 degrees and avoidance of prophylactic antibiotic therapy has been safe and effective. If profuse or persistent (longer than 10 to 14 days), CSF leaks may require surgical repair.

Monitoring of Intracranial Pressure. Although intracranial pressure monitoring has not been proved to improve outcome in head injury, the use of monitoring facilitates the rational care of the severely head-injured patient (GCS of 7 or less). In the more severely head-injured patient, the risk-to-benefit ratio favors the careful use of invasive monitoring of intracranial pressure. Four different types of monitoring systems exist, each with benefits and limits (Table 3).

Management of Intracranial Pressure. Initial measures are outlined in Table 4.

Fluid Management. Normal hydration is the goal of fluid management in serious acute head trauma. Recommendations for initial fluid restriction are more appropriate to metabolic cerebral edema. In trauma, blood loss from associated injuries may cause volume depletion and hypotension. Hypotension, rarely seen as a result of head injury alone, can be extremely deleterious to the injured brain. Lack of cerebral perfusion will result in cerebral ischemia. An ischemic brain will develop cerebral edema and increased intracranial pressure.

Objective evaluation of hydration status by central venous pressure or pulmonary artery wedge pressure is appropriate in those with serious head injuries and increased intracranial pressure. Fluids may then be managed to optimize cerebral perfusion without over hydration. The cerebral perfusion pressure (CPP) is equal to the mean arterial pressure minus the intracranial pressure. CPP should be above 60 mm Hg.

Table 4 Treatment of Increased Intracranial Pressure

Goal: ICP < 15 mm Hg

- Maintain head and neck neutral and unflexed
- Avoid jugular obstruction
- Hyperventilation:
  Pco_2, 25–30 mm Hg, Po_2
  Po_2, 100 mm Hg, Pco_2
- Mannitol, 0.25–2 g/kg q4–6h
  Adult initial dose, 12.5–25 g; maintain serum osmolality between 300–320 osmols
- Lasix, 10–20 mg IV prn

Positioning and Sedation. Optimal patient positioning was once thought to include elevation of the head to 30 degrees. More recent studies have shown that optimal position varies. Position should be individualized for the lowest intracranial pressure. Whenever possible, the use of tape or ties that encircle the neck should be avoided, as they may occlude venous return, which may increase intracranial pressure. Efficient venous return is also facilitated by a neutral position without flexion of head and neck.

Sedatives and muscle relaxants can be effective adjuvants for the control of intracranial pressure. The intracranial pressure of a coughing, struggling patient will increase. The loss of ability to follow a physical examination is compensated for the use of intracranial pressure monitoring.

Ventilation. Hyperventilation is the cornerstone of the initial management of head trauma. Decreasing the carbon dioxide partial pressure (PCO_2) results in vasoconstriction and decreased cerebral blood flow. The diminution of blood flow allows the intracranial contents and intracranial pressure to decrease. Adequate cerebral perfusion and control of intracranial pressure is maintained when the PCO_2 is greater than 25 mm Hg, but less than 30 mm Hg. Hypoxia should be avoided. The fractional inspired oxygen (FIO_2) should be adjusted to keep the partial pressure of oxygen (PO_2) approximately 100 mm Hg.

Positive end-expiratory pressure (PEEP) can be used even when the intracranial pressure is elevated. PEEP may add to intracranial pressure but does so only when the lungs are noncompliant. The benefits of improved oxygenation may outweigh the risks of increased intracranial pressure. Hyperventilation should be reduced gradually after intracranial pressure is under control.

Pulmonary dysfunction resulting in hypercarbia and hypoxia may be harmful to the compromised brain and must be aggressively managed. Neurogenic pulmonary edema is a rare but serious cause of declining pulmonary function usually seen early in the patient's course and heralded by the sudden onset of frothy pink sputum. A rapid increase in intracranial pressure is thought to trigger pulmonary edema. Therapy should focus on relieving the increased intracranial pressure and improving oxygenation by treating the pulmonary edema.

Adult respiratory distress syndrome (ARDS) has been discussed in another chapter. Patients with other injuries associated with head trauma, especially those who have required significant volume resuscitation, are at risk for ARDS. Pneumonia in the patient with head trauma patient is often heralded by a drop in PO_2 long before changes are evident in the physical examination or chest film. A balance must be achieved between the benefits of aggressive pulmonary toilet and the risk of increasing intracranial pressure. Vigorous sedation may help to protect the brain during necessary suctioning and postural drainage.

Mannitol. Mannitol, an osmotic diuretic, is widely used for lowering intracranial pressure. Its action depends on an intact blood-brain barrier and adequate renal function. The usual dose is 0.25 to 2 g per kilogram, given every 4 to 6 hours. The serum osmolality should be checked about 2 hours after dosing. The dose should be adjusted to keep the serum osmolality between 300 and 320 osmols. Higher levels are associated with metabolic complications, including azotemia and metabolic acidosis. The initial dose of mannitol should be the lowest possible to achieve the desired effect. Evidence exists that a lower dose (0.25 g per kilogram) is just as effective as a higher dose and has fewer side effects.

If the patient is volume-depleted, the administration of mannitol may result in hypotension after the therapeutic diuresis, which is often brisk. Mannitol should be used in a setting where blood pressure can be closely monitored and in a patient who has been adequately fluid-resuscitated.

The action of mannitol depends on an intact blood-brain barrier. Mannitol may theoretically cause expansion of areas of blood-brain barrier breakdown, such as hematomas. This phenomenon is not usually a problem in clinical practice.

Cessation of mannitol should be gradual by lengthening the dose interval and decreasing dose to prevent rebound cerebral edema and allow for the rapid reinitiation of therapy if intracranial pressure increases.

Glycerol and urea are pharmacologic agents that have been useful in the past for control of increased intracranial pressure, but they are no longer usually used now in the treatment of head trauma.

Lasix. Lasix can be helpful in controlling cerebral edema. Usually used as an adjunct to mannitol, lasix is given at low doses (0.5 to 1 mg per kilogram or 10 to 20 mg in adults) as needed. As with mannitol, diuresis may result in hypotension.

Anticonvulsants. A single seizure at the time of head injury or shortly after injury is not uncommon. Early post-traumatic epilepsy (one or two seizures within the first 24 hours) does not imply future seizures. Maintenance of oxygenation is paramount during seizures. Vigorous pharmacologic treatment with diazepam derivatives may cause respiratory depression, necessitating intubation.

Multiple seizures and status epilepticus should be treated vigorously, as seizures increase cerebral metabolic demands. In the compromised injured brain, such metabolic demands are poorly tolerated. Treatment for status epilepticus is outlined in another chapter. Postictal depression of the central nervous system may temporarily worsen the GCS.

In the patient with severe head injury, diphenylhydantoin (Dilantin) may be used to prevent seizures. Patients particularly at risk are those with acute subdural hematoma, cerebral edema, parenchymal hematomas, and depressed skull fractures. Loading doses of 20 mg per kilogram (1,000 to 1,500 mg in adults) are appropriate. Rapid administration (faster than 50 mg per minute), which may cause hypotension, should be avoided. Decadron has no role in the treatment of post-traumatic cerebral edema.

Barbiturate coma does not have proven clinical efficiency in improving outcome in increased intracranial pressure. When conventional methods have failed, however,

Table 5 Management of Elevations in Intracranial Pressure

1. ICP monitor: check transducer level and function
2. Check patient position
3. Check ABGs, electrolytes, glucose
4. Repeat CT: exclude mass lesions and hydrocephalus
5. EEG or empiric therapy for subclinical seizures
6. Consider use of ventricular catheter to drain CSF
7. Pentobarbital/barbiturate coma: load with 3–5 mg/kg; maintenance, 0.5–3 mg/kg/hr

this treatment can be tried. The dose of pentobarbital (Nembutal), a readily available short-acting barbiturate, is 3 to 5 mg per kilogram intravenously as a bolus. The maintenance dose, given every 1 to 2 hours, is 0.5 mg to 3 mg per kilogram. Electroencephalographic monitoring may be helpful in assessing cortical suppression. Blood levels should be between 30 and 60 μg per deciliter.

At doses sufficient to maintain barbiturate coma, hypotension from direct cardiac effects may occur. Inotropic agents and fluids should be utilized as needed to improve cardiac output. Phenobarbital may be substituted for pentobarbital. Phenobarbital has less cardiac effect but a much longer half-life. This longer half-life will lengthen the time needed to assess patients clinically once the dose has been terminated.

If intracranial pressure remains high or increases after initial control is achieved, the steps outlined in Table 5 should be considered.

SUGGESTED READING

Crutchfield J, Stuart N, Raj K, et al. Evaluation of a fiberoptic intracranial pressure monitor. J Neurosurg 1990; 72:482–487.
Gennarelli TA, Spielman, GM, Langfitt TW, et al. Influence of the type of intracranial lesion on the outcome from severe head injury. J Neurosurg 1982; 56:26–32.
Langfitt TW, Gennarelli TA. Can the outcome from head injury be improved? J Neurosurg 1982; 56:19–25.
Teasdale G, Jennett B. Assessment of coma and impaired consciousness: a practical scale. Lancet 1974; 2:81–84.

COMA

DAVID E. LEVY, M.D.

Coma is one of several serious disorders of consciousness frequently faced in an intensive care setting. Clinically, coma is an eyes-closed state of unarousal without any learned responses to internal or external stimuli (Table 1). By contrast, in the vegetative state, to which coma often leads, the eyes open spontaneously, and sleep-wake cycles frequently develop. Nonetheless, the vegetative patient fails to exhibit any of the learned responses that characterize consciousness. The vegetative state must be distinguished in turn from the locked-in state, in which patients may superficially appear to be unconscious but on careful examination are found to retain the ability to respond to commands that involve eye movements (usually vertical, sometimes horizontal) and thus are conscious. Because their cerebral hemispheres are usually intact, communication can be established with locked-in patients through codes that involve movements of the eyes or eyelids.

Being a symptom rather than a specific disease entity, unconsciousness requires that management be directed to the underlying cause and to the prevention of complications. Moreover, the inherent seriousness of coma means that the physician's responsibility extends beyond diagnosis and treatment to include humane and ethical considerations about potentially prolonged support in helpless situations.

Table 1 Disorders of Consciousness

	Conscious	Locked-in	Vegetative	Coma	Brain Dead
Wakefulness Present	+	+	+	−	−
Eyes open	+	+	+	−	−
Awareness Present	+	+	−	−	−
Motor better than withdrawal	+	−	−	−	−
Verbal better than groans	+	−	−	−	−
Eyes move to command	+	+	−	−	−
Other Brain-Stem Signs					
Present	+	±	±	±	−

+ = yes; − = no; ± = only some.

DIAGNOSIS

Operationally, *coma* is recognized by failure to open the eyes in response to any stimulus; by the absence of any motor response to commands or pain (usually pressure applied to the supraorbital ridge or the nail bed) or by primitive posturing responses only (e.g., abnormal extensor posturing or abnormal flexor posturing, often called decerebrate or decorticate posturing, respectively); and by the absence of any vocalizations more complex than moaning (see Table 1). The patient in a *vegetative state* is similar except that the eyes open spontaneously and blink. To determine that the vegetative patient is truly incapable of responding in a learned fashion to external stimuli, it is helpful to provide both aural and written commands (in the patient's language), to make certain that the patient does not obey commands with the eyes or eyelids (as seen in the *locked-in state*), to observe the patient for spontaneous movements reflecting prior learning (e.g., pulling bed sheets up), and to determine whether there is any emotional response (e.g., crying or laughing) to appropriate verbal input. The presence of any of these behaviors excludes a diagnosis of the vegetative state. Both comatose and vegetative patients exhibit at least some evidence of brain-stem function (e.g., retained pupillary or corneal reactions or preserved spontaneous respiration). When all brain-stem function is absent on clinical examination, a diagnosis of *brain death* must be considered, and apnea testing should be undertaken.

Localization

For patients presenting in acute coma, the physician's immediate role is to provide cardiorespiratory support while rapidly reaching an accurate diagnosis, particularly when coma results from a potentially treatable cause. It is helpful first to localize the site of dysfunction causing coma. Although there are occasional exceptions, a good rule is that unilateral cerebral hemispheric lesions by themselves do not cause coma. Coma is generally seen only with dysfunction of both cerebral hemispheres or of the reticular activating system in the upper brain stem. A few easily recognized clinical syndromes underlie most cases of coma (Table 2). One way in which both cerebral hemispheres and/or the upper brain stem can be affected is by diffuse or multifocal processes. For a focal lesion to produce coma other than by directly affecting the upper brain stem (e.g., pontine hemorrhage), the process must cause brain swelling, which in turn causes more extensive dysfunction, a process called herniation. These processes can be characterized as originating in the supratentorial or subtentorial spaces.

Herniation Syndromes

There are several different types of herniation. One that is not recognized as frequently as it occurs is central herniation, where dysfunction successively affects the hypothalamus and diencephalon but spares the uncus. These patients do not exhibit unilateral pupillary dilatation (as in uncal herniation) but instead develop bilateral pupillary constriction as sympathetic influences in the hypothalamus are lost. Usually stupor and Cheyne-Stokes (periodic) respirations develop concurrently. If allowed to progress, irreversible damage to the upper brain stem can occur rapidly. Recognizing central herniation requires that the clinician note the pupillary size so that subsequent changes can be appreciated.

By contrast, in uncal herniation the tip of the temporal lobe is pushed over the tentorial edge, leading to ipsilateral pupillary dilatation (because of parasympathetic interruption from compression of the adjacent third cranial nerve) and if not already present, contralateral hemiparesis (from compression of the cerebral peduncle). Uncal herniation is more readily recognized than central herniation, but the urgency for prompt intervention is no less. Unilateral supratentorial masses can also push the medial cerebral hemisphere beneath the falx cerebri into the space normally occupied by the contralateral hemisphere, a process termed subfalcine herniation. Although not so easily recognized clinically, the nearly invariable occurrence of uncal along with subfalcine herniation makes identification easy.

Table 2 Localizing the Cause of Coma

Type	Recognition	Representative Causes
Supratentorial	Progressive rostrocaudal deterioration (herniation)	Subdural or epidural hematoma; brain tumor; abscess; intracerebral hemorrhage
Subtentorial	Signs of primary brain-stem or cerebellar dysfunction	Cerebellar hemorrhage or infarction; pontine hemorrhage
Diffuse or Multifocal	No consistent focal signs	Poisoning; hypoglycemia; anoxia with cardiac arrest; hepatic or renal failure; meningitis; subarachnoid hemorrhage

Two other forms of herniation should be recognized. When the cerebellar tonsils are shifted by a mass of the posterior fossa through the foramen magnum at the base of the skull, passive neck flexion is usually resisted. This "nuchal rigidity" from tonsillar herniation may mimic the meningismus seen in meningitis and subarachnoid hemorrhage. Since a lumbar puncture (usually mandatory for meningitis) could aggravate this tonsillar herniation, it is essential that the physician make certain that there are no signs or symptoms suggesting primary disease of the posterior fossa before doing a lumbar puncture for meningitis or subarachnoid hemorrhage. Much less common is upward transtentorial herniation, also from a mass in the posterior fossa. This can usually be detected by loss of vertical eye movements (spontaneously or in response to oculocephalic or doll's eyes maneuver) because of tectal compression. This might be important if ventricular drainage is contemplated in patients who develop hydrocephalus from a posterior fossa process.

Treatment of Herniation. If a focal mass causing herniation is suspected clinically, an emergency computerized tomography (CT) scan or magnetic resonance imaging (MRI) test is indicated, and the neurosurgeon should also be called, since craniotomy to treat a subdural hematoma, acute hydrocephalus, or a cerebellar hemorrhage might be required. The immediate treatment of herniation, however, is hyperventilation, which by reducing the arterial carbon dioxide tension also reduces intracranial blood volume and thus provides extra space within the cranial vault. Intravenous osmotic agents (e.g., 250 ml of a 20 percent solution of mannitol in water) works more slowly. Although corticosteroids (e.g., dexamethasone, up to 100 mg intravenously), which also work slowly, are effective for edema caused by cancer, they may even be harmful when given to stroke patients.

Psychogenic Unresponsiveness

Psychologic factors can at times produce a coma-like state that persists despite painful stimuli, including invasive interventions. Whenever psychogenic unresponsiveness is suspected, it is wise to perform ice-water caloric testing by instilling up to 50 ml of ice water in an ear with an intact tympanic membrane. The normal response in conscious patients is nystagmus, with the rapid phase directed away from the irrigated ear; when more than a few, desultory beats of nystagmus are observed, the clinician can be assured that the patient is not truly unconscious and that he or she should undergo psychiatric evaluation.

Diffuse or Multifocal Causes of Coma

When the clinical examination fails to reveal an area of focal dysfunction and subsequent signs of pressure, attention must shift to diffuse or multifocal causes of coma. The list is long, but determination of arterial blood gases can help distinguish among the possible causes (Table 3).

Table 3 Abnormal Ventilation and Coma From Diffuse Causes

Pattern	Causes
Hyperventilation and metabolic acidosis	Diabetic ketoacidosis; diabetic hyperosmolar coma; lactic acidosis (anoxia); uremia; poisons (paraldehyde, methyl alcohol, ethylene glycol)
Hyperventilation and respiratory alkalosis	Hepatic failure; sepsis, psychogenic unresponsiveness
Hypoventilation and metabolic acidosis	Diuretics (heart disease); gastric loss (vomiting); Cushing's disease; primary hyperaldosteronism
Hypoventilation and respiratory acidosis	Sedative drugs; chronic pulmonary disease

MANAGEMENT

Although the management of subarachnoid hemorrhage usually includes urgent angiography to identify aneurysms that might be clipped, surgery is usually contraindicated in comatose patients; thus angiography is used primarily to confirm the clinical (or radiologic) diagnosis. Intravenous nimodipine (90 mg every 4 hours) is now used to limit ischemic complications in subarachnoid hemorrhage.

Whenever meningitis is suspected, immediate administration of antibiotics is essential; accordingly, some would question the common practice of obtaining a CT scan and then a lumbar puncture if this sequential testing will significantly delay the institution of antibiotics. Although several different regimens are used, a reasonable choice for patients without immunocompromise is ampicillin (2 g every 2 hours) and sometimes chloramphenicol (1 g every 6 hours).

If hypoglycemia is suspected, prompt intravenous administration of thiamine (100 mg, to treat Wernicke's disease, which can coexist) and then glucose (50 ml of a 50 percent solution of glucose in water) can be lifesaving. Coma caused by Wernicke's disease has recently been reported in patients with chronic renal failure on hemodialysis, and thus in these patients too, thiamine might reverse coma. Recently, the benzodiazepine antagonist flumazenil (up to 15 mg intravenously over 3 hours) along with lactulose was associated with substantial clinical improvement in patients with hepatic encephalopathy; the possibility of using this and related inhibitors clinically is currently being explored.

For exogenous poisoning from opiates and related compounds, intravenous naloxone (start with 0.4 mg) is mandatory, but it is also essential in patients who respond to naloxone to observe them closely since additional naloxone may be needed as the initial dose is metabolized. A recent report that intravenous 4-methylpryazole (9.5 mg per kilogram every 12 hours) improved the clinical state and acidosis of ethylene glycol poisoning suggests a possible clinical use for this compound in methanol and ethylene glycol poisoning once additional confirmatory studies have appeared.

All comatose patients require scrupulous nursing care with good fluid, electrolyte, and acid-base management; adequate oxygenation and good pulmonary toilet usually via an endotracheal tube early in the course; good skin care with turning every 2 hours; stool softeners and frequent rectal examinations so that impactions can be relieved promptly; and eyelid closure to protect the corneas. If possible, sedatives should not be used to control agitation. Seizures may be difficult to control, but intravenous diazepam (5 to 10 mg slowly) followed by phenytoin or barbiturates will often help. Phenytoin should be started with 1,000 mg by nasogastric tube or slow intravenous infusion at 50 mg per minute, followed by 300 mg daily, adjusted to maintain therapeutic levels of 10 to 20 μg per milliliter. Myoclonus is even more difficult to control, but clonazepam (0.5 mg by nasogastric tube every 8 hours) can be tried.

Comatose and vegetative patients deserve respectful treatment at all times. When in doubt, the safe course is to say nothing around the bed that the patient ought not to hear. For locked-in patients, who can repeat conversations months later, this warning is even more important, for these patients are conscious.

PROGNOSIS

Intensivists are by nature involved in triage decisions, and unconscious patients pose particularly thorny problems, as so few of them are likely to do well. Nonetheless, rather than moving comatose patients out of intensive care units regardless of their clinical condition, intensivists should be aware of efforts to improve outcome prediction based on clinical signs. Several groups have been involved in this work, and results are summarized below.

Nontraumatic Coma

For nontraumatic coma, age appears not to be related to outcome, possibly because so many patients in nontraumatic coma have complicated medical conditions and are therefore elderly. There is disagreement on whether seizures or myoclonus implies a poor prognosis; they certainly do not help matters. For many metabolic causes of coma, aggressive treatment of seizures is unsatisfactory, and thus one might reserve treatment for situations in which (1) the metabolic demands of continuous seizures might place unacceptable demands on the heart and (2) the seizure itself might suppress consciousness (e.g., "psychomotor status epilepticus").

In nontraumatic coma, the absence of multiple brain stem signs for several days, not otherwise explained by medications or pre-existing conditions, portends a very poor chance of recovery. In one study, only one of 87 patients lacking two or more of the following brain stem signs ever regained independence: corneal reflex, pupillary reactions to light (observed with a hand lens), any response to caloric stimulation, and any motor response to pain. Other investigators have reported similar observations, with one adding that patients comatose from cardiac arrest who have high initial blood glucose levels (above 300 mg per deciliter) are less likely to do well than those with lower levels. A study of thiopental-induced coma in survivors of cardiac arrest showed no benefit, and thus barbiturate coma cannot be recommended in this setting.

Traumatic Coma

For traumatic coma, the approach has been somewhat different, with most groups relying on the Glasgow Coma Score. This is the sum of three subscores for eye opening (1 to 4), verbal responses (1 to 5), and motor responses (1 to 6), with 3 being the worst possible score and 15 the best. In one study, no patient with scores of 3 or 4 at 3 days regained independence within 6 months. As with nontraumatic coma, the absence of pupillary reactions predicted a poor outcome, but there were some exceptions (4 percent based on observations within the first day). Also, age is related to outcome for these patients: in the same study, there was a continuous inverse relationship between age and the chance of regaining independence. Finally, the presence of an intracranial hemorrhage reduced the chance of recovery, especially in younger patients, who might otherwise have been expected to do well.

The Vegetative State

Prolonged coma is rare. Most patients open their eyes and become vegetative (see Table 1) within a short time, but without return of awareness, the simple presence of wakefulness does not predict recovery. Once the vegetative state has lasted more than a few weeks, the chance of regaining independent function falls precipitously. Of 12 patients who were vegetative 2 weeks after the onset of nontraumatic coma, none ever regained independent function. By contrast, independent function was reported in 14 of 140 patients who were vegetative 1 month after the onset of traumatic coma, but no patient in this series who was still vegetative at 3 months ever regained the ability to live independently.

Isolated case reports of "recovery" (usually only partial) after more prolonged durations of the vegetative state have appeared in the literature and are sometimes cited by families asking that all measures be continued. To put these reports in perspective, a highly conservative estimate of 10,000 new vegetative patients in the United States each year (based on a Japanese survey) would suggest that these few reports over the last 10 to 15 years may be derived from as many as 100,000 patients. The chance that an individual patient who was vegetative for several months will recover any meaningful function is thus probably less than one in 10,000.

Needless to say, decisions about the care of unconscious patients cannot be reached unilaterally but require discussion with families and sometimes with hospital ethicists. Withdrawal of care, whether in an intensive care unit or on a ward, places difficult demands on families and requires understanding and tact from physicians and nurses.

SUGGESTED READING

Jennett B, Teasdale G, Braakman R, et al. Prognosis of patients with severe head injury. Neurosurgery 1979; 4:283–289.
Levy DE, Bates D, Caronna JJ, et al. Prognosis in nontraumatic coma. Ann Intern Med 1981; 94:293–301.
Plum F, Posner JB. The diagnosis of stupor and coma. 3rd ed. Philadelphia: FA Davis, 1980.

NEUROLOGIC CRITERIA FOR DEATH

ALISON WICHMAN, M.D.
SUSUMU SATO, M.D.

The traditional medical definition of death is the permanent cessation of heartbeat and respiration. Cessation of heart and lung function is easily observable and usually sufficient basis for a declaration of death. With the routine use of cardiopulmonary resuscitation (CPR) and more effective artificial cardiopulmonary support systems, it is possible to restore and maintain cardiopulmonary function. The development of these medical technologies, however, has led to recognition of the brain's unique vulnerability to anoxia. It is this characteristic of the brain that is a major factor in the outcome of CPR. The irreversible failure of the brain normally precludes the continued function of the heart and lungs and vice versa. The clinical reality of being able to maintain circulation and respiration artificially in patients who have lost all brain function necessitated reevaluation of the traditional definition of death.

DEFINITION OF DEATH: LEGAL CONSIDERATIONS

Progress in organ transplantation was a major impetus for reconsideration of the accepted definition of death. In response to the need to increase the availability of donor organs, the Uniform Anatomical Gift Act (UAGA) was drafted and in 1968 received rapid acceptance and implementation. The UAGA did not define death, since death was considered a matter of medical judgment, not statutory law. In 1970 Kansas became the first state to give judicial approval to a statutory definition of death, which included both cardiovascular and brain criteria. Since then, 29 states have adopted statutory definitions of death that include brain-based criteria. The diversity of the proposed and enacted laws from state to state has created substantial confusion. Consequently, the American Bar Association, the American Medical Association, and the President's Commission for the Study of Ethical Problems in Medicine and Biomedical and Behavioral Research have proposed that each jurisdiction adopt the following model statute:

Uniform Determination of Death Act: "An individual who has sustained either (1) irreversible cessation of circulatory and respiratory functions or (2) irreversible cessation of all functions of the entire brain, including the brain stem, is dead. A determination of death must be made in accordance with accepted medical standards."

The wording "functions of the entire brain, including the brain stem" may be redundant but was intentionally formulated to distinguish brain death from other severe irreversible brain injuries, including persistent vegetative state, in which the cerebral cortex is irreversibly destroyed, but all or some of the brain stem still functions. The wording was meant to ensure that declarations of death would not be confused with the poor prognosis of those who are comatose but do not meet neurologic criteria for death.

Since brain death statutes vary widely, we suggest that physicians familiarize themselves with the situation in their states. Case law has uniformly approved the use of brain criteria, and medical-legal experts have concluded that physicians in states without such statutes or case law precedent can feel secure in using accepted neurologic criteria as a means of determining death.

NEUROLOGIC CRITERIA FOR THE DETERMINATION OF DEATH

The President's Commission has specified that the criteria physicians use in determining death should (1) eliminate errors in classifying a living individual as dead, (2) allow as few errors as possible in classifying a dead body as alive, (3) allow the determination to be made without unreasonable delay, (4) be adaptable to a variety of clinical situations, and (5) be explicit and accessible to verification. Several medically accepted guidelines for the neurologic determination of death have been published. These include the "Harvard criteria," the "Minnesota criteria," and criteria known as the "U.S. Guidelines," which were formulated by the Medical Consultants to the President's Commission. Because there is some variation in these standards, local, state, and national institutions and professional organizations are encouraged to examine and publish their practices. The Warren G. Magnuson

Clinical Center of the National Institutes of Health has had a policy on brain death since 1979, based on the U.S. Guidelines.

Neurologic criteria for the determination of death must document irreversible cessation of functions of the entire brain (Table 1). Brain functions relevant to the determination are those that are clinically observable. When indicated, the clinical determination is subject to confirmation by laboratory tests. While law generally requires that physicians declaring death be licensed, standard medical practice also requires that physicians be familiar with the neurologic criteria and experienced in the neurologic examination. At the Clinical Center, declarations of brain death based on neurologic criteria require consultation with a board-certified neurologist who is a member of the senior medical staff. When the patient is a potential organ donor, most hospital policies require independence between the physician declaring death and the transplant team. The physician declaring death should not be the patient's primary physician.

There must be deep coma—that is, cerebral unreceptivity and unresponsivity. Decerebrate or decorticate posturing or seizures are inconsistent with the declaration of death. Peripheral nervous system and spinal cord reflexes may persist, however, and complex muscle movements emanating from the spinal cord have been reported in individuals meeting the neurologic criteria for death. Brain stem reflexes must be absent (Table 2). When there are no pupillary, oculocephalic, oculovestibular, corneal, or oropharyngeal reflexes, performance of a respiratory (apnea) test is indicated. The apnea reflex is the last to be tested and is tested only if the other reflexes are absent. Apnea is defined as the absence of spontaneous respiration without assistance of the respirator. There are several accepted methods of performing an apnea test. Regardless of the method, avoiding significant hypoxemia while creating hypercarbia is the goal. The method used at the Clinical Center is to ventilate the patient with 100 percent fraction of inspired oxygen (FiO_2) for 10 minutes. Ventilation is discontinued and oxygen is delivered by passive flow (4 to 6 L per minute) through a cannula placed in the endotracheal tube.

Hypercarbia adequately stimulates respiratory effort within 30 seconds when the arterial carbon dioxide pres-

Table 1 Neurologic Criteria for the Determination of Death (U.S. Guidelines)

I. Cessation of all functions of the entire brain (that are clinically observable)
  (a) Deep coma
  (b) Absence of the following brain stem reflexes:
    (1) Pupillary light reflex
    (2) Oculocephalic reflex
    (3) Oculovestibular reflex
    (4) Corneal reflex
    (5) Oropharyngeal reflexes (gag and cough)
    (6) Respiratory (apnea) reflex
  (c) When indicated (e.g., when reflexes in (b) cannot be adequately assessed or if conditions in II(b) exist) confirmatory tests are recommended

II. Cessation of all functions of the entire brain must be irreversible
  (a) The cause of coma is established and sufficient to account for the loss of all brain functions
  (b) The possibility of recovery of any brain function is excluded. Rule out:
    (1) Drug and metabolic intoxication
    (2) Hypothermia
    (3) Shock
  (c) Period of observation:
    (1) Period of observation may be a matter of clinical judgment
    (2) When cause of coma is established in presence of electrocerebral silence (EEG)
      • Two clinical examinations separated by 6 hours
    (3) When cause of coma is established but no EEG performed
      • Two clinical examinations separated by 12 hours
    (4) For anoxic brain damage
      • Observation for 24 hours
      • May be decreased if confirmatory tests performed
  (d) Confirmatory tests
    (1) EEG
    (2) Studies to document cessation of intracranial blood flow
      • Four-vessel cerebral angiogram
      • Cerebral radionuclide angiogram

Table 2 Absence of Brain-Stem Reflexes

Pupillary Light Reflex: Absence of change in pupil size when a strong light is directed to each pupil sequentially. Pupils need not be equal or dilated but must be nonreactive to light. Clinical testing may not be adequate if patient has received scopolamine, opiates, neuromuscular blocking agents, atropine, glutethimide, or mydriatic eye drops, or in the presence of ocular trauma.

Oculovestibular Reflex: Absence of movement of the globe within the orbit when the patient's head is moved quickly from side to side. Clinical assessment may not be possible in patients with trauma of the cervical spine.

Corneal Relfex: Absence of eyelid movement when each cornea is touched lightly with cotton. Clinical testing is not adequate in the presence of severe facial weakness.

Oculovestibular Reflex: Head is elevated 30 degrees, and each ear is irrigated sequentially with 50 cc of ice water. There is absence of movement of the globes toward the irrigated ear. Clinical testing may not be possible in patients with trauma to the inner ear or basilar skull fracture.

Oropharyngeal Reflexes (cough and gag): No movement of the uvula or retching when back of the pharynx is stimulated with a tongue depressor or endotracheal tube is moved. No cough is elicited when a suction catheter is passed into the tracheobronchial tree.

If *all* of these reflexes are absent, then the apnea test is performed.

Respiratory (apnea) Reflex: Ventilate with 100% FiO_2 for 10–15 minutes. Discontinue ventilation and oxygenate through cannula in endotracheal tube at 4–6 L/minute. Continue test until $PCO_2 \geq 60$ mm Hg.

Table 3 Conditions Complicating Declaration of Death

Sedative or anesthetic drugs

Neuromuscular blocking agents, aminoglycoside antibiotics, and diseases such as myasthenia gravis

Some severe metabolic illnesses (hepatic encephalopathy, hyperosmolar preterminal uremia)

Hypothermia (core temperature below 32.2°C)

Shock

---

sure (Pco_2) is greater than 60 mm Hg. Generally, 10 minutes is adequate to reach a Pco_2 of 60 mm Hg. Measurement of arterial blood gases to document hypercarbia is recommended. In patients with lung disease who may be dependent on a hypoxic stimulus for respiration, the arterial oxygen tension must be less than 50 mm Hg at the end of the test. Spontaneous breathing efforts during the performance of the apnea test indicate that part of the brain stem is functioning and the declaration of death cannot be made.

Several complicating conditions make it impossible to rely solely on the clinical examination (Table 3). When adequate clinical assessment is not possible, or when drug or metabolic intoxication is present, confirmatory tests may be required. Drug intoxication is the most serious problem in the determination of death, especially when multiple drugs are used. Cessation of brain functions caused by drugs such as barbiturates, benzodiazepines, meprobamate, methaqualone, trichloroethylene, narcotics, and alcohol may be fully reversible, even though the drugs may produce clinical cessation of brain functions and electrocerebral silence on the electroencephalogram (EEG). A determination of death by neurologic criteria must not be made until intoxicants are metabolized or a confirmatory test reveals the absence of intracranial blood flow.

The absence of blood flow to the cerebrum and brain stem is a decisive indicator of total destruction of the brain. Four-vessel angiography or cerebral radionuclide angiography can document the absence of brain perfusion and allow for the declaration of death. When paralysis, unresponsiveness, and apnea may be caused by neuromuscular blocking agents, aminoglycoside antibiotics, or diseases such as myasthenia gravis, a careful review of the patient's medical history is indicated. There may be indications for performing electromyography, peripheral nerve stimulation, EEG, or tests of intracranial circulation.

Extreme caution should be used if patients are in shock because the reduction in cerebral circulation may render clinical examination and perfusion tests unreliable.

The Clinical Center death criteria do not require an EEG, although some attending neurologists prefer to obtain an EEG to aid their evaluation. We adopted the 1980 guidelines of the American EEG Society for electrocerebral silence. Testing of evoked potentials, such as brain-stem auditory or somatosensory evoked responses, is sometimes used to study the integrity of the nervous system. These tests are helpful but must be interpreted cautiously; the presence of an experienced and competent EEG technologist and interpreter is essential for a proper examination.

The period of observation before death is declared may vary. When the cause of coma is known and there is electrocerebral silence on the EEG, two examinations separated by 6 hours suffice. When the cause of coma is known and no EEG has been performed, two examinations separated by 12 hours should be performed. In cases of anoxic damage, in which the extent of damage is more difficult to ascertain, observation for 24 hours is generally desirable, unless cessation of intracranial blood flow or electrocerebral silence is demonstrated in an adult patient who is without drug intoxication, hypothermia, or shock. When absence of blood flow to the brain is documented by confirmatory tests, no further observation period is necessary before declaring death.

Guidelines for the determination of death by neurologic criteria in children have been drafted by a task force with wide representation from the legal, neurologic, and pediatric communities. In children older than 1 year of age, the guidelines are the same as for adults (see Table 1). For term infants 1 week to 1 year of age, the guidelines are the same as for adults except for the period of observation and the use of confirmatory tests. In term infants 7 days to 2 months of age, two examinations and two EEGs performed 48 hours apart are required. For children 2 months to 1 year of age, two examinations and two EEGs separated by 24 hours are required. However, repeated examinations and EEGs are not necessary in either age group if confirmatory tests show the absence of intracranial blood flow. There are no guidelines for infants younger than 7 days old because neurologic evaluations are considered unreliable in very young infants.

EFFECTIVE COMMUNICATION WITH THE FAMILY

The reality of death and communication with the family about death may be difficult experiences for intensive care unit personnel. Honest communication with the family about the clinical determination of death and the nature of and rationale for confirmatory tests is important. The time required to perform and interpret the confirmatory tests gives family members an opportunity to begin to cope with the imminent death of their loved one.

The declaration of death by neurologic criteria is a medical act and is made when death is confirmed, not when ventilation is discontinued or the heart ceases to beat. Once death has been determined, it is mandatory for the patient to be pronounced dead and for all treatment to be stopped. There are three major circumstances in which life-support systems may be justifiably continued after death has been pronounced: (1) to allow the family a reasonable length of time to decide whether transplantation is appropriate, (2) to allow adequate time to remove the organs when organ donation is approved, and (3) in a pregnant woman, when there is a possibility of delivering a viable fetus if treatment is continued.

Although consent is not required for the declaration of death by neurologic criteria, physicians have an obligation to communicate the medical facts to families in a clear and sensitive manner. They should address any of the concerns, reservations, or objections the family may have. Family members will have several decisions to make, including whether to donate organs. However, it is important to help them understand that they are not being asked to decide to discontinue mechanical ventilation. The determination of death and decision to discontinue ventilation are medical decisions and should not be left to the family. As in other situations in clinical medicine, the physician's role is to present the family with the medical information, help them understand what it means, and clarify the physician's responsibilities.

SUGGESTED READING

American Electroencephalographic (EEG) Society. Minimum technical standards for EEG recording in suspected cerebral death. J Clin Neurophysiol 1986; 3:144–149.
Chatrian GE. Electrophysiologic evaluation of brain death: a critical appraisal. In: Aminoff MJ, ed. Electrodiagnosis in clinical neurology. New York: Churchill Livingstone, 1986:669.
Special Task Force. Guidelines for the determination of death in children. Pediatrics 1987; 80:298–300.
Medical Consultants on the Diagnosis of Death to the President's Commission for the Study of Ethical Problems in Medicine and Behavioral Research. Guidelines for the determination of death. JAMA 1981; 246:2184.
Oro JJ. Determination of death by neurologic criteria. Mo Med 1989; 86:628–631.
Outcalt D. Brain death: medical and legal issues. J Fam Pract 1984; 19:349–354.

ASCENDING POLYNEURITIS (GUILLAIN-BARRÉ SYNDROME)

MICHAEL RUBIN, M.D.

Guillain-Barré syndrome (GBS) is an acute, inflammatory, demyelinating polyradiculoneuropathy thought to be autoimmune in nature. Disease usually begins with leg weakness that tends to be more proximal than distal. Sensory symptoms and signs are frequent accompaniments. The weakness may plateau and resolve or may progress to complete flaccid quadriplegia with respiratory failure. Great advances have been achieved in recent years in the treatment of these patients.

APPROACH TO THE PATIENT

Patients who when first seen are suspected of having GBS should be admitted to the hospital for observation. Until a patient has been stabilized (i.e., no change in clinical status over 72 hours), the clinical course can be highly unpredictable with rapid deterioration over hours. For this reason, any patient suspected of having GBS requires close medical and nursing observation. When the patient is first seen, if the course appears to be rapidly progressive or if respiratory difficulties and bulbar compromise appear inevitable, admission to an intensive care unit (ICU) is indicated. If the admitting institution does not have facilities for plasmapheresis, the patient should be transferred promptly to one that does.

On admission, work-up for the various diagnostic possibilities may be undertaken (Table 1). In present-day circumstances, patients with GBS should undergo human immunodeficiency virus (HIV) testing.

THERAPY

Plasmapheresis

Once the diagnosis of GBS has been made, the first question that faces the physician is: At what point along the course should plasmapheresis begin? The Johns Hopkins University Multi-Center Trial of Plasmapheresis in GBS demonstrated that plasmapheresis has a significant beneficial effect in the treatment of patients with GBS. The

Table 1 Differential Diagnosis of Guillain-Barré Syndrome

Infections
    Epstein-Barr virus (infectious mononucleosis)
    Diphtheria
    Botulism
    Tick paralysis
    Polio
    Human immunodeficiency virus (HIV)
Collagen vascular disease
    Lupus
Toxicity
    Arsenic
    Thallium
    Hexacarbon abuse (glue sniffing)
    Tri-ortho-cresyl phosphate
    Lead
    Antibiotics (nitrofurantoin)
Porphyria
Paraneoplastic syndromes
Periodic paralysis
Transverse myelitis

New York Hospital experience with the treatment has been similar. Improvement was seen for all endpoints tested: status at 4 weeks, time to improve one clinical grade, time to independent walking, and status at 6 months. Plasmapheresis was particularly effective if started within 7 days of the onset of disease. This trial, as well as the French Cooperative Trial on Plasma Exchange in GBS, demonstrated the value of plasmapheresis in GBS. Thus, all patients with GBS at least deserve consideration for plasma exchange.

The design of the Johns Hopkins trial was such that no conclusion could be drawn regarding whether patients with *mild* GBS should undergo plasmapheresis. It is reasonable, therefore, to observe and *not* initiate plasma-exchange in patients with only mild weakness that is neither progressive nor associated with respiratory or bulbar compromise. Patients whose condition remains stable and improves will not need pheresis. By contrast, patients who show progression of weakness or respiratory or bulbar symptoms should be started on plasma exchange as quickly as possible. Obviously plasmapheresis should begin immediately for those who demonstrate severe weakness, a rapidly progressive course, or respiratory or bulbar compromise early in the course. At the New York Hospital we tend to treat all patients, even in the early stages of GBS, within 12 to 24 hours of admission unless contraindications exist.

Plasma exchange is done to a volume of 200 to 250 ml per kilogram body weight usually as five treatments over 10 to 14 days. Plasmanate or 5 percent salt-poor albumin is used as the replacement solution. Continuous- rather than intermittent-flow machines are preferred.

The complications of plasmapheresis are those of obtaining venous access, maintaining venous access with an indwelling catheter, and possibility of hypotension due to the large volume of fluid exchanged. If hypotension does occur, lower volume of fluid may be exchanged.

Only two small controlled trials have been performed to investigate the possible benefit of steroid use in acute GBS, and they arrived at opposite conclusions. Currently, large doses of steroids and intravenous gamma-globulin are being evaluated in the management of acute GBS, but there is no evidence, at present, that these drugs influence the course of the acute disease.

Respiratory Control

Another major problem in acute GBS is when the patient should be intubated and ventilated. The current trend is to ventilate before, rather than after, the patient develops classical signs of respiratory failure. Although some patients will be intubated who otherwise might not have required it, overall morbidity and mortality are decreased by early ventilatory support.

In deciding when to intubate or extubate a patient, I generally follow the recommendations of the *Washington Manual of Medical Therapeutics*. Two indicators can be used: clinical status and inspiratory pressures. Early signs of impending ventilatory failure include tachycardia, sweating of the brow, and inability to finish a sentence without taking a breath of air. This is followed only later by confusion, disorientation, hyperpnea, respiratory alternans (alternating rib cage and abdominal breathing) and paradoxical abdominal breathing (inward movement of the abdomen during inspiration). Respiratory efforts usually maintain normal or near-normal arterial blood gases during early respiratory failure, and they cannot be relied upon as an early warning signal of the need for respiratory support. Patients who demonstrate the signs noted above are in imminent danger of ventilatory failure and should be prophylactically intubated and ventilated. Additional useful parameters to follow as guidelines for elective intubation and mechanical ventilation include inspiratory pressure of less than 25 cm H_2O, vital capacity of less than 15 ml per kilogram, and respiratory rate over 30 to 40 breaths per minute.

Intermittent mandatory ventilation (IMV) is preferred for patient comfort. Initial ventilator settings include FIO_2 of 1.0, which can be adjusted downward by following the arterial blood gases. An arterial PaO_2 of over 60 mm Hg should be the goal, with an FIO_2 of less than 0.6. Initial tidal volume may be set at 10 to 15 ml per kilogram, with a rate of 8 to 14 breaths per minute, the higher settings being used as the patient gets progressively weaker.

Weaning is best performed by lowering the IMV rate slowly, usually not more than 1 to 2 breaths per day. This may begin when the patient has a vital capacity of over 10 ml per kilogram and climbing, with a respiratory rate of less than 25 breaths per minute, and inspiratory pressure of 20 cm H_2O and climbing.

Autonomic Dysfunction

Autonomic instability is common in GBS. Cardiac arrhythmias potentially are the most dangerous complication. Relative tachycardia occurs in almost all patients. Bradycardia is rare but may require a cardiac pacemaker in the short term. Patients with autonomic dysfunction should be monitored to anticipate these possibilities.

Hypertension and hypotension also occur in GBS. The physician's tendency to overtreat hypertension must be resisted. In the usual young patient with GBS who is otherwise well, I would not treat a blood pressure lower than 200/110. Such levels are usually without complication, and the risks of therapy outweigh the benefits. When treatment is indicated, such as in patients with extremely high blood pressure or with unstable angina or heart disease, short-acting agents are preferred because of the rapid swings in blood pressure that may occur with this disorder. Labetalol is a good choice, acting as it does as both an alpha- and a beta-blocker. It can be given intravenously, initially as a 5-mg bolus. Maximum action is within 5 minutes. If precipitous fall of blood pressure does not occur, this initial dose may be followed by 20 mg IV and then with further doses as needed. A maximum of 300 mg of labetalol may be given in doses of up to 80 mg every 10 minutes for rapid control of blood pressure. The patient must be adequately hydrated before administration of this medication. If hydration is contraindicated, other agents such as nitroprusside may be used. Side effects of labetalol include postural hypotension; therefore, treatment should be given with the patient in a supine position.

Hypotension in GBS is best managed with fluid replacement, which again should be administered cautiously because of the rapid fluctuations in blood pressure that can occur.

The syndrome of inappropriate ADH secretion (SIADH) is seen in GBS, possibly due to impaired parasympathetic function of the vagal afferents. Hyponatremia is the signal that SIADH may be developing. Appropriate fluid restriction and electrolyte monitoring are usually all that is needed to restore serum sodium to the normal range.

Urinary retention is rare, but constipation can occur. If present at all, urinary retention usually resolves in a few days and is easily managed with Foley catheterization. It is imperative that aseptic technique and strict closed urinary drainage system be utilized to prevent urinary tract infection from setting in. Constipation should be prevented with stool softeners. The physician should be alert to the possibility of fecal impaction in severely paralyzed cases.

Pain

Up to 75 percent of patients with GBS experience pain at some point during the course of their illness. This is described most frequently as an aching discomfort in the hands and feet or in the muscles of the thigh or back. Analgesics including codeine and Percodan (with added stool softener to prevent constipation) give the best relief. Quinine (300 mg twice a day) or Solu-Medrol (20 to 40 mg intravenously as a single bolus) may be useful alternatives. However, Solu-Medrol should not be used in the setting of infection.

Deep Venous Thrombosis

Five percent of patients with GBS develop deep venous thrombosis (DVT). Heparin should be given subcutaneously, 5,000 units every 12 hours, to all patients who are not ambulatory. Tight-fitted stockings (Jobst leotard) are useful in addition.

Infections

Many patients with GBS develop pulmonary and urinary tract infections. Chest physiotherapy and good respiratory toilet are important in preventing lung infection. Early intubation and ventilation also decrease this possibility. Mild fevers in patients with GBS most frequently are caused by atelectasis and pneumonia. Antibiotic therapy should not be instituted for pneumonia unless there is strict evidence of pulmonary infection in the form of an abnormal chest film or purulent sputum. Cultures should be secured before therapy is started.

Urinary tract infections are best avoided by strict adherence to aseptic technique. There is no place for prophylactic bladder irrigation with antibiotics or other antiseptics. A closed urinary drainage system must be maintained.

An important point to prevent infection is to assure handwashing by all physicians and nurses coming in contact with the patient.

Nutrition

Patients with GBS may experience bulbar symptoms in the form of dysphagia with the risk of aspiration. At this point, the patient will usually be intubated, and feeding can be done either by insertion of a nasogastric tube or, if parenteral nutrition will be required for longer than 3 to 4 weeks, by percutaneous endoscopic gastrostomy (PEG).

Nursing Care

Good nursing care comprises the most important element of sustained treatment in patients with GBS, especially those who are paralyzed. These patients must be turned regularly to avoid developing bedsores. Soft, eggcrate mattresses, sheepskins, and water mattresses are useful as well.

Patients with eye-closure weakness require either eye-patching or methyl cellulose eye drops applied to the eyes every 2 to 4 hours. Oral care should be maintained for the general well-being of the patient. The mouth may be swabbed every 4 to 6 hours, using iced gauze rinsed in mild lemon juice.

Passive range-of-motion exercises should start early on immobile patients to prevent contractures. Stretching exercises are not needed unless contractures have already begun to set in or the patient has started to improve. At this point a full physical therapy program may be initiated.

PROGNOSIS

Overall, 80 to 85 percent of patients with GBS recover completely. Mortality, however, remains at 1 to 3 percent, even at major university centers. Respiratory support will be required by 20 to 25 percent of patients at some point during their illness. In addition to the therapeutic measures noted above, the importance of psychological support for the patient and family, with repeated encouragement that recovery is likely, is of great benefit.

SUGGESTED READING

Arnason BGW. Acute inflammatory demyelinating polyradiculoneuropathies. In: Dyck PJ, Thomas PK, Lambert EH, Bunge R, eds. Peripheral neuropathy. Vol. 2. Philadelphia: WB Saunders, 1984.

French Cooperative Group on Plasma Exchange in Guillain-Barré Syndrome. Efficiency of plasma exchange in Guillain-Barré Syndrome: role of replacement fluids. Ann Neurol 1987; 22:753–761.

Guillain-Barré Syndrome Study Group. Plasmapheresis and acute Guillain-Barré Syndrome. Neurology 1985; 35:1096–1104.

McKhann GM, Griffin JW. Plasmapheresis and the Guillain-Barré Syndrome. Ann Neurol 1987; 22:762–763.

Pollard JD. A critical review of therapies in acute and chronic inflammatory demyelinating polyneuropathies. Muscle Nerve 1987; 10:214–221.

Ropper AH, Shahani BT. Diagnosis and management of acute areflexic paralysis with emphasis on Guillain-Barré Syndrome. In: Asbury AK, Gilliatt RW, eds. Peripheral nerve disorders: a practical approach. London: Butterworths, 1984.

SEIZURES IN THE INTENSIVE CARE UNIT

THOMAS P. BLECK, M.D.

Seizures complicate the care of approximately 3 percent of patients with critical non-neurologic disease. For some of them, the seizures (or their therapy) precipitate admission to the intensive care unit (ICU); in others, the seizures are comorbid events that stress both the patient and the staff. A small but important group of patients are admitted solely for the management of serial seizures or status epilepticus.

A seizure is of great concern both for its own management as a marker of possible abnormality of the central nervous system (CNS). In our ICU, the most common proven etiologies of seizures, in order of incidence, are postanoxic, metabolic, cerebrovascular, infectious, and neoplastic. Many patients have more than one potential cause of ictal activity; only the rare intensive care patient acquires the diagnosis of "idiopathic" seizures. Making an etiologic diagnosis is an essential part of planning the diagnostic evaluation and making therapeutic decisions. As part of this process, the seizure(s) must be classified as *partial* (with or without secondary generalization) or *primary generalized* (i.e., having no focal component, which in the ICU, is usually synonymous with a generalized convulsion). Postanoxic and metabolic encephalopathies tend to produce generalized seizures, whereas cerebrovascular and neoplastic disorders commonly result in seizures with focal components. Seizures in infectious diseases tend to reflect the geography of the underlying process. Some notable exceptions are the focal seizures associated with nonketotic hyperglycemia and the convulsions that occasionally herald a subarachnoid hemorrhage.

DIAGNOSTIC STUDIES

The most important diagnostic measure in the patient with a seizure is the description of the ictus. The intensive care patient, in contrast to others in the hospital, is usually observed by a staff member from the onset of the event. Because a focal onset is so strongly predictive of localized CNS pathology, this observation alone usually determines the direction of diagnosis and treatment. Focal findings on neurologic examination, especially the immediate postictal examination, have similar importance. Assessing the return of awareness to the patient's baseline is crucial, as subclinical status epilepticus remains an overlooked cause of coma.

Important historical data may be difficult to obtain from the patient and therefore must be sought from others. The most crucial overlooked factor is abuse of alcohol or hypnosedative drugs, which often results in withdrawal convulsion when critical illness interrupts habitual use.

Of the diagnostic studies usually applied to a patient with seizures, only electroencephalography (EEG) is always indicated at the new onset of seizures. While the electrically hostile environment of the ICU commonly produces artifacts, the findings of concern after a seizure are rarely obscured. Muscle and movement artifact are a more serious problem, and the patient may require sedation or neuromuscular blockade to obtain the necessary information. The EEG is most useful for (1) determining the presence of focal dysfunction, (2) assessing the degree of a diffuse disorder, (3) excluding subclinical status epilepticus in the formerly conscious patient who remains unresponsive after a seizure, and (4) gauging the treatment of status epilepticus or serial seizures.

Neuroradiologic studies are essential for patients in whom the clinical evaluation and EEG raise the suspicion of localized pathology. The benefit of these procedures must be weighed against the risk to the patient entailed by transportation, and the added interference with observation and care posed by magnetic resonance imaging (MRI) equipment. In most patients, a computed tomographic (CT) scan will suffice. Decisions regarding the administration of radiocontrast material should be individualized. Patients whose cardiorespiratory status will not permit transportation may benefit from a bedside nuclear brain scan if a chronic subdural hematoma, brain abscess, or metastatic tumor is suggested. A negative scan does not exclude these treatable entities.

In patients with impaired mentation or focal neurologic findings, lumbar puncture is best postponed until a CT scan can be obtained to exclude the risk of herniation. Lumbar puncture is usually indicated in the patient who has had a seizure without a definite etiology, as CNS infections often lack classic findings in these commonly immunoincompetent hosts. To reduce the risk of an epidural hematoma, coagulopathy should be partially corrected prior to the puncture.

THERAPEUTIC ALTERNATIVES

The various anticonvulsant agents differ markedly in their spectrum of activity, pharmacokinetics, pharmacodynamics, and adverse effects. In critical-care practice, the most useful agents are lorazepam, phenytoin, phenobarbital, pentobarbital, and paraldehyde.

Lorazepam

The parenteral benzodiazepines (lorazepam, diazepam, midazolam) are equally efficacious for terminating status epilepticus and for the short-term prevention of seizures. Lorazepam is pharmacokinetically superior, with an anticonvulsant action lasting from 4 to 14 hours. By contrast, a single dose of diazepam is effective against status epilepticus for only 20 minutes, and midazolam requires both a loading dose and a constant infusion to maintain anticonvulsant activity. Lorazepam is administered in 2-mg increments every 2 to 3 minutes for the treatment of status epilepticus; if control is not achieved with a total dose of 8 mg, a higher dose is unlikely to be effective. Because all of these agents may produce apnea when given intravenously, intubation equipment must be available.

Phenytoin

Phenytoin is a very useful agent in selected settings. Its major advantages are ease of administration, the preservation of awareness during a loading dose, and the ubiquitous availability of serum concentration measurements ("blood levels"). The parenteral form of phenytoin is dissolved in propylene glycol and must have a pH greater than 11 to stay in solution. Therefore, it should not be given intramuscularly, as it precipitates in muscle and is slowly and erratically absorbed. When given intravenously, it must be injected into a line containing only normal saline. It should be administered by injection from a syringe and not given as a rider (where its dissolution in saline appears to lower its bioavailability).

The commonly recommended rate of administration of 50 mg of phenytoin per minute is poorly tolerated by elderly patients and by anyone with cardiovascular instability or hypoxemia. Except in the treatment of status epilepticus, it is rarely necessary to deliver the total dose in 30 minutes. We therefore recommend a rate of 25 mg per minute, with continuous electrocardiographic monitoring and blood pressure measurement no less often than every 2 minutes during the loading dose. Subsequent doses should be given in 100-mg increments over 5 to 10 minutes. Loading doses of phenytoin should be varied with the weight and metabolic status of the patient. An initial dose of 18 mg per kilogram will produce a level of about 20 μg per milliliter for the next 24 hours. This dose may be given orally (in 300-mg doses every 30 to 60 minutes) if rapid treatment is not required and gastrointestinal function is normal. The habitual "gram of phenytoin" loading dose is inadequate for patients weighing more than 55 kg. The drug is normally 90 percent protein-bound; thus, patients with markedly depressed albumin levels should receive modestly lower loading doses (reduced by about half of the percentage decrease of serum albumin). The maintenance dose (normally, 5 to 7 mg per kilogram per day) need not be changed unless hepatic function is markedly impaired. With a low albumin level, the target total level of phenytoin should be reduced to about 7 to 15 μg per milliliter (usually, 10 to 20 μg per milliliter is considered therapeutic). In renal failure, the metabolism of phenytoin is normal, but the drug is displaced from albumin so the total level is reduced. Levels of unbound ("free") phenytoin are now commonly available and are occasionally helpful in these settings.

Because of phenytoin's unusual pharmacokinetics and the wide range of drugs with which it interacts, blood levels should be obtained frequently during the first week of treatment. Once a steady state is reached, levels may be obtained every 3 to 4 days during a period of critical illness when many other drugs are given and metabolic fluctuations are common. These measurements are used primarily to ensure that an adequate dosage of phenytoin is being given; the symptomatic toxicity of slightly elevated levels is mild and easily recognized. Some patients may require levels above 20 μg per milliliter for seizure control; one need not stop tolerated therapy purely on the basis of a level.

Phenobarbital

Phenobarbital can be administered by mouth, vein, or muscle. While it is not the drug of first choice for seizures in the ICU, it is useful and very commonly employed adjunct. The usual loading dose is 10 to 15 mg per kilogram, but smaller doses are sometimes effective in terminating status epilepticus or when the drug is used in combination with other agents. Although the therapeutic range in chronic use is 20 to 40 μg per milliliter, higher levels may be useful in patients with acute intracranial pathology.

Paraldehyde

For status epilepticus that resists lorazepam, phenytoin, and phenobarbital, paraldehyde is still employed. Because the parenteral form of this drug is no longer manufactured, it is given rectally. Conscious patients may take it orally in milk or juice. Because of its propensity to dissolve plastics, it cannot be given through nasogastric tubes unless they are Teflon-coated. The initial dose is 4 to 12 g, followed by 4 g every 3 hours thereafter.

Barbiturate Coma

Status epilepticus that remains uncontrolled by the preceding agents is an indication for barbiturate coma. This therapy is undertaken, at great risk to the patient, in hope of terminating status epilepticus and preserving viable neurons. Although a loading dose of 10 to 12 mg of pentobarbital per kilogram is commonly recommended, this is often not sufficient to control seizures. The optimal loading dose is probably that which stops seizures and produces a suppression-burst EEG pattern. The optimal duration of this treatment is unknown; we attempt to maintain the EEG pattern for 12 hours, then wean the drug over 24 to 48 hours. Before weaning, therapeutic phenytoin and phenobarbital levels are established. If status epilepticus recurs, another course of pentobarbital coma is instituted. While we suggest pentobarbital because of its superior calcium antagonist effect (which presumably decreases excitotoxic neuronal destruction), others use high doses of phenobarbital.

SELECTION OF THERAPEUTIC OPTIONS

A single seizure is more important as a sign of CNS dysfunction than as an indication for emergent treatment. This philosophy must be tempered for those in whom the metabolic demands of another convulsion may push myocardial oxygen requirements to unattainable levels (e.g., the unstable angina patient). For the majority, however, the risks of overly aggressive anticonvulsant treatment appear to outweigh the potential benefits.

After a second seizure or a series of seizures, intervention is warranted to reduce the likelihood of subsequent spells. The likely etiology serves as the best guide to treatment. Seizures caused by hypoxic-ischemic encephalopathy are difficult to treat but are most likely to respond to benzodiazepines. Myoclonus in the comatose posthypoxic patient does not appear to be ictal and probably requires treatment only if it discomfits the family or staff. Myoclonus is exceptionally drug-resistant but may respond to benzodiazepines. Neuromuscular blockade will prevent the expression of myoclonus.

Convulsions consequent to withdrawal of alcohol or hypnosedatives commonly occur in a cluster within the first 3 days of abstinence. They rarely benefit from treatment but may herald the onset of delirium tremens. Benzodiazepines may be used as a short-term therapy, but chronic anticonvulsant therapy is not indicted.

Seizures due to metabolic disorders (e.g., renal failure) are best managed by correction of the systemic disorder and the exclusion of intercurrent toxins (e.g., normeperidine, the epileptogenic metabolite of meperidine that accumulates in renal failure). When the underlying problem cannot be quickly corrected, benzodiazepines may be tried. While phenytoin has the advantage of relatively light sedation, it is unlikely to be effective.

When repeated seizures occur as a consequence of acute cerebrovascular disease or neoplasms, phenytoin is a reasonable first agent but is often successful only at preventing secondary generalization. Adding phenobarbital will usually control the remaining partial seizures. It is important to make an attempt at monotherapy, however, so that one does not lose the use of two drugs should an adverse reaction occur. A similar approach is useful in meningitis, subdural empyema, brain abscess, and herpes simplex encephalitis. Even if seizures have not occurred, many physicians begin prophylactic anticonvulsant treatment prior to surgery for focal brain infections.

Status epilepticus requires immediate and definitive treatment because it can produce permanent cerebral damage and occasional fatalities. Even some nonconvulsive forms carry the risk of irreversible memory loss. The brain damage is probably mediated by excessive intracellular free calcium, which activates a variety of second messenger systems, phosphorylases, and lysozymes. When

Table 1 Suggested Protocol for Managing Status Epilepticus (SE)

1. Basic life support
   a) Attempt airway control by repositioning of head suctioning, and intubation if needed. Blind nasotracheal intubation may be possible. If orotracheal intubation is necessary, use vecuronium (0.1 mg/kg) for transient neuromuscular blockade. Avoid longer-acting agents, as they render clinical assessment of SE impossible.
   b) Start two intravenous lines, one with normal saline.
   c) Administer dextrose (1 g/kg) and thiamine (1 mg/kg).
   c) Monitor blood pressure, respiration, and ECG throughout drug administration. *Elapsed time: 3 minutes* (not including intubation, which should proceed simultaneously with medication).

2. Terminate status epilepticus
   a) Administer lorazepam (0.05–0.2 mg/kg at 2 mg/min; dilute in equal volume of IV solution); maximal suggested adult dose 8 mg. *Elapsed time: 10 minutes.*
   b) If lorazepam fails, begin *phenytoin* (18 mg/kg at a rate no higher than 50 mg/min in saline; slower if hypotension or arrhythmias occur). Institute EEG monitoring. *Elapsed time: 40 minutes.*
   c) If phenytoin fails, intubate patient, if this has not already been done. Administer *phenobarbital* (5–10 mg/kg IV), and/or *paraldehyde* (0.1–0.2 ml/kg per rectum, in oil).
   d) If SE continues, begin *pentobarbital* (about 12 mg/kg IV at 50 mg/min; less if recently loaded with phenobarbital) to terminate all seizures *and* obtain burst-suppression EEG. Place arterial line and central venous catheter or pulmonary artery catheter as indicated. Use saline infusions, *dopamine, dobutamine,* or *norepinephrine* infusions to maintain blood pressure. Use external temperature control to maintain body temperature. *Elapsed time: 80 minutes.* Continue pentobarbital at 0.25–1.0 mg/kg/hr, as needed to maintain EEG control for 12 hours; then administer appropriate dose of phenytoin and phenobarbital to obtain levels of 20 µg/ml and wean pentobarbital over 12–24 hours. If seizures recur during weaning, reinstitute pentobarbital and repeat sequence.

3. Prevent recurrence of SE, using phenytoin, phenobarbital, divalproex, or carbamazepine.

4. Prevent or treat complications
   a) Rhabdomyolysis: use neuromuscular-junction blockade during treatment (e.g., pancuronium or vecuronium; requires EEG monitoring) and saline diuresis. If renal faiure occurs, institute dialysis as dictated by volume status, acidosis, or hyperkalemia.
   b) Hyperthermia: use external cooling. If severe, consider cool peritoneal dialysis or extracorporeal blood cooling.
   c) Cerebral edema: consider hyperventilation, *dexamethasone,* and/or *mannitol* as needed.

status epilepticus continues for more than about 20 minutes, local oxygen and glucose delivery fails despite hypertension and increased cerebral blood flow. Thus, seizures lasting for more than 20 minutes must be stopped immediately. In addition, the recurrence of seizures must be prevented, and complications must be managed. Table 1 presents a suggested protocol for managing generalized convulsive status epilepticus.

SUGGESTED READING

Aminoff MJ, Simon RP. Status epilepticus: causes, clinical features and consequences in 98 patients. Am J Med 1980; 69:657–666.

Bleck TP. Therapy for status epilepticus. Clin Neuropharmacol 1983; 6:255–269.

Bleck TP, Klawans HL. Neurologic emergencies. Med Clin North Am 1986; 70:1167–1184.

Delgado-Escueta AV, Wasterlain CG, Treiman DM, Porter RJ, eds. Status epilepticus: mechanism of brain damage and treatment. New York: Raven Press, 1983.

Levy R, Mattson R, Meldrum B, et al. Antiepileptic drugs. 3rd ed. New York: Raven Press, 1989.

Ropper AH, Kennedy SF. Neurological and neurosurgical intensive care. Rockville MD: Aspen Publishers, Inc., 1988.

INCREASED INTRACRANIAL PRESSURE

THOMAS P. BLECK, M.D.

Increased intracranial pressure (ICP) is the result of many pathologic processes injuring the central nervous system (CNS). In our medical intensive care unit, life-threatening or fatal elevations of ICP develop in about 6 percent of patients. The etiologies of intracranial hypertension are numerous but can be divided into the following categories: those due to mass lesions (e.g., abscess), hyperemia (post-traumatic), and edema (after cerebral infarction). Many processes (such as metastatic tumors) raise ICP by more than one mechanism and may require treatment with several modalities.

Three types of brain edema can be distinguished, again with considerable therapeutic import. *Vasogenic edema* arises in areas where the blood-brain barrier is disturbed; this allows relatively unrestricted transudation of plasma. *Cytotoxic edema* occurs when brain cells are metabolically deranged, imbibing fluid (and solute) from the extracellular space. *Interstitial edema* follows obstruction of cerebrospinal fluid (CSF) flow within the ventricular system, forcing the CSF out into the surrounding brain.

Increased ICP is recognized by history (headache, confusion, nausea, vomiting, neck pain, coma), physical examination (papilledema, nuchal rigidity, bulging fontanelle in infants), and laboratory procedures. Neuroradiologic studies are paramount; computed tomography (CT) is most easily obtained in the critically ill patient and usually suffices to answer the three most immediate questions: (1) what is the etiology of the ICP elevation, (2) is surgical treatment indicated, and (3) should a lumbar puncture be performed? Contrast-enhanced CT is sometimes necessary to determine etiology but, because of the potential toxicity of the contrast agent, should not be performed until the plain scan has been reviewed. Magnetic resonance imaging (MRI) is becoming an increasingly useful option in critically ill patients as nonferrous ventilatory and monitoring technology improves.

Lumbar puncture remains important in the diagnosis of some conditions raising ICP. In particular, lumbar puncture may be needed to prove a subarachnoid hemorrhage in a patient with a normal CT scan. Meningitis may raise ICP either directly or by producing communicating hydrocephalus. The patient with pseudotumor cerebri ("benign" intracranial hypertension) usually requires lumbar puncture as the first treatment modality to preserve vision and relieve headache. Conversely, patients with mass lesions only rarely have conditions diagnosable by CSF analysis and are at an increased risk of herniation if lumbar puncture is performed.

Intracranial pressure monitoring is becoming increasingly accepted as a guide to managing these patients. Three major techniques are employed in children and adults: the ventricular catheter, the subarachnoid bolt, and the fiberoptic sensor. Catheter systems are indicated when the disease process requires ventricular drainage as well as control of ICP (e.g., intracerebral hemorrhage with ventricular obstruction). Subarachnoid bolts are more easily placed than catheters when the ventricles are small or markedly displaced but are more prone to failure by obstruction. Both of these systems involve a fluid-filled column and a transducer, which carry the risk of infection. The fiberoptic sensor system has earned increasing use because of its ease of insertion (intraparenchymal, subdural, or intraventricular), stability of recording, and minimal risk of infection. During the next decade, this system should markedly expand the availability of ICP measurement.

Not all patients require monitoring of ICP. Certain physical findings (e.g., level of alertness, signs of compression of the third cranial nerve may be followed in selected cases as approximate guides to the degree of ICP elevation and the adequacy of its treatment. However, since the response to treatment is often unpredictable (or, as with hyperventilation, may actually be counterintuitive) and patients with the most serious elevations of ICP tend not to have reliable signs of follow, monitoring of ICP should be strongly considered whenever one attempts to manage intracranial hypertension. To date, the value of ICP monitoring is generally acknowledged in Reye's syndrome and in head trauma and remains debatable in other conditions. The greater reliability and lower infection rate of newer monitoring systems should shift the risk-to-benefit ratio strongly in favor of monitoring all patients in whom therapy for increased ICP is attempted.

PHYSIOLOGIC CONSIDERATIONS

Three variables are paramount in treating ICP elevation; the ICP itself, the cerebral perfusion pressure (CPP), and the geometry of the intracranial fossae.

ICP is normally below 15 mm Hg, although transient peaks of 20 to 30 mm Hg are common (e.g., during coughing). Acute sustained increases in ICP to high levels (40 mm Hg or greater) may produce coma or sudden death, but the same pressure achieved chronically may produce only a headache. Periodic normal fluctuations in ICP reflect pulse, respiration, and changes in carbon dioxide partial pressure (Pco_2) during sleep. Loss of fluctuation (plateau waves) is usually an ominous sign. Treatment is usually aimed at keeping ICP below 25 mm Hg.

CPP is defined as the difference between mean arterial pressure (MAP) and ICP (or jugular venous pressure, should it transiently exceed ICP). CPP is normally greater than 60 mm Hg. When it falls below 40 mm Hg, early symptoms of diminished cerebral blood flow appear; below 30 mm Hg, coma supervenes; and below 20 mm Hg, substrate delivery at the capillary level fails. Treatment usually attempts to keep CPP at 50 mm Hg or greater, either by lowering ICP or raising MAP. At times, these attempts are antagonistic. Furthermore, reducing CPP below acceptable levels produces ischemia, which triggers vasodilation and raises ICP.

The intracranial geometry determines the risk and consequences of herniation due to mass lesions. Reducing ICP usually diminishes the driving force for herniation.

THERAPEUTIC ALTERNATIVES

Airway Management

Because hypoxemia, hypercarbia, and elevated intrathoracic pressures all raise ICP, control of the airway is the first step in managing intracranial hypertension. The indications for intubation are the same as for other patients: preventing or relieving obstruction, avoiding aspiration, maintenance of pulmonary toilet, and the need for mechanical ventilation. In addition, therapeutic hyperventilation is often indicated.

Intubation is a potent elevator if ICP. This effect is blunted by intravenous lidocaine (1 mg per kilogram) or pentobarbital (0.5 to 1 mg per kilogram) immediately preceding the procedure. Intratracheal lidocaine is not an adequate substitute.

In the setting of head trauma, care must be taken to avoid aggravating a potential cervical spine injury during intubation. The neck must be kept straight, and care taken not to flex or severely hyperextend it. Most trauma centers recommend two attempts at blind nasotracheal intubation if the patient is moving air. If the patient is apneic or cannot be intubated nasotracheally, laryngoscopic (preferably fiberoptic if immediately available) orotracheal intubation is preferred over an emergency cricothyrotomy.

Airway suction often results in arterial desaturation, raising ICP. The patient should be well oxygenated (e.g., bag ventilated with 100 percent oxygen) prior to suctioning. Coughing will also elevate ICP; sedation or transient neuromuscular junction blockade (e.g., vecuronium, 0.1 mg per kilogram) may be required to prevent this. Since the intrathoracic pressure primarily affects ICP via the jugular venous system, the patient should be kept sitting up in bed between 30 and 45 degrees. Because the optimal airway management and posture varies among patients and may change over time, ICP monitoring is a useful guide.

Hyperventilation

Reducing the Pco_2 to 25 to 30 mm Hg will decrease the cerebral blood volume and lower ICP without markedly affecting oxygen and substrate delivery at the capillary level. This effect is seen within minutes, making it the most rapid of the initial ICP therapies. However, the increase in mean intrathoracic pressure necessary to achieve the requisite minute ventilation may raise jugular venous pressure and hence actually elevate ICP, even with the usually recommended Pco_2 range. Thus, if the physical examination deteriorates, or the measured ICP rises, the minute ventilation should be decreased.

Patients with problems of ICP may develop neurogenic pulmonary edema. The pulmonary capillary wedge pressure (PCWP) is usually normal, and the edema fluid is rich in protein. Brain stem–triggered pulmonary venoconstriction appears to be the mechanism. Fluid shifts with the lung are often quite abrupt, with a time course of minutes. Treatment of the primary CNS disorder, lowering ICP, increasing the inspired oxygen fraction, and judicious use of diuretics are appropriate treatments. While afterload reduction could be helpful, nitroprusside will dilate cerebral vessels and may thereby raise ICP; trimethaphan is a useful alternative. Since these agents lower CPP, they should be reserved for patients in whom ICP can be measured. Positive end-expiratory pressure (PEEP) may be helpful but can also alter ICP in these patients.

In contrast to patients with neurogenic pulmonary edema, those with adult respiratory distress syndrome (ARDS) or other causes of decreased pulmonary compliance can transmit only a fraction of their intrathoracic pressure to the jugular venous system. This latter group can thus tolerate more PEEP without substantial ICP elevations. If PEEP adversely affects their systemic hemodynamics, CPP will suffer.

The effective duration of hyperventilation remains controversial. Since it does not alter the underlying intracranial process, ICP often rises in the hours after an initial fall. This has been misinterpreted as an escape phenomenon. However, if hyperventilation is terminated abruptly, the ICP rises further as vessels dilate. Most workers in the field will maintain hyperventilation for 1 to 3 days, and then decrease minute ventilation as tolerated over a few days.

Since hyperemia is a major cause of elevated ICP after head trauma, some recommend hyperventilation as the preferred treatment modality in this setting. Hyperventilation does not induce the osmotic difficulties of mannitol but may not be adequate as the sole treatment of the head-injured person.

Osmotic Agents and Other Diuretics

Osmotic agents extract extracellular fluid from areas where the blood-brain barrier is intact, thereby decreasing brain volume and ICP. They cannot remove fluid from edematous regions. Mannitol is the most commonly employed agent and should be given intermittently (e.g., 0.25 gm per kilogram every 4 hours). Some administer a loading dose of 1 mg per kilogram, but its efficacy is uncertain. The initial target serum osmolality should be about 320 mOsm per liter but may be raised to 330 mOsm per liter if a greater effect is needed. Because some mannitol will cross the blood-brain barrier and exert osmotic pressure in the brain, the drug should be tapered over 1 to 2 days to prevent a rebound elevation of ICP. Loop diuretics (e.g., furosemide) may be given 15 to 30 minutes later to enhance the effect of mannitol. Mannitol can be removed by peritoneal dialysis if necessary. Other osmotic agents (such as urea) are of limited value in the critical-care setting.

Mannitol is commonly used as the initial treatment for the elevation in ICP that commonly complicates acute hepatic failure. Earlier concerns about a deleterious effect of hyperventilation in these patients were probably incorrect, however, and both modalities should be used as needed.

Steroids

When vasogenic edema contributes to ICP elevation, steroids should be considered. Therefore, these agents are most useful in the settings of intracranial tumors or abscesses. Although the edema that develops around an intracerebral hemorrhage is vasogenic, it does *not* respond to steroids (in two controlled studies, the steroid-treated patients fared worse owing to infectious and metabolic complications). The most commonly employed steroid is dexamethasone (10 mg initially, followed by 4 mg every 6 hours; the dose may be escalated almost indefinitely with increasing efficacy and increasing complications). The antiedema effect of dexamethasone takes several hours to become manifest.

Because of the lympholytic effect of steroids, many choose to initiate the treatment of CNS lymphoma with 100 mg or more of dexamethasone.

High-Dose Barbiturates

When the preceding modalities are insufficient, high-dose barbiturate therapy should be considered. The mechanism of action is uncertain but at least in part may reflect diminished metabolic demands with a concomitant decline in cerebral blood volume. Pentobarbital and thiopental have been used most extensively. We employ pentobarbital at a loading dose of 4 to 10 mg per kilogram (at a rate no greater than 50 mg per minute), with subsequent doses of 5 to 20 mg per hour as needed to control ICP. A pressure monitor is almost mandatory if this therapy is to be used. If direct monitoring is contraindicated because of a severe coagulopathy, electroencephalographic (EEG) monitoring may be substituted. However, the dose required to produce the recommended burst-suppression EEG is usually greater than that producing the desired effect on ICP.

These agents are potent vasodilators and can also decrease cardiac inotropism. Patients are at high risk for many complications, including hypothermia, infection, and pulmonary embolism.

The large doses used result in saturation of body stores for barbiturates, producing coma that lasts a day or more after tapering has begun. EEG monitoring is useful for assessing patients during this period. In acute hepatic failure, the recovery time is markedly prolonged (unless transplantation occurs).

Surgery

The most effective means of reducing ICP in the setting of an acute intracerebral mass is resection of the lesion. Medical control of ICP should be attempted prior to surgery and is usually required afterwards. Depending on the deficit anticipated from the nature and location of the lesion, some surgeons believe that death from herniation may represent an outcome preferable to the postoperative deficit. Such decisions are always difficult and require discussion with the patient's family.

Most extracerebral masses causing intracranial hypertension, such as chronic subdural hematoma, routinely have an excellent postoperative outcome.

Radiation Therapy

Neoplastic disease often responds rapidly to external radiation. Steroid treatment should precede radiation by several hours to help prevent an acute (and rarely fatal) increase in ICP with the first treatment, especially in the setting of multiple metastases. It is usually continued through the course of radiation.

Ventricular Drainage

Processes that obstruct the flow of CSF result in hydrocephalus; even if a mass lesion is resected, local edema often continues to interfere with flow and requires shunting. External ventricular drainage can be performed at the bedside; a definitive shunting procedure may be accomplished later.

SUGGESTED READING

Bleck TP, Klawans HL. Neurologic emergencies. Med Clin North Am 1986; 70:1167–1184.

Forbes A, Alexander GJM, O'Grady JG, et al. Thiopental infusion in the treatment of intracranial hypertension complicating fulminant hepatic failure. Hepatology 1989; 10:306–310.

Hamill JF, Bedford RF, Weaver DC, et al. Lidocaine before endotracheal intubation: intravenous or endotracheal? Anesthesiology 1981; 55:578–581.

Ostrup RC, Luerssen TG, Marshall LF, Zornow MN. Continuous monitoring of intracranial pressure with a miniaturized fiberoptic device. J Neurosurg 1987; 67:206–209.

Plum F, Posner JB. The diagnosis of stupor and coma. 3rd ed. Philadelphia: FA Davis, 1980.

Ropper AH, Kennedy SF. Neurological and neurosurgical intensive care. Rockville MD: Aspen, 1988.

RENAL, GASTROINTESTINAL, HEMATOLOGIC, AND METABOLIC THERAPEUTICS

ACUTE RENAL FAILURE

MARGARET JOHNSON BIA, M.D.

Acute renal failure (ARF) can be defined as an abrupt decrease in glomerular filtration rate (GFR), which becomes manifest in patients as a rise in serum creatinine and blood urea nitrogen (BUN) concentration or a decrease in urine output. Serum creatinine is actually an unreliable guide to GFR early in the course of ARF, when GFR can be minimal before the creatinine has risen to high levels, but it remains the most clinically useful test for renal function that we have. The frequency of ARF in critically ill patients is quite high, occurring in approximately 10 to 20 percent of all patients admitted to intensive care units (ICUs). Causes of ARF are divided into prerenal, intrinsic renal, and postrenal etiologies (Table 1), with prerenal azotemia and acute tubular necrosis (ATN) constituting the majority of cases. For patients in the intensive care unit (ICU), shock, sepsis, nephrotoxins, and surgery are the most likely precipitating causes since the combination of simultaneously renal hypoperfusion and toxic insults, so frequent in this setting, act synergistically to increase the probability of ARF.

Acute tubular necrosis (ATN) accounts for most cases of ARF associated with intrinsic renal injury. Patients with certain diseases and medical conditions can be identified as being at increased risk for developing ATN, should a precipitating factor occur. For example, patients with advanced age, diabetes mellitus, multiple myeloma, and pre-existing renal disease have an increased risk of ATN after the administration of contrast agents and/or aminoglycosides. Similarly, volume depletion, advanced age, cirrhosis, nephrosis, and congestive heart failure are all conditions that predispose patients to ARF after administration of nonsteroidal antiinflammatory agents. Recognition of these risk factors should allow a physician to treat high-risk patients more cautiously in an attempt to avoid ARF when a nephrotoxic agent or maneuver is required.

Table 1 Causes of Acute Renal Failure*

Prerenal Azotemia	*Intrinsic Renal Failure*	*Postrenal Failure*
Hypovolemia	Acute tubular necrosis	Ureteral obstruction
True volume losses	Postischemic, postsurgery,	Bladder obstruction
Redistribution	postshock, sepsis	Bladder rupture
Cardiac failure	Toxic Causes	
Hepatorenal syndrome	Contrast media	
	Drugs	
	Heme pigment	
	Heavy metals	
	Acute glomerulonephritis	
	Acute interstitial nephritis	
	Allergic	
	Infectious	
	Vascular causes	
	Vasculitis	
	Malignant hypertension	
	Intrarenal thrombosis	
	Hemolytic uremic,	
	thrombotic thrombocytopenic purpura	
	Crystal precipitation	
	Acute uric acid nephropathy	
	Myeloma kidney	

*Republished with permission from Ellison DH, Bia MJ. Acute renal failure in critically ill patients. J Intens Care Med 1987; 2: 8–24.

APPROACH TO THE PATIENT

The following five steps should always be taken when a patient presents with renal failure:

1. Decide if the renal failure is acute or chronic: A sudden decrease in urine output always represents ARF, but a patient admitted with an elevated serum creatinine could have either acute or chronic renal failure.
2. Determine the etiology
3. Ascertain whether specific treatment is necessary.
4. Determine optimal management of fluids, electrolytes, drugs, and dialysis.
5. Estimate the prognosis and prospects for survival.

Once it is established that the patient's renal failure is acute, the etiology should be determined since possibilities for therapeutic intervention depend on the specific cause. For instance, prerenal azotemia due to volume contraction can be readily reversed with fluid administration. It is also critical to consider a postrenal cause for the ARF since this can frequently be reversed by relief of obstruction. Distinction between the main categories of ARF can frequently be made by following the simple work-up outlined in Table 2. These steps should be taken mainly to exclude prerenal or postrenal causes of azotemia as well as causes for intrinsic ARF other than ATN.

SPECIFIC TREATMENT

When prerenal or postrenal causes of azotemia are present, specific therapeutic interventions as outlined above can lead to rapid improvement in renal function. When allergic interstitial nephritis has been documented, usually with a kidney biopsy, therapy should be directed at discontinuing the offending agent and possibly using corticosteroids to speed renal recovery and improve long-term prognosis. Specific therapies—such as corticosteroids, cytotoxic agents, antiplatelet drugs, and plasma exchange—are also recommended for certain kinds of glomerulonephritis.

Table 2 Evaluation of Acute Renal Failure

- Physical examination and evaluation of volume input and ouput.
- Check for nephrotoxic drugs (e.g., aminoglycosides, nonsteroidal anti-inflammatory agents or angiotensin-converting enzyme inhibitors) or a nephrotoxic event (e.g., hypotension, septicemia, contrast load).
- Urinalysis: looking for significant proteinuria, pyuria, or hematuria more consistent with acute glomerulonephritis or interstitial nephritis than with acute tubular necrosis.
- Examine urinary indices: high U_{osm} with low U_{Na} and fractional sodium excretion (FE_{Na}) are consistent with prerenal azotemia or glomerulonephritis, whereas isotonic urine and $U_{Na} > 40$ with $FE_{Na} > 1\%$ more consistent with ATN or obstruction.
- Rule out obstruction (most easily done with renal ultrasonography)

Table 3 Prevention and Treatment of Acute Tubular Necrosis

Prevention
  Avoid volume contraction
  Establish a solute diuresis (urinary output, 150–400 ml/hr) with mannitol, saline, furosemide, or saline plus furosemide.
  Administer a calcium-channel blocker (e.g., nifedipine, 10 mg sublingually).

Treatment
  Mannitol
  Loop diuretics (furosemide or ethacrynic acid)
  ? Essential amino acids
  ? Thyroxine

Unfortunately, despite its frequency as a cause of ARF, no specific treatment has proved to be effective for established ATN. Over the years, published protocols have been directed at preventing ATN, shortening its course, or increasing urinary output (converting oliguric to nonoliguric ATN). Prophylactic maneuvers that have been reported to reduce the incidence or severity of ATN when given before a toxic or ischemic insult include the use of mannitol, saline, or furosemide to produce a solute diuresis and the use of calcium-channel blockers (Table 3). Intravenous administration of mannitol (12.5 to 25 g) saline (200 to 400 ml per hour, depending on the patient's size and renal and cardiac function), or furosemide (80 to 400 mg intravenously) before a contrast load or before surgery may be useful in preventing ATN in high-risk patients. What seems to be more important here is the establishment of a solute diuresis with a urine output of 150 to 400 ml per hour, regardless of which drug is utilized. Mannitol should be avoided in patients with significant renal failure or congestive heart failure since, if not excreted, it can remain in the extracellular fluid and exacerbate volume expansion. The dose can be repeated every 1 to 3 hours, however, in patients responding with a diuresis. Attention to volume status must also be maintained with the use of saline or furosemide, which are perhaps best used together to avoid potential problems of overexpansion or volume depletion. The rate of saline administration and/or the dose of furosemide administered should be increased until the desired urine output is obtained. The diuresis should be continued until surgery is completed or until the contrast load is excreted, several hours after its administration.

Alternatively, calcium-channel blockers can be used prophylactically to avoid ATN. Experimentally, these drugs have been demonstrated to decrease the incidence of ischemia- or contrast-induced ATN. Based on these findings, we frequently administer nifedipine (e.g., 10 mg sublingually) to diabetic and other high-risk patients before a contrast load.

Although no intervention has been shown to alter the course of ATN once it is established, a number of maneuvers continue to enjoy widespread clinical use (see Table 3). First, the use of loop diuretics (e.g., furosemide, 200 to 400 mg intravenously) or, less commonly, mannitol (12.5

to 25 g intravenously) sometimes increases urine output when administered early in the course of oliguric ATN. Because nonoliguric patients have a better prognosis than oliguric ones and are easier to manage, it may be of some benefit to increase urine output, even without improving GFR. Furosemide appears less ototoxic than ethacrynic acid and has been the drug of choice for high-dose diuretic challenges. Although there is no clear evidence that diuretics shorten the duration of azotemia or reduce its complications, a cautious trial of furosemide seems warranted in patients in whom oliguric renal failure develops. Furosemide can be started at a dose of 200 mg IV and then doubled if no response occurs. To avoid ototoxicity and permanent deafness (its major side effect in patients with limited renal function), its rate of administration should never exceed 15 mg per minute. For the same reason, repeated challenges with high doses during the course of renal failure should be avoided, especially in patients in whom no response occurs with its initial use. Early addition of low-dose dopamine infusion (2 to 5 μg per kilogram per minute) to the diuretic challenge has been reported to improve the efficacy of this form of therapy, although controlled trials are lacking.

Reduction in the incidence and severity of ATN with the use of essential amino acids has also been reported, although results from clinical trials are controversial regarding its true benefit. The unresolved issue concerning more rapid improvement in renal function of nutritional care in the critically ill patient with ARF. Another agent with potential importance is thyroxine, which has been shown to accelerate healing of renal insufficiency in experimental animals. The value of this agent is currently being investigated in appropriate clinical trials.

Clinical Management of Established Acute Renal Failure

General management of the patient with ARF should emphasize the prevention of infection, which is the leading cause of death in these patients. Unnecessary use of catheters, especially Foley catheters in oliguric patients, should be avoided. Urine output can be monitored with daily intermittent bladder catheterization, if necessary, with lower risk of infection.

Attention should be paid on daily basis to the points outlined in Table 4. Not every patient requires volume or sodium restriction, but oliguric patients (urine output of less than 600 ml per day) certainly do. Potassium and phosphate restriction will be necessary in most patients. Kayexalate (25 to 50 g in 50 ml of 50 percent sorbitol) and phosphate-binding drugs (calcium carbonate- or aluminum-containing antacids) may be required to control potassium and phosphate levels, respectively, especially in catabolic patients. Limitations to the use of these drugs, however, often exist in patients with ileus and poor intestinal function. To control hyperkalemia before or between dialysis treatments, insulin can be given through a peripheral intravenous site (10 percent dextrose in water plus 40 U insulin at 50 ml per hour) or a beta$_2$-adrenergic agonist (e.g., salbutamol) can be given in-travenously or by inhalation. Dose adjustment of all drugs must be considered and ulcer prophylaxis begun. In addition to gastrointestinal bleeding, uremic patients have an increased risk of bleeding from other sites as well because of uremia-induced platelet dysfunction. If such bleeding does occur or if better hemostasis is required for an invasive procedure, the prophylactic use of desmopressin acetate (0.3 μg per kilogram intravenously) or cryoprecipitate (10 bags), both of which can shorten the prolonged bleeding time of uremia, is recommended. Lastly, since most patients with ARF are catabolic, caloric needs may increase to 50 kcal per kilogram per day. Patients should receive at least 100 g of glucose daily and 30 to 40 g of high-biologic-value protein (or 20 to 25 g of protein supplemented with essential amino acids or ketoacids). This regimen helps keep BUN below 100 mg per deciliter while providing adequate caloric intake. Parenteral alimentation should be considered early in patients who are unable to eat or are catabolic. Likewise, dialysis or hemofiltration should also be considered early both to make room for the volume necessary for adequate nutrition and remove nitrogenous waste products and allow greater protein intake without precipitating uremic symptoms.

Table 4 Management of Acute Renal Failure

- Adjust volume and electrolyte (especially Na, K, Mg, PO$_4$) intake.
- Adjust all drugs to renal-failure doses where necessary.
- Initiate ulcer prophylaxis (avoid Mg-containing antacids).
- Establish adequate nutrition.
- Decide when and how to dialyze, or use hemofiltration.

Dialysis and Continuous Arterial Hemofiltration

Hyperkalemia and volume overload are the most common indications for urgent dialysis. Acidosis, seizures or uremic serositis occur less frequently. In the absence of these complications, dialysis or hemofiltration is usually initiated to keep BUN and creatinine below 100 and 10 mg per deciliter respectively. In practice, one of these techniques is usually started sooner, especially in oliguric patients, to remove volume and allow for adequate nutrition. Peritoneal dialysis is the most simple form of dialytic therapy, provided that an adequate peritoneal space is available and toxin removal (e.g., ethylene glycol or uric acid) is not a primary consideration. To minimize its most common complication, peritonitis, an indwelling catheter (e.g., Tenckhoff) is usually utilized and continuous exchanges are initiated. Patients with respiratory difficulty who are not on a ventilator must be watched carefully for further respiratory compromise once the abdomen is distended with 1 to 2 L of peritoneal fluid. Hemodialysis, a more efficient form of dialysis, is preferred in patients who are severely catabolic and in those in whom toxin removal is required. Hemodynamic instability during and after treatment, and bleeding when heparin is used for anticoagulation in the machine, are its major drawbacks. When

Table 5 Continuous Arteriovenous Hemofiltration

Advantages
  Better tolerated in hemodynamically unstable patients
  Allows for removal of large volumes of fluid
  Does not require pumps, machines, or continuous monitoring by dialysis nurses
  Can be done continuously at bedside in the ICU

Disadvantages
  Need for arterial access
  Demands *intense* ICU nursing care (can lose 3–900 ml/hr)
  Clotting in cartridge leads to decreased efficiency

the risk of bleeding is high, regional anticoagulation with citrate or dialysis without anticoagulation can be utilized.

Continuous arteriovenous hemofiltration (CAVH) is an increasing popular technique that has proved to be quite useful in critically ill patients. It is indicated in patients in whom volume overload is a major manifestation of acute renal failure, in whom vascular instability increases the risk of conventional hemodialysis, or in whom aggressive parenteral nutrition will necessitate large amounts of volume administration. During CAVH, blood is given past a highly permeable membrane by the patient's own blood pressure rather than by a pump causing formation of an ultrafiltrate of plasma. Solute clearance (and removal of nitrogenous waste products) during CAVH is primarily via convection and is less efficient than during dialysis, when solute is cleared by diffusion. However, adequate solute clearance can be achieved in many patients with CAVH alone because treatment is continuous throughout the day. Alternatively, solute clearance can be enhanced by running dialysis bath fluid (approximately 1 L per hour) in the outer chamber of the cartridge, thus initiating slow continuous dialysis (CAVHD). The major advantage of CAVH (Table 5) derives from the large volumes of fluid that can be removed in a manner that is better tolerated by the patient than hemodialysis. In addition, it does not require special pumps, machines, or continuous use of dialysis nurses. However, it does require access to both artery and vein (unlike hemodialysis, which can be performed with only venous access), which can usually be obtained either by placement of a Scribner shunt or by femoral artery and vein catheterization. Intense ICU nursing is also required to monitor the patient, to maintain an hourly balance of input and output, and to administer the large volumes of fluid (frequently lactated Ringer's solution). In experienced hands, however, the technique has proved quite useful in managing ARF in critically ill patients.

PROGNOSIS

Despite improved therapeutic measures, ARF is still associated with high mortality, ranging from 20 to 58 percent for nonoliguric patients and from 41 to 72 percent for oliguric patients. Infection remains the most common cause of death, especially in ICU patients. Mortality depends primarily on the severity of the underlying illness and on the number of associated complications (i.e., number of organ failed systems). Prognosis for recovery of renal function is, however, excellent in patients who survive the underlying illness and leave the ICU and the hospital.

SUGGESTED READING

Brezis M, Rosen S, Epstein FH. Acute renal failure. In: Brenner BM, Rector FC, eds. The kidney. Philadelphia: WB Saunders, 1986:735.
Ellison DH, Bia MJ. Acute renal failure in critically ill patients. J Intens Care Med 1987; 2:8–24.
Ellison D, Bia MJ. Renal, fluid and electrolyte disorders in the critically ill immunosuppressed patient. In: Parillo JE, Masur H, eds. The critically ill immunosuppressed patient. Rockville, MD: Aspen, 1987:81.
Meyers BD, Moron SM. Hemodynamically mediated acute renal failure. N Engl J Med 1986; 314:97–105.
Rasmussen HH, Ibels LS. Acute renal failure: multivariate analysis of causes and risk factors. Am J Med 1982; 73:211–218.

LIFE-THREATENING ELECTROLYTE AND METABOLIC DISORDERS

MARGARET JOHNSON BIA, M.D.

HYPERKALEMIA

Causes

Before searching for causes of hyperkalemia, it is necessary to exclude pseudohyperkalemia, due to either hemolysis from release of potassium during blood drawing or potassium release from white cells or platelets (with levels greater than 500,000 per cubic millimeter). While any factor listed in Table 1 can cause hyperkalemia, severe life-threatening hyperkalemia is usually due to a decrease in renal excretion (from intrinsic renal disease, drugs or hormone deficiencies affecting renal excretion) often in association with an increased input into the extracellular fluid (ECF), either from cell lysis or from an external source. Cell destruction from severe catabolism in a patient with acute renal failure would be a common example. Severe hyperkalemia is particularly common in sick diabetic patients in whom selective hypoaldosteronism and hypertonicity from hyperglycemia frequently coexist with insulin deficiency.

Dangers

Hyperkalemia is perhaps the most serious of electrolyte emergencies because of its potentially fatal effect on

Table 1 Causes of True Hyperkalemia

Alterations in external potassium balance
  Excess input
  Decreased renal excretion
    Renal failure (GFR < 20 ml/min)
    Impaired renin-aldosterone axis (Addison's disease, selective hypoaldosteronism)
    Primary renal tubular secretory defects (obstruction, renal transplantation, systemic lupus erythematosus, amyloidosis)
    Drugs: potassium-sparing diuretics, nonsteroidal anti-inflammatory drugs, angiotensin-converting enzyme inhibitors

Alterations in internal potassium balance
  Cell lysis (hemolysis, rhabdomyolysis, tumor lysis, catabolism)
  Acidemia
  Hypertonicity
  Hormonal defects (decreased insulin, aldosterone, or epinephrine activity)
  Drugs: digitalis overdose, beta-adrenergic blockers

*Adapted from Ellison DH, Bia MJ. Renal, fluid and electrolyte disorders in the critically ill immunosuppressed patient. In: Parrillo JE, Masur H, eds. The critically ill immunosuppressed patient. Rockville, MD: Aspen, 1987:103.
GFR = glomerular filtration rate.

the myocardium. Ventricular arrhythmias, conduction disturbances, and cardiac standstill can all occur. Rapidity of onset and concomitant hypocalcemia or hyponatremia are factors known to exacerbate the effect of hyperkalemia on the myocardium. Speed of correction should depend on the height of the serum elevation and the magnitude of the anticipated release of potassium. Serum potassium levels greater than 6.5 mEq per liter should be treated aggressively, especially if electrocardiographic changes are present; levels greater than 7 mEq per liter should be treated as a true emergency even if electrocardiographic changes are absent.

Treatment

Treatment consists of (1) cessation of all drugs that can cause or exacerbate hyperkalemia; (2) driving K into cells (with insulin, bicarbonate, or beta$_2$-adrenergic agonists), and (3) enhanced removal of potassium with diuretics, or if renal function is poor, with Kayexalate or dialysis (Table 2). We have found an insulin drip to be particulary helpful in patients in whom dialysis cannot be performed or in whom more prolonged treatment of hyperkalemia is required. Plasma glucose and potassium must be checked every 2 to 4 hours during this infusion, and the amount of glucose and insulin in the solution must be adjusted to maintain optimal levels of both. Recent reports have indicated that beta$_2$-adrenergic agonists (such as salbutamol or terbutaline) are also effective for treatment of severe hyperkalemia when administered intravenously or by inhalation. Although tachyarrhythmias have not been reported with the clinical use of these drugs, they have the potential to develop because beta$_2$-adrenergic agonists are not entirely beta$_2$-specific. In addition, resistance to the potassium-lowering effects of these agents has been reported in patients with renal failure. Additional clinical studies are needed before widespread clinical use of beta$_2$-adrenergic agonists can be recommended as standard treatment for severe hyperkalemia.

Most patients with life-threatening hyperkalemia will not be responsive to diuretics and will require use of Kayexalate (orally or rectally) or dialysis to remove potassium from the body. Hemodialysis is much more efficient than peritoneal dialysis for this purpose and is preferred for rapid treatment of life-threatening hyperkalemia.

HYPOKALEMIA

Causes

Mild-to-moderate hypokalemia is very common in critically ill patients because factors that lead to this disorder (Table 3) are often present in this patient population. Life-threatening hypokalemia (serum potassium less than 2 or 2.5 mEq per liter with symptoms) is uncommon, however, and is virtually always due to potassium losses through the gastrointestinal tract (as in diarrhea) or through the urine (e.g., use of diuretics). Decreased potassium intake and/or shift of potassium into cells (al-

Table 2 Treatment of Severe Hyperkalemia

Drug	Mechanism	Dose	Onset	Duration
Calcium gluconate (10% solution)	Membrane antagonism*	10–20 ml IV	1–3 min	30–60 min
Sodium bicarbonate	Shifts potassium intracellularly	50–100 mEq IV	5–10 min	2 hours
Glucose and insulin	Shifts potassium intracellularly	5:1 ratio for bolus	30 min	4–6 hr with bolus; indefinite with drip†
Salbutamol‡	Shifts potassium intracellularly	0.5 mg IV§; 10 or 20 mg nebulized	<30 min; <30 min	>2 hours; >2 hours
Kayexalate	Gut excretion	20–50 g	1–2 hours	4–6 hours
Hemodialysis	Removes potassium	4–6 hr treatment	<30 min	Variable

*Doesn't alter serum potassium concentration but alters its effect on cardiac cell membrane.
†Insulin drip: begin with 40 U regular insulin in 10% aqueous dextrose solution at 50 ml/hr (delivers 2 U insulin/hour).
‡Requires further study before widespread use is recommended.
§0.5 mg IV diluted in 100 ml of 5% aqueous dextrose solution over 25 minutes.

Table 3 Causes of Hypokalemia*

Alterations in external potassium balance
  Decreased intake
  Nonrenal losses
    Gastrointestinal (vomiting, diarrhea, laxatives)
    Skin
  Renal losses
    With hypertension
      Primary hyperaldosterone, Cushing's disease, ectopic ACTH, renin-secreting tumor, renovascular hypertension, malignant hypertension
    Without hypertension
      Drugs (diuretics, amphotericin B, penicillin drugs), renal tubular acidosis, Bartter's syndrome, hypomagnesemia, hypercalcemia

Alterations in internal potassium balance
  Alkalemia
  Periodic paralysis
  Rapid cell growth (e.g., acute myelogenous leukemia or treatment of megaloblastic anemias)
  Drugs (beta$_2$-adrenergic agonists, insulin)

Republished with permission from Ellison DH, Bia MJ. Renal, fluid and electrolyte disorders in the critically ill immunosuppressed patient. In Parillo JE, Masur H, eds. The critically ill immunosuppressed patient. Rockville, MD: Aspen, 1987:103. With permission of Aspen Publishers, Inc., © 1987.

tering internal potassium balance) may exacerbate the disturbance, but these are rarely causes for severe hypokalemia by themselves. Hospitalized patients will frequently have more than one cause. For example, a patient with acquired immunodeficiency syndrome (AIDS) may have severe hypokalemia due to a combination of anorexia (decreased intake), amphotericin B treatment (increased urinary losses), and diarrhea (increased gut losses).

Dangers

The manifestations of hypokalemia, which rarely occur unless levels fall below 2.5 mEq per liter, are primarily due to its effect on muscles, which can be fatal if cardiac muscle becomes involved and conduction disturbances or arrhythmias occurs. The adverse effects of hypokalemia on the heart can be exacerbated by digitalis use or by hypercalcemia. Significant morbidity can also occur when skeletal muscle is involved, resulting in ileus, urinary retention, or paralysis. Hypokalemia can be fatal when respiratory muscles become affected.

Treatment

Hypokalemia should be treated as a true medical emergency if cardiac toxicity is present or respiratory muscle function is compromised. Persistent but less aggressive treatment is warranted when other symptoms are present. Decreases in serum potassium of 1 or 2 mEq per liter usually represent deficits of 300 or 600 mEq. Below a serum level of 2 mEq per liter, however, total deficits are harder to predict. Replacement of potassium chloride too rapidly can lead to cardiac arrhythmias, a risk that can be minimized by adhering to the guidelines listed in Table 4. First, oral potassium therapy is always the preferred route, even in sick patients. Newer potassium preparations with potassium embedded in a slow-release capsule or pill are often better tolerated by patients than are the liquid preparations. Second, if intravenous therapy is necessary, there is a limit to the rate of potassium replacement and to its concentration in solution. Thus, to avoid dangerous hypokalemia, potassium should not be administered faster than 40 to 60 mEq per hour and, to avoid pain, peripheral intravenous solutions should not contain more than 40 to 60 mEq of potassium chloride per liter. Rapid administration of potassium chloride in small quantities should be avoided, as it is unphysiologic and runs a higher risk of producing hypokalemia than does a constant infusion. Potassium should be administered as quickly as possible so that the patient is taken out of immediate danger, after which the remainder of the deficit can be replaced more slowly. Finally, it is important to ascertain that the patient has a good urine output. Intravenous potassium therapy should rarely be given to an oliguric patient.

Potassium is usually administered as chloride salt, potassium chloride. There are times, however, when potassium bicarbonate is the preferred salt, as in cases of renal tubular acidosis (RTA), in which replacement of both bicarbonate and potassium are required. When patients with RTA present in crisis with severe acidosis and life-threatening hypokalemia, aggressive treatment of the acidosis with bicarbonate will aggravate the hypokalemia by causing an intracellular shift of potassium. This complication can be avoided with the use of potassium bicarbonate.

HYPONATREMIA

Causes

Several factors predispose the critically ill patient to hyponatremia, including the presence of conditions that generate salt loss (e.g., vomiting and diarrhea), conditions that stimulate release of antidiuretic hormone (ADH), and

Table 4 Treatment of Life-Threatening Hypokalemia

- Treat as an emergency only if life-threatening signs (e.g., arrhythmia, conduction disturbance, paralysis) are present.
- If possible, always choose the oral route for potassium replacement, even in very sick patients.
- Potassium concentration in a peripheral IV is limited by pain (keep concentration 40–50 mEq/L).
- Speed of potassium correction is limited by the danger of transient hyperkalemia (keep delivery rate <40–60 mEq/hour).
- Mix potassium chloride in saline solutions, where possible, to avoid a further decrease in potassium with glucose solutions.
- Be sure that urine output is adequate. It can be fatal to give potassium chloride intravenously to an oliguric patient.

Table 5 Causes of True Hyponatremia

Decreased ECF volume
  (e.g., renal losses with diuretics or gastrointestinal losses with diarrhea or vomiting)
Normal ECF fluid volume
  (e.g., SIADH or reset osmostat)
Increased ECF fluid volume
  (e.g., cirrhosis, nephrosis, or congestive heart failure)

ECF = extracellular fluid volume; SIADH = syndrome of inappropriate ADH secretion.

the need to administer large volumes of water to deliver drug therapy. Causes of true hyponatremia (i.e., hyponatremia associated with hypoosmolality) are divided into categories according to the ECF status of the patient (Table 5). Classification into one of these categories is determined by history, physical examination, urine sodium concentration (U_{Na}), and urine osmolality (U_{osm}). The reason for this classification is that specific treatment depends on the diagnostic category. Life-threatening hyponatremia is usually the result of water intake in association with salt losses (as with thiazide diuretics) and/or with continued ADH secretion (e.g., syndrome of inappropriate secretion of antidiuretic hormone [SIADH]).

Dangers

Morbidity and mortality from hyponatremia and hypoosmolality occur because of the neurologic damage that results from brain cell swelling in the closed space of the skull. Disorientation, somnolence, seizures, and coma can occur with subsequent death or permanent neurologic damage. The development of signs and symptoms depends on both the rate of the decrease in the serum sodium concentration as well as the severity of the hyponatremia itself.

Treatment

Aggressive therapy for hyponatremia depends more on the presence of symptoms and the rapidity of onset than on the level itself. Treatment principles are listed in Table 6. Therapy is indicated for any patient who is significantly symptomatic and for most patients in whom serum sodium is less than 110 mEq per liter. In these cases, the goal is to achieve a serum sodium concentration of 120 mEq per liter, with slower correction toward normal over the subsequent 24- to 48-hour period. The combination of furosemide (to promote free water loss) plus saline is particulary effective. Furosemide should be administered at a dose large enough (40 to 240 mg IV) to initiate diuresis. The subsequent urine sodium losses (which will appear in the urine at a sodium concentration of 40 to 70 mEq per liter) should be measured every 6 hours and replaced with normal saline (sodium concentration, 154 mEq per liter). The diuretic can be administered every 4 to 6 hours until the desired serum sodium concentration is achieved. It is important that saline replacement be calculated to replace urinary sodium losses, not urinary volume, or else dangerous volume expansion will occur. Treatment with hypertonic saline (e.g., 3 percent saline) may also be utilized when rapid correction is desired but has the disadvantage of requiring special preparation and inducing excess volume expansion if too much is administered. The dose utilized should be based on the number of milliequivalents of sodium needed to raise serum sodium to approximately 120 mEq per liter in a space of distribution of total body water (60 percent body water).

Considerable controversy has appeared in the literature concerning the speed of correction of severe hyponatremia. Some authors believe that rapid correction reduces the morbidity of hyponatremia, whereas others believe that rapid correction may exacerbate central nervous system toxicity and lead to central pontine myelinolysis. Data from the literature seem to indicate that it is safe to raise serum sodium by 5 to 6 mEq in the first few hours, with the total rise not to exceed 12 mEq on the first day. Thereafter, slower correction toward normal is advised.

In patients who are asymptomatic or who are mildly symptomatic but whose hyponatremia has developed more slowly, it is safer to avoid aggressive therapy and to allow correction of the sodium concentration to proceed more slowly. Water restriction remains a cornerstone of therapy for hyponatremia and may in fact be sufficient in patients with reversible defect in water excretion (e.g., in a patient whose thiazide diuretic has been discontinued). Specific treatment directed at the underlying cause is also indicated. Thus, according to the diagnostic categories listed in Table 5, group I patients with volume depletion should be volume-expanded with normal saline to turn off the volume stimulus for ADH and allow correction of hyponatremia. In group II patients with SIADH, demeclocycline (300 mg three times daily) can be added to antagonize ADH action in the distal nephron. For group III patients, many of whom have a nonosmotic stimulus for secretion of ADH, improvement of cardiac function or recovery of liver function will often improve the hyponatremia.

Table 6 Treatment of Life-Threatening Hyponatremia

- Reserve aggressive therapy for symptomatic cases.
- Aim to bring serum sodium up to 120–125 mEq/L with slow correction thereafter.
- Raise the serum sodium by no more than 12 mEq in the first 24 hours.
- Raise serum sodium concentration with:
  Normal saline*
  Normal saline and furosemide
  3% saline with or without furosemide†
- Restrict water intake and treat a defect in water excretion where possible.

*Preferred treatment if patient is volume-contracted.
†Use with caution and watch for signs of fluid overload.

HYPERNATREMIA

Causes

Hypernatremia is observed much less frequently than hyponatremia because thirst is a potent stimulus that can, by itself, increase oral water ingestion and lower serum sodium concentration and osmolality. Thus, hypernatremia occurs primarily in patients who are too old, too young (i.e., infants), or too sick to drink. As with hyponatremia, causes are categorized as those associated with contraction of ECF volume (from renal or gastrointestinal losses), with normal ECF volume (as in diabetes insipidus), and with expanded ECF volume (as with administration of sodium bicarbonate or infant formula). Most cases are associated with some amount of salt loss. Causes associated with sodium excess and ECF volume expansion are uncommon.

Dangers

Morbidity is again mainly confined to neurologic signs and symptoms due to brain cell shrinkage from the hyperosmolality. Confusion, lethargy, and coma can occur, as well as hemorrhage into the central nervous system. Signs and symptoms such as syncope and hypotension may be present in patients who are also volume-contracted. Again, symptomatology is related to the speed of onset of the disturbance.

Treatment

Two concepts must be remembered when treating hypernatremia. First, the body's defense of ECF volume takes precedence over the defense of osmolality; thus, in patients with both volume contraction and hypernatremia, normal saline (not water) is the most appropriate therapy until salt losses are corrected. Second, replacement of water deficits too quickly carries the risk of cerebral edema as brain cells begin to swell with treatment. It is therefore prudent to calculate the amount of water needed to return the serum sodium level to normal, using total body water (60 percent body weight) as the space of distribution. Approximately half of this replacement should be given during the first 12 to 24 hours, with the remaining fluid administered over the next 1 to 2 days. Hypotonic saline and 5 percent aqueous dextrose solutions are preferred, as in the oral route for replacement.

In addition to replacing water (as in a patient with diabetes insipidus) or water and salt deficits (as in a patient with diarrhea or vomiting), it is important to try to stop any further water losses. In patients with ADH deficiency from central diabetes insipidus, desmopressin (DDAVP) (10 to 20 μg intranasally or intravenously) is the treatment of choice.

SEVERE HYPOPHOSPHATEMIA

Causes

Life-threatening hypophosphatemia occurs when levels drop below 1 mg per deciliter. The most common causes for this disturbance include conditions that cause an intracellular shift of phosphate (e.g., hyperalimentation or use of other glucose-containing solutions, recovery from starvation or burns, respiratory alkalosis, or treatment of diabetic ketoacidosis and alcoholism). Many times these conditions coexist with those that cause phosphate depletion, such as use of antacids, diabetic ketoacidosis, or alcoholism. Gastrointestinal phosphate losses (from vomiting, diarrhea, or malabsorption) as well as renal phosphate losses (from hyperparathyroidism or renal tubular defects) can also cause hypophosphatemia, but usually not by themselves, to levels below 1 mg per deciliter. Severe hypophosphatemia in patients admitted for diabetic ketoacidosis or alcoholism frequently occurs not on admission but by the second or third day of hospitalization.

Dangers

Muscle weakness is the outstanding finding and can precipitate or exacerbate congestive heart failure or respiratory failure if cardiac or respiratory muscles become significantly affected. Paralysis and rhabdomyolysis can also occur in severe cases. Neurologic manifestations include paresthesias, encephalopathy, seizures, and coma. Dysfunction of red cells (leading to decreased survival or hemolysis), platelets (leading to decreased survival), and white cells (predisposing to infection) also occurs.

Treatment

Since many of the conditions that precipitate life-threatening hypophosphatemia occur in the treatment phase of a patient's illness, it is important to anticipate the phosphate shifts that will occur with refeeding and the use of glucose-containing solutions to provide adequate phosphate supplementation early. Intravenous therapy (Table 7) is hazardous but is warranted for symptomatic

Table 7 Treatment of Severe Hypophosphatemia

- Give intravenously if level <1 mg/dl. Use phosphate as potassium or sodium phosphate (each containing 93 mg of phosphorus and 4 mEq of sodium or potassium/ml). Administer 2.5–5.0 mg/kg every 6–8 hr until serum phosphate rises >2 mg/dl.
- Watch for hypocalcemia; follow serum calcium every 8–12 hours.
- Follow serum phosphate every 6–8 hours and avoid hyperphosphatemia, which can precipitate metastatic calcification.
- After serum phosphate >2 mg/dl, continue phosphate repletion for 5–10 days in phosphate-depleted patients, choosing oral phosphate therapy, if possible.
- Remove offending drug (e.g., antacids)

cases as well as for all cases with serum phosphate levels below 1 mg per deciliter. Hazards of therapy include hypotension, hypocalcemia (especially if hyperphosphatemia develops). Intravenous therapy should be avoided as much as possible in patients with hypercalcemia, as metastatic calcification is a real risk in this situation. After serum levels reach 2 mg per deciliter, oral therapy (with Neurtra-Phos, potassium phosphate, or Phospho-Soda) is preferred to avoid the risks associated with intravenous therapy. Treatment of phosphate-depleted patients is usually required for at least 5 days to replenish intracellular stores, since these stores can remain low even after serum levels return to normal.

SEVERE HYPERCALCEMIA

Causes

Causes for severe hypercalcemia include malignancy, granulomatous diseases (e.g., sarcoidosis), hyperparathyroidism, thyrotoxicosis, milk alkali syndrome, and immobilization. Drugs such as thiazide diuretics, adrenal insufficiency, vitamin D and A intoxication, and renal failure may also cause hypercalcemia. Many of these conditions involve an increase in bone reabsorption relative to bone formation. The renal tubular damage caused by hypercalcemia leads to volume contraction and a depression in the glomerular filtration rate, both of which diminish renal calcium excretion and exacerbate the disturbance even further.

Dangers

Symptoms related to hypercalcemia depend on speed of onset, degree of elevation, and associated medical problems. Early symptoms include anorexia, nausea, vomiting, and constipation; mental confusion can also be an early symptom. If left untreated, hypercalcemia can lead to obtundation, coma, and death. Significant morbidity or mortality can also arise from cardiac toxicity with arrhythmias, conduction disturbances, and cardiac arrest.

Treatment

Any symptomatic elevation in serum calcium concentration should be treated aggressively. Even if the etiology of the disturbance is not known, measures should be taken to lower the level (Table 8).

If renal function is adequate, calcium excretion can be increased by volume expansion with normal saline delivered at 200 to 500 ml per hour to establish a urine output of 200 to 1,000 ml per hour. Although there is no proof that adding furosemide to this regimen further increases calcium excretion, it is common practice to do so to avoid excess volume expansion. Careful monitoring of other electrolytes at this time, particularly potassium and magnesium, is essential. Furosemide administration can be repeated every 2 to 6 hours to maintain the diuresis until the calcium level returns to normal. Forced diuresis with

Table 8 Emergency Treatment of Hypercalcemia

Increase Calcium Excretion
 Expand volume with saline
 Add furosemide every 2–6 hours
 Dialysis

Decrease bone reabsorption

Drug	Dose	Onset	Duration
Calcitonin	4 units/kg IV* or IM†	<4 hours	6–10 hours
Didronel	7.5 mg/kg IV‡	3–5 days	7–10 days
Mithramycin	25µg/kg IV§	12–24 hours	3–7 days
Hydrocortisone	1 mg/kg IV#	1–3 days	1 day

*Given by continuous infusion.
†Given IM b.i.d. to q.i.d.
‡Mixed in 500 ml of 5% aqueous dextrose or saline solution and delivered over 3 hr daily for 3–5 days.
§Delivered over 6 hours.
#Given every 8 hours for the first few days.

saline and furosemide is considered a front-line measure to treat hypercalcemia emergently and can produce a net excretion of 1 to 2 g of calcium in 24 hours.

If a vigorous diuresis cannot be established easily, early consideration should be given to hemodialysis against a zero-calcium bath to relieve the patient of any danger and possibly to improve renal function so that a diuresis can be established.

In many patients, it will also be necessary to decrease the bone reabsorption rate in order to bring serum calcium concentration into the normal range. Drugs available for this purpose are listed in Table 8. Calcitonin is the safest drug to use but loses efficacy in many patients after a few days. Didronel (EHDP), the only diphosphonate currently available, can be very effective, but its effect is often not apparent for 3 to 5 days (although it can last for more than 1 week). Because of its renal excretion, it should be used with caution in patients with renal impairment. Newer diphosphonate preparations that can be given orally are currently under investigation. Mithramycin is effective in most patients and has a long duration of action but should be avoided in those with significant renal or hepatic dysfunction because of its nephrotoxic and hepatotoxic side effects. Glucocorticoids are particularly effective in lowering serum calcium concentration in patients with hematologic malignancies, sarcoidosis, and breast cancer. Phosphate therapy can also lower serum calcium concentration, but its use should be limited to patients with a serum phosphate level below 3 mg per deciliter (e.g., those with hyperparathyroidism) to avoid metastatic calcification. For the same reason, it should be given orally, and never intravenously, to treat hypercalcemia.

In addition to measures taken to lower the serum calcium concentration, every effort should be made to mobilize the patient and prevent further increases in serum calcium concentration that result from immobilization. Even in seriously ill patients, attempts should be made to promote weight-bearing activity several times daily, even simple quiet standing. Finally, there is experimental evidence to indicate that calcium-channel blockers may ameliorate some of the cardiotoxic effects of hypercalcemia. Clinical studies are needed to substantiate this finding.

SEVERE HYPOCALCEMIA

Causes

Severe hypocalcemia is always associated with a lowering of the ionized calcium level and not just a lowering of total calcium concentration due to a decrease in serum albumin concentration. Common causes include pancreatitis, hypomagnesemia, vitamin D deficiency (usually associated with malabsorption or liver disease), and hyperphosphatemia (associated with cell lysis). Renal failure (chronic more often than acute) is another cause in which case phosphate values are quite high. Primary parathyroid deficiency is unusual, but cases secondary to surgery, trauma, or radiation therapy are more common cases of hypocalcemia.

Dangers

Neuromuscular irritability, paresthesias, and twitches are common, with frank tetany occurring in the most severe cases. A positive Chvostek or Trousseau sign can often be elicited before these events occur. Contraction of respiratory muscles can lead to laryngospasm and eventual respiratory arrest. Mental irritability, confusion, and seizures can also occur. Manifestations of cardiac toxicity include congestive heart failure, arrhythmias, hypotension, and insensitivity to pressor agents.

Treatment

If hypocalcemia is symptomatic, it should be treated as a medical emergency. Aggressive treatment is also appropriate in hypocalcemic patients being treated for acidosis (e.g., a patient with RTA), as bicarbonate therapy could lower ionized serum calcium even further and precipitate symptoms. Acute treatment begins with a bolus (10 ml) of 10 percent calcium gluconate over 10 minutes (delivering approximately 100 mg of calcium). This is followed by a calcium drip designed to deliver 100 mg of elemental calcium per hour until the serum level reaches 8 to 9 mg per deciliter. Calcium gluconate or calcium chloride can be utilized and mixed in 5 percent aqueous dextrose solution. When the volume of delivery must be limited (as in a hypocalcemic patient with renal failure), calcium chloride may be preferred because it contains a larger amount of elemental calcium per gram of salt than does calcium gluconate. In such cases, we prefer to deliver the solution through a central line to avoid the irritative effects of the salt in peripheral veins and to avoid extravasation, which can produce extensive soft tissue damage. Replacement should be done extremely cautiously in patients on digitalis, as hypercalcemia can precipitate digitalis toxicity.

In all cases in which intravenous replacement is utilized, serum calcium levels should be followed every 4 to 6 hours to avoid treatment-induced hypercalcemia. Urine output, renal function, and serum phosphate values should also be monitored. Serum magnesium levels should be checked initially and then followed daily, as it is impossible to maintain correction of hypocalcemia until magnesium depletion is also corrected. Once hypocalcemic symptoms have abated and levels remain above 8 mg per deciliter, oral therapy with or without vitamin D supplementation is preferred where possible.

SUGGESTED READING

Ellison DH, Bia MJ. Renal, fluid, and electrolyte disorders in the critically ill immunosuppressed patient. In: Parillo JE, Masur H, eds. The critically ill immunosuppressed patient. Rockville, MD: Aspen, 1987:81.
Montoliu J, Lens XM, Revert L. Potassium-lowering effect of albuterol for hyperkalemia in renal failure. Arch Intern Med 1987; 147:713–717.
Stewart AF, Broadus AE. Mineral metabolism. In: Felig P, Baxter JD, Broadus AE, Frohman LA, eds. Endocrinology and metabolism. New York: McGraw-Hill, 1987:1317.

NUTRITION IN THE CRITICALLY ILL

JOHANE P. ALLARD, M.D.
KHURSHEED N. JEEJEEBHOY, M.B.B.S., Ph.D.

The critically ill patient often suffers from a combination of injuries, sepsis, and specific organ (kidney, liver, lung, and heart) failure. The results of injury, sepsis, and enforced bed rest are alterations in nitrogen handling and energy requirements. At a clinical level, these patients waste rapidly and lose muscle bulk. They often have metabolic abnormalities and abnormal liver function and depressed glomerular filtration. The metabolic abnormalities are characterized by an increase in gluconeogenesis, accelerated production of urea, and an enhanced turnover of free fatty acids. These abnormalities are believed to be partly mediated by an increase in the so-called counter-regulatory hormones, cortisol, catecholamines, and glucagon, which together oppose the action of insulin. Therefore, despite high circulating levels of insulin, the presence of continuing hyperglycemia, high free fatty acid, and leucine levels suggests a resistance to the action of insulin.

Our studies in these patients have indicated that such patients will metabolize both fat and carbohydrate equally well, provided that higher insulin levels are achieved when carbohydrate is the infused substrate. Under these circumstances protein balance was achieved with either carbohydrate or fat. However, with carbohydrate infusions and insulin administration, the production of carbon dioxide was higher than with fat and may contribute to ventilatory demand.

Recently it has been suggested that an increased level of cytokines released by the presence of sepsis may increase muscle proteolysis and increase the metabolic rate. Finally, some patients develop multiple organ failure, which is associated with a reduced metabolic rate and an inability to utilize nutrients, including glucose and fatty acids. In this situation, the provision of energy substrates causes marked hyperglycemia and hyperlipidemia.

Thus, the critically ill patient appears to have increased energy demands with reduced ability to handle nutrient substrates. This problem is accentuated by hepatic and renal failure.

NUTRITIONAL ASSESSMENT

A good nutritional assessment in the critically ill patient is difficult to make. Its goal is to identify patients at risk for morbidity and mortality from malnutrition. Traditional methods rely heavily on objective anthropometric measurements and laboratory test results that are often difficult to interpret in the critically ill.

Anthropometric Measurements

Among anthropometric measurements, body weight is the most commonly used. However, in the critically ill, it fluctuates widely with the degree of hydration. Thus, the actual body weight of the patient should not be used to calculate caloric requirements or to judge the nutritional status. The same problem will render skin-fold thickness and arm circumference as poor indices of the true fat and muscle mass.

Immunologic Functions

Protein-calorie malnutrition is known to depress humoral and cellular immunity. However, numerous factors such as peripheral edema, uremia, hepatic failure, and ongoing sepsis can blunt or eliminate the response to skin testing and lower the lymphocyte count. Thus indices of immune deficiency in these patients do not uniquely reflect the nutritional status.

Biochemical Tests

Many biochemical tests have been proposed for assessing nutritional status. Serum proteins unfortunately are an inaccurate criteria in the critically ill patient. They show great variability independent of nutritional status, mainly because they are influenced by dilution, gastrointestinal or wound protein loss, and reduced hepatic synthesis because of sepsis. In this situation, low serum protein levels do not reflect an inadequate nutrient intake but are due to disease-related hypercatabolism and rate of synthesis. Even in the absence of such factors, low serum protein levels may not respond promptly to refeeding. Serum albumin (normal half-life is 20 days) concentration can decline during rapid intravenous hydration, and the plasma level will not respond to nutritional repletion before 4 to 5 weeks. Transferrin (half-life is 8 to 9 days) is reasonably sensitive, and the plasma level rises about 2 weeks after repletion. However, the transferrin level is influenced also by anemia and inflammation, and it is not specific. Thyroxine-binding prealbumin (half-life is 2 days) and retinol-binding protein (half-life is 12 hours) are definitely more sensitive to changes in nutritional status but are less responsive during critical illness. More recently, fibronectin (half-life is 12 hours) has been reported to be sensitive to nutritional changes even in stressed patients and can rise within 1 week of parenteral nutrition. However, it can fall rapidly if there is accelerated consumption secondary to acute illness. The last on the list, somatomedin C, is under investigation in the critically ill.

Creatinine-Height Index

This test is a reasonable measure of muscle mass in chronic nutritional depletion but may not be accurate in the critically ill because of artifactual reduction of creatinine excretion due to renal failure.

Nitrogen Balance

This test is useful for grossly measuring protein intake and breakdown. Urinary urea nitrogen (UUN) can be measured with a 24-hour urinary collection. Because amino acids and ammonia account for approximately 15 percent of total urinary nitrogen loss, it is recommended to divide the 24-hour UUN value by 0.85. Nitrogen intake is estimated by dividing the quantity of protein administered by 6.25, which is the number of grams of high-biologic-value protein that contain a gram of nitrogen. The nitrogen balance is the difference between the intake and the loss. It has been recommended that 4 g be added to the nitrogen loss to account for fecal losses in patients fed enterally. However, our own data have rarely indicated losses of more than 2 g per day. It is near zero to 1 g when they receive total parenteral nutrition (TPN) even when there is diarrhea. If there is renal failure, then nitrogen, instead of being excreted, accumulates in the body water and renders the normal balance data inaccurate. To estimate the UUN loss, in this situation the following equation may be used.

$$\text{24-hr UUN loss} = \text{UUN} + (\text{BUN at 24 hr} - \text{BUN at 0 hr}) \times \text{body weight} \times 2/3$$

Indirect Calorimetry

Energy expenditure is determined by the method of indirect calorimetry. Mobile metabolic carts are now available to measure oxygen consumption and carbon dioxide production in critically ill patients. The basal energy expenditure (BEE) is obtained when the measurements are performed early in the morning on a subject who remains in bed, in a thermoneutral environment, at least 12 hours postprandially. The resting energy expenditure (REE) is obtained when the measurements are done in a thermoneutral environment, after resting for at least 30 minutes in a supine position at least 2 hours postprandially. Because several factors such as position, procedure, caloric intake, and exercise influence the energy expenditure, it is important to follow a strict protocol for routine monitoring. In nonambulatory critically ill patients, we have determined that there is a 10 percent increase in metabolic rate caused by "bed activity" (position changes, procedures, receiving visitors) and approximately another 10 percent increase caused by diet-induced thermogenesis. Thus measurements of metabolic rate in the fasting state need to be adjusted by 20 percent for bed activity and diet-induced thermogenesis to get the full requirements. If the patient has been fed, then 10 percent needs to be added to account for bed activity only. The respiratory quotient (RQ) is also monitored. A value of 0.7 is encountered primarily in starvation and reflects fat oxidation. A value higher than 1.0 may suggest lipogenesis from excessive caloric intake. We try to maintain the RQ around 0.9 during the fed state.

TYPE OF NUTRITION

A patient who is unable to take oral diet for the next 3 to 5 days after the start of acute illness or who has been starved or underfed for a week or more should be considered for enteral or parenteral feeding. Whenever possible, the enteral route should be the first choice. Parenteral nutrition is indicated in patients who have severely compromised bowel function such as with paralytic ileus, short gut, peritonitis, abdominal abscesses, intractable diarrhea, and acute pancreatitis.

Enteral Feeding

Access

Enteral feeding can be infused into the stomach, duodenum, or jejunum. Infusion can be given through a nasogastric or nasoduodenal tube, a percutaneous gastrostomy, or a jejunostomy. Because the stomach is more likely to become atonic than the small intestine, gastric infusion is not indicated if there is decreased gastrointestinal motility. With this site of infusion, gastric residual volume should be monitored frequently (each 3 to 4 hours), while one keeps in mind that the volume can increase abruptly if there is clinical deterioration. At such time, as pulmonary aspiration may become a serious problem, it is mandatory to discontinue the feeding. Duodenal feeding is the preferable type of infusion and avoids gastric intolerance and delayed nutrition. The feeding tube is inserted through a nostril or through a gastrostomy and is usually advanced into the duodenum under fluoroscopic guidance. Sometimes with gastric atony, it is necessary to add a nasogastric tube in order to aspirate the residual content or to administer sucralfate for stress ulcer prophylaxis. Jejunal feeding via jejunostomy has been used in patients with surgery and multiple trauma, because nutrients are well absorbed in the small intestine despite the ileus involving the stomach and large bowel. However, technically, tubes advanced through the pylorus into the small bowel avoid a number of problems associated with direct jejunal intubation and achieve the same results.

Type of Feeding Solution

The feeding products on the market are numerous and each hospital has its own formulary. They can be classified in four groups: standard (polymeric), elemental (monomeric), modular, and specialized solutions (Table 1).

Standard Solutions. These solutions are composed of nutrients that are whole protein (sodium and calcium caseinate), triglycerides (corn and soybean oil), and complex carbohydrates (corn syrups, sucrose). They are generally lower in osmolarity, contain 1 kcal per milliliter, and are less expensive than other specialized formulae. A few others are more concentrated and contain 1.5 to 2 kcal per milliliter (hypertonic). Most of them are now lactose-free and contain about 14 to 16 percent of the total kilocalories as protein. These solutions are indicated in patients who are unable to eat because of underlying disease but who have a normal intestine with the capacity to digest and absorb.

Elemental Solutions. The protein source of these solutions is composed of amino acids alone or in combination with small peptides from partially hydrolyzed whey, soy, and meat proteins. The carbohydrate source is generally in the form of oligosaccharides and monosaccharides from hydrolysis of corn starch. The fat content of these products is three to four times less than in the standard solutions and may contain 50 percent of the fat as composed of medium-chain triglyceride (MCT). These formulae are hyperosmolar and contain 1 kcal per milliliter and 14 to 17 percent of the total kilocalories as protein. They are more expensive. However, their advantage is that prior to absorption, they do not require digestion (proteolysis and lipolysis). For this reason, they are indicated in states like chronic pancreatitis, the recovery phase of acute pancreatitis, acute inflammatory bowel disease, short bowel, some enterocutaneous fistulae, and other states that require low residue. In long-term feeding, safflower oil supplementation may be required to avoid essential fatty acid deficiency.

Modular Feeding. This is a feeding that is supplied as separate units of protein, lipid, and carbohydrate sources and micronutrients that are mixed in desired proportions prior to administration. It is used in patients who have

Table 1 Examples of Enteral Nutrition Formulae

Product	Calories/ml	Protein Source	g/L(%)	Cholesterol Source	g/L(%)	Fat	Osmolarity
Elemental							
Vital HN (Ross)	1	Partially hydrolyzed whey and meat, soy, free amino acids	41.7 (16.7)	Hydrolyzed cornstarch, sucrose	185 (73.9)	MCT (45%) safflower (55%)	460
Vivonex TEN (Norwich Eaton)	1	Free amino acids	38.2 (15.3)	Maltodextrins, modified starch	206 (82.2)	Safflower	630 630
Standard							
Enrich (Fiber) (Ross)	1.1	Sodium and calcium caseinates, soy protein isolate	39.7 (14.5)	Hydrolyzed cornstarch, sucrose, soy, polysaccharide	162 (55.0)	Corn	480
Ensure (Ross)	1.06	Sodium and calcium caseinates soy protein isolate	37.2 (14.0)	Corn syrup, sucrose	145 (54.5)	Corn	450
Ensure Plus (Ross)	1.5	Sodium and calcium caseinates, soy protein isolate	54.9 (14.7)	Corn syrup, sucose	200 (53.3)	Corn	600
Isocal (Mead Johnson	1.06	Calcium and sodium caseinates, soy protein isolate	34.2 (13.0)	Maltodextrin	133 (50.0)	Soy (80%) MCT (20%)	300
Osmolite HN (Ross)	1.06	Sodium and calcium caseinates, soy protein isolate	44.4 (16.7)	Hydrolyzed cornstarch	141 (53.3)	MCT (50%) corn, soy (50%)	300
Compleat Modified (Sandoz)	1.07	Beef calcium caseinate	43 (16)	Hydrolyzed cereal, solids, fruits and vegetables	141 (54)	Beef corn oil	300
Magnacal (Chesebrough-Pond)	2	Sodium and calcium caseinates	70.0 (14.0)	Maltodextrin, sucrose	250 (50.0)	Hydrogenated soybean oil	590
Modular							
Pro-Pac (Chesebrough-Pond)	4/g	Whey	(76.0)	—	(8.0)	—	—
MCT oil (Mead Johnson)	7.7	—	—	—	—	Coconut Oil	—
Polycose Liquid (Ross)	2	—	—	Glucose polymers	(100)	—	900
Polycose Powder (Ross)	3.8/g	—	—	Glucose polymers	(100)	—	
Specialized							
Hepatic Aid (Kendal McGaw)	1.2	EAA + NEAA	44.1 (15.0)	Maltodextrin, sucrose	169 (57.3)	Hydrogenated soybean oil	560
Amin Aid (Kendal McGaw)	2	EAA + Histidine	194.0 (4.0)	Maltodextrin, sugar	366 (74.8)	Hydrogenated soybean oil	1095
Pulmocare (Ross)	1.5	Sodium and calcium caseinate	82.4 (16.7)	Hydrolyzed cornstarch, sucrose	105 (28.1)	Corn oil	490

special needs not met by commercial solutions. Multiple nutrients can be combined to make a nutritionally complete feeding or can be used to enhance the nutritive value of a commercial formula. Vitamin supplementation and electrolytes need to be added.

Specialized Solutions. *Hepatic-Aid.* Some investigators have suggested that the decreased ratio of branched-chain amino acids (BCAAs) to aromatic amino acids (AAAs) found in patients with chronic liver disease may be of etiologic importance in hepatic encephalopathy. Therefore, an enteral solution with high BCAAs and low AAAs has been created. This formula is hyperosmolar, with 1.6 kcal per milliliter and 10 percent of the total calories as protein. The ratio of carbohydrate to fats (70 percent to 20 percent of total calories) is higher than in the standard formulae (50–55 percent to 30–35 percent). This solution does not have minerals and vitamins.

Amin Aid. This formula has been designed for patients with renal failure. It is hyperosmolar and contains 2 kcal per milliliter. The amino acid content is restricted to eight essential amino acids plus histidine. The vitamins and minerals must be added on an individual basis. The ratio of carbohydrate to fat is 65 percent to 32 percent of total calories.

Pulmocare. This formula has been designed for patients with respiratory insufficiency to avoid excess production of carbon dioxide. In this solution, the fat content is 55 percent of total calories. It is isotonic and contains 1.5 kcal per milliliter and 16.7 percent protein.

Administration

Enteral solutions should be started at 25 ml per hour and increased as tolerated by no more than 25 ml per hour per day until the requirements are reached. The maximum rate should be 100 ml per hour in order to avoid the risk of high gastric residue and pulmonary aspiration. The cause of diarrhea is among other factors an imbalance between the rate of infusion and absorption. There is no need to dilute feeds. However, the total load of osmoles infused needs to be increased gradually as tolerated. For the same reason, bolus feeding is likely to cause diarrhea, and continuous infusion with a pump is the best way of giving enteral feeds.

Complications

The mechanical complications are rare and related to tube placement and positioning. More frequent are the adverse gastrointestinal reactions. Gastric retention, emesis, and aspirations are common when the feeding is given into the stomach. Diarrhea is also frequent and its etiology multifactorial. When confronted with this problem, we generally take these steps:

1. Collect stools for ova, parasites, *C. difficile* toxin. If positive, specific treatment is given.
2. Decrease the rate of feeding by half and replace fiber-free solutions with Enrich (which contains fiber). Resume rate slowly. Bolus feeding is avoided, and lactose-free solutions are mandatory.
3. If a hyperosmotic solution is infused into the duodenum, the rate of infusion is decreased. If the diarrhea remains, the hyperosmotic solution can be replaced empirically by an iso-osmolar formula (for example, Ensure Plus replaced by Isosource).
4. In patients with a short bowel, Imodium may be used cautiously to control the diarrhea. Some are using instead 30 ml of Kaopectate along with 10 ml of paregoric per liter of solution for 3 to 4 days.
5. Polymeric formulae can be replaced by elemental solutions if there is evidence of reduced digestion or absorption (based on the clinical picture or documented by fecal fat measurement). In the case of chronic pancreatitis, it may be indicated to give pancreatic enzymes along with polymeric solutions.
6. In the case of prolonged antibiotherapy, administration of lactinase granules (Lactinex) three times over the course of 1 day can be tried. However, no studies were done to suggest the usefulness of this regimen.
7. If these measures have failed, albumin can be infused to raise the serum albumin to 25 mg per deciliter. However, this approach is empirical and no controlled studies have been done to confirm its benefit.
8. To try to improve absorption through the sodium-glucose pump, 5 ml of salt (about 2 g of sodium chloride) can be added to each liter of enteral solution.
9. If diarrhea persists for one week or more and caloric requirements cannot be met, parenteral nutrition is indicated for total or partial nutritional support.

Parenteral Nutrition

Access

Parenteral nutrition can be administered via a peripheral or a central line. The peripheral route is indicated when the insertion of the central line is delayed, unnecessary, or impossible because of danger or technical difficulty. It can also be used temporarily (about 1 week) as a complement to oral feeding when intake is not sufficient. Several peripheral veins must be available for the perfusion, since the catheter needs to be rotated each 48 hours to avoid thrombosis. Caloric intake is also limited, compared with TPN. Co-infusion of amino acid–dextrose solution and lipid emulsion is mandatory to avoid hypertonicity and to inhibit endothelial procoagulant activity; it is best given by pump. A central line is more often used in an intensive care setting for parenteral nutrition. The subclavian site is the first choice, mainly because insertion is better protected by occlusive dressings, which are

Table 2 Amino Acid Solutions and Lipid Emulsions

Amino acid solutions

Standard	High EAA	High BCAA
Aminosyn 8.5% (Abbott)	Aminosyn RF 5.2% (Abbott)	Hepatamine 8% (McGaw)
Freamine 8.5% (McGaw)	Nephramine 5.4% (McGaw)	Freamine HBC 6.0% (McGaw)
Travasol 8.5% (Travenol)	Renamine (Travenol)	

Lipid emulsions

Product	Oil	kcal/ml	% Linoleic	% Oleic	% Palmitic	% Linolenic
Intralipid 10% (Kabi Vitrum)	Soybean	1.1	54.0	26.0	9.0	8.0
Intralipid 20% (Kabi Vitrum)	Soybean	2.0	50.0	26.0	10.0	9.0
Liposyn II 10% (Abbott)	Safflower and soybean	1.1	65.8	17.7	8.8	4.2
Liposyn II 20% (Abbott)	Safflower and soybean	2.0	65.8	17.7	8.8	4.2

not adequate in lines inserted through the jugular route. Complications, although more serious than for enteral or peripheral nutrition, are fortunately rare. After catheter placement, a chest film is mandatory to check for pneumothorax and for the position of the catheter tip, which should lie just above the right atrium.

Type of Solutions (Table 2)

Dextrose. Commercially available dextrose solutions are in the form of dextrose monohydrate, 3.4 kcal per gram. Therefore, 1 liter of 10 percent dextrose solution provides 340 kcal. Dextrose solutions with an osmolarity higher than 300 mOsm per liter are defined as hyperosmolar. When mixed with amino acid solutions, most standard formulae have a final concentration of dextrose of 25 to 35 percent, which results in an osmolarity of 1200 to 1700 mOsm per liter. The pH of dextrose solutions is between 3.5 and 5.5.

Lipid Emulsion. Fat emulsions have a high caloric density (9 kcal per gram) and are rendered isotonic by the addition of glycerol. The source of fatty acids is soybean with or without safflower, and 50 to 66 percent of its content is provided as linoleic acid and 4 to 9 percent as linolenic acid. In general, commercial emulsions are all equivalent nutritionally.

Crystalline Amino Acid Solutions. These synthetic amino acids have replaced the previous hydrolysates of naturally occurring proteins (fibrin, casein). The standard formulae contain a combination of 40 to 50 percent essential amino acids (EAAs) and 50 to 60 percent nonessential amino acids (NEAAs). There are several solutions on the market that differ in their available concentrations (3.5 to 10 percent) and amino acid and electrolyte profiles. However, clinically no difference has been found between the products. There are also solutions designed specifically for certain disorders. The ones for renal failure supply concentrated EAAs and L-histidine. Their clinical advantages over the standard solutions remain controversial, and they are not currently recommended for use in the intensive care unit. There are also solutions for patients with hepatic encephalopathy. They contain a high concentration of BCAAs (valine, leucine, isoleucine). Their ability to achieve the claimed clinical advantages is also controversial.

Administration

When dextrose and amino acid solutions are mixed, the final concentration is 25 to 35 percent dextrose and 3.5 to 5 percent amino acids, with an osmolarity of 1200 to 1500 mOsm per liter. The maximum concentration tolerated in peripheral veins is 10 percent dextrose and 4.25 percent amino acids. Higher concentrations are infused centrally. In the past we infused separately over 12 hours a 10 or 20 percent fat emulsion with the amino acid–dextrose solution, via a "Y" connector. Currently, we are using the three-in-one admixture, in which amino acids, dextrose, and lipids are mixed with additives in the same bag and infused over 24 hours. The total daily dose of lipids should not exceed 4 g per kilogram body weight.

Complications

The complications are rare but serious and can be divided into two groups: catheter-related and metabolic.

Sepsis complicates TPN in about 1 to 2 percent of patients. Primary catheter sepsis is present when no other source is found and when it is resolved by catheter removal. In most cases, organisms cultured from the tip of the catheter are the same as those found in the peripheral blood. Secondary catheter infection may develop when there is seeding from another infected site. When a patient becomes septic the catheter should not be removed immediately unless sterility has been clearly violated and a culture obtained through it by retrograde withdrawal of blood. TPN is temporarily stopped while awaiting culture. If the blood is sterile, the catheter can be left in place and TPN resumed. However, if the patient remains febrile and no source of infection has been found, the catheter should be changed over a wire and the tip of the catheter removed for culture. In some cases the catheter should be changed.

The most frequent metabolic complication in septic patients receiving TPN is hyperglycemia. Careful monitoring of blood glucose is mandatory in order to prevent a hyperglycemic, hyperosmolar, nonketotic state. Regular insulin, given according to a sliding scale is initially infused separately. Insulin infusion not only improves the glycemia but also has a positive effect on the nitrogen balance. If the requirements for insulin remain constantly high, 10 U of regular insulin per bag can be added. However, it should be kept in mind that with clinical improvement, insulin requirements will decrease and this may produce hypoglycemia. We rarely add insulin in the three-in-one admixture bag infused to critically ill patients because of this variation in glucose intolerance and the interruption of nutrition support if hypoglycemia develops.

Complications reported with lipid emulsions are rare and related to excessive rates of infusion. If lipid clearance is decreased, the emulsion can be given over 24 hours or two to three times a week to avoid essential fatty acid deficiency.

Liver function tests are often mildly increased in patients with TPN. In critically ill patients, the increase can be multifactorial and TPN, using the glucose-lipid system, is generally not the most important cause. In the case of progressive cholestasis, an abdominal ultrasound is generally indicated in order to exclude biliary obstruction, acalculous cholecystitis, or liver steatosis; the latter condition is now less frequent since the use of this glucose-lipid system.

NUTRITIONAL REQUIREMENTS

Once the decision has been made to feed the patient through a chosen route of infusion, the nutritional requirements are estimated. Whether it is enteral or parenteral, the same quantities and relative proportion of nutrients are delivered (Table 3).

Nonprotein Energy

Number of Calories

In general, an energy intake between 30 and 40 kcal of nonprotein energy per kilogram ideal body weight (IBW) per day should be administered, depending on the degree of catabolism. The weight is the one taken before the acute illness or estimated according to the height in order to give a body mass index (BMI) of 23 (normal is between 20 and 25).

$$BMI = \frac{weight\ (kg)}{[height\ (m)]^2}$$

In obese patients (weight over 10 percent of IBW), the same rule is used and the REE and nitrogen balance is followed to prevent excessive weight loss. In malnourished patients (under 10 percent of IBW), we give half the estimated caloric need for the first 3 to 4 days to prevent refeeding edema. If tolerated, caloric intake is progressively increased until it reaches the estimated requirements and patients are monitored with nitrogen balance and REE. Another way to calculate the caloric requirement is by using the Harris-Benedict (HB) formula multiplied by a stress factor:

Males: HB = 66.5 + 13.75W + 5H − 6.8A
Females: HB = 665 + 9.6W + 1.85H − 4.7A
where W = weight, H = height, and A = age.

We usually use this formula, especially in the case of elderly patients. The stress factor is derived from Long's observation and is 1.3 × HB for sepsis alone or uncomplicated major surgery; 1.5 × HB for complicated sepsis (with organ failure) and burns of less than 20 percent; and 2 × HB for burns over 20 percent. However, if an indirect calorimeter is available, it is the most practical method for accurate determination of caloric requirement. Several investigators have shown that the 24-hr energy expenditure of critically ill, ventilated patients is only 5 to 10 percent higher than the REE (fed state). Therefore, in these patients, we give 1.1 × REE (if measured in the fed state) or 1.2 × REE (if measured in the fasting state).

Glucose Versus Fat

Generally for TPN the glucose-to-fat ratio varies between 60:40 and 40:60. Larger amounts of glucose can be detrimental to the patient for the following reasons: (1) It significantly increases norepinephrine excretion, which further increases the energy expenditure, stimulates glucagon secretion, and enhances insulin resistance. (2) Excess glucose will be converted to fat in the liver and produce liver steatosis. (3) In the acutely ill, the use of glucose as the only source of nonprotein energy has been shown to increase production of carbon dioxide by up to 75 percent, increasing the pulmonary work load and sometimes delaying weaning from the ventilator. (4) Lipid emulsion is as good as hypertonic glucose in improving protein synthesis in catabolic patients.

Protein Energy

It is desirable to start with an intake that is between 1.2 and 1.5 g per kilogram per day. The most catabolic patients, such as those with major burns, will require up to 2 g per kilogram per day. We then monitor the patients

Table 3 Nutritional Requirements

	Enteral Nutrition	*Parenteral Nutrition*	
Electrolytes			
Sodium	1.3–3.3 g/day 56.5–143.3 mmol/day	90–120 mmol/day	Increase with gastrointestinal loss; 50 mmol/day in elderly or heart-failure patients
Potassium	1.9–5.6 gm/day 48.6–143.2 mmol/day	80–120 mmol/day	Decrease in renal failure; increase with amphotericin B
Magnesium	350 mg/day 14–15 mmol/day	8–12 mmol/day	Increase with gastrointestinal loss and cyclosporine
Phosphorus	800 mg/day 25–26 mmol/day	14–16 mmol/day	Increase when glucose alone is infused; decrease with renal failure
Calcium	800 mg/day 20 mmol/day	7–10 mmol/day	Decrease with renal failure
Trace Metals			
Iron		1–2 mg/day	
Zinc	2.5–4.0 mg/day	2.5 mg/day	+12 mg/L of small bowel fluid loss; +17 mg/L stool loss
Copper	0.5–1.5 mg/day	0.3 mg/d	0.5 mg/day if diarrhea; none with abnormal liver function test
Chromium	10–15 μg/day	10–20 μg/day	
Selenium		120 μg/day	
Iodine		120 μg/day	
Manganese	0.15–0.8 mg/day	0.2–0.8 mg/day	
Molybdenum		48–96 mg/day	
Vitamins			
Vitamin A	4000–5000 IU	3300 IU/day	
Vitamin D	200–400 IU	None	
Vitamin E	10–20 IU	10 IU/day	
Vitamin K		10 mg/wk IM; none if anticoagulation used	
Thiamine	—	5 mg/day	
Riboflavin	—	5 mg/day	
Niacin	13–19 mg	40 mg/day	
Pantothenic Acid	4–7 mg	15 mg/day	
Pyridoxine	—	5 mg/day	
Folic Acid	400 μg	400 μg/day	
Vitamin B_{12}	—	12 μg/day	
Vitamin C	50–60 IU	100 IU/day	
Biotin	100–200 μg	60 μg/day	
Cyanocobalamin	3 μg	5 μg	

with nitrogen balance. Standard feeding formulae or dextrose–amino acid solutions are used.

Water and Electrolytes

In general, adequate nutrition results in weight gain. In fasting individuals, refeeding with carbohydrate results in a reduction of sodium and water excretion. When sodium is provided simultaneously, the weight gain is rapid through expansion of extracellular space. In addition, injury further reduces urinary sodium and water excretion. It is therefore advisable to be aware of possible fluid overload following the initiation of TPN and to monitor closely the fluid balance and hemodynamics. The most important electrolytes to follow in the initial period are potassium, phosphorus, and magnesium. Daily or twice-daily monitoring is required.

Trace Elements

Seven trace elements have been shown to be necessary to human beings: iron, zinc, copper, chromium, selenium, iodine, and cobalt. They are present in the commercial enteral formulae in amounts recommended by the

FDA, and they are added to the TPN solutions. Most of these elements can be lost through the gastrointestinal tract, and requirements may be increased in the case of severe diarrhea. Renal disease does not reduce the need for these elements. In chronic liver disease, however, we reduce or avoid giving manganese and copper, which are excreted in the biliary tract.

Vitamins

Vitamins are also provided in recommended amounts by the standard commercial formulae; they are added to the TPN solutions. The optimal doses for TPN have not been studied in detail.

SPECIAL NEEDS

Renal Failure

Nutritional support in this type of patient increases the risk of uremia and fluid overload, which may require dialysis or hemofiltration. In the hypercatabolic patient, the decision must be made to give nutritional support after 1 week of inadequate intake even if it implies starting dialysis. If there is hemodynamic instability precluding dialysis, continuous hemofiltration or peritoneal dialysis are other alternatives for controlling fluid overload and uremia.

In patients with progressive renal failure, but who are not hemodialyzed, the caloric requirements are calculated as recommended. Protein intake is restricted to 0.5 to 0.75 g per kilogram IBW per day, and standard solutions are used. Fluid is restricted to 1.5 to 2 L per day if urine output is low. If after 1 week there is no clinical improvement, dialysis or hemofiltration in the case of fluid overload should be considered in order to be able to give an appropriate nutritional intake. With improvement of the condition or the start of dialysis, protein intake is increased up to 1.5 g per kilogram IBW per day, and fluid balance is monitored. If enteral nutrition is given, it may be necessary to prepare a modular feeding in order to adjust the amount of protein and the volume. A carbohydrate-to-fat ratio of 60:40 can be used as a start. Glucose intolerance and hyperlipemia, especially in chronic renal failure, is prevented by frequent monitoring. The addition of insulin and modification of the glucose-to-fat ratio is generally sufficient to treat these conditions. During the process of dialysis or hemofiltration, there is loss of nutrients, especially amino acids (Table 4), and the recommended increase in protein intake should compensate for that. In peritoneal dialysis, the loss of protein can be more important during episodes of peritonitis. In addition, in this type of dialysis, glucose is absorbed significantly and this can account for hyperglycemia. In this situation, we usually estimate that about 150 g of glucose is absorbed daily and subtract that amount from the nutritional supplementation.

The use of EAA formulae remains controversial, and such formulae should be used only under certain circumstances. Its rationale is that endogenous nitrogen can then be reused to synthesize NEAA, therefore slowing the rate of rise of blood urea nitrogen (BUN). EAAs can be prescribed only when a patient suffering severe renal failure is a poor candidate for dialysis and has a rapid rise of BUN with standard formulae. The EAA solution is utilized twice as efficiently as a standard solution. However, it still requires the same volume because the concentration of the solution is half that of the standard ones, when mixed with glucose. Therefore, fluid overload remains a problem. In critically ill patients, we give no more than 0.5 to 0.75 g per kilogram IBW. In less catabolic patients, as low as 0.3 g per kilogram IBW per day can be given.

Hepatic Failure

If there is no encephalopathy, the patient should receive between 1 and 1.5 g of protein per kilogram per day from standard solutions. If there is a history of encephalopathy, or if encephalopathy occurs or progresses, most patients will tolerate an intake of about 0.5 g of pro-

Table 4 Effects of Renal Therapy On Nutrients

Therapy	Amino Acids	Protein	Glucose
Hemodialysis	Loss of 6–12 g/treatment	No loss	Loss of 28 g/6 hours treatment with glucose-free dialysate
Peritoneal Dialysis	Loss of 0.5–0.3 g/exchange (up to 3.5 g/d)	Loss of 0.1 to 1 g/hr of treatment; increase if peritonitis (up to 9 g/day)	Gain of 120–240 g/day when continuous, varies with volume and glucose concentration
Ultrafiltration	Loss of 4 g/day		

tein per kilogram IBW per day of standard solution, which can be increased progressively according to the clinical state. Infusion of BCAA, either enterally (Hepatic-Aid) or parenterally (Hepatamine), should be considered only when the encephalopathy does not improve after 7 to 10 days of optimal treatment on the low-protein regimen. In hypercatabolic patients, it is then essential to increase the protein intake. We usually start by providing 0.5 to 0.75 g of amino acids per kilogram IBW per day and we increase the intake progressively, by 0.25 to 0.5 g per kilogram per day to a goal of 1.5 g per kilogram IBW. The initial glucose-to-fat ratio should be around 60:40 and adjusted according to glucose and lipid monitoring. Caloric intake is as recommended above.

Pulmonary Failure

Carbohydrates should be restricted when the patient suffers from chronic pulmonary disease and is a carbon dioxide retainer. This is especially important during the weaning process from mechanical ventilation. Caloric and protein intake are as recommended previously. However, glucose-to-fat ratio should be 50:50 to 30:70 in parenteral or enteral nutrition. If enterally fed, modular feeds or Pulmocare can achieve these goals. In adult respiratory distress syndrome, we usually use the standard TPN with a glucose-to-fat ratio of 60:40 and with the three-in-one system, the lipid is infused over 24 hours. If lipid is given separately, it should be infused over at least 12 hours and ideally over 24 hours in order to prevent possible arterial desaturation. In these situations, arterial blood gases can be monitored before and during the infusion to see if there is a significant change.

Heart Failure

The major concern with heart failure is fluid and sodium intake, and these should be adjusted on an individual basis. Diuretic therapy may be required to avoid fluid overload. However, it can produce hypokalemia and hypomagnesemia; these electrolytes along with sodium should be monitored closely. The caloric and protein intake is as recommended. A glucose-to-fat ratio of 60:40 can be given initially. TPN is usually started with half the caloric requirement for a period of 3 to 4 days in order to avoid pulmonary edema secondary to refeeding and increased metabolic rate. It is then progressively increased up to the patient's requirements.

SUGGESTED READING

Cerra FB. Hypermetabolism, organ failure, and metabolic support: clinical review. Surgery 1987; 101:1–14.
Jeejeebhoy KN: Nutrition in critical illness. In: Shoemaker WC, Ayres S, Grenvik A, et al, eds. Textbook of critical care. 2nd ed. Philadelphia: WB Saunders, 1989:1093.
Lemoyne M, Jeejeebhoy KN. Total parenteral nutrition in the critically ill patient. Chest 1986; 89:568–575.
Marshall DK, ed. Nutritional support of the critically ill. Chicago: Year Book Medical Publishers, Inc., 1988.

HEPATIC FAILURE

PAUL MISKOVITZ, M.D.

Hepatic failure can result as a complication of most clinically significant liver diseases. The hepatic pathology seen is variable, making this syndrome a functional rather than a histopathologic entity. For clinical convenience it is best to think of hepatic failure as either chronic or acute (sometimes fulminant). Etiologies include viral, drug and toxic hepatitis, cirrhosis from any cause, inborn errors of metabolism, hepatic neoplasms both primary and metastatic, circulatory or vascular insult to the liver, and chronic cholestatic liver disease of varying etiologies. Although the etiologies and clinical aspects of hepatic failure may differ, the treatment is quite uniform, depending upon the manifestations of disordered function that are present (e.g., portosystemic encephalopathy, cerebral edema, ascites, infection, gastrointestinal hemorrhage, renal failure, and hypoglycemia). In recent years, aggressive treatment in the form of liver transplantation has become available for patients for whom there is no specific alternative therapy.

APPROACH TO THE PATIENT

The treatment of the patient with hepatic failure is predicated on the premise that liver function can be accurately quantitated and followed to measure the success or failure of therapy. Measurements of function may be made independently of those tests done to determine diagnosis in the patient with liver disease, but accurate diagnosis is essential to anticipate the natural history of the illness and to offer specific therapy where available. Biochemical tests such as bilirubin and its fractions, alkaline phosphatase, gamma glutamyl transpeptidase, and serum transaminases are useful in the initial evaluation of jaundice. Ultrasound examination, endoscopic retrograde cholangiography, computerized axial tomography (CT), and magnetic resonance imaging (MRI) often provide additional useful information in the jaundiced patient. The biochemical assessment of the severity of hepatocyte damage is estimated by serial determinations of bilirubin, albumin, transaminases, and prothrombin time after vitamin K replenishment. This estimate can be further enhanced by radioisotope scanning and needle liver biopsy, particularly in chronic liver disease. Quantitative determinations of hepatic function (galactose elimination capacity, the aminopyrine breath test, the intravenous Bromosulphalein clearance test, and the indocyanine green clearance test) in both compensated and decompensated patients can be made serially using various techniques, but these tests are complex, may not be readily available, and may lack standardization.

As the treatment of hepatic failure is the supportive therapy of derangements involving multiple organ systems, the need to intervene should be anticipated. In patients with chronic liver disease, the following signs and symptoms will be encountered: jaundice, ascites, gastrointestinal hemorrhage, circulatory embarrassment, neurologic changes including encephalopathy, fever, dermatologic, endocrine, renal, electrolyte, hematologic, pulmonary, infectious, and psychiatric abnormalities. In acute hepatic failure the same systems may be involved and the prognosis is generally much worse, but the hepatic pathology remains potentially reversible, with survivors often recovering completely. In either situation, liver transplantation will have to be considered, although often with more urgency in the acute setting. It can be anticipated that patients will require monitoring in the intensive care unit (ICU), possible blood and enteric isolation precautions, ventilatory support, and renal, neurologic, and infectious disease consultations.

ACUTE LIVER FAILURE

General Measures

Improvement in survival in this population in large measure results from attention to the details of good supportive care coupled with the judicious use of hepatic transplantation. Ideally the patient should be cared for in an ICU by a staff experienced in the care of comatose patients with liver disease. Attending staff should have received hepatitis B vaccination. The wearing of gloves, gowns, and masks should be routine when ministering to the patient or when handling specimens from the patient. Daily weights should be obtained, and fluid intake and output balance recorded. Pulmonary artery pressure monitoring via Swan-Ganz catheter should be performed, and an indwelling urinary bladder catheter placed. A nasogastric tube should be utilized to administer hourly antacids, to maintain the intragastric pH over 5. Flow sheets should be maintained at the bedside with continuous recordings of temperature, pulse, blood pressure, fluid intake, and output, and weights. The liver should be palpated and percussed daily, with the lower edge marked on the abdominal wall. In the presence of ascites, the abdominal girth should be measured and recorded daily. Preventative care for decubitus ulcers should be instituted. Seizure precautions should be observed.

CHRONIC LIVER FAILURE

General Measures

Chronic liver failure is characterized by loss of the patient's general sense of well-being, jaundice, ascites, circulatory and pulmonary changes, neurologic deterioration, and endocrine, dermatologic, nutritional, hematologic, infectious, electrolyte, and renal derangements. Symptoms and findings in this setting may be insidious in onset, and there may at any time be unexpected acute deterioration, necessitating active intervention. As the liver retains regenerative capacity, some compensation in function may be attained with appropriate supportive measures. Bed rest may be of value in some patients, but most should be allowed moderate activity. In general an 80- to 100-g-protein diet that provides in excess of 2,000 calories is desirable provided that portosystemic encephalopathy is not present. Sodium restriction may have to be instituted. Folic acid may have to be specifically replaced, particularly in the alcoholic patient. Abstinence from alcohol should be maintained, and the use of sedatives should be avoided. There is no proven benefit from the administration of corticosteroid hormones or testosterone. Regular medical follow-up appointments should be scheduled and necessary care provided.

COMPLICATIONS

Portosystemic Encephalopathy

Precipitating factors should be sought and eliminated. These include a good response to the administration of potent diuretics, large-volume paracentesis, diarrhea, vomiting, gastrointestinal hemorrhage, alcohol ingestion, the intake of a large protein meal, infection, constipation, and surgical procedures requiring anesthesia. Sedation should be avoided. If the portosystemic encephalopathy was precipitated by drug administration, particular antagonists should be sought and/or the drug discontinued. Dietary intake of protein should cease. Glucose can be administered intravenously or intragastrically via continuous drip and will thus supply some calories. When protein is reintroduced into the diet, this should be done gradually with the utilization of vegetable rather than animal sources.

Neomycin (4 to 6 g per day given orally in divided doses) or metronidazole (250 mg four times per day) is effective in decreasing formation gastrointestinal ammonia. Hearing impairment is a possible complication of the former, and dose-related central nervous system toxicity has been related to the latter. Lactulose (10 to 30 ml orally three times per day) may be given in an attempt to produce two to three acidic semisolid stools per day. Its mode(s) of action in improving portosystemic encephalopathy is controversial. Neutral or acidic enemas (including those made of lactulose) should be considered in the constipated patient. Levodopa may be of transient benefit in some patients with acute hepatic encephalopathy. Bromocriptine has been of extremely limited success in the patient with chronic portosystemic encephalopathy and is not to be recommended for use in the patients with an acute neuropsychiatric syndrome. Studies of the use of intravenous and oral branched-chain amino acid therapy have yielded conflicting results. If portosystemic encephalopathy has resulted acutely from the surgical creation of a portosystemic anastomosis, surgical or radiologic occlusion of the shunt may be used to reverse the encephalopathy. Frequent neurologic examination and electroencephalograms should be used to monitor the patient.

Cerebral Edema

Cerebral edema, often with associated brain stem and cerebellar involvement, is a frequent finding at autopsy in patients with acute hepatic failure. Clinically its presence is heralded by poorly reacting pupils, papillary changes, episodes of hypertension, and occasionally decerebrate posturing. CT or MRI of the head is helpful in excluding intracranial hemorrhage. Extradural intracranial pressure monitors, while not providing direct therapy of hepatic failure, can provide useful information that may lead to earlier treatment and may be helpful in selecting appropriate patients for hepatic transplantation. At the earliest signs of brain stem dysfunction, an infusion of a 20 percent solution of mannitol (100 g of mannitol in 500 ml of 5 percent aqueous dextrose solution) should be given intravenously (utilizing a filter to exclude crystals) over 10 to 20 minutes. Repeated infusions can be given at intervals of 4 to 6 hours as necessary, but a rebound increase in intracranial pressure may be seen. In the anuric patient arteriovenous hemofiltration may have to be performed.

Ascites

In the setting of liver disease, ascites forms as a result of portal hypertension, the exact mechanism of formation being unknown. All patients with recent-onset ascites should undergo diagnostic paracentesis. After the diagnosis of cirrhotic ascites is made based upon clinical evaluation and analysis of ascitic fluid, the urinary sodium concentration should be measured and the patient started on a sodium-restricted diet (1 g of sodium per day for inpatients and 2 g of sodium per day for outpatients). A dietician should be involved in the patient's care. Spironolactone in a dose of 100 mg per day orally and furosemide 40 mg per day orally should be initiated. In nonedematous patients, a daily weight loss of 1 kg per day should be achieved. Furosemide may be increased to 80 mg per day, and spironolactone to 200 mg per day during the first week of treatment. Chronic mild hyponatremia (serum sodium 125 to 133 mEq per liter) is expected and should not necessitate fluid restriction. Prostaglandin inhibitors should be avoided in these patients. This regimen should be discontinued if patients develop a serum creatinine level over 2 mg per deciliter, serum sodium level under 120 mEq per liter, or encephalopathy.

For patients who fail inpatient diuretic therapy, therapeutic paracentesis should be considered. Large-volume paracentesis of 5 L is usually tolerated surprisingly well and may be considered a "second-line" therapy. The need for infusions of albumin during such procedures is controversial. Peritoneovenous shunting should be considered only for those patients who fail both diuretic and paracentesis therapy. This technique may be helpful in controlling ascites in selected patients but is associated with many complications, including operative mortality, failure to maintain shunt patency, disseminated intravascular coagulation, ascitic fluid leak, bacterial peritonitis, pulmonary edema, and esophageal variceal hemorrhage.

Infection

Spontaneous bacterial peritonitis, pneumonia, urinary infections, and catheter-related infections are common in patients with hepatic failure. "Routine" use of antibiotics is to be avoided, but all opportunities to obtain cultures in the appropriate clinical settings should be utilized.

Spontaneous bacterial peritonitis, a largely monomicrobial blood-borne infection of ascites in the absence of secondary causes of peritonitis, is common in patients with hepatic failure. The onset of infection characteristically occurs after admission to the hospital, requires sampling of the ascitic fluid to diagnose, and is associated with a grave prognosis. The selection and use of appropriate antibiotics depends upon the results of culture and sensitivity testing of the isolates (commonly gram-negative coliforms or streptococci) and the degree of impairment of renal function. The recurrence rate may run as high as 50 percent.

Gastrointestinal Hemorrhage

Gastrointestinal hemorrhage frequently complicates hepatic failure and is often due to esophageal varices but may be due to other causes such as duodenal ulcer, gastric ulcer, stress ulcer, and Mallory-Weiss tears. Esophagogastroduodenoscopy should be the primary modality of evaluating these patients for the cause of bleeding. Prophylaxis for stress ulcer bleeding should be considered in all such patients in an ICU, particularly those who require mechanical ventilation for 5 days or more or those who have a platelet count of less than 50,000 per microliter or show a prolonged prothrombin time or partial thromboplastin time. This can be accomplished with H_2-antagonists or hourly antacids given by nasogastric tube to titrate the intragastric pH to over 5. Adjustments in these regimens may have to be made for renal insufficiency and the development of diarrhea.

It is difficult to predict when and why esophageal varices bleed, but the effect is injurious to hepatic parenchymal cells. In patients with cirrhosis, the mortality associated with each episode of bleeding may reach 40 percent. Despite controversy, primary therapy for variceal hemorrhage remains 100 U of vasopressin in 250 ml of 5 percent aqueous dextrose solution given intravenously at an initial dose of 0.3 U per minute, with a range of 0.1/minute to 0.6 U per minute. The concurrent use of nitrates to diminish the likelihood of coronary artery vasoconstriction has been advocated. In centers with experienced personnel, the use of the Sengstaken-Blakemore tube and its variations to effect balloon tamponade of both esophageal and gastric varices has proved successful. This technique is good for initially stopping bleeding, but long-term results are not good. Complications include those due to improper balloon positioning, balloon migration, and aspiration.

The acute use of endoscopic sclerotherapy is associated with a high likelihood of initial control of hemorrhage and a reduction in the incidence of rebleeding. The experience of the group performing the procedure seems to be a major factor affecting these results. Chronic sclerotherapy to obliterate esophageal varices is less costly than surgery and does reduce the incidence of rebleeding from varices but has not been shown to prolong survival. Complications of sclerotherapy include hemorrhage, fever, dysphagia, chest pain, esophageal stricture requiring dilatation, pneumonia, pleural effusions, bacteremia, and mediastinitis.

Surgical approaches to variceal hemorrhage include esophageal transection and stapling and portosystemic shunting. In experienced hands, esophageal transection is associated with control of bleeding, short operative time, and few complications. Many of these patients, however, die of hepatic failure during the admission and for those who survive varices often recur and rebleed. The aim of portosystemic shunts is to reduce portal venous pressure while maintaining portal blood flow. In general, hepatic reserve is a major determinant of survival after shunting, as hepatocellular function deteriorates to some degree after all shunting procedures. Patients selected for shunting procedures should have had gastrointestinal hemorrhage from proven esophageal varices. They should have no history of hepatic encephalopathy and for best results should be Child's grade A or B. Both the end-to-side or side-to-side portocaval shunts are effective in reducing portal pressure but are associated with postshunt encephalopathy. The mesocaval shunt made between the superior mesenteric vein and the inferior vena cava using a Dacron graft is technically easy to perform, but the incidence of shunt occlusion high. The selective "distal" splenorenal shunt may be particularly helpful in patients with gastric varices, but it has not lived up to early expectations, probably because of variable surgical expertise. After portosystemic shunting patency has been confirmed by ultrasonography, CT scan, or angiography. Postoperative jaundice is due to hemolysis and decreased hepatic function. Encephalopathy may be transient or, particularly in older patients, chronic. Shunt closure, regardless of the cause, may lead to further hepatic failure and death.

Portal pressure and flow can be reduced by lowering cardiac output, by causing splanchnic vasoconstriction or venodilation, or by reducing intrahepatic vascular resistance. Although propranolol has been used to regulate portal pressure and flow, its efficacy for prophylaxis or to prevent recurrent bleeding from varices is unproven. At the present time no pharmacologic agent can be recommended for the long-term reduction of portal pressure and flow.

The coagulopathy associated with hepatic insufficiency may in part be corrected by the administration of 10 mg of vitamin K per day subcutaneously or intravenously and by the administration of fresh frozen plasma and platelets where indicated. Disseminated intravascular coagulation should be suspected in the setting of thrombocytopenia when fibrin-splint products are detected in the blood.

Renal Failure

Renal failure in patients with hepatic failure may have multiple etiologies. Drug injury, acute tubular necrosis in the setting of hemorrhage, hypotension, infection, or hepatorenal syndrome may be responsible. Hepatorenal syndrome is the most common and is marked by renal failure, with normal tubular function occurring in patients with severe liver disease and portal hypertension. Seldom precipitating admission, this syndrome occurs in the hospital, often in response to fluid restriction or fluid shifts and sometimes precipitated by paracentesis or diuresis. It is characterized by avid sodium resorption by the kidney, resulting in urinary sodium levels of less than 10 mEq per liter. It may be difficult to differentiate renal failure from prerenal azotemia, thus warranting a cautious trial of volume expansion. There is no effective treatment for this syndrome. Conservative management includes the restriction of fluids, sodium, potassium, and protein, coupled with the monitoring of weights and fluid intake and output on a daily basis, as well as withdrawal or avoidance of potentially nephrotoxic drugs. Dialysis does not prolong survival. Levodopa and metaraminol have not proved successful in altering the impaired renal cortical circulation seen in patients with this syndrome.

Hypoglycemia

Hypoglycemia rarely complicates chronic liver disease but may be seen in acute hepatocellular failure from a variety of etiologies including Reye's syndrome in children. In patients with fulminant hepatitis, it may be severe and recurrent and has been associated with sudden death. This is one aspect of acute hepatic failure that can be adequately treated through the use of continuous infusions of 10 percent glucose with potassium chloride supplementation.

Table 1 Indications for Hepatic Transplantation

Primary biliary cirrhosis
Cryptogenic cirrhosis
Chronic active hepatitis
Primary biliary cirrhosis
Primary sclerosing cholangitis
Budd-Chiari syndrome
Biliary atresia
Wilson's disease
Hemochromatosis
Alpha-1-antitrypsin deficiency
Fibrolamellar hepatocellular carcinoma
Fulminant hepatic failure

Table 2 Some Contraindications for Hepatic Transplantation

Acquired immunodeficiency syndrome (AIDS)
Advanced age
Advanced cardiopulmonary disease
Advanced renal disease
Active alcoholism
Metastatic cancer
Sepsis
HBsAg + HBeAG + patients
Extensive previous abdominal surgery
Portal vein thrombosis

HBeAg = hepatitis Be antigen; HBsAg = hepatitis B surface antigen.

TRANSPLANTATION

Patients with irreversible and progressive hepatic disease either unresponsive to treatment or in cases where treatment is unavailable should be considered for orthotopic liver transplantation (Table 1). The preferred candidate is a stable outpatient, with acutely ill ICU patients representing the other end of the spectrum. Absolute contraindications for liver transplantation at the present time include sepsis, metastatic malignancy, advanced cardiopulmonary disease, acquired immunodeficiency syndrome, and active or recent alcoholism (Table 2). Previous portocaval shunts, portal vein thrombosis, prior upper abdominal surgery, and age greater than 60 years are often cited as relative contraindications. The pretransplantation medical evaluation may take up to 1 week to complete, and the patient may wait additional time for a suitable donor. Children generally fare better than adults, but donor livers are more difficult to obtain for children. The patient and family should be made aware of the magnitude of the undertaking, the likelihood of success, and the need for life-long immunosuppression.

SUGGESTED READING

Schiff L, Schiff E, eds. Diseases of the liver. Philadelphia: JB Lippincott, 1987.
Sherlock S. Diseases of the liver and biliary system. Oxford: Blackwell, 1989.
Zakim D, Boyer T, eds. Hepatology. Philadelphia: WB Saunders, 1989.

ACUTE PANCREATITIS

DONALD M. JENSEN, M.D., F.A.C.P.
SEYMOUR M. SABESIN, M.D., F.A.C.P.

Regardless of its cause, acute pancreatitis is a poorly understood condition of uncertain pathogenesis for which no specific therapy exists. Nonetheless, much is known about the clinical syndrome of acute pancreatitis and the recognition and management of its complications, both local and systemic. The clinical spectrum of acute pancreatitis may range from a relatively benign, self-limited condition to a fulminant, often lethal form, complicated by multiorgan failure.

PATHOGENESIS

No single unifying mechanism for the pathogenesis of acute pancreatitis has been demonstrated. However, recent work in experimental pancreatitis in animals suggests that fusion of zymogen granules with lysosomes could lead to the intrapancreatic activation of trypsin, a necessary intermediate that would lead to the subsequent activation of other pancreatic proenzymes and the cascade of biochemical reactions resulting in cellular necrosis. Improved understanding of the pathogenesis is certainly necessary before significant advances in medical treatment are forthcoming.

ETIOLOGY

Although there are multiple etiologies for acute pancreatitis, alcohol and biliary tract are the most common. Epidemiologic studies suggest that alcoholic pancreatitis is associated with consumption of 150 to 175 g of alcohol daily, but may occur with smaller amounts.

Gallstones presumably cause pancreatitis by traversing the sphincter of Oddi rather than impaction, since stones are seldom recovered at the time of surgery. In support of this concept, Acosta has demonstrated that gallstones could frequently be recovered from the stool of patients with acute gallstone pancreatitis. Inspection of duodenal bile may occasionally prove useful to identify microstones and crystals when other etiologic clues are absent. Table 1 lists many of the conditions associated with acute pancreatitis.

DIAGNOSIS

In general, the diagnosis of acute pancreatitis is straightforward. A high-risk individual (e.g., a patient who is an alcoholic or has gallstones) with abdominal pain, nausea and vomiting, in conjunction with hyperamylasemia, most likely has pancreatitis. However, neither the clinical signs and symptoms nor the biochemical tests are specific. In patients presenting with severe pancreatitis, the diagnostic dilemma may be more profound and the differential diagnosis might include bowel obstruction, ruptured aortic aneurysm, cholecystitis, perforated pep-

Table 1 Etiology of Acute Pancreatitis

Biliary tract disease
Alcohol
Peptic ulcer disease
Trauma, surgery
Pregnancy (third trimester)
Hyperlipoproteinemia (types I, IV, V)
Hypercalcemia
Drugs:
    Azathioprine   Methyl alcohol
    Estrogens   L-asparaginase
    Corticosteroids   Furosemide
    Thiazides   Sulfonamides
Hereditary pancreatitis
Infection
    Bacterial
    Viral: Coxsackie, ECHO, Mumps, CMV
Scorpion bites (Trinidad)
Carcinoma of the pancreas
Hypotensive shock
Cardiac bypass surgery
ERCP
Post-transplantation

Table 2 Conditions Associated with Hyperamylasemia*

	Type of Isoamylase
Pancreas	
Pancreatitis of any etiology	P
Carcinoma of pancreas	P
Obstruction of pancreatic drainage	P
Trauma	
Blunt or penetrating abdominal injury	
ERCP	
Complications of pancreatitis:	
pseudocyst, ascites, or abscess	P
Salivary glands	
Trauma	S
Infection (e.g., mumps)	S
Radiation	S
Duct obstruction	S
Salivary-type hyperamylasemia of	
unknown origin	S
Renal insufficiency	P,S
Intra-abdominal conditions (nonpancreatic)	
Perforated peptic ulcer	P
Mesenteric infarction	P
Bowel obstruction	?
Acute appendicitis	?
Lung disease	
Pneumonia?	S
Tuberculosis?	S
Carcinoma	S
Malignant tumors	
Ovary	S
Prostate	S
Lung	S
Pancreas	S
Miscellaneous	
Diabetic acidosis	Usually S
Cerebral trauma	?
Thermal burns	P and S
Postoperative	P and S
Ruptured ectopic pregnancy	S
Ovarian cyst	S

P = pancreatic isoamylase; S = salivary isoamylase.
Reproduced with permission from Levitt M. Diagnostic assays for acute pancreatitis. American Gastroenterology Associate Postgraduate Course, 1985.

tic ulcer, or infarcted bowel. In fact, in one study of 118 patients with well-evaluated severe acute pancreatitis, five (4.2 percent) were later discovered to have other intra-abdominal conditions, including aortic aneurysm, ruptured gallbladder, and perforated duodenal ulcer.

An increase in the serum amylase activity has long been considered the hallmark of the diagnosis of acute pancreatitis. The serum amylase activity is elevated in over 75 percent of patients with this disease but increased levels may be observed in other conditions (Table 2). The magnitude of the serum amylase activity does not correlate with the severity of the pancreatitis and usually normalizes within 3 to 5 days in an uncomplicated attack. Recent advances in amylase isoenzyme technology have led to the development in isoamylase assays, which have proved clinically useful. Although pancreatic isoamylase accounts for only 40 percent of normal serum amylase activity, appreciable increases in this fraction enhance the diagnostic accuracy of the serum amylase test. False-positive tests may occur, however, particularly in the case of perforated viscus, bowel obstruction, and intestinal infarction.

Serum lipase activity is derived almost exclusively from the pancreas and therefore should be a very specific test for pancreatitis. However, serum lipase is subject to the same problems of specificity as is pancreatic isoamylase. In fact, both of these enzymes appear to be comparable in terms of diagnostic sensitivity and specificity.

Tests of pancreatic enzymes must be interpreted with caution in the presence of renal insufficiency and metabolic acidosis, both of which may be associated with significant hyperamylasemia in the absence of acute pancreatitis. Likewise, hyperlipidemia may cause the serum amylase activity to be spuriously normal in the presence of pancreatitis.

CLINICAL MANIFESTATIONS

Abdominal pain is the most common presenting symptom, and occurs in 85 to 100 percent of patients. It is often located in the epigastrium but may be in the left upper quadrant or periumbilical area. The pain is typically dull in character, radiating to the back. Nausea and vomiting occur in over half the patients and may be due to ileus of inflammation of the serosal surfaces of the stomach and duodenum. Fever is common and occurs in 27 to 80 percent of patients but is usually low-grade in the absence of infection. Orthostatic hypotension, induced by third-space fluid sequestration, frequently occurs.

COMPLICATIONS

The severity and, hence, the mortality associated with acute pancreatitis is directly related to the local and systemic complications of the disease. For the most part, these are related (directly or indirectly) to the release and bloodstream absorption of activated pancreatic enzymes, particularly trypsin and lipase. It is often useful to think of the complications as being either local (intra-abdominal) or systemic (Table 3).

Table 3 Complications of Acute Pancreatitis

Local Complications
  Pancreatic
    Phlegmon
    Pseudocyst
    Abscess
    Hemorrhage
    Peripancreatic fat necrosis
    Splenic vein thrombosis
  Hepatobiliary
    Hyperbilirubinemia (indirect)
    Obstructive jaundice
    Cholecystitis
    Portal hypertension
  Gastrointestinal
    Ileus
    Gastritis/duodenitis
    Bowel obstruction
    Bowel infarction
    Gastrointestinal bleeding

Systemic Complications
  Metabolic
    Acidosis
    Hypocalcemia
    Hyperglycemia
    Hyperkalemia
    Hypertriglyceridemia
  Circulatory
    Hypovolemia/shock
    Arrhythmias
    Pericarditis/effusions
    Vascular thrombosis
  Renal
    Oliguria/anuria
    Cortical or tubular necrosis
    Renal vein thrombosis
  Respiratory
    Atelectasis
    Pneumonitis
    Adult respiratory distress syndrome
    Mediastinal abscess
  Hematologic
    Anemia
    Disseminated intravascular coagulation
    Leukocytosis
  Neurologic
    Psychosis/encephalopathy
    Cerebral emboli
    Purtscher's retinopathy
  Musculoskeletal
    Tetany
    Lytic bone lesions
    Arthritis/joint effusions

Local complications are common in patients with severe pancreatitis. Failure to improve in the hospital with fluids and bowel rest after 48 to 72 hours should alert one to possible presence of these conditions. In addition, evidence of a palpable abdominal mass, anemia, and ecchymoses (Grey Turner's or Cullen's sign) may also indicate a local complication such as hemorrhage, phlegmon, pseudocyst, or abscess. Splenic vein thrombosis and variceal hemorrhage have been reported as late complications of pancreatitis. The unique anatomic relationship between the pancreas and the transverse mesocolon may give rise to infarction, gastrointestinal bleeding, or bowel obstruction. Extrahepatic cholestasis due to compression of the intrapancreatic portion of the common bile duct may occur and requires differentiation from an impacted gallstone or periampullary tumor.

Systemic complications include those due to fluid sequestration (hypotension, shock, prerenal azotemia), metabolic derangements, and specific end-organ problems. Hypocalcemia is due, in part to saponification of calcium soaps in the abdomen but may also involve an inadequate parathyroid hormone response. Hyperglycemia is typically mild, but cases of nonketotic hyperosmolar coma have been reported in association with pancreatitis. Both metabolic and respiratory acidosis may occur as a result of tissue hypoperfusion and respiratory compromise.

Pulmonary complications are often the most devastating of the extra-abdominal manifestations. Hypoxemia, often unrecognized clinically, is present on admission in 50 percent of patients. Adult respiratory distress syndrome is a particularly troublesome development and may be further complicated by pleural effusions, atelectasis, or pneumonitis.

Cardiac difficulties are probably underappreciated as a cause of morbidity and mortality. Although arrhythmias and pericardial effusions occur, autopsy studies have revealed a surprisingly high incidence of coronary artery thrombosis in patients dying of severe pancreatitis.

DETERMINANTS OF PROGNOSIS

Although several valid protocols have been developed in an attempt to assess prognosis in acute pancreatitis, the one produced by Ranson has gained the widest acceptance (Table 4). Ranson's criteria are based upon eleven clinical parameters: five assessed on admission to the hospital and six others assessed during the initial 48 hours of hospitalization. Although this protocol was developed for use in cases of presumed alcoholic pancreatitis, minor modifications make it applicable to other types. It should be kept in mind that over 60 percent of all episodes of acute pancreatitis are mild and associated with a good short-term prognosis.

APPROACH TO MEDICAL MANAGEMENT

Since there is no recognized specific therapy to inhibit pancreatic inflammation and necrosis, the goal of medical management is largely supportive. The recogni-

Table 4 Ranson's Prognostic Criteria

At admission
 Age >55 years
 WBC >16,000/cu mm
 Glucose >300 mg/dl
 LDH >350 IU/L
 SGOT >250 SF U

During initial 48 hours
 Hematocrit fall >10%
 BUN rise >5 mg/dl
 Calcium <8 mg/dl
 PaO$_2$ <60 mm Hg
 Base deficit >4 mEq/L
 Fluid sequestration >6 L

Interpretation of results:

No. of positive signs:	0-2	3-4	5-6	7-8
No. of Patients	347	67	30	6
Mortality	0.9%	16%	40%	100%

tion and prompt treatment of complications play a particularly important role.

Initial management includes meticulous attention to fluid resuscitation with monitoring and maintenance of intravascular volume status. In the severely ill patient, this may imply hemodynamic studies in an intensive care setting. Blood and colloid replacement may be necessary to treat shock or hemorrhage. Pain relief may usually be accomplished with intravenous meperidine; morphine should be avoided.

Bowel rest is somewhat controversial, but nasogastric tubes should be placed in patients with ileus, nausea, or vomiting. Oral feeding should be avoided until the pancreatitis has been completely resolved; too early refeeding has been associated with clinical relapse. Total parenteral nutrition should be considered for episodes lasting more than 5 to 7 days.

Monitoring and aggressive correction of metabolic and electrolyte disturbances require diligent attention. Serum magnesium calcium, and phosphorus levels should also be assessed and replaced appropriately. Arterial blood gases should be obtained upon admission and repeated every 12 hours. Hypoxemia is frequently present in severe cases, even in the absence of cyanosis or obvious dyspnea. If arterial oxygen desaturation exists, early intubation may prove beneficial.

Prophylactic H$_2$-receptor antagonist therapy may be instituted to prevent gastroduodenal erosions and ulcerations. All febrile patients should be cultured, but antibiotics reserved for those with choledocholithiasis or proven septic complications.

Peritoneal lavage has been largely abandoned as a therapeutic modality but may be quite useful diagnostically. Controlled trials have recently demonstrated that therapeutic peritoneal lavage, although associated with an improvement in early mortality, predisposes to an increase in late septic complications and no improvement in overall mortality.

The role of early endoscopic retrograde cholangiopancreatography (ERCP) and sphincterotomy for gallstone pancreatitis is somewhat controversial. Several recent series, however, support this approach in patients who have not improved after 24 hours of conservative management and in whom gallstones are the likely etiology. Early ultrasound examinations are particularly useful to identify potential candidates for this therapy.

Finally, radiographic studies, particularly dynamic-enhanced computed tomography, play an important role in the diagnosis of local complications of acute pancreatitis: pseudocysts, phlegmons, abscesses, infected necrosis, and hemorrhagic necrosis. In selected cases, thin-needle aspiration biopsy (avoiding overlying bowel) may be combined with these studies to assist in determination of bacterial infection of a pancreatic mass. These investigations have proved quite useful to the surgeon in timing drainage or debridement operations.

SUGGESTED READING

Acosta JM, Pellegrini CA, Skinner DB. Etiology and pathogenesis of acute biliary pancreatitis. Surgery 1980; 88:118-125.

Jensen DM, Royse VL, Newell J, Schaffner J. Use of amylase isoenzymes in the laboratory evaluation of hyperamylasemia. Dig Dis Sci 1987; 32:561-568.

Mayer DA, McMahon MJ, Corfield AP, et al. Controlled clinical trial of peritoneal lavage for the treatment of severe acute pancreatitis. N Engl J Med 1985; 312:399-404.

Ranson JHC. Etiological and prognostic factors in human acute pancreatitis: a review. Am J Gastroenterol 1982; 77:633-638.

Steer ML, Meldolesi J. The cell biology of experimental pancreatitis. N Engl J Med 1987; 316:144-150.

Steinberg W, Goldstein S, Davis N, et al. Diagnostic assays in acute pancreatitis: a study of sensitivity and specificity. Ann Intern Med 1985; 102:576-580.

Weir GC, Lesser PB, Drop LJ, et al. The hypocalcemia of acute pancreatitis. Ann Intern Med 1975; 83:185-188.

UPPER GASTROINTESTINAL HEMORRHAGE

EAMONN M. M. QUIGLEY, M.D.

Because gastrointestinal (GI) hemorrhage may result from a number of underlying disease states, regardless of whether the upper or lower GI tract is involved, it is necessary to perform diagnostic and therapeutic strategies simultaneously. Diagnostic and therapeutic studies are inextricably intertwined and should proceed in parallel in the evaluation and management of the individual patient.

Various estimates have reported the incidence of upper GI hemorrhage to be between 50 and 150 episodes per 100,000 population per year in the developed world. Overall, approximately 85 percent of patients stop bleeding spontaneously within 48 hours of admission, 25 percent rebleed during the same admission, 25 percent require surgical intervention, and 10 percent die. Though this overall mortality rate is similar to that of 30 years ago, it needs to be stressed that since that time there has also been a large increase in the proportion of patients who are older than 60 years of age; well over 50 percent of all GI bleeders now fall into this age group. By virtue of their advancing years, many of these patients will have advanced cardiac disease, respiratory insufficiency, or disseminated malignancy, which may play a more significant role in determining eventual outcome than does the GI hemorrhage that precipitated admission to the hospital. Table 1 depicts the relative incidence and mortality rates of the major causes of upper GI hemorrhage in the United States.

Bleeding from the upper GI tract (i.e., hemorrhage occurring from a lesion(s) at or above the ligament of Treitz) manifests in one or more of the following four ways:

1. Hematemesis: vomiting of fresh or altered (coffee-ground) blood.
2. Aspiration of fresh or altered blood via a nasogastric tube.
3. Melena: the passage of altered blood (black/tarry) in the stool. It should be emphasized, however, that massively bleeding upper GI lesions may result in the passage of either bright red or maroon blood rectally.
4. Chronic low-grade GI hemorrhage may present with anemia and the detection of occult blood in the stool.

On occasion, major acute bleeding may not be frank and present instead with symptoms such as faintness, dizzy spells, worsening angina, or dyspnea. In elderly patients or those with cerebrovascular disease, mental confusion resulting from cerebral hypoxia may be the presenting symptom and will, in itself, further obscure the underlying problem which can be revealed by the routine performance of a rectal examination in the acutely confused elderly patient.

GENERAL APPROACH

Initial Clinical Assessment and Resuscitation

The aims of the initial assessment of a patient presenting with upper GI hemorrhage are fourfold: (1) to determine the severity of the bleeding and its hemodynamic consequences; (2) to identify those patients at greatest risk of complications and death from the hemorrhage and to institute management protocols aimed at minimizing such morbidity and mortality; (3) to define the relative risk of recurrent hemorrhage and prevent its occurrence in those most likely to rebleed; and (4) to define the precise cause of the bleed and institute appropriate therapy.

Definition of the Severity of the Bleeding and Its Hemodynamic Consequences. This relies primarily on the correct assessment of vital signs. The presence of postural hypotension (orthostasis) is an early and sensitive sign of blood loss; a postural drop in blood pressure in excess of 10 mm Hg signifies a loss of at least 1 L of blood. Similarly, a pulse rate of over 100 beats per minute suggests a 20 percent reduction in blood volume; a rise, above baseline, in excess of 20 beats per minute indicates a blood loss in excess of 1 L. It should be emphasized, however, that these simple cardiovascular signs may not be reliable in the elderly, in the presence of autonomic neuropathy, and in patients receiving medications such as beta-blockers or anticholinergics. Assessment of skin perfusion, and more objectively, of urine output provides an index of vital organ perfusion. Some assessment of the severity of the hemorrhage can also be obtained by inspection of the vomitus, nasogastric aspirate, and stool, with presence of fresh blood indicating more rapid blood loss.

Laboratory investigations play a secondary role. In the acute situation, hemoglobin or hematocrit estimations are poor indicators of blood volume loss; changes in these parameters take 24 to 48 hours to reach stable and meaningful levels.

Identification of High-Risk Patients. Table 2 lists several clinical and endoscopic features that have been associated with poor prognosis in upper GI bleeding. The following have proved to be the most reliable predictors of mortality: advanced age; a hemorrhagic episode recurring during the same hospital admission; the presence of significant cardiac, respiratory, hepatic, or renal disease;

Table 1 Major Causes of Upper Gastrointestinal Hemorrhage

	Incidence	Mortality Rate
Esophageal varices	10%	30–40%
Mallory-Weiss tear	7%	3–4%
Erosive gastritis	23%	1.5–10%
Gastric ulcer	21%	8–10%
Duodenal ulcer	24%	3–7%

Table 2 Features Indicating Poor Prognosis in Upper Gastrointestinal Bleeding

History
   Age over 60
   No recent alcohol or NSAID ingestion
   No previous GI bleed or known GI disorder
   Presents with hematemesis
   Hemorrhage occurs in hospital (especially in ICU)
   Recurrent hemorrhage

Clinical Observations
   Cardiac or respiratory disease (especially heart failure)
   Renal failure
   Cirrhosis
   Shock or anemia on presentation
   Hemorrhage severe and persistent
   Blood transfusion requirements >6 units
   Red blood on nasogastric aspirate

Investigations
   Increased blood urea or creatinine on admission
   Abnormal EKG

Endoscopic Findings
   Esophageal varices
   Peptic ulcer
   Active bleeding from ulcer (spurting more than oozing)
   Visible vessel in ulcer base

the presence of hypovolemic shock on admission; the need for large transfusions; and the delineation of stigmata of recent hemorrhage at endoscopy.

Definition of Risk of Rebleed. The clinical feature that has proved most predictive of rebleeding is the severity of the initial hemorrhage; patients in shock or anemic on admission and who require large volumes of blood are most likely to rebleed. Endoscopic findings can also predict rebleeding, not only by defining high-risk lesions such as varices or peptic ulcer but also by defining stigmata of recent hemorrhage. Thus, the presence of an actively spurting vessel in an ulcer base is associated with a rebleeding rate of between 75 to 85 percent; a visible, but not actively bleeding, vessel has a rebleeding rate of 50 percent; flat red or black spots have an 8 to 10 percent rebleeding rate; and upper GI lesions with none of these stigmata have very low rebleeding rates of between 0 to 5 percent.

Defining the Cause. While differentiation between upper and lower sources of bleeding is straightforward in most instances, difficulties may arise in the patient who presents with melena or hematochezia alone. The presence of hyperactive bowel sounds or a disproportionate elevation in the blood urea level suggest an upper-tract lesion. Where doubt exists, a nasogastric tube should be passed and upper endoscopy performed.

With respect to the diagnosis of specific upper-tract lesions, though history and clinical examination may prove most helpful in predicting prognosis, they are far less useful in indicating the correct diagnosis (overall accuracy being approximately 40 percent). A history of liver disease is important, however; given the high mortality of variceal hemorrhage, such patients should be presumed to be bleeding from esophageal varices until proved otherwise. In most situations delineation of the underlying problem will depend on the performance of specific investigations.

Blood should be drawn for complete blood count, platelet count, prothrombin time, and partial thromboplastin time to define any underlying coagulation problem or myeloproliferative disorder. The presence of abdominal pain or evidence of possible peritonitis necessitates performance of erect and supine abdominal films as well as estimation of serum amylase (the latter in view of the occasional patient with acute pancreatitis who presents with GI bleeding).

Once the patient's status has been determined, adequate resuscitation has been instituted, and the patient is hemodynamically stable, upper GI endoscopy should be performed. In over 90 percent of patients who are scoped within 24 hours of hemorrhage, endoscopy will provide a positive diagnosis. Furthermore, many lesions can be treated directly at endoscopy. Endoscopy is not without hazard; the American Society of Gastrointestinal Endoscopy survey reported a 0.9 percent complication rate and an incidence of one death per 700 examinations in the acutely bleeding patient. These examinations should be performed by endoscopists who have specific experience in GI hemorrhage. Where aspiration is a major risk, endoscopy should be performed under anesthesia with an endotracheal tube in situ.

Further studies may be necessary in three particular circumstances: when (1) the patient is actively bleeding but endoscopy is negative; (2) there is blood in the upper gut at endoscopy but a responsible lesion is not identified; (3) the patient is a recurrent obscure bleeder.

Both radioisotopic scanning techniques and arteriography are useful only if the patient is actively bleeding (at rates in excess of 0.1 ml per minute for technetium-sulfur colloid scan and in excess of 0.5 ml per minute for angiography). Of the available nuclear medicine techniques, technetium-sulfur colloid scan is the most useful in acute massive bleeding; technetium pertechnetate-labeled red blood cell scans are of greater value in the slow or intermittent bleeder. The usefulness of both techniques is limited by liver and spleen uptake and by false localization due to aboral propulsion of extravasated contrast material by gut peristalsis. Scans cannot, therefore be relied upon to direct surgical resection accurately; their real value lies in detecting active bleeding and providing some general guidelines to the angiographer. Given their greater sensitivity to detect bleeding, scans should, however, precede angiography; angiography is unlikely to be useful if a scan has been unequivocally negative. Widespread use of the angiography has been limited by availability of experienced radiologists; the precise identification of bleeding sites in many cases requires superselective catheterization of minuscule vessels, a technique within the scope of only the most expert. If patients are selected according to the aforementioned guidelines, then a positive diagnosis can be expected in over 80 percent of patients at angiography, either temporary or permanent control of bleeding can be achieved in many instances by angiographic therapy.

If clinical examination, endoscopy, isotope scans, and arteriography have been carefully performed, only a small proportion of patients will remain undiagnosed (the so-called "obscure" bleeders). As blind laparotomy may often prove fruitless in such patients, several diagnostic techniques have been developed to guide the surgeon. If the responsible lesion is not obvious after careful inspection and palpation of abdominal contents at laparotomy, vascular abnormalities can be sought by transillumination, use of a Doppler probe, or local injection of methylene blue. Intraoperative endoscopy, using a colonoscope passed orally and over which the entire small bowel has been telescoped, may prove extremely fruitful.

MANAGEMENT

Major GI bleeds should be managed by physicians with expertise in this area, preferably by a joint gastroenterology/surgery team. While many patients with minor bleeds can be safely managed on a general ward, certain patient groups should be cared for in an intensive care situation: the elderly; those who present with massive hemorrhage resulting in a clinical state of shock and requiring large volume transfusions; patients with bleeding esophageal varices; individuals with serious cardiac, respiratory, renal, or hepatic disease; and those who demonstrate endoscopic stigmata predictive of recurrent hemorrhage.

On admission, blood should be drawn for baseline hematologic and biochemical parameters and crossmatching, a large-bore venous cannula inserted, and oxygen administered. Continuous electrocardiographic monitoring is indicated in patients with known cardiac disease or those who exhibit an abnormal 12-lead tracing at the time of admission; arterial blood gas samples should be obtained on patients with known respiratory disease. Central venous pressure monitoring or Swan-Ganz catheter placement is essential for adequate hemodynamic monitoring in patients who require large volumes of blood transfusion and in those with poor cardiac reserve. A nasogastric tube should be placed, primarily to maintain gastric decompression and therefore to prevent aspiration.

Gastric lavage should be performed using a wide-bore Edlich-type tube. Tap water at room temperature is instilled and aspirated until the aspirate is clear. There is no evidence that iced saline lavage is more effective; indeed it may be injurious to the gastric mucosa. Although evidence to support direct benefit in arresting or reducing hemorrhage for lavage is lacking, its performance certainly facilitates endoscopy. Transfusion is indicated in those patients who develop shock or in whom the stable hematocrit is less than 25 percent. Transfusion should aim, in the acute phase, to restore circulation and not to replace all lost volume. Indeed, overtransfusion with resultant cardiac overload and pulmonary edema is the most common complication of blood transfusion. For this reason, packed red blood cells rather than whole blood is preferred. One unit of fresh frozen plasma should be administered for every 2 to 3 units of packed red cells; platelet transfusions are necessary only with massive (over 10 units) transfusions.

Several therapeutic modalities have been proposed either to arrest hemorrhage in those who continue to bleed or to prevent recurrent hemorrhage in those destined to rebleed.

Drug Therapy. Despite numerous studies, results of various forms of drug therapy have proved disappointing. Antacids alone appear to confer little benefit on patients who have actually bled. Several trials have failed to show significant benefit in terms of either overall mortality, operation rates, or likelihood of rebleeding with administration of any of the available histamine$_2$ (H$_2$)-receptor antagonists. Consistent benefit has also not been shown for either the antifibrinolytic agent tranexamic acid, vasopressin (in nonvariceal hemorrhage), or somatostatin. Pharmacologic agents are, therefore, unlikely to prove beneficial in the immediate management of acute upper GI hemorrhage. This is not to say that appropriate therapy of underlying lesions such as peptic ulcers, with H$_2$-receptor antagonists, for example, should be delayed.

Endoscopic Methods. Available endoscopic techniques fall into four principal categories: injection methods, laser, electrocoagulation (monopolar and bipolar), and heater probe. All of these techniques rely on the passage of either an injection needle, laser probe, electrode, or heater probe through the biopsy channel of the endoscope and its application to or around the bleeding point. Injection techniques have not enjoyed universal success. Trials of both argon and neodymium-YAG lasers have proved inconclusive, and their widespread use has also been limited by expense and lack of portability. Electrocoagulation and heater probe techniques appear to be effective in controlling bleeding, and some studies, at least, suggest that they may reduce rebleeding rates and even overall mortality. Use of these systems by experienced operators is associated with a low risk of perforation, and we believe that application of a bicap-electrocoagulation or heater probe to actively bleeding lesions should be attempted, where possible, at the time of diagnostic endoscopy. Coagulation of the high-risk, visible-vessel lesions should also be attempted, but we are not convinced that adherent clots should be washed off to uncover visible vessels; more severe hemorrhage may be precipitated.

Angiographic Methods. Angiographic therapy, whether in the form of direct intra-arterial vasoconstrictor infusion or arterial embolization, while not especially successful in peptic ulcer hemorrhage, may prove particularly valuable in certain circumstances, particularly in those massively hemorrhaging patients who are poor surgical risks.

Surgery. Approximately 25 percent of all patients will require an operation during the first hospitalization. Most of those who require surgery will be bleeding from duodenal and gastric ulcers; operation rates for gastric ulcers are slightly greater than for duodenal ulcers.

Regardless of whether carried out immediately on presentation to hospital or following a recurrent hemorrhage, emergency operations of patients with bleeding ulcers are associated with a high operative mortality of between 15 and 28 percent; in contrast, mortality for elective ulcer surgery is between 0.4 and 3 percent. Generally accepted indications for surgery are as follows:

1. Persistent hemorrhage leading to hypotension and shock; endoscopic or angiographic techniques either unavailable, unsuccessful, or inappropriate.
2. Loss of over 30 percent of estimated blood volume and/or requirement of over 1.5 L of blood transfusion in first 24 hours.
3. Rebleed during the same admission.
4. Age over 60 years with bleeding peptic ulcer or stigmata at endoscopy and endoscopic treatment unsuccessful.
5. Age under 60 years with active bleeding ulcer at endoscopy and endoscopic therapy unsuccessful.

In those patients who are massively bleeding and rapidly exsanguinating, emergency surgery may be the only option. Wherever possible, endoscopy should be performed before laparotomy to rule out varices. As the sole aim of emergency laparotomy is to stop bleeding, then first priority should be to undersew responsible vessels should they be at the base of an ulcer, feeding an arteriovenous malformation, or on the surface of a neoplasm. The decision of whether to proceed to more definitive antiulcer or resective surgery must again be based on the clinical state of the patient. If bleeding has now been arrested, the hemodynamic stability has been established, and the patient is otherwise fit, it seems reasonable to proceed and perform the appropriate procedure, especially as the risk of rebleeding without so doing remains high. Available data suggest that vagotomy and drainage procedures are associated with a lower postoperative mortality, yet no greater rebleeding rate than for more extensive gastric resection operations. A conservative approach—i.e., oversewing of bleeding point of duodenal ulcer, or excision of gastric ulcer together with vagotomy plus drainage procedure—would therefore seem the most logical.

Specific Disorders

Esophageal Varices and Portal Hypertension. Given a high immediate and long-term mortality, a high rebleeding rate, and the fact that the initial and long-term management of esophageal varices is quite different from that for other bleeding lesions, it is of vital importance that the correct diagnosis be made. Immediate endoscopy is, therefore, essential. Because up to one-third of bleeding episodes may be from other lesions, it is important to document not only that varices are present but that they are the source of hemorrhage. These patients should be managed in an intensive care unit by individuals with specific experience in the management of liver disease and esophageal varices. The advent of successful liver transplantation now provides hope of long-term survival for patients with end-stage liver disease and has made the acute management of variceal bleeding episodes all the more important. Salvage of these patients from an episode of hemorrhage may allow them to proceed to liver transplantation with long-term survival.

In most centers, variceal injection sclerotherapy is the first-line emergency treatment for bleeding varices. This is performed by injection of a sclerosing agent via a needle passed through the biopsy channel of a standard endoscope, either into (intravariceal technique) or around (paravariceal technique) the varices; the aim, with either method, is to produce variceal thrombosis and sclerosis. Where continuing hemorrhage obscures the endoscopist's view, temporary control to permit performance of sclerotherapy can be achieved with intravenous metoclopramide. The balance of evidence seems to favor the intravariceal route, but regardless of the technique chosen, immediate control of hemorrhage can be achieved in up to 90 percent of patients with a single injection session. Prevention of recurrent bleeding is dependent on complete obliteration of all columns of varices. This may require several sessions, usually performed at weekly intervals. Complications of sclerotherapy include local ulceration, esophageal perforation, mediastinitis, pleural effusions, and systemic embolic events. Local ulceration is common and may progress to the formation of esophageal strictures, but this can usually be managed by simple bougienage, in the same manner as for benign peptic esophageal strictures. Extension of ulceration into the muscularis or submucosa may result in erosion of large submucosal arteries and torrential hemorrhage. This and other serious complications are fortunately rare. Control of hemorrhage prior to performance of sclerotherapy or following its failure can be attempted by use of vasopressin and/or balloon tamponade. Vasopressin, administered by intravenous infusion, has an overall efficacy of approximately 50 percent. Serious side effects include peripheral ischemia and myocardial infarction. To prevent such occurrences sublingual nitroglycerin can be administered simultaneously. Balloon tamponade should be performed only with a four-lumen assembly (i.e., one that incorporates an esophageal aspiration port). Wherever impaired consciousness increases the risk of aspiration, adequate airway protection should first be instituted by placement of an endotracheal tube. The assembly is passed by mouth and advanced into the stomach. The gastric balloon is then inflated and the assembly withdrawn until the gastric balloon is felt to jam at the level of the lower esophageal sphincter. Inflation of the gastric balloon alone is sufficient to control hemorrhage in the vast majority of patients. Major complications of balloon tamponade, which include esophageal perforation and pulmonary aspiration, occur in as many as 15 percent of patients and are associated with a significant mortality. Both vasopressin infusion and balloon tamponade should be looked upon as temporary stand-by procedures; tachyphylaxis occurs with prolonged vasopressin infusion, and prolonged balloon tamponade (i.e., longer than 12 hours) is associated with an ever-increasing risk of complications, especially aspiration.

Several surgical options are available for those patients who fail sclerotherapy. The least invasive, yet effective, technique is esophageal transection using a staple gun. In the emergency situation, end-to-side or side-to-side total portacaval shunts have been preferred over selective shunts, and though associated with a high operative mortality rate, result in a low rebleeding rate among survivors. A major problem with these shunt procedures is their precipitation of portosystemic encephalopathy. Currently, liver transplantation offers a further therapeutic option in appropriate patients.

Patients with portal hypertension may also bleed from gastric varices. In the emergency situation, these can also be controlled by vasopressin and balloon tamponade, but results of sclerotherapy have been disappointing. Persistent hemorrhage will therefore require some form of operative therapy, either a gastric devascularization procedure or a formal shunt.

Recently, it has become clear that patients with portal hypertension may also bleed from a diffuse abnormality of the gastric mucosa, a condition called portal hypertensive gastropathy. Some success in the long-term control of hemorrhage from this condition has been reported with propranolol.

Mallory-Weiss Tear. This lesion, which usually takes the form of a single tear, is most commonly found not in the esophagus but along the lesser curvature of the stomach immediately below the esophagogastric junction. It occurs most commonly in young males, between 75 and 90 percent of whom will give a history of vomiting, retching, coughing, or straining immediately preceding the hematemesis. Contrary to popular belief, less than 50 percent will give a history of recent excessive alcohol intake. Accurate diagnosis relies upon a careful endoscopy. Up to 90 percent of tears stop bleeding spontaneously. For those who continue to bleed, immediate control can be achieved with balloon tamponade, endoscopic electrocoagulation, or direct infusion of vasopressin into the left gastric artery. Endoscopic electrocoagulation, angiographic embolization, or surgical oversew may provide long-term control.

"Stress" Ulceration. This syndrome involves the development of multiple superficial mucosal lesions in seriously ill patients. Despite a high incidence of such lesions in critically ill patients, frank hemorrhage is relatively rare but when it does occur it is associated with a poor outcome. The key, therefore, to this condition is prevention. Patients at risk from these lesions (i.e., patients with major burns, multiple trauma, head injury, acute liver failure, acute renal failure, gram-negative sepsis, and coagulopathy, as well as those requiring mechanical ventilatory support) should receive stress ulcer prophylaxis. This can be achieved either by intragastric administration of antacid titrated to maintain intragastric pH above 4 or by intravenous infusion (rather than repeated bolus administration) of an H_2-receptor antagonist. Although some studies suggest that antacid administration may be more effective, this technique is time-consuming and may result in troublesome diarrhea. Many institutions, therefore, prefer intravenous H_2-receptor antagonists. Some concern has been expressed lately regarding an increased incidence of nosocomial pneumonia in patients receiving these forms of stress ulcer prophylaxis. Suppression of gastric acidity by antacids or H_2-antagonists is thought to lead to bacterial proliferation in the stomach with subsequent colonization of the respiratory tract. For this reason, some prefer to use a mucosal protective agent such as sucralfate for stress ulcer prophylaxis, though consistent evidence of its efficacy is not yet available.

Should stress ulcer hemorrhage occur, every effort should be made to avoid surgery, as it is associated with an extremely high mortality. Angiographic therapy, either in the form of vasopressin infusion into, or embolization of, the left gastric artery offers a highly effective and much safer alternative.

Aortoenteric Fistula. While instances of spontaneous rupture of the aorta into adjacent bowel have been recorded, most aortoenteric fistulae occur in those who have aortic grafts in situ. Indeed, the diagnosis of aortoenteric fistula should be suspected in any individual with an aortic prosthesis who presents with upper GI hemorrhage. Such fistulae usually arise in the context of graft-related sepsis, and rupture most commonly occurs into the third part of the duodenum. Endoscopy should be performed to rule out other more proximal lesions. A CT scan may prove diagnostic by demonstrating the presence of gas in the retroperitoneal tissues. The communication may not be evident at aortography, and many would recommend proceeding directly to laparatomy at this stage. Treatment is surgical and necessitates removal of the infected graft, repair of the intestinal defect, and performance of an axillofemoral bypass.

Recurrent Obscure Bleeder. Some of the important causes of "obscure" upper gastrointestinal hemorrhage are listed in Table 3. Many of these lesions are more likely to cause lower-tract than upper-tract hemorrhage and will be discussed in detail elsewhere in this text. In most series, gastroduodenal erosions figure prominently. As erosions are frequently evanescent, and other conditions such as the Dieulafoy lesion (which results from erosion of an unusually large submucosal artery on the high lesser curve of the stomach) will be diagnosed only when actively bleeding, endoscopy should be repeated as soon as possible after a hemorrhage recurs. Nowadays, hemobilia is

Table 3 Causes of "Obscure" Gastrointestinal Hemorrhage

Gastroduodenal erosions
Dieulafoy's lesion
Watermelon stomach
Duodenal duplication
Hemobilia
Vascular malformations
Small bowel tumors
Jejunal diverticula
Small bowel ulcers
Meckel's diverticulum

seen most commonly in the context of liver trauma or instrumentation, and the responsible lesion is often amenable to angiographic therapy.

SUGGESTED READING

Editorial. The role of endoscopy in the management of upper gastrointestinal hemorrhage. Guidelines for clinical application. Gastrointest Endosc 1988; 34(suppl):44–55.
Fromm D. Endoscopic coagulation for gastrointestinal bleeding. N Engl J Med 1987; 316:1652–1654.
Gostout CJ. Acute gastrointestinal bleeding—a common problem revisited. Mayo Clin Proc 1988; 63:596–604.
Peterson WL. Gastrointestinal bleeding. In: Sleisenger MH, Fordtran JS, eds. Gastrointestinal disease: pathophysiology, diagnosis and management. 4th ed. New York: WB Saunders, 1989:397.
Peterson WL. Pharmacotherapy of bleeding peptic ulcer—is it time to give up the search? Gastroenterology 1989; 97:796–797.
Quigley EMM. Acute upper gastrointestinal hemorrhage. In: Turnberg LA, ed. Clinical gastroenterology. Oxford: Blackwell Scientific, 1989:54.
Terblanche J, Burroughs AK, Hobbs KEF. Controversies in the management of bleeding esophageal varices. N Engl J Med 1989; 320:1393–1398, 1469–1475.

LOWER GASTROINTESTINAL HEMORRHAGE

EAMONN M.M. QUIGLEY, M.D.

Perhaps in part because of its lower incidence, epidemiologic data with respect to lower gastrointestinal (GI) hemorrhage are scanty in comparison with that regarding upper GI hemorrhage, and its true incidence, morbidity, and mortality are not known. In the past, before the advent of endoscopy and interventional radiology, it was generally believed that most episodes of lower GI tract hemorrhage originated from diverticula in the left colon and that most stopped spontaneously; a relatively low level of investigation and expectant conservative management were therefore employed. For those patients who continued to bleed massively, an empiric left hemicolectomy or total colectomy was often carried out but was accompanied by a high mortality and rates of recurrent bleeding of up to 50 percent. Modern diagnostic techniques—most notably, colonoscopy and angiography—have revolutionized our understanding of lower GI hemorrhage. Most important is the recent realization that perhaps up to 75 percent of episodes of colonic hemorrhage originate not from diverticula but from arteriovenous malformations, polyps, tumors and other colonic lesions. Furthermore, it would appear that those diverticula that do give rise to hemorrhage are as likely to be located on the right as on the left side of the colon, thus explaining the poor results of left hemicolectomy. Finally, many of the responsible lesions can now be treated at the time of either colonoscopy or angiography, thus avoiding the need to proceed to colonic resection on what is often a high-risk patient.

CLINICAL FEATURES AND GENERAL APPROACH

The overall approach to the patient with lower GI hemorrhage should be based primarily on the definition of the severity of the hemorrhage, thus leading to appropriate resuscitation, and then on the definition of the cause of the lesion, thus directing specific therapy.

Bleeding from the lower GI tract—i.e., from lesions distal to the ligament of Treitz—may present in one of three ways:

1. Acute, massive hemorrhage, the presenting symptom being the passage of bright red blood or maroon stool rectally (hematochezia).
2. Intermittent, recurrent bleeding. Depending on the location of the bleeding lesion, these patients may present with the intermittent passage of bright red blood rectally (usually signifying a lesion distal to the cecum) or the passage of melena (lesion in small bowel or cecum). Whether or not blood in the stool appears as bright red or as melena depends ultimately on its degradation by intraluminal enzymes, the extent of which depends not only on the site of the lesion but also on the rapidity of its transit through the intestine.
3. By the detection of occult blood in the stool.

Several recent studies have consistently demonstrated that these patients are usually elderly, their mean age being between 60 and 65 years of age. Significant concomitant cardiac and respiratory disorders are therefore to be expected and will place many in a high-risk category from the outset. Figures for overall mortality vary considerably, from as low as 5 percent to as high as 21 percent.

With appropriate investigation the cause of most episodes of lower GI hemorrhage can now be defined. Table 1 depicts the relative incidence of the more common causes of lower GI hemorrhage in recent surveys. In these and other modern series, the precise definition of cause permitted specific therapy and resulted in a very low rate of recurrent hemorrhage. It stands to reason, therefore, that patients with significant lower GI tract hemorrhage should be cared for only in institutions in which facilities for complete investigation and appropriate therapy are available. Delayed diagnosis and management consequent on the nonavailability of these resources will be associated with increased morbidity and mortality.

Table 1 Causes of Lower Gastrointestinal Hemorrhage

	Incidence
Unsuspected upper-tract or small-bowel lesions	13–20%
Colon	
Diverticula	17–26%
Arteriovenous malformations	24–30%
Polyps and cancer	7–11%
Ischemia, colitis, and miscellaneous lesions	5–10%
Anorectal lesions	5%

MANAGEMENT

Initial Clinical Assessment and Resuscitation. While between 80 and 90 percent of all episodes of acute lower GI tract hemorrhage will stop spontaneously, those patients with massive acute hemorrhage (i.e., continued bleeding for several hours, hypotension, requiring greater than 4 units of blood transfusion) usually do not. Several studies have now shown that up to 70 percent of this latter group may ultimately require surgery or some other invasive therapeutic intervention. It is clear, therefore, that the initial assessment of the patient must be directed toward identifying that group at greatest risk for initial mortality and recurrent hemorrhage. The clinical definition of such risk is based on the accurate definition and monitoring of basic vital signs and simple laboratory data. The principal risk factors for mortality in lower GI hemorrhage appear to be large volume transfusion requirements, hypotension at presentation, the presence of significant multisystem disease, and a history of a prior episode of lower-tract hemorrhage.

As in the case of upper GI hemorrhage, resuscitation should be the first priority, and no attempt should be made to proceed to invasive procedures until the patient has been adequately resuscitated. Resuscitation should be carried out on exactly the same lines as defined previously for upper GI hemorrhage. Thus those patients who have massive bleeding, are hemodynamically unstable, or who have significant multisystem disease should be managed in an intensive care unit with appropriate hemodynamic monitoring.

Some clues with regard to etiology may also be obtained from the patient's history and physical examination: e.g., a past history of inflammatory bowel disease is of particular importance. Historical or clinical evidence of diffuse arteriosclerosis, particularly in association with the symptom of abdominal pain, should suggest the possibility of colonic or small bowel ischemia. A history of a recent colonoscopy with polypectomy should lead one to assume that the bleeding is occurring from a polypectomy site until proved otherwise.

Apart from determining the hemodynamic status of the patient, the physical examination should place emphasis on the definition of serious multisystem disease and should include careful examination of the abdomen for evidence of perforation or local peritonitis. The anal region should be carefully inspected and a digital rectal examination performed.

Blood should be drawn for hemoglobin, hematocrit, white blood cell count, platelet count, prothrombin time, partial thromboplastin time, electrolytes, urea, and creatinine. Study of the colonic gas outline on a plain abdominal film (flat plate) may provide important information in instances of toxic megacolon or ischemic colitis. Where any suspicion of colonic perforation exists, an abdominal perforation series should be obtained.

Further Assessment and Management Following Resuscitation. Most would recommend proceeding immediately to performing anoscopy and proctoscopy at the bedside at this stage. A number of caveats need to be emphasized with respect to these procedures, however. First, the visualization of anorectal lesions such as hemorrhoids does not, of course, mean that these are the cause of the hemorrhage. Second, one recent study has suggested that a retroflexion view of the anorectal region obtained during colonoscopy is more accurate than either anoscopy or rigid proctoscopy in defining bleeding anorectal lesions. Finally, the visualization of blood in the colonic lumen at a level above the anorectum does not mean that a higher lesion is causing the bleeding. Several instances of blood from bleeding hemorrhoids tracking all the way round to the cecum have been well documented.

If, as in most instances, the cause of the hemorrhage is not evident at this stage, additional invasive procedures will now be necessary. Before attempting procedures to evaluate the small intestine and colon and even in those patients who do not have any upper GI symptoms and in whom a nasogastric aspirate has proved negative, an upper GI endoscopy should always be performed. Thus, one recent study found unsuspected upper GI lesions in 13 percent of patients presenting with massive hematochezia. Once an upper-tract lesion has been ruled out, further diagnostic steps will be determined by the clinical status of the patient.

Patient Stable, Bleeding Has Stopped Spontaneously. As both radioisotope studies and angiography rely on the definition of extravasation to document a bleeding lesion, neither is indicated in these patients, and all would agree that early colonoscopy is the first-line investigation of choice. If the cause of the bleeding is identified, it is treated appropriately by colonoscopic or other methods. If colonoscopy proves negative, attention should be directed to the small intestine. In younger (i.e., under 50 years of age) individuals, a Meckel's diverticulum should be sought by a technetium pertechnetate scan and, if found, surgical excision performed. In all age groups, other small bowel lesions should be sought by a barium follow-through study or enteroclysis (small bowel enema). Alternative approaches include extended upper GI endoscopy using a pediatric colonoscope, enteroscopy, and elective angiography (to define arteriovenous malformations or tumor circulation).

Continuing Massive Hemorrhage. The further management of these patients remains controversial. Some have suggested that these patients should immediately undergo *mesenteric angiography*, citing the accuracy of this modality and also its therapeutic potential. However, several large series have reported a rather low diagnostic yield from angiography and also a significant incidence of serious complications such as mesenteric infarction and systemic embolic events. These techniques are also time-consuming and dependent on the availability of a highly skilled and specialized radiologist. Others have supported a role for *nuclear medicine studies*, in particular, either a technetium-sulfur colloid or a technetium-tagged red blood cell study. These modalities have the advantage of being able to detect bleeding at rates as low as 0.1 ml per minute but are limited by poor localization. However, a technetium-sulfur colloid scan, which can demonstrate immediate extravasation of dye at the bleeding point, may prove useful in providing the surgeon or radiologist with a rough guide to the locality of the bleeding site. The technetium-tagged red blood cell scans, in contrast, are of particular value in the investigation of the intermittent or recurrent bleeder and have little role in the assessment of the acutely hemorrhaging patient.

Initial attempts at performing *colonoscopy* in the patient acutely bleeding from the lower GI tract were fraught with problems of visualization and achieving access to the right colon. The recent description of a technique for rapid cleansing of the colon in these patients has greatly enhanced its usefulness. In this method, patients consume a sulfate purge solution over a period of 2 to 7 hours until the rectal effluent is clear. This can be performed in most patients by the oral route, and complications of fluid overload are rare. Following this preparation, full examination of the entire colon is possible in the vast majority, provided that the procedure is performed by an experienced colonoscopist. Accurate diagnosis can be achieved in the vast majority of patients and definitive therapy carried out in a majority. Endoscopic therapeutic approaches include electrocoagulation biopsy, laser, heater probe, or monobipolar electrocoagulation of vascular malformations and bleeding vessels, and endoscopic polypectomy. The choice of technique will depend on local expertise and availability of equipment. Laser systems suffer from high cost and lack of portability; heater probe and mono-polar or bipolar electrocoagulation systems are relatively inexpensive, readily portable on an endoscopy cart, and are easier to use, yet appear at least as effective. We currently use a heater probe system in our practice. Furthermore, complications such as perforation, secondary hemorrhage, and sepsis are extremely rare.

Another approach to the massively bleeding patient that is advocated by some is *early laparotomy* with intraoperative colonoscopy, upper GI endoscopy and, where indicated, enteroscopy. Advocates argue that if bleeding is severe enough to merit emergency surgery, angiographic therapy is unlikely to arrest the hemorrhage and is no better at identifying the bleeding site than intraoperative colonoscopy; the delay involved in performing angiography exposes the patient to an increased risk. We would suggest, however, that in the patient who is hemodynamically stable, colonoscopy should be performed preoperatively, given that many lesions, such as polyps and vascular malformations, can be definitively treated at colonoscopy and laparotomy therefore avoided. The concept of *intraoperative endoscopy* prior to small bowel or colonic excision at the time of surgery is entirely appropriate, however, as empiric local or total colonic resection has been associated with a high rate of recurrent bleeding and a high mortality.

No mention has been made of the *barium enema* examination in the assessment of lower GI hemorrhage. This omission has been deliberate, as we believe today that this study does not have a place in the assessment of major lower GI bleeding. Furthermore, the introduction of barium into the colon may make subsequent endoscopic visualization difficult and angiographic interpretation impossible.

Based on this assessment of the current literature and on our own experience, our approach to the patient with a major lower GI hemorrhage is as follows:

1. Resuscitate and determine risk status.
2. Look for local anorectal causes.
3. Perform esophagogastroduodenoscopy to rule out upper GI source.
4. If bleeding has stopped spontaneously and patient is stable, proceed to early colonoscopy with colonoscopic therapy of appropriate lesions. Lesions not amenable to colonoscopic electrocoagulation, laser, or heater probe therapy may require surgical excision. If negative, study the small bowel.
5. If patient continues to bleed massively and remains unstable, proceed to surgery and perform intraoperative endoscopy prior to resection.
6. If patient continues to bleed and is stable, proceed to urgent colonoscopy following sulfate purge. If colonoscopy proves negative, proceed to sulfur colloid scan and follow with angiography, if positive. If expertise is available, temporary or short-term control of hemorrhage can be attempted by local intra-arterial vasopressin infusion or angiographic embolization. If scan negative, study the small bowel. If all tests negative and patient continues to bleed, consider laparotomy and intra-operative endoscopy. However, in those instances where bleeding has already stopped spontaneously at the end of the diagnostic evaluation and the diagnosis is still not clear, it may be more prudent to wait for rebleeding to occur on the strict understanding that definitive diagnostic procedures (scan, colonoscopy, endoscopy, angiography) will be immediately performed at the first sign of further bleeding.

Specific Lesions

Diverticula. The high frequency of diverticula in the elderly population accounts for the frequent incorrect attribution of bleeding to a diverticulum. A diverticulum should be assumed to be the cause of bleeding *only* if active bleeding is seen to originate from it (at colonoscopy or angiography) or if in the presence of diverticula no other potential bleeding source can be defined despite exhaustive search. It is evident from a number of recent studies that right-sided diverticula account for a disproportionate number of those diverticula that may give rise to bleeding. In those patients who bleed from a diverticulum, bleeding will stop spontaneously and not recur in approximately 60 percent. In those other patients with persistent hemorrhage, angiography may serve not only to define the source of the bleeding (and is more accurate than colonoscopy in the case of diverticula) but may have definite therapeutic potential. Temporary control of bleeding may be obtained with intra-arterial infusion of vasopressin locally at the site of the lesion; more long-term control may be obtained by embolization. While this approach has been advocated by interventional radiologists, its overall efficacy and long-term results remain unclear; others therefore recommend a surgical approach with local excision of the responsible area. Which option to choose should be guided in the first instance by local experience and expertise; angiographic therapy should be attempted only by expert interventional radiologists with surgical help at the ready at all times.

Vascular Malformations. The widespread use of colonoscopy has led to the definition of many vascular abnormalities in the colon. These lesions may also occur in the small intestine or indeed anywhere in the GI tract. In some rare occasions, they may form part of a systemic syndrome such as hereditary hemorrhagic telangiectasia (Rendu-Osler-Weber syndrome), the blue rubber bleb nevus syndrome, and the acquired CRST (calcinosis, Raynaud's phenomenon, sclerodactyly, telangiectasia) syndrome. They are also common in patients with portal hypertension and advanced renal failure and may result from radiation therapy. The precise definition of what, on either macroscopic or microscopic grounds, represents a truly pathologic vascular malformation remains somewhat unclear, and there has been a tendency to overdiagnose these lesions with any tortuous or prominent vessel seen in the right colon in an elderly person being described as angiodysplasia. Colonic vascular malformations are most common in the right colon and may appear as bright, erythematous, homogenous spots; as flat, bright red, and fern-like lesions; as a loose network of ectatic vessels; as spider-like configurations (similar to spider nevi on the skin); or as prominent dendritic arms of grossly ectatic vessels. Given the variable appearance of these lesions and the fact that they frequently occur in large numbers, the accurate definition of the bleeding site assumes utmost importance. Caution needs to be exerted, therefore, as in the case of diverticula, in ascribing a bleeding episode to a vascular malformation, in the absence of definite stigmata. These lesions can be treated at the time of colonoscopy using either diathermy forceps ("hot biopsy" forceps), mono/bipolar electrocoagulation, heater probe, or laser. Several sessions may be necessary to eliminate all lesions, however. Given its thin wall, care must be taken with any form of heating or coagulation therapy in the right side of the colon. Bleeding from these lesions can also be arrested by angiographic embolization and, in instances of continuing massive hemorrhage and endoscopic or angiographic failure, by surgery. Given the predilection of these lesions to involve the right colon, a right hemicolectomy is usually indicated.

Polyps and Cancer. While surgical therapy is the ultimate therapeutic modality for patients with colonic or small bowel cancer in all patients in whom surgery is feasible, control of hemorrhage in the acute situation may be temporarily achieved by either colonoscopic or angiographic techniques. This may allow for a more complete evaluation of the patient prior to resection. Most polyps can be dealt with colonoscopically by either diathermy biopsy (if less than or equal to 7 mm in diameter) or snare-diathermic removal of the whole polyp. Risks related to colonoscopic polypectomy include postpolypectomy bleeding and perforation; the incidence of these complications is directly related to the size of the polyp.

Small Bowel Lesions. Small intestinal lesions represent a small proportion of all causes of gastrointestinal hemorrhage but often prove particularly difficult to diagnose; the more common of these lesions are listed in Table 2. Most, it should be noted, will ultimately require surgical excision as definitive therapy.

The small intestine is, of course, relatively inaccessible to conventional endoscopes, although use of a pediatric colonoscope may permit careful examination of the entire duodenum and even proximal jejunum, and the very distal reaches of the terminal ileum can frequently, and with experience, be visualized at the time of colonoscopy. As some of these lesions may be visualized by conventional radiographic techniques, a barium study of the small intestine should be the first line of investigation in those patients who are stable and who have stopped bleeding. There is some evidence to suggest that small bowel enema may be more accurate in detecting small lesions than a conventional small bowel follow-through examination. For those patients who continue to bleed, a nuclear medicine study should be the initial investigation; first, to define the point of extravasation, and second, to thereby guide angiography or surgery. If extravasation is seen, angiography may be performed to define the site and nature of the bleeding lesion more accurately. By maintaining a catheter in situ and performing selective injection of a dye

Table 2 Small Intestinal Lesions That May Cause Acute Lower or Recurrent Gastrointestinal Hemorrhage

Vascular malformations
Hamartomas
Carcinomas
Lymphomas
Regional enteritis
Ulcerative jejunoileitis
Solitary jejunal ulcers
Meckel's diverticulum
Enteric duplication cyst
Jejunal diverticula
Vasculitis
Aorto-enteric fistula

marker at the bleeding site at surgery, the radiologist can further guide appropriate resection.

An alternative approach and the next step in those in whom angiography has proved negative or nondiagnostic is to proceed with laparotomy. Careful palpation and transillumination of the entire small bowel may reveal the causative lesion. In most instances, however, some form of intraoperative study will be necessary. It is our opinion that the optimal technique in this situation is intraoperative endoscopy performed jointly by the surgeon and endoscopist. A colonoscope is passed either orally or anally, and the entire small intestine is telescoped over it by the surgeon. By the coordinated actions of the surgeon and endoscopist, the entire small intestine can be examined, and when performed by experienced operators, a high diagnostic yield is to be expected.

SUGGESTED READING

Berry AR, Campbell WB, Kettlewell MGW. Management of major colonic hemorrhage. Br J Surg 1988; 75:637–640.
Gostout CJ, Bowyer BA, Ahlquist DA, et al. Mucosal vascular malformations of the gastrointestinal tract: clinical observations and results of endoscopic neodymium-yttrium-aluminum-garnet laser therapy. Mayo Clin Proc 1988; 63:993–1003.
Jensen DM, Machicado GA. Diagnosis and treatment of severe hematochezia: The role of urgent colonoscopy after purge. Gastroenterology 1988; 95:1569–1574.
Leitman IM, Paull DE, Shires GT. Evaluation and management of massive lower gastrointestinal hemorrhage. Ann Surg 1989; 209:175–180.
Peterson WL. Gastrointestinal bleeding. In: Sleisenger MH, Fordtran JS, eds. Gastrointestinal disease: pathophysiology, diagnosis and management. 4th ed. New York: WB Saunders, 1989:397.

HEMORRHAGIC AND THROMBOTIC DISORDERS

MARGARET E. RICK, M.D.

Acquired disorders of hemostasis and thrombosis are common in patients in the intensive care unit. These disorders often result from the underlying disease state, secondary organ failure, or the necessary treatment.

APPROACH TO THE PATIENT

It is important to obtain a history of past bleeding, hemostatic challenges, and thrombotic disease from either the patient, a relative, or available records. Occasionally a history of an inherited disorder (such as von Willebrand's disease) or an acquired disease (such as chronic immune thrombocytopenic purpura) will be discovered, which will alter treatment. Previous coagulation studies and platelet counts are also extremely helpful for comparison with current values. A medication history is particularly important in assessing platelet function, since a large number of nonprescription drugs impair platelet function; these include not only aspirin-containing compounds but also ibuprofen. Antihistamines and the semisynthetic penicillins also inhibit platelet function. Tables 1 and 2 list many of the medications that cause quantitative or qualitative platelet defects. Although very few medications cause decreases in coagulation factor levels or functions, there are several cephalosporins that impair the production of vitamin K–dependent coagulation factors, including cefamandole, moxalactam, and cefoperazone. Obviously patients taking oral anticoagulants (warfarin) or heparin are expected to have coagulation abnormalities. L-asparaginase causes hypofibrinogenemia, and certain disease states can be associated with characteristic coagulation factor abnormalities: nephrotic syndrome with factor IX deficiency; amyloidosis with factor X deficiency; and sepsis, metastatic malignancy, and obstetrical complications with disseminated intravascular coagulation (DIC).

Table 1 Causes of Quantitative Platelet Defects (Thrombocytopenia)

Cause	Treatment	Time to Rise in Platelet Count
Decreased Production		
Bone marrow disorders Infiltrative diseases, aplasia	Treat underlying disease	variable
Chemotherapy and radiotherapy	Discontinue	10–24 days
Megaloblastic anemias	Folic acid or vitamin B_{12}	4–7 days
Ethanol	Discontinue	3–5 days
Thiazides	Discontinue	2–8 weeks
Increased Destruction		
Autoimmune states ITP, SLE, lymphoproliferative	Prednisone, IV IgG, splenectomy, other	2–15 days
HIV-1 infection	Prednisone, IV IgG	2–15 days
Sepsis	Treat infection	hours–days
DIC	Treat underlying disease ±heparin	hours–days
Extracorporeal circulation	Discontinue	1–3 days
Medications	Discontinue	variable
Antibiotics (penicillins, cephalothin, sulfamethoxazole), analgesics (ASA, acetaminophen), heparin, thiazides, aldomet, gold salts, quinine/quinidine, others		

ITP, idiopathic thrombocytopenic purpura; SLE, systemic lupus erythematosus; HIV, human immunodeficiency virus; DIC, disseminated intravascular coagulation

Table 2 Qualitative Platelet Defects

Disease States
 Uremia
 Primary bone marrow diseases
  Myeloproliferative
  Myelodysplastic
  Acute leukemias
 Dysproteinemias
 Extracorporeal circulation

Drugs
 Prostaglandin inhibitors
  ASA, nonsteroidal anti-inflammatory agents
 Drugs increasing cAMP in platelets
  Dipyridamole, methylxanthines
 Membrane-stabilizing agents
  Tricyclics, phenothiazines, anesthetics
 Others
  Dextrans, propranolol, nitroprusside, furosemide, antihistamines, ethanol

Physical Examination

Petechiae, bleeding around catheters or drains, and mucous membrane bleeding (gastrointestinal and genitourinary) are most likely to be associated with thrombocytopenia or platelet dysfunction. Coagulation factor abnormalities will also contribute to bleeding in these areas but are more likely to lead to soft tissue and retroperitoneal bleeding. The presence of petechiae, ecchymoses, or frank bleeding in sites of the body that have not sustained invasive procedures suggests a more generalized hemostatic impairment. It is important to perform appropriate diagnostic procedures to evaluate possible localized lesions when gastrointestinal and genitourinary bleeding occurs; both an anatomic and a hemostatic abnormality may be contributing to the bleeding. Thrombotic processes are often clinically silent, but careful examinations of extremities and skin should be carried out daily.

Laboratory Evaluation

Routine coagulation screening tests—prothrombin time (PT), activated partial thromboplastin time (PTT), thrombin time (TT), fibrinogen concentration, and a platelet count—are often diagnostic in patients with bleeding. Table 3 indicates the expected abnormalities in these tests in several of the common acquired hemorrhagic disorders. There are currently no widely used screening laboratory tests for evaluation of hypercoagulability states or thrombosis.

MANAGEMENT OF HEMORRHAGIC DISORDERS

The specific management of these patients depends on the correct diagnosis. One cannot overemphasize the importance of a correctly drawn blood sample for coagulation assays, if possible, from a peripheral venipuncture by a two-syringe technique, or if necessary, from an indwelling catheter. To ensure an uncontaminated specimen in the latter situation, an initial sample of 20 to 25 ml of blood should be withdrawn for other tests or for reinjection (if a closed system is used) before blood is drawn for coagulation studies. General management of patients with hemostatic disorders includes thoughtful nursing care and no intramuscular injections.

Table 3 Common Hemostatic Disorders*

	Screening Coagulation Test Abnormalities	Confirmatory Test	Treatment
Vitamin K deficiency	PT (early) PT, PTT (late)	Decrease factor II, VII, IX, X; TT and Fib normal	Vitamin K_1 5–10 mg IV or SQ
Liver disease			
Early	PT, PTT	Decrease factor II, VII, IX, X	Plasma
Late	PT, PTT, TT, Fib	Decrease fluid volume, plasminogen; increase FDP	Plasma or factor IX concentrate‡
DIC	PT, ± PTT, TT Fib, platelets	Decrease factor II, V ±VIII; increase FDP	Treat underlying disease ±Heparin + blood products
Massive transfusion	Platelets, PT, PTT ± TT	General decrease in coagulation factors; FDP normal†	Platelets and fresh frozen plasma or cryoprecipitate
Heparin administration	TT, PTT PT 1–2 sec	Reptilase time normal; toluidine blue or protamine correct; long TT in vitro	Discontinue or decrease heparin; rarely administer protamine sulfate

Fib, fibrinogen; FDP, fibrinogen degradation products.
*Republished with permission from Gralnick HR. Hemorrhagic and thrombotic disorders. In Parrillo JE, ed. Current therapy in critical medicine. Philadelphia: BC Decker, 1987: 275.
†Some patients with massive transfusion have concomitant intravascular coagulation, and the FDP level is elevated.
‡Contraindicated in the presence of intravascular coagulation; may cause thrombosis and carry a risk of blood-borne infections.

Platelet Disorders

In the absence of accompanying qualitative platelet or coagulation factor defects, patients usually do not bleed spontaneously unless platelet counts are less than 20,000 per microliter. Platelet counts of 40,000 to 70,000 per microliter usually support minor invasive procedures (i.e., intravenous line changes), whereas platelet counts of 70,000 to 100,000 per microliter are generally recommended for surgery, during the immediate postoperative state (12 to 24 hours), and during episodes of active bleeding. When thrombocytopenia occurs, any medications that are not absolutely necessary should be discontinued. Although a bone marrow examination may ultimately be indicated to assess platelet production, this is often delayed while medications are discontinued or switched to alternatives and while other causes for thrombocytopenia (consumption, splenomegaly) are sought. If platelets are administered, a platelet count should be obtained 1 to 4 hours after; this will be helpful in planning further platelet therapy. One expects an increment in the platelet count of 5,000 to 10,000 per microliter in an adult recipient for each unit administered. If this increase is not seen, platelets obtained by apheresis from HLA-matched donors, other single donors, or family donors may be given. Intravenous IgG (1 g per kilogram for 2 days) may also be administered, although this is helpful in fewer than 50 percent of alloimmunized patients. Prophylactic transfusion of platelets may be appropriate for patients who are not bleeding if they have platelet counts of less than 20,000 per microliter. Platelet transfusions usually have no role in treating autoimmune thrombocytopenia (except when there is active life-threatening bleeding) when prednisone (1 mg per kilogram) and/or intravenous IgG are also indicated.

We recommend transfusion of platelets to patients with qualitative defects only for episodes of active bleeding or when invasive procedures are planned. In these situations, platelet counts cannot be used as a guideline, and the patient must be followed clinically. Five or six single donor units or equivalent numbers of platelets obtained by apheresis comprise a common dose in an adult.

Heparin-induced thrombocytopenia, which can occur with any heparin dose, can cause either hemorrhage or arterial and venous thrombosis. The latter is thought to result from heparin-induced platelet aggregates. When heparin causes severe thrombocytopenia (less than 50,000 per microliter) or thrombosis, heparin should be discontinued and an oral anticoagulant should be substituted. In patients with thrombosis who cannot tolerate oral anticoagulation, a mechanical filter such as a Greenfield or "bird's nest" filter may be inserted. Platelets should not be administered until after the heparin is cleared from the circulation, except in instances of life-threatening bleeding.

Uremia causes both a qualitative platelet defect and a coagulation abnormality. Transfused platelets are helpful only transiently but may be lifesaving in certain instances of active bleeding (gastrointestinal, central nervous system) in uremic patients. An additional defect in von Willebrand factor appears to cause a defect in platelet adhesion to subendothelium. Both cryoprecipitate (which supplies von Willebrand factor) and desmopressin (DDAVP, which causes release of von Willebrand factor into the circulation) have been used to decrease the bleeding associated with uremia. The bleeding time usually decreases between 1 and 2 hours after infusion of 10 U of cryoprecipitate. Desmopressin (0.3 μg per kilogram, not to exceed 20 μg) usually shortens the bleeding time within 1 to 4 hours after the infusion. High doses of conjugated estrogens (0.6 mg per kilogram per day) given intravenously over 30 minutes for 5 days) have also decreased the bleeding times in patients with uremia. Bleeding times are also decreased in uremic patients by transfusion of red cells to maintain hematocrits at 30 percent or higher.

Coagulation Disorders

As shown in Table 3, the coagulation screening tests may allow one to make a presumptive diagnosis in a given clinical setting and to initiate treatment while confirmatory tests are being performed.

Vitamin K Deficiency. Vitamin K deficiency may occur within 1 week in chronically ill patients who discontinue their oral intake and are on broad-spectrum antibiotics. Because of the short half-life of factor VII (4 to 6 hours), the PT is the first test to prolong; ultimately the PTT will be prolonged because of low levels of factors IX and X. Both PT and PTT will be corrected in vitro when the patient's plasma is mixed with an equal volume of normal plasma. If the patient's liver function is normal, vitamin K_1 (not vitamin K_2), given by intravenous infusion over 15 minutes, will normalize the PT within 6 to 24 hours. Correction of the PTT may take 24 to 48 hours. Parenteral vitamin K_1 will reverse the effect of warfarin in the same period of time. If correction does not occur, liver function abnormalities must be suspected. In patients who are actively bleeding, plasma can be administered in addition to vitamin K to provide the coagulation factors, but one cannot expect to correct the PT completely because of the large volume of plasma required.

Liver Disease. Patients with acute severe liver disease have low levels of vitamin K–dependent factors; as hepatocellular function worsens, they have additional decreases in factor V and fibrinogen. Thus, the PT alone or the PT, PTT, and thrombin time may be abnormal. These patients cannot utilize vitamin K and will not respond to it. They may also have poor clearance of activated coagulation factors and decreased levels of protein C, another vitamin K–dependent factor, which predisposes them to developing DIC. Splenomegaly, which occurs in chronic liver disease, may cause thrombocytopenia. Treatment of bleeding episodes in patients with liver disease must be individualized but usually requires factor replacement with fresh frozen plasma (FFP); in acute bleeding situations in which the patients cannot tolerate the volume of FFP necessary, exchange transfusion with FFP replacement may be lifesaving. Platelet transfusions may also be necessary, although one cannot expect an increment in platelet count if the patient has significant splenomegaly.

Factor IX concentrates (prothrombin complex concentrates), which are rich in the vitamin K–dependent factors, have been used, but they carry the risk of blood-borne viruses and have been associated with thrombotic complications, including DIC. Patients with liver disease who are not actively bleeding do not require treatment unless an invasive procedure is anticipated.

Disseminated Intravascular Coagulation. DIC presents as a clinical spectrum ranging from thrombosis to bleeding. The syndrome has diverse causes that all lead to abnormal activation of the coagulation cascade and secondarily to activation of the fibrinolytic system. Screening coagulation studies may be normal in low-grade DIC when synthesis of coagulation factors and platelet production keeps pace with the increased utilization; the only laboratory abnormality may be an increase in fibrinogen and fibrin-degradation products. In this situation, thrombi in the microvasculature may cause central nervous system, hepatic, and renal dysfunction and skin lesions. With increasing rates of consumption, the screening studies become abnormal as the coagulation factor levels fall and platelet levels drop, and bleeding ensues. These patients usually have multiple bleeding sites, including areas covered by mucous membrane surfaces and venipuncture sites. One must begin treatment for the underlying disease and decide whether specific treatment is necessary for the DIC. If treatment of the underlying disease is likely to increase the rate of intravascular coagulation as in acute promyelocytic leukemia, or if the patient has epistaxis or bleeds from venipuncture sites and skin wounds or manifests signs of organ impairment from ischemia due to intravascular thrombi, heparin should be considered. Contraindications to heparin include active gastrointestinal bleeding, central nervous system lesions, or thrombocytopenia that cannot be supported to the level of 50,000 per microliter. A commonly used heparin dosage is 30 units per kilogram as a loading dose, followed by a constant infusion of 500 to 700 units per hour. Cryoprecipitate may also be given after heparin is started if the fibrinogen is less than 70 to 100 mg per deciliter. The patient should be followed clinically and with laboratory studies, which should show increases in the level of fibrinogen and platelets over 12 to 24 hours if the treatment is successful.

Massive Transfusion. Patients who lose large volumes of blood will develop thrombocytopenia and a decrease in coagulation factors if they receive replacement with only packed red blood cells, colloid solutions, and stored whole blood, none of which contains platelets or the labile coagulation factors. Intensive plasmapheresis with colloid solution replacement can also cause similar abnormalities. After replacement of two blood volumes, less than 15 percent of the patient's original blood remains, platelet counts decrease, and screening coagulation studies become prolonged. Platelets are administered to maintain platelet counts above 80,000 to 100,000 per microliter and fresh frozen plasma (FFP) is given to replace coagulation factors, especially factors V and VIII, which are labile factors. If necessary, cryoprecipitate can be given to maintain fibrinogen levels at 70 to 100 mg per deciliter. Guidelines for prophylactic administration of platelets and FFP vary, but usually one unit of FFP is given after every 5 U of packed red blood cells and a 4- to 6-unit platelet pack after 10 U of packed red blood cells. Platelet counts and coagulation studies should be monitored frequently during the bleeding and replacement therapy. If the patient continues to bleed after adequate replacement, the patient should be evaluated for an anatomic lesion or for other causes for bleeding. DIC is not uncommon after trauma and in shock states with poor tissue perfusion.

Heparin. Heparin is administered to maintain intravascular catheter patency and is a common cause of abnormal coagulation studies. It may be given inadvertently in doses that will cause bleeding in patients with pre-existing hemorrhagic conditions. The PTT can be prolonged, but usually the only abnormality is a prolonged thrombin time. The diagnosis is made when the prolonged coagulation test is corrected in vitro by heparin antagonists (toluidine blue, protamine sulfate, or cationic resins). Usually treatment consists of simply decreasing or stopping the heparin. Rarely protamine is needed to reverse the heparin effect: the dose is 1 mg for each 100 units of heparin given within the previous hour; the protamine dose is reduced by 50 percent if the heparin was given 2 hours previously or by 75 percent if the heparin was given 3 hours previously.

MANAGEMENT OF THROMBOTIC DISORDERS

Thrombolytic Therapy. The monitoring and treatment of patients with venous thromboembolism, acute myocardial infarction, and peripheral arterial thromboembolism are often carried out in the intensive care unit; thrombolytic drugs are frequently part of the therapy. The systemic fibrinolytic agents streptokinase and urokinase, and the more fibrin- or "clot-specific" tissue plasminogen activator and single-chain urokinase plasminogen activator (as well as other agents) are given to enhance dissolution of clots. These patients must have baseline coagulation studies and subsequently have coagulation tests within 2 or 3 hours after starting therapy to establish that a lytic state has been achieved. The thrombin time, which is sensitive to fibrinogen/fibrin degradation products, and the fibrinogen level can be used to indicate the presence of a fibrinolytic state. Because hemorrhagic complications have not correlated with the degree of abnormalities in the coagulation tests, laboratory monitoring should not be relied on to prevent hemorrhage. The patients should be followed clinically and their hemoglobin levels measured frequently. Local hemorrhage can be treated with pressure dressings, but major bleeding requires discontinuing therapy and administering cryoprecipitate and/or FFP and packed red blood cells as necessary. Epsilon-aminocaproic acid can be given to neutralize the effects of the thrombolytic agent, though this is rarely necessary because of the short half-lives of the thrombolytic agents. In general, heparin and antiplatelet agents should not be given during the treatment period, and heparin should not be started until after the fibrinogen levels are at least 50 to 100 mg per deciliter. Meticulous nursing care is necessary to prevent unnecessary hemorrhage in these patients. Absolute contraindications to the use of lytic agents include central nervous system lesions, surgery or trauma within 2 weeks, uncontrolled hypertension, and concurrent gastrointestinal bleeding.

Prevention of Venous Thrombosis. Patients in the intensive care unit who do not have pre-existing hemorrhagic disease should be considered for prophylactic subcutaneous heparin (5,000 U every 12 hours) or pneumatic stockings to prevent the development of deep vein thrombosis.

SUGGESTED READING

Marder VJ, Sherry S. Thrombolytic therapy: current status. N Engl J Med 1988; 318:1512–1520, 1585–1594.
Ratnoff OD, Forbes CD, eds. Disorders of hemostasis. New York: Grune & Stratton, 1990.
Williams WJ, Beutler E, Erslev AJ, Lichtman MA, eds. Hematology. 4th ed. New York: McGraw-Hill, 1989.

BLOOD PRODUCT THERAPY

RICHARD J. DAVEY, M.D.

Blood products, when used properly, are one of the most powerful therapeutic tools in the critical care setting. As with any therapeutic intervention, however, the risks and benefits of these products must be carefully weighed before they are administered. Blood should be viewed as a drug, and its use should be subjected to the same medical analysis as any pharmaceutical. Specific blood products are appropriate for specific clinical situations.

The increased awareness of some of the hazards of blood transfusion, especially the transmission of viral diseases such as hepatitis and acquired immunodeficiency syndrome (AIDS), has resulted in greater scrutiny being focused on transfusion. Blood is now screened for the antibodies to human immunodeficiency virus (HIV-I) and human T-cell leukemia virus (HTLV-I), hepatitis B surface antigen, and syphilis. An assay has been recently developed for screening blood for the agent of non-A, non-B hepatitis (hepatitis C). These advances, coupled with careful donor screening, have resulted in a blood supply that is as safe as it has ever been. Complete safety cannot be achieved, however, and small risks remain for the transmission of disease as well as for a range of other hazards of transfusion, such as hemolytic transfusion reactions. The following discussion reviews the currently available blood products and the indications for their use (Table 1).

RED BLOOD CELLS

Red blood cells are prepared by removing most of the plasma from a unit of whole blood. This component is the product of choice when increased oxygen-carrying capacity is desired in an anemic patient. Each unit contains 200 to 225 ml of red cells, which, in an adult, should raise the hematocrit about 3 percent. In the bleeding patient, red cells may have to be supplemented with crystalloid or colloid volume expanders. The decision to transfuse red cells should be based on the clinical condition of the patient, not on a predetermined laboratory value (e.g., hematocrit below 30 percent). Parameters such as the volume and rapidity of blood loss, the patient's age, and pre-existing cardiac or pulmonary disease should be considered in determining the need for transfusion. For example, a patient with cardiac disease who has rapidly lost blood should be transfused more aggressively than a person with chronic anemia of kidney failure. In the acutely hemorrhaging patient, uncrossmatched O-negative red cells may be used until blood can be prepared that is type-specific and crossmatched for the patient. Red cells should not be used to correct anemias responsive to specific therapies such as iron, vitamin B_{12}, folate, or recombinant human erythropoietin.

WHOLE BLOOD

Whole blood contains both the red cells and the plasma of the donor unit. It therefore provides both oxygen-carrying capacity and volume. Platelets and the labile coagulation factors V and VIII are not well maintained in whole blood. In the massively bleeding patient, whole blood is often the product of choice. "Reconstituting" whole blood from separate units of red cells and plasma only serves to increase the number of donor exposures for the patient. The use of whole blood for patients who are not massively bleeding, however, not only exposes the patient to unnecessary plasma but prevents the donor unit from being processed into other blood components. Whole blood must be ABO identical with the recipient.

LEUKOCYTE-POOR RED CELLS

This red cell product must be prepared by a method that reduces the leukocytes in the unit to less than 5×10^8 with retention of at least 80 percent of the original red cells. While centrifugation and washing can achieve these results, various methods of filtration are now most widely used. Leukocyte-poor red cells are used for patients with recurrent febrile reactions to standard red cell products. These reactions are thought to be caused by sensitization to human leukocyte antigen (HLA) and other

Table 1 Major Blood Components

Component	Major Indications	Hazards/Precautions
Red blood cells	Restoration of oxygen-carrying capacity	Disease transmission, alloimmunization, transfusion reactions
Whole blood	Restoration of oxygen-carrying capacity, restoration of blood volume	Disease transmission, alloimmunization, transfusion reactions, volume overload
Leukocyte-poor red cells	Restoration of oxygen-carrying capacity, prevention of febrile transfusion reactions	Disease transmission, alloimmunization (red cell)
Platelets	Bleeding from thrombocytopenia or thrombocytopathy	Disease transmission, alloimmunization (HLA), transfusion reactions
Granulocytes	Neutropenia with sepsis	Disease transmission, transfusion reactions
Fresh frozen plasma	Replacement of coagulation factor deficiencies	Disease transmission
Cryoprecipitate	Hemophilia A, von Willebrand's disease, hypofibrinogenemia	Disease transmission
Factor VIII concentrate	Hemophilia A	Disease transmission (minimal risk with new preparations)
Prothrombin complex concentrate	Deficit of factors II, VII, IX, or X	Disease transmission, disseminated intravascular coagulation (DIC)
Albumin and plasma protein fraction (PPF)	Plasma volume expansion	Volume overload

antigens on white cells and platelets and occur most commonly in multiply transfused patients. Reducing the number of leukocytes and platelets may also lessen the incidence of HLA-alloimmunization caused by blood products and may also decrease the transmission of cytomegalovirus, although neither of these complications is completely prevented by leukocyte-poor red cells.

FROZEN/DEGLYCEROLYZED RED CELLS

Red cells can be frozen and stored for up to 10 years if an intracellular cryoprotectant such as glycerol is used. The glycerol must be removed by extensive washing after the red cells are thawed, a process that removes almost all plasma, leukocytes, and platelets. This product is useful, therefore, in the unusual patient who is sensitized to small amounts of plasma, such as the IgA-deficient patient. Rare types of red cells and autologous red cells for planned elective surgery can be stored by this method. An inventory of common blood types, such as O-negative, can be stockpiled for use in an emergency. However, as this product is expensive to prepare and store and requires considerable time to prepare, it is not recommended for routine use.

PLATELET TRANSFUSIONS

Platelet transfusions are indicated to control or prevent bleeding in patients with severe thrombocytopenia or with functional platelet defects. The platelets prepared from one unit of whole blood (0.5 to 1.0×10^{11}) can raise the platelet count about 10,000 per microliter per square meter of body surface area, or about 5,000 to 7,000 per microliter in a 70-kg adult. The usual dose of platelets is about 6 to 8 units, prepared either from pooling the platelets from individual units of whole blood or from a single donor by an automated apheresis procedure. The 1-hour and 24-hour post-transfusion platelet counts are essential to measure accurately the effectiveness of the platelet transfusion. Fever, sepsis, splenomegaly, drugs, uremia, and alloimmunization can impair the ability of transfused platelets to survive and function normally.

The indication for platelet transfusions varies depending on the clinical situation. The actively bleeding patient usually achieves adequate hemostasis with a platelet count above 50,000 per microliter if thrombocytopenia is the only hemostatic abnormality. Many clinicians prefer to keep the platelet count above 80,000 per microliter for 24 hours following major surgery. Prophylactic platelet transfusions can prevent life-threatening hemorrhage in severely thrombocytopenic patients, such as the oncology patient or the marrow transplant recipient. Although a platelet count of less than 20,000 per microliter is frequently used as an indication for prophylactic platelet transfusions, there is evidence that lower counts (10,000 to 15,000 per microliter) can be tolerated in many patients without a significant increase in the risk of hemorrhage. Platelet transfusions are not required to correct dilutional thrombocytopenia after massive transfusion in the absence of abnormal bleeding, or prophylactically after cardiac surgery.

An inadequate response to random platelets, documented by poor 1-hour post-transfusion increments in platelet count, is often an indication of alloimmunization to platelet antigens, usually in the HLA system. Partial or complete HLA matching can improve post-transfusion platelet increments in about 70 percent of alloimmunized patients. Obtaining HLA- matched platelets, however, often can be difficult due to the marked heterogeneity of the HLA system.

Platelet transfusions are not useful to correct thrombocytopenia due to autoimmunization to platelet antigens, such as is seen in idiopathic thrombocytopenic purpura (ITP). Transfused platelets are destroyed rapidly by the autoantibody, with no post-transfusion increment observed. Patients with ITP often do quite well with very low platelet counts (e.g., 5,000 per microliter), presumably because the normal marrow is producing large quantities of young "sticky" platelets that are hemostatically effective during their brief lifespan.

A trial of platelets may be given to the seriously bleeding patient with platelet autoantibodies or alloantibodies for whom compatible platelets cannot be found. An increment in the platelet count should not be expected, however, and long-term platelet support is impractical. Some clinicians have found that platelets given by slow intravenous drip may be beneficial in these situations. Desmopressin acetate (DDAVP), which increases the level of von Willebrand's factor, has proved to be useful in improving platelet function in uremic patients and in patients on cardiopulmonary bypass.

LEUKOCYTE TRANSFUSIONS

Granulocytes for transfusion are prepared almost exclusively by centrifugation-apheresis techniques. Granulocyte donors are usually given a red cell sedimenting agent such as hydroxyethyl starch and a granulocyte demarginating agent such as dexamethasone. The final product contains 0.5 to 2.0 × 10^{10} granulocytes in 300 to 500 ml of plasma. The product contains large numbers of lymphocytes, platelets, and red cells, and it can be stored for only 24 hours. Fever, chills, and other allergic reactions are common in the recipient.

The indications for granulocyte transfusions are quite limited. They are used in support of neutropenic patients who meet the following criteria: (1) fewer than 500 neutrophils per microliter, (2) fever for 24 to 48 hours that is unresponsive to antibiotics, (3) bone marrow demonstrating myeloid hypoplasia, and (4) potential for clinical recovery. This product is also used to support infected patients with qualitative disorders of granulocyte function, such as chronic granulomatous disease.

FRESH FROZEN PLASMA

A unit of fresh frozen plasma (FFP) is prepared from whole blood and is frozen within 6 hours of the donation of the unit. Each unit of FFP contains about 250 ml of plasma and has near-normal amounts of all the clotting factors, including about 400 mg of fibrinogen. FFP is indicated for the treatment of bleeding patients with documented deficiencies in the level of the multiple clotting factors. Patients with severe liver disease, dilutional coagulopathy following massive transfusion, and disseminated intravascular coagulation (DIC) are often candidates for transfusion with FFP.

One unit of FFP will increase the level of the clotting factors by about 3 percent per unit in an adult. Complete correction of clotting factor deficiencies is rarely necessary, however, and may be difficult to achieve. Adequate hemostasis is usually attained when individual clotting factor levels are over 30 percent, or when the prothrombin time (PT) and partial thromboplastin time (PTT) are less than 1.5 times the control values. The adequacy of a course of FFP must be monitored by close attention to coagulation assays, primarily the PT and PTT, and by the clinical course of the patient. Specific factor deficiencies are often treated with specific factor replacement, as described below. FFP is useful in reversing the coagulopathy associated with warfarin therapy and may be beneficial in treating thrombotic thrombocytopenic purpura and antithrombin III deficiency.

FFP is often used inappropriately. It should not be given routinely in a predetermined ratio to red cell transfusions, nor should it be given prophylactically following cardiac bypass or other surgery. It is not the product of choice for volume expansion (albumin or crystalloids are preferred), and it should not be transfused as a nutritional supplement.

CRYOPRECIPITATE

One unit of cryoprecipitate, prepared from a unit of FFP, contains about 250 mg of fibrinogen, 80 to 100 units of factor VIII:C (factor VIII procoagulant), 40 to 70 percent of the original factor VIII:vWF (von Willebrand factor), and 30 percent of the original factor XIII. It does not contain the vitamin K–dependent factors II, VII, IX, and X, or other components of hemostasis. Single units of cryoprecipitate are usually combined into a 6- to 10-unit pooled product in about 200 to 250 ml of plasma. Cryoprecipitate is used for the treatment of hemophilia A, von Willebrand's disease, factor XIII deficiency, and fibrinogen deficiency. Desmopressin acetate (DDAVP) is also useful in patients with hemophilia A and von Willebrand's disease.

In the bleeding patient with hemophilia A, the factor VIII level should be kept above 30 percent. The amount of cryoprecipitate necessary can be calculated by the following formula

$$\frac{\text{Desired factor VIII level}(\%) \times \text{patient's plasma volume (ml)}}{<100 \times 80 \text{ (average units of cryo per bag)}} = \text{Number of bags of cryo necessary}$$

Bleeding from fibrinogen deficiency can occur in consumptive states such as DIC and obstetrical complications but rarely occurs with fibrinogen levels above 100 mg per deciliter.

CLOTTING FACTOR CONCENTRATES

Factor VIII concentrate and factor IX concentrate (prothrombin complex concentrate) are prepared by fractionation and lyophilization of pooled plasma. Factor VIII concentrate contains factor VIII procoagulant (VIII:C) in a specific dose indicated on the medication vial. It is used for the treatment of hemophilia A. It is not useful for treating von Willebrand's disease or for the correction of fibrinogen deficiency. This produce is now prepared by several methods, all of which inactivate the human immunodeficiency virus (HIV-1) and lessen the likelihood of transmission of non-A, non-B hepatitis. Patients with acquired inhibitors to factor VIII:C can be treated with porcine factor VIII concentrate or with activated prothrombin complex concentrates that bypass the activation step of factor VIII:C in the coagulation pathway.

Factor IX concentrate contains coagulation factors II, VII, IX, and X and is used for the treatment of deficiencies of these factors. This material can transmit viral infections and may be thrombogenic in certain patients, such as those with liver disease.

OTHER BLOOD PRODUCTS

Immunoglobulin Preparations. These products are prepared by commercial fractionation of large pools of plasma. Intravenous immunoglobulin (IVIG) is used to treat congenital immunoglobulin deficiency and certain immune-mediated diseases such as ITP and autoimmune hemolytic anemia. Its value in the treatment of platelet or red cell alloimmunization is less well established. Standard immune serum globulin (ISG, gamma globulin), given intramuscularly, provides passive antibody protection to patients exposed to certain diseases, such as hepatitis A.

Specific immune globulin preparations are available for the prevention of treatment of selected disorders. Rh immune globulin is used to prevent hemolytic disease of the newborn, hepatitis B immune globulin (HBIG) for prophylaxis following exposure to the hepatitis B virus, varicella immune globulin (VZIG) to prevent chickenpox in certain immunosuppressed patients, and cytomegalovirus (CMV) immune globulin to prevent CMV infection in certain high-risk patients.

Albumin and Plasma Protein Fraction (PPF). These products are prepared from pooled plasma that has been heat-treated to inactivate transfusion-transmitted viruses. Human serum albumin (HSA) contains about 96 percent albumin and 4 percent globulin and other proteins. It is supplied in either 5 percent or 25 percent solutions. PPF contains 83 to 88 percent albumin and 12 to 17 percent globulin and other proteins. Albumin is preferred over PPF. PPF contains less albumin than HSA and has caused hypotension if infused rapidly. Albumin is indicated to support blood pressure when hypovolemia occurs without the loss of red cells. It is useful in the treatment of burns and to support blood pressure in patients with protein-losing nephropathies or enteropathies. It should not be used solely to raise serum albumin levels or for nutritional support.

Departments of Transfusion Medicine can provide other products and services to patients in critical care situations. Gamma-irradiated blood products are necessary for selected immunosuppressed patients to prevent transfusion-related graft-versus-host disease. Therapeutic apheresis procedures have proved beneficial in a variety of neurologic, rheumatologic, renal, and hematologic diseases. Rare blood products, such as IgA-deficient plasma and red cells of rare phenotype, can usually be obtained for patients requiring such support.

ADVERSE EFFECTS OF TRANSFUSION

Transfusion Reactions. The transfusion of blood products involves certain risks that must be weighed against the potential benefits to the patient. About 5 percent of transfusions will be associated with an adverse reaction. The major types of acute, immune-mediated transfusion reactions are summarized in Table 2.

Disease Transmission. There has been major progress in screening the blood supply to eliminate units of blood that may transmit viral disease. Blood donors are carefully evaluated to identify and eliminate donors from high-risk groups. Essentially all blood donated in the United States is from volunteer donors, a group clearly more safe than paid blood donors. All blood is now screened for hepatitis B surface antigen (HBsAg), antibody to HTLV-I, and antibody to HIV. Surrogate tests for non-A, non-B hepatitis are performed, and a specific test for the hepatitis C virus has been developed.

This screening effort has resulted in a blood supply that is very safe. The risk of disease transmission is not zero, however, and must be considered in any decision to

Table 2 Acute Transfusion Reactions

Category	Etiology	Treatment
Urticarial: hives, pruritus	Antibodies to donor plasma proteins (mild)	Slow transfusion, administer antihistamines
Anaphylactic: anxiety, chest pain, shock	Antibodies to donor plasma proteins (severe); often anti-IgA	*Stop* transfusion and notify blood bank; treat shock (pressors, steroids, fluids)
Febrile, nonhemolytic: fever, chills	Antibodies to donor leukocytes or plasma proteins	*Stop* transfusion and notify blood bank; antipyretics, evaluate for possible hemolysis. If repeated reactions, use leukocyte-poor blood products
Acute hemolytic: fever, flank pain, hematuria, shock	Antibodies to donor red cell antigens	*Stop* transfusion and notify blood bank; monitor and support renal function and coagulation status, treat DIC and shock

transfuse blood. Recent data indicate that the risk of transmission of HIV is between 1 in 40,000 and 1 in 200,000 per unit of blood. The risk of hepatitis transmission is higher, estimated at about 2 to 3 percent per unit of blood, including cases detected by laboratory abnormalities alone. The introduction of the hepatitis C screening test should reduce this risk further.

The elective donation of autologous units of blood before elective surgery and the use of cell-saver devices for the salvage and reinfusion of blood shed during surgery can reduce the number of donor exposures for a blood recipient. Directed or designated donors, however, have not proved to be more safe than volunteer blood donors.

SUGGESTED READING

Mollison PL. Blood transfusion in clinical medicine. 8th ed. Oxford: Blackwell, 1987.
Petz LD, Swisher SN. Clinical practice of blood transfusion. 2nd ed. New York: Churchill Livingstone, 1989.
Pisciotto PT, ed. Blood transfusion therapy: a physician's handbook. 3rd ed. Arlington, VA: American Association of Blood Banks, 1989.
Walker RH, ed. Technical Manual. 10th ed. Arlington VA: American Association of Blood Banks, 1989.

THE CANCER PATIENT

JOHN W. SMITH II, M.D.
DAN L. LONGO, M.D.

With improvements in early diagnosis, surgery, and adjuvant therapy, over 50 percent of patients diagnosed with cancer can be cured of their malignancy. While patients with prevalent cancers like lung, colorectal, or breast carcinoma cannot be cured with current therapies once their disease has metastasized, the following types of cancer are curable even in the presence of clinically overt metastases: acute lymphoblastic leukemia, acute myelogenous leukemia, chronic myelogenous leukemia (with high-dose chemotherapy and allogeneic bone marrow transplantation), Hodgkin's disease, aggressive and high-grade lymphomas, gestational choriocarcinoma, testicular cancer, Wilms' tumor, embryonal rhabdomyosarcoma, Ewing's sarcoma, small-cell lung cancer, and ovarian cancer. In addition, the survival of patients with certain types of cancer, such as metastatic colon cancer, can be extended by current therapy even when the potential for cure from such therapy is low.

Antineoplastic chemotherapy and radiation therapy are treatments that are toxic to normal host tissues as well as the malignant tissue. The basis of their effectiveness is the ability of normal host tissues to repair the damage quicker or more completely than the tumor cells. These treatments are usually given in a manner that causes significant but reversible host toxicity. In animal tumor models, the efficacy of therapy is generally inversely proportional to tumor burden and directly proportional to the dose-intensity of the treatment. For this reason, considerable emphasis has been placed on treating cancer patients with dose-intensive regimens that frequently result in periods of granulocytopenia and thrombocytopenia that increase the likelihood of infection and/or bleeding.

Over the last decade, biological therapy has begun to make its way into the standard treatment of certain malignancies. Biological agents are either those that stimulate a host response (e.g., levamisole) or are the mediators of such responses (e.g., interferons, tumor necrosis factor, or interleukin-2). Biological mediators, now produced in large quantities by recombinant genetic engineering, are physiologic molecules that regulate host defense and may exert antitumor effects directly or indirectly. They are normally produced locally in small quantities, but in the clinical trials to date usually have been administered systemically in much higher doses, with significant resultant toxicity that may require intensive care management.

The following clinical presentations or treatment-related complications require intensive care unit (ICU) care: cardiac tamponade, tumor lysis syndrome, perforation of a viscus, respiratory failure, uncontrolled seizures, encephalopathy or coma, congestive heart failure, superior vena cava syndrome, hyperviscosity syndrome, hemorrhage or disseminated intravascular coagulopathy (DIC), septic shock or severe infections, increased intracranial pressure, anaphylaxis, and cardiac arrhythmias. Many conditions that are considered oncologic emergencies and demand immediate treatment do not necessarily require intensive care, especially if detected early (e.g., spinal cord compression, hypercalcemia, hyponatremia, or obstructive uropathy).

METABOLIC COMPLICATIONS

Patients with rapidly proliferating tumors that are sensitive to chemotherapy can develop a syndrome of hyperuricemia, hyperkalemia, hyperphosphatemia, and hypocalcemia with rapid lysis of malignant cells. Although classically identified with Burkitt's lymphoma patients, the tumor lysis syndrome has been reported with other malignancies such as non-Hodgkin's lymphoma, acute lymphoblastic leukemia, acute nonlymphoblastic leukemia, chronic myelogenous leukemia in blast crisis, and rarely with small-cell lung cancer, metastatic breast cancer, and metastatic medulloblastoma. Management guidelines for tumor-lysis syndrome are listed in Table 1.

Although frequently detected before symptoms become severe, the syndrome of inappropriate secretion of antidiuretic hormone (SIADH) can cause seizures, coma, and even death. It occurs in 1 to 2 percent of patients with cancer and can be caused by the tumor (e.g., small-cell lung cancer) or be due to chemotherapy (cyclophosphamide or vincristine). While mild cases of hyponatremia can be successfully treated with fluid restriction or therapy with demeclocycline (600 mg/day), severe cases require treatment with normal saline and furosemide diuresis. The rate of rise in serum sodium should be limited to 0.5 to 1.0 mEq per liter per hour to minimize the risk of central pontine myelinolysis.

Hypercalcemia is the most commonly diagnosed metabolic complication of malignancy, occurring in 10 percent of cancer patients. It frequently occurs in patients with multiple myeloma and HTLV-I–associated adult T-cell leukemia as well as several solid tumors (e.g., lung, breast, head and neck, and renal cell cancer). While many pa-

Table 1 Management of Patients at Risk for Tumor-lysis Syndrome

When no metabolic aberration exists
  Allopurinol: 500 mg/m^2/day; reduce to 200 mg/m^2/day after 3 days of chemotherapy
  Hydration: 3,000 ml/m^2/day
  Initiate chemotherapy within 24–48 hr of admission
  Monitor serum chemistries every 12–24 hr

When metabolic aberration exists
  Allopurinal as above; reduce dose if hyperuricemia controlled or for renal insufficiency
  Hydration as above; add nonthiazide diuretics as needed
  Urinary alkalinization (urine pH ≥ 7)
    NaHCo$_3$: 100 mEq/L IV initially, then adjust as needed
    Discontinue when uric acid is normal

Postpone chemotherapy until uric acid controlled or dialysis begun
Monitor serum chemistries every 6–12 hr until stable
Replace calcium with slow IV infusion of calcium gluconate when symptomatic or for severe ECG changes
Treat hyperkalemia with exchange resins, bicarbonate

Criteria for hemodialysis in patients unresponsive to the above
  Serum potassium ≥ 6 mEq/L
  Serum uric acid ≥ 10 mg/dl
  Serum phosphorus rapidly rising or ≥ 10 mg/dl
  Fluid overload
  Symptomatic hypocalcemia

tients with hypercalcemia are diagnosed and treated out of the ICU setting, the condition can have a rapid onset, producing confusion, agitation, psychosis, lethargy, obtundation, or stupor. Initial treatment consists of restoring intravascular volume with aggressive hydration: 5 to 8 L of normal saline the first 24 hours and 3 to 4 L daily thereafter. After the patient has been rehydrated, frequent doses of furosemide (40 to 80 mg intravenously) should be given to maintain a urine output of 3 to 4 L per day. Overdiuresis should be avoided, and potassium and magnesium losses should be replaced. Hypophosphatemia should be corrected, if present, with oral neutral phosphate salts in doses of 500 to 1,500 mg of elemental phosphorus per day. Mobilizing the patient, avoiding thiazide diuretics, and eliminating supplemental vitamins A and D are important adjunctive measures. Mithramycin, corticosteroids, calcitonin, and diphosphonates are all agents that decrease hypercalcemia by reducing bone resorption. One of the few randomized studies of this condition assigned patients to treatment with diphosphonate, mithramycin, or a combination of corticosteroids and salmon calcitonin. The latter regimen reduced the serum calcium to quickest, but seldom to normal. Mithramycin's effect was better but not sustained. The diphosphonate had a slower onset of action but the effect was more complete and sustained. Doses and schedules for these agents are listed in Table 2.

Patients with cancer who have received treatment with cisplatin can develop hypomagnesemia, hypocalcemia, and

Table 2 Agents to Decrease Bone Resorption in Treatment of Hypercalcemia

Drug	Dosage
Corticosteroids (prednisone)	1–2 mg/kg/day PO
Salmon calcitonin	100–400 U every 6–12 hr SQ
Mithramycin	25 µg/kg IV once or twice/wk
Diphosphonates (etidronate disodium)	7.5 mg/kg/day IV for 7 days

hypokalemia from the tubular damage caused by this chemotherapeutic agent. Severe hypomagnesemia (below 1.0 mEq per liter) requires parenteral therapy with 1.0 to 1.5 mEq of magnesium sulfate per hour for several days followed by oral therapy. The renal damage may require chronic therapy.

CARDIAC COMPLICATIONS

Cardiac tamponade in cancer patients is most often caused by accumulation of fluid containing malignant cells in the pericardial sac but can also be secondary to encasement of the heart by tumor or due to constrictive pericarditis from irradiation. Although primary tumors involve the heart, metastatic tumors, especially carcinomas of the breast and lung, melanoma, lymphomas, and leukemias, account for the majority of cases of cardiac tamponade. As discussed elsewhere in this text, management includes hemodynamic support with a 500-ml intravenous bolus of saline solution followed by an infusion of 100 to 500 ml per hour. Pericardiocentesis usually reverses the hemodynamic abnormalities, but long-term management depends on preventing the reaccumulation of fluid. Of the several ways this can be accomplished (sclerosis, local radiation therapy, or surgery), we favor the surgical procedure of subxiphoid pericardiotomy that can be performed under local anesthesia with high control rates and a low incidence of complications. In the patients for whom effective antineoplastic treatment exists, initiation of that therapy postpericardiocentesis may obviate further measures to control the malignant effusion.

Superior vena cava syndrome is an oncologic problem that demands swift treatment but rarely necessitates admission to the intensive care unit for management. In recent series, over 80 percent of the cases of superior vena cava syndrome were secondary to malignancies, with the two most common tumors being small-cell lung cancer and lymphoma. These tumors can be effectively treated with combination chemotherapy and/or irradiation; however, because the treatments are different, it is important to attempt to make a tissue diagnosis before instituting therapy. The incidence of benign causes of this syndrome should caution one against instituting presumptive toxic therapy. Treatment includes palliative measures such as bed rest with elevation of the head of the bed, diuretics, and corticosteroids for relief of laryngeal or cerebral edema. Patients with small-cell lung cancer or lymphoma should be treated promptly with chemotherapy. Radiation therapy is effective for other malignancies. With the increased use of indwelling venous catheters, superior vena cava syndrome due to thrombosis has become more common. Our preference is to treat these patients with a 24- to 48-hour infusion of urokinase directed right into the clot by means of a catheter. Tissue plasminogen activator plus heparin may also be effective but is more expensive.

Congestive heart failure from a cardiomyopathy induced by chemotherapeutic agents such as doxorubicin (Adriamycin) or high-dose cyclophosphamide (Cytoxan) should be managed in a manner similar to other causes of dilated cardiomyopathy. Patients receiving doxorubicin should have baseline and serial radionuclide cardiac scintigraphy to detect decreases in left ventricular function and permit discontinuation of the chemotherapeutic agent before overt manifestations of heart failure appear.

Over the last 5 years, clinical experience with the use of biological agents has grown significantly. These agents can cause profound hypotension as well as precipitate arrhythmias.

PULMONARY COMPLICATIONS

Respiratory failure can be due to a variety of clinical syndromes. Table 3 lists the respiratory problems common to cancer patients and their suggested treatment.

White blood cell counts over 100,000 cells per cubic millimeter in patients with acute myelogenous leukemia (AML) or with chronic myelogenous leukemia (CML) in blast phase are likely to cause leukostasis with obstructed blood flow in small pulmonary and central nervous system vessels, leading to poor gas exchange, hypoxemia, and respiratory failure as well as cerebromeningeal hemorrhage. Some patients with adenocarcinoma of the breast, lung, prostate, pancreas, or stomach develop respiratory failure due to lymphangitic carcinomatosis. Massive hemoptysis can occur in patients with non–small-cell lung cancer, especially with squamous cell histology. Central airway obstruction may result from tumor involvement of the upper airways or from enlarged mediastinal or hilar lymph nodes.

Respiratory failure may also result from the treatments a cancer patient receives. Several chemotherapy agents, especially bleomycin and mitomycin, can cause chronic pneumonitis that leads to pulmonary fibrosis. Similarly,

Table 3 Respiratory Complications in Cancer Patients

Problem	Treatment
Pulmonary leukostasis	Leukapheresis, chemotherapy
Lymphangitic carcinomatosis	Chemotherapy
Hemoptysis	YAG laser, bronchial artery embolization, surgery
Airway obstruction	YAG laser, interstitial irradiation
Chemotherapy induced pneumonitis/fibrosis	Stop drug if DLCO decreases Avoid RBC transfusions (mitomycin) Keep FiO$_2$ as low as possible Steroid prophylaxis (mitomycin) Limit total doses given
Radiation-induced pneumonitis/fibrosis	Prednisone, 1–1.5 mg/kg/day
Interstitial pneumonitis post-transplantation	Use CMV-negative blood products High-titer CMV immune globulin Ganciclovir (DHPG)
Non-cardiogenic pulmonary edema from interleukin-2	Limit IV fluids Keep CVP low Furosemide Avoid high FiO$_2$

radiation therapy can produce pneumonitis and fibrosis especially if large volumes of lung are irradiated, a large total dose of irradiation is given, or chemotherapy is given with the radiation therapy. It is important to note that radiation and the chemotherapeutic agents that damage the lung induce injury through free radical oxygen formation. The pathophysiology is similar to oxygen toxicity and can be exacerbated by oxygen. For this reason, cancer patients requiring oxygen therapy either by mask or by endotracheal tube should receive the lowest possible FiO$_2$ that produces 90 percent oxygen saturation of hemoglobin. The most common error in management we see is the delivery of high FiO$_2$, which virtually assures the irreversibility of the lung damage.

Certain malignancies (e.g., acute leukemia, Hodgkin's disease, malignant lymphoma, and chronic myelogenous leukemia) are being treated with high-dose chemotherapy and/or radiation therapy plus bone marrow transplant up front or in relapse in an attempt to produce long-term disease-free remissions or cure. Some solid-tumor patients with a high risk of recurrence after standard treatment, such as patients with stage III breast cancer, are also being treated with these aggressive regimens with curative intent. This treatment results in prolonged periods of neutropenia and thrombocytopenia that can predispose a patient to the development of severe pneumonia and occasionally pulmonary hemorrhage. In addition, a number of patients develop diffuse interstitial pneumonitis post-transplantation from cytomegalovirus (CMV) or idiopathic pneumonia. While the incidence is less frequent in patients receiving an autologous transplant, the mortality associated with this diagnosis in any patient is very high (75 percent) in spite of vigorous supportive care. These patients may have additional problems such as veno-occlusive disease of the liver or graft versus host disease (with allogeneic bone marrow transplants) that often complicate management.

In addition to the significant cardiovascular side effects mentioned above, biologic agents (especially interleukin-2) can cause severe pulmonary compromise secondary to noncardiogenic pulmonary edema.

NEUROLOGIC COMPLICATIONS

Although intracranial metastases are usually detected and managed outside the ICU, they occasionally cause a significant increase in intracranial pressure leading to brain herniation that requires immediate intensive management. Therapy includes intubation with mechanical ventilation to maintain the arterial PCO$_2$ between 25 and 30 mm Hg, mannitol (1 to 1.5 g per kilogram intravenously as a 20 percent solution), and high-dose steroids. Definitive therapy with radiation therapy and possibly surgery should follow quickly.

Severe metabolic encephalopathy can be caused by hypercalcemia and hyponatremia associated with malignancy and requires ICU care. High doses of antineoplastic drugs such as cytarabine, etoposide, methotrexate, or ifosfamide can also cause encephalopathy. Newer biological agents such as interferon-alpha and interleukin-2 have been associated with somnolence and confusion; with interleukin-2, even paranoid psychosis, combative behavior, seizures, and coma have occurred. Treatment of these drug-induced neurologic problems is mainly supportive, with discontinuation of the offending agent being the most essential action.

GASTROINTESTINAL COMPLICATIONS

While bowel perforation can be seen as a presenting feature of some malignancies, it can also result from neutropenic enterocolitis (typhlitis, ileocecal syndrome), a condition that most often occurs in patients with hematologic malignancies who have received chemotherapy. Treatment depends on the severity of the syndrome. Medical management consists of bowel rest, nasogastric suction, antibiotics, and total parenteral nutrition. Surgery is required for perforation, severe bleeding, abscess, or failure to improve with medical treatment.

Obstruction may complicate certain tumor types. Since surgery, radiation therapy, or intraperitoneal treatments may be accompanied by adhesions or bowel damage leading to obstruction, usually it is difficult to discern whether obstruction is related to progressive tumor. The decision to operate must be guided by an estimate of the reversibility of the process.

HEMATOLOGIC COMPLICATIONS

DIC has been associated with a variety of cancers but especially with acute promyelocytic leukemia; carcinoma of the prostate, lung, breast, gastrointestinal tract; and melanoma. Patients may have one or more episodes of thrombophlebitis (migratory thrombophlebitis), and some also will have nonbacterial thrombotic endocarditis with arterial embolization. Bleeding associated with hypofibrinogenemia can be treated with intravenous infusions of cryoprecipitates, one bag per 2 kg body weight initially followed by one bag per 15-kg body weight daily. With life-threatening bleeding, patients will require transfusions of platelets, plasma, and packed red blood cells. Although full-dose intravenous heparin therapy is sometimes effective in restoring normal hemostasis, it should be used cautiously, especially in patients with severe renal or hepatic failure. Low-dose subcutaneous heparin (50 U per kilogram body weight every 6 to 12 hours) is often effective in the patient with overt bleeding or a recent operative wound. Antifibrinolytic agents such as epsilon-aminocaproic acid should be avoided because they may block the normal dissolution of thrombi and enhance tissue damage. The underlying cause of the DIC must be reversed for these therapies to be effective.

BIOLOGICAL THERAPY REQUIRING INTENSIVE CARE MANAGEMENT

Medical oncologists have been comfortable with the management of cancer patients who become profoundly neutropenic as a result of their treatment; however, it is likely that oncologists will need to become more familiar with the acute toxicities that accompany biological agents and encompass a different set of ICU problems. Studies with interleukin-2 (IL-2) over the last 5 years have shown that significant toxicities accompany treatment, but most are short-lived and reversible. With aggressive supportive care in an ICU or ICU-like setting, hundreds of patients have been treated with acceptable toxicity and a mortality of under 5 percent. The treatment is labor-intensive and costly but, in some cancers such as renal cell carcinoma and melanoma, it produces response rates that are superior to other treatment modalities. Even partial responses can be durable enough to prolong survival. IL-2 is licensed for use in Europe and is available in the United States through the National Cancer Institute group-C mechanism. In addition, other biological agents with clinical promise (e.g., tumor necrosis factor, IL-1) have similar dose-limiting toxicities that require ICU management, so it behooves the physicians taking care of cancer patients to familiarize themselves with the unique toxicities associated with these biological agents and their correct management.

IL-2 is a naturally occurring protein that supports the growth of T cells and has been shown to activate large granular lymphocytes (LGLs) to become cytotoxic to a broad range of fresh tumor targets and tumor cell lines. This activity is termed lymphokine-activated killer (LAK) cell activity, and it occurs in vitro when patients' peripheral blood mononuclear cells are incubated with IL-2. In some clinical trials, these ex vivo activated cells have been infused (adoptively transferred) into the cancer patient from whom they originated. LAK activity can also be induced in vivo with the administration of IL-2 alone. The mechanism of tumor regression in patients undergoing this treatment is not definitely known. Originally, it was thought that the adoptively transferred cells trafficked to the tumor sites, where they killed the cancer cells. Now, it is believed that LAK cells may not be necessary for the antitumor effect of the treatment and that IL-2 is causing the tumor regression by activating cells in situ or causing the secretion of secondary cytokines that are toxic to the cancer cell. Therefore, when IL-2 is approved for clinical use, it may not need to be used with LAK cells (which have their own unique toxicities). It many be used alone or in combination with other cells such as tumor-infiltrating lymphocytes or anti-CD3 activated cells. Regardless of the ultimate form of successful treatment, any IL-2–containing regimen will produce a predictable spectrum of toxicities, some of which will require management in the intensive care setting.

The two most common severe toxicities of IL-2 are hypotension and noncardiogenic pulmonary edema. Invasive monitoring of patients undergoing high-dose IL-2 treatment has indicated that they experience a profound decline in their systemic vascular resistance. The hypotension and underperfusion of vital organs that this causes results in a reflex tachycardia, but frequently the systolic blood pressure falls below 90 mm Hg. Patients are peripherally vasodilated, resembling the "warm shock" state seen with gram-negative sepsis. Although one might be inclined to support the blood pressure in these patients with increased intravenous fluids, experience has shown that this is not the best approach. These patients develop a capillary-leak phenomenon as a result of the IL-2 treatment and extravasate fluid into the extravascular spaces, including the lungs, where it causes respiratory compromise from interstitial edema and pulmonary edema. Because of this tendency to leak fluid into the lungs and because blood pressure support is often required for several days on IL-2 treatment, it is better to support the blood pressure with intravenous pressors, especially alpha-adrenergic agents. Phenylephrine is the one best suited to reverse the pathophysiology of IL-2 therapy. It is a pure alpha-adrenergic agonist (postsynaptic alpha-receptor stimulant) and works by increasing the systemic vascular resistance without exerting any inotropic or chronotropic effects on the heart. In the clinical setting where the patient already has reflex tachycardia, it is ideally suited to raise the blood pressure and in turn eliminate the increased heart rate. We mix 50 mg of phenylephrine (Neo-Synephrine) in 250 ml of 5 percent aqueous dextrose solution and start treatment with 20 to 40 μg per minute administered with an IMED pump to maintain a systolic blood pressure of 90 mm Hg or above. If the patient requires more than 200 μg of phenylephrine per minute to maintain this pressure, IL-2 is discontinued.

Although most patients with hypotension secondary to IL-2 can be successfully managed in this way, it must be noted that some patients, especially after several days of treatment, can develop a decline in left ventricular function, which can contribute to the hypotension. This is clinically difficult to detect because many of these patients also have noncardiogenic pulmonary edema from the treatment; however, it must be considered in any patient who is not responding to the usual management of hypotension. Swan-Ganz catheterization and bedside echocardiography can confirm the diagnosis. These patients need inotropic support with either dopamine or dobutamine. Finally, the severe cardiovascular effects of IL-2 often reverse within hours, and sometimes the best decision is to stop the IL-2 temporarily and resume with a 25 percent dose reduction when the patient is medically stable.

Special attention must be paid to the respiratory status of patients receiving IL-2. As fluid leaks into the interstitium and alveoli, gas exchange is impeded. To compensate, the respiratory rate increases and frequently is sufficient to maintain an oxygen saturation of over 90 percent. However, one must not be comfortable with an oximetry reading in the low 90s if the patient's respiratory rate is increased. Although the physical examination may not reveal any abnormalities and an early chest radiography may be unremarkable, the patient is leaking fluid into the interstitium of the lungs and efforts must be made to minimize the problem. One of the most important first steps is to eliminate excessive intravenous hydration and to support any hypotension with pressors as noted above. If this respiratory compromise occurs early in the course of IL-2 therapy, patients will often respond to intravenous furosemide. If the central venous pressure (CVP) is elevated, the lymphatic drainage from the lungs that can remove excess fluid will be impeded, so attempts should be made to keep the CVP in the low normal range. Oxygen therapy is supportive only. If a patient is not maintaining an adequate oxygen saturation on a 40 percent FIO_2 face mask, serious consideration should be given to stopping the IL-2 treatment. Unfortunately, the respiratory toxicity induced by IL-2 is not usually as quickly reversible as the hypotension, so careful attention must be paid to prevent it from progressing too far.

Patients who have received adoptively transferred LAK cells can develop acute respiratory failure in addition to the underlying respiratory compromise caused by the IL-2. Between 10^{10} and 10^{11} cells are routinely administered intravenously to these patients and can cause sludging in the pulmonary capillary bed accompanied by an acute decline in gas exchange. Occasional patients also develop bronchospasm with the cell infusion. The respiratory decompensation with LAK cells is frequently transient and begins to improve within 4 to 6 hours. If the patient's respiratory status fails to improve within this time, then serious consideration should be given to stopping the interleukin-2. Acute pulmonary edema associated with LAK cells can sometimes be reversed with the use of continuous positive airway pressure administered by face mask. Occasional patients will need to be intubated, but in most series this represents only 5 to 10 percent of patients.

Attempts to design IL-2 regimens with comparable efficacy but reduced toxicity have largely been unsuccessful. Future regimens might incorporate the addition of other cytokines with similar side effects, making it unlikely that the need for ICU management will be eliminated. While the toxicities of high-dose IL-2 are severe, they are generally reversible and with proper aggressive management are associated with a low treatment-related mortality. Although these toxicities are relatively novel for cancer therapeutic agents, they need not prevent us from the ongoing investigation of this important new class of agents.

Cancer and its treatment can result in a broad range of physiologic derangements. The vast majority of treatment-related problems are reversible and merit aggressive intervention. Certain tumor-related complications are also reversible. The use of intensive care unit support for a cancer patient hinges on the clinical judgment of the reversibility of the pathophysiology. Problems judged irreversible should be managed with palliation as the primary goal.

SUGGESTED READING

Berger NA, ed. Oncologic emergencies. Semin Oncol 1989; 16:461–593.
Lee RE, Lotze MT, Skibber JM, et al. Cardiorespiratory effects of immunotherapy with interleukin-2. J Clin Oncol 1989; 7:7–20.
Margolin KA, Rayner AA, Hawkins MJ, et al. Interleukin-2 and lymphokine-activated killer cell therapy of solid tumors: analysis of toxicity and management guidelines. J Clin Oncol 1989; 7:486–498.

DIABETES AND DIABETIC COMA

DAVID BALDWIN, Jr., M.D.

Uncontrolled diabetes mellitus encompasses a wide range of diagnostic and therapeutic challenges. Diabetic ketoacidosis (DKA) in young patients has a low mortality (under 5 percent), and in the absence of complications its management is generally straightforward. The mortality of uncontrolled diabetes (usually nonketotic) in older patients is high and correlates closely with age (30 to 40 percent for patients over age 70 years). Elderly patients typically have multiple complicating medical and surgical problems. An aggressive initial approach and careful attention to a myriad of details are critical to patient survival.

DKA generally occurs in severely insulinopenic type I diabetics. DKA may be the initial presentation of type I diabetes. Most episodes are provoked by infection or cessation of insulin therapy. DKA is particularly common in adolescents and in patients using continuous pumps to deliver insulin subcutaneously. Hyperglycemia leads to osmotic diuresis, dehydration, and worsened hyperglycemia. Potassium losses are proportionate to the degree and duration of this osmotic diuresis. Free fatty acids are released peripherally and are hepatically oxidized to the organic acid beta-hydroxybutyrate. A progressively severe metabolic acidosis then ensues. A variable amount of beta-hydroxybutyric acid is converted to acetoacetate and acetone, which are easily detected in serum and urine. Most patients have both severe hyperglycemia and ketoacidosis. However, a small subgroup of patients will present with normal or only minimally elevated serum glucose values (80 to 300 mg per deciliter) accompanying severe ketoacidosis. This presentation, known as "euglycemic" DKA, is often confusing and must be distinguished from alcoholic ketoacidosis. Proximate vomiting is common to both groups. Diabetic patients usually have continued to take insulin while not eating. Alcoholic patients may have serum glucose levels ranging from hypoglycemic up to 300 mg per deciliter. Usually the patient's history will help to differentiate "euglycemic" DKA from alcoholic ketoacidosis. The alcoholic patient requires only intravenous hydration with dextrose and 0.9 percent saline solution; insulin is not required. Euglycemic DKA must be treated similarly to hyperglycemic DKA.

The hyperosmolar syndrome usually occurs in older type II diabetic patients. It is common for this to be the first presentation of hyperglycemia. Osmotic diuresis leads to severe dehydration, but production of ketoacids is inhibited by residual insulin secretion. Inspection of the main determinants of serum osmolarity

$$2[NA^+] + \frac{glucose}{18} + \frac{BUN}{2.8}$$

reveals that in the face of hyperglycemia, the development of hypernatremic dehydration results in an often neurologically disastrous elevation in serum osmolarity. Patients who are able to compensate and lower serum sodium concentration (1.6 mEq per liter for each elevation in serum glucose of 100 mg per deciliter), maintaining a normal "corrected" serum sodium, usually avoid coma, seizures, and hyperosmolar brain death. Serum sodium or osmolarity is closely correlated with the patient's sensorium. The typical symptoms of the syndrome are listed in Table 1. The acute precipitating etiologies of the hyperosmolar syndrome fall into three groups (Table 2). Clearly many are preventable.

The initial therapeutic approaches to DKA and the hyperosmolar syndrome are similar. The first step is a rapid but thorough history and physical examination with attention to intravascular volume assessment, neurologic status, and potential sites of infection. Any patient with a history of diabetes or suggestive of hyperglycemia and all patients with neurologic abnormalities should have a fingerstick blood glucose measured as soon as possible. Severe hypoglycemia will be rapidly detected and can be treated usually with reversal of neurologic manifestations (hemiplegia, seizures, coma). Virtually all patients with significant hyperglycemia (glucose over 400 mg per deciliter) will appear hypovolemic and may begin immediately on intravenous 0.9 percent normal saline solution at 500 to 1,000 cc per hour, depending on the systolic blood pressure. Serum electrolytes, BUN, creatinine, glucose, acetone, complete blood count, differential, platelets, arterial blood gas analysis, and blood cultures should be promptly sent. Urine (preferably catheterized) should be sent for urinalysis and culture, and a Foley catheter left indwelling in all comatose and hypotensive patients. Upright chest film, electrocardiogram, and initiation of continuous electrocardiographic monitoring are important. It is my view that most comatose young patients with DKA should have continuous nasogastric suction. Similarly, most comatose elderly patients with the hyperosmolar syndrome should have elective endotracheal intubation for control of ventilation, oxygenation, and protection from aspiration of gastric contents. After cultures are obtained, younger patients with clinical or laboratory evidence of infection should be prescribed appropriate intravenous antibiotics. It is my view that all elderly patients with the hyperosmolar syndrome, whether or not infection is immediately obvious, should be given empiric broad-spectrum intravenous antibiotics to cover most meningeal, pulmonary, abdominal, urinary, and soft tissue bacterial pathogens. In a patient population whose incidence of in-

Table 1 The Hyperosmolar Syndrome: Presenting Symptoms

Weakness
Polyuria
Vomiting
Lethargy
Focal seizures
Epilepsia partialis continua
Generalized seizures and coma

Table 2 Etiology of the Hyperosmolar Syndrome

Infection (~50%)
  Pneumonia
  Pyelonephritis
  Cellulitis/fasciitis
  Meningitis
  Cholangitis
  Otitis externa

Iatrogenic causes (~30%)
  Withdrawal of insulin
  Withdrawal of oral hypoglycemic agent
  Corticosteroids
  Thiazide diuretics
  Phenothiazines
  Hyperalimentation

Miscellaneous causes (~20%)
  Myocardial infarction
  Cerebrovascular accident
  Gastrointestinal hemorrhage
  Severe burns
  Surgical abdomen

fection and whose mortality both approach 50 percent, a 24- to 48-hour delay in initiation of needed antibiotics may have severe adverse consequences.

Once the patient has received the first liter of intravenous 0.9 percent normal saline solution and has begun to stabilize hemodynamically, the initial laboratory evaluation should be available to guide further intravenous fluid replacement as well as initiation of insulin therapy and potassium replacement.

INTRAVENOUS FLUID REPLACEMENT

For patients with hyperglycemic DKA, 0.9 percent normal saline is given at 500 ml per hour until serum glucose is less than 300 mg per deciliter. Then the solution is changed to 5 percent dextrose in 0.45 percent saline, at 100 ml per hour.

For patients with euglycemic DKA, 5 percent dextrose in 0.9 percent normal saline is given at 250 ml per hour, and a simultaneous bag of 0.9 percent normal saline is given at 250 cc per hour until the volume deficit is largely repleted. Then the solution is changed to 5 percent dextrose in 0.45 percent normal saline, at 100 ml per hour.

When treating the hyperosmolar syndrome in elderly patients, I recommend that central access be established and central venous pressure be monitored. Patients with heart failure may benefit from direct monitoring of pulmonary capillary wedge pressure. Patients should receive 0.9 percent normal saline at 500 ml per hour until right- or left-sided filling pressures are normalizing. Exceptions to this approach are elderly patients who present with or subsequently develop the combination of hyperglycemia and hypernatremia. If 0.9 percent normal saline is continued after the first 1,000 ml at 500 cc per hour, these patients often develop serious worsening of elevated serum sodium and osmolarity with adverse neurologic consequences. I recommend changing to 0.45 percent normal saline if the serum sodium is 145 to 160 mEq per liter or a 5 percent aqueous dextrose solution if the serum sodium is greater than 160 mEq per liter. In severely dehydrated and hypernatremic patients 0.45 percent normal saline or 5 percent aqueous dextrose solution may be given at 500 to 1,000 ml per hour. I recommend that severe tissue hypoperfusion and shock be additionally treated with rapid infusions of salt-poor 25 percent albumin, instead of 0.9 percent normal saline. Of course, anemic patients may also be volume-expanded with packed red blood cells. Patients initially given high rates of 5 percent aqueous dextrose solution will require higher rates of intravenous insulin infusion than the usual patient hydrated with 0.9 percent normal saline or 0.45 percent normal saline. For all patients the fluid should be changed to 5 percent dextrose-containing solutions once the serum glucose is less than 300 mg per deciliter, and the infusion rates may be decreased to 100 ml per hour once hemodynamic parameters are normalizing.

INSULIN REPLACEMENT

A continuous intravenous insulin infusion is appropriate for all patients with DKA and the hyperosmolar syndrome. The plasma half-life of insulin in patients without profound renal or hepatic failure is about 5 minutes. Thus, steady-state plasma levels are rapidly reached and rapidly respond to changes in the infusion rate. One hundred units of human regular insulin may be added to 100 ml of 0.9 percent normal saline and the first 10 ml flushed through the tubing and wasted. I have not found it necessary to add protein to the solution to counter insulin binding to the plastic tubing. Given the pharmacokinetics of intravenous insulin, a loading bolus of intravenous insulin is unnecessary.

Hyperglycemic patients with ketoacidosis may be started at 0.1 unit per kilogram per hour on an intravenous infusion pump. Patients whose plasma glucose has not decreased or whose acidosis has not begun to improve in 2 to 4 hours should have the infusion rate increased to 0.2 to 0.3 unit per kilogram per hour. Once serum glucose has been lowered (in 12 to 18 hours) and 5 percent dextrose has begun, the insulin infusion rate may be halved to 0.05 unit per kilogram per hour. The paired dextrose-insulin infusions should be continued for another 12 to 24 hours until ketones are cleared and blood pH has normalized. Each of their rates may be adjusted to "clamp" the serum glucose at about 200 mg per deciliter during this period. It is my convention to resume NPH and regular insulin subcutaneously before breakfast and supper once the patient is tolerating oral calories. Continuous intravenous insulin infusions must never be discontinued until 2 hours after the first injection of NPH and regular insulin; otherwise, recurrent ketoacidosis may develop. NPH and regular insulin are then continued subcutaneously twice a day, with adjustment of doses as guided by preprandial and bedtime blood glucose values.

Patients with euglycemic DKA may be treated similarly except that an initial infusion rate of 0.05 units per kilogram per hour may be used.

Elderly patients with the hyperosmolar syndrome are also most safely and efficaciously treated with a continuous intravenous infusion of insulin. Since ketoacidosis is not present and hydration alone will have a significant plasma glucose–lowering effect, the lower rate of 0.05 unit per kilogram per hour usually is appropriate. This may be reduced further when plasma glucose approaches normal. Many of these patients may not require chronic subcutaneous insulin therapy once the precipitating cause of decompensation is corrected.

POTASSIUM REPLACEMENT

Most patients with uncontrolled diabetes have had a subacute or chronic osmotic diuresis and have developed significant total body potassium deficits. Exceptions to this rule are patients with euglycemic DKA as well as patients who develop DKA quite rapidly, such as patients using subcutaneous insulin pumps. However, most patients with ketoacidosis initially will have serum potassium levels in the upper range of normal or frankly elevated. Patients who present with hypokalemia have profound total body potassium deficits. Elevated hydrogen-ion concentration shifts potassium into the extracellular compartment in exchange for intracellular hydrogen-ion buffering. Once insulin therapy and hydration are begun, potassium transport is stimulated and serum potassium levels fall. Patients who present with hyperkalemia, therefore, need no potassium-lowering therapy unless the elevation is severe and associated with electrocardiographic changes. Given the respiratory and cardiac dangers of both hyperkalemia and hypokalemia, I believe that potassium replacement should be carefully guided by frequent measurements of serum potassium (Table 3). Continuous electrocardiographic monitoring is recommended but is not an adequate substitute for frequent direct measurement of potassium concentration.

MISCELLANEOUS LABORATORY ABNORMALITIES

Studies have failed to show benefit from intravenous bicarbonate supplementation in typical young patients with DKA and blood pH values greater than 7.0. The use of

Table 3 Potassium Replacement

Serum Potassium mEq/L	IV Potassium Infusion Rate (mEq/hr)
<3.0	40
3–4	30
4–5	10
>5.0	0

Table 4 Treatment Flow Sheet

Parameter	Interval
Vital signs and blood glucose by fingerstick	qh
Venous plasma Na^+, K^+, glucose, pH	q2h
Serum Na^+, K^+, Cl^-, CO_2, acetone	q6h
Serum BUN/creatinine	a12h
Complete blood count	q24h
Urine ketones	q6h
Arterial blood gas as needed for assessment of PO_2 and PCO_2	
IV intake and urine output documentation	q2h
Continuous electrocardiographic monitoring	

bicarbonate in young patients with more severe ketoacidosis or older patients with severe lactic acidosis is controversial. However, I believe that the administration of 50 to 100 mEq of sodium bicarbonate to raise the blood pH not higher than 7.2 is reasonable while initiating therapy to correct the underlying cause. Comatose patients with an inadequate respiratory compensation are helped by controlled mechanical ventilation as well.

Hypophosphatemia is a common laboratory abnormality that develops during the treatment of DKA. However, controlled trials have not shown phosphate replacement to be beneficial, and I do not recommend it. Malnourished chronic alcoholic patients with ketoacidosis, however, often develop profound hypophosphatemia (serum phosphate less than 1 mg per deciliter) and are at risk for hemolysis, rhabdomyolysis, and respiratory embarrassment. These patients may be given sodium or potassium phosphate, 40 mEq intravenously every 12 hours, until the serum phosphate level is above 2.0. Empiric administration of intravenous phosphate may cause hypocalcemia and should be avoided. Transient hyperamylasemia and proteinuria are commonly present in DKA and are usually without significance. Careful documentation of treatment and laboratory and clinical variables in a flow sheet is critical and a suggested format is shown in Table 4.

COMPLICATIONS

Potential complications of DKA and hyperosmolar syndrome must be diligently sought during the evaluation and treatment of all patients with uncontrolled diabetes mellitus.

Among the complications of DKA are hyperkalemia, hypokalemia, hypoglycemia, cerebral edema (rare, usually in children; may be more common if plasma glucose is lowered faster than 50 mg per deciliter per hour), and rhinocerebral mucormycosis.

The complications of hyperosmolar syndrome are seizures, adult respiratory distress syndrome, lactic acidosis, rhabdomyolysis, vascular thrombosis, and aspiration pneumonia.

SUGGESTED READING

Arieff AI, Carroll HJ. Nonketotic hyperosmolar coma with hyperglycemia: clinical features, pathophysiology, renal function, acid-base balance, plasma-cerebrospinal fluid equilibria and the effects of therapy in 37 cases. Medicine 1972; 52:73–94.

Daugirdas JT, Kronfol NO, Tzamaloukas AH, Ing TS. Hyperosmolar coma: cellular dehydration and the serum sodium concentration. Ann Intern Med 1989; 110:855–857.

Keller U. Diabetic ketoacidosis: current views on pathogenesis and treatment. Diabetologia 1986; 29:71–77.

Kreisberg RA. Diabetic ketoacidosis: new concepts and trends in pathogenesis and treatment. Ann Intern Med 1978; 88:681–695.

Maccario M. Neurological dysfunction associated with nonketotic hyperglycemia. Arch Neurol 1968; 19:525–534.

Munro JF, Campbell IW, McCuish AC, Duncan LJP. Euglycaemic diabetic ketoacidosis. Br Med J 1973; 2:578–580.

ADRENAL INSUFFICIENCY

D. LYNN LORIAUX, M.D., Ph.D.

Adrenal insufficiency can be either primary, from adrenal gland destruction, or secondary, from ACTH deficiency. The clinical picture resulting from primary adrenal insufficiency will reflect the deficiency of both glucocorticoid and mineralocorticoid (the dominant findings being hypotension), weight loss in association with salt wasting, hyponatremia, and hyperkalemia. The clinical picture associated with secondary adrenal insufficiency is that of hypotension leading to the syndrome of inappropriate secretion of antidiuretic hormone (SIADH), resulting in water intoxication and hyponatremia. Both the primary and secondary forms of adrenal insufficiency can become manifest as an acute syndrome very akin to cardiovascular shock, so-called acute adrenal insufficiency. The diagnosis of adrenal insufficiency is confirmed by demonstrating that the adrenal glands are unable to respond normally to an ACTH challenge. Synthetic ACTH, 25 U intravenously, is the usual test. The plasma cortisol should exceed 20 μg per deciliter 45 minutes after administration. With the suspicion of acute adrenal insufficiency, treatment must be initiated before this test can be done. A good guide to the diagnosis in this circumstance is a plasma cortisol concentration under 20 μg per deciliter during the acute illness.

THERAPEUTIC ALTERNATIVES

The treatment of adrenal insufficiency consists of replacing the missing hormones. Primary adrenal insufficiency requires the replacement of both glucocorticoid and mineralocorticoid, whereas secondary adrenal insufficiency requires only the replacement of glucocorticoid. There is only one convenient mineralocorticoid preparation, Florinef, available for general clinical use. This is not so for glucocorticoids, as many synthetic preparations are available, which vary in potency and activity. For replacement therapy, it is best to employ the natural hormone hydrocortisone. Dose is determined by the production rate of the hormone in the given circumstance. Hydrocortisone is secreted at a rate of about 6 mg per squared meter per day under basal conditions, and up to 10 times that during times of physical stress. Aldosterone, the primary mineralocorticoid in humans, is secreted at a rate of about 100 μg per day under most conditions. The biologic potency of orally administered hydrocortisone is about 50 percent. The biologic potency of orally administered Florinef approaches 100 percent, as does the biologic potency of intravenously administered hydrocortisone.

PREFERRED APPROACH

Chronic Adrenal Insufficiency

Hydrocortisone should be given at a dose of 12 to 15 mg per squared meter per day as a single daily dose in the morning. Florinef should be given as a 100-μg dose daily at the same time. Should the oral route of administration be contraindicated or otherwise impractical, intramuscular and intravenous preparations are available for hydrocortisone. Florinef is available only as an oral preparation, but deoxycorticosterone, an intramuscular preparation, can be substituted at a dose of 2 to 5 mg per day. Because this treatment represents replacement of a deficiency with quantities of hormone that reconstitute the normal production rates of these hormones, side effects and complications of therapy are not expected and do not occur. Therapeutic response is manifested in the correction of salt and water metabolism and restoration of appetite and sense of well-being. Some evidence of this response should be evident by 12 hours after the initiation of therapy.

Acute Adrenal Insufficiency

Acute adrenal insufficiency is managed by the intravenous administration of hydrocortisone at a dose of 400 mg per day (100 mg every 6 hours). The mineralocorticoid activity of this amount of hydrocortisone is enough to render unnecessary the concomitant administration of a mineralocorticoid. Until this therapy has time to reverse the adrenal-insufficient state, which may be as long as 12 hours, other measures to support the vital signs should be employed. The condition, for therapeutic purposes, can be conceptualized as impaired cardiac output. (A few cases presenting with the picture of decreased peripheral resistance have been reported, but this is the exception rather than the rule.) As the crisis passes, treatment appropriate for the chronic management of primary or secondary adrenal insufficiency, whichever underlies the process, should be implemented as rapidly as possible to avoid the untoward consequences of the excessive administration of glucocorticoids, Cushing's syndrome medicamentosus.

SUGGESTED READING

Aron DC. Endocrine complications of the acquired immunodeficiency syndrome. Arch Intern Med 1989; 149:330-333.

Clayton RN. Diagnosis of adrenal insufficiency. Br Med J 1989; 298:271-272.

Dorin RI, Kearns PJ. High output circulatory failure in acute adrenal insufficiency. Crit Care Med 1988; 16:296-297.

Jurney TH, Cockrell JL Jr, Lindberg JS, et al. Spectrum of serum cortisol response to ACTH in ICU patients: correlation with degree of illness and mortality. Chest 1978; 92:292-295.

Lindholm J, Kehlet H. Re-evaluation of the clinical value of the 30 min ACTH test in assessing the hypothalamic-pituitary-adrenocortical function. Clin Endocrinol 1987; 26:53-59.

Walker C, Butt W. A case of cardiovascular collapse due to adrenal insufficiency. Aust Paediatr J 1988; 24:197-198.

THERAPEUTICS FOR PHYSICAL INJURY

INITIAL TRAUMA MANAGEMENT

H. DAVID REINES, M.D.

Trauma continues to be the number-one killer of patients in the 2- to 40-year age group. Automobiles are responsible for the majority of blunt trauma, while the increasing use of firearms has been especially decimating to the young male minority population. Therefore, the most important treatment of trauma is prevention, education, and legislation on seat belts, guns, and drunk driving.

The mortality and morbidity of trauma depend on several variables, which can be ascertained by a concise but adequate history. Mechanism of injury helps to determine outcome: the more force from speed, the height of a fall, and the load of the bullet, the more probable the damage. The presence or absence of safety restraints is becoming more important as "seat belt injuries" are seen with increasing frequency. The age of the patient and underlying disease have a direct impact on outcome, whereas a knowledge of previous surgeries, allergies, and medications becomes important to the diagnostic and therapeutic approach. Finally the time from the trauma until treatment may alter the therapeutic approach, (i.e., primary closure versus packing of a wound more than 6 hours old).

The classification of a patient's prehospital condition also determines diagnostic and therapeutic approaches. Table 1 shows several categorization scores already in place, including CRAMS (Circulation, Respiration, Abdomen, Motor Speech) and TS (Trauma Score). Both give rapid objective physiologic data in the field to help triage patients. The trauma score consists of three components: cardiovascular and respiratory factors and neurologic in the form of the Glasgow Coma Scale. A score of 12 or less means significant morbidity, while 10 or less is associated with a 33 percent mortality.

Rapid initial survey and simultaneous resuscitative efforts require adequate personnel and ancillary services. While obtaining a history, the ABCs of resuscitation should be implemented immediately when confronted with a multiply injured patient.

AIRWAY

Airway control must be obtained immediately at the scene or in the emergency department. Because spinal column injury may occur in the cervical area without evident neurologic impairment, it is extremely important to assume an unstable cervical spine in anyone with a possible injury. The trauma patient's airway must be secured without flexion or extension of the neck. The jaw thrust or chin lift is the first maneuver if the patient is unable to maintain an airway. Failure to respond to this by an unconscious or hypoxic patient should immediately be followed first by an attempt to bag mask with 100 percent oxygen and to preoxygenate prior to an attempt at blind nasal intubation. Nasal intubation should be performed only in the patient making some attempt at ventilation and in the absence of obvious severe midfacial trauma. If there is significant blood from the nose, crepitus suggesting a fracture, evidence of cerebrospinal fluid (CSF) leak, or a midfacial fracture with bilateral "raccoon eyes," nasal intubation should be avoided.

If nasal intubation is unsuccessful, an attempt at two-person oral intubations with a skilled operator and paralysis is warranted. One individual should hold in-line traction to prevent the cervical spine from moving while another attempts orotracheal intubation with a styletted endotracheal tube. The dangers of this technique are loss of the airway secondary to paralysis and the potential for injuring the spinal column. Intubation either orally or nasally should be confirmed with the presence of equal breath sounds, the absence of abdominal breath sounds, and a chest film to confirm the position of the tube. Newer devices to determine end-tidal carbon dioxide content and pulse oximetry can also help confirm position of the tube in the trachea.

If intubation fails or is obviously impossible secondary to major facial trauma, then a surgical cricothyrotomy should be performed. Needle cricothyrotomy in a trauma patient using jet ventilation is not usually an option, although percutaneous placement of a No. 8 French catheter introducer and bag ventilation may be successful.

Surgical cricothyrotomy should be performed rapidly by a knowledgeable individual. After palpating up from the sternal notch to the cricothyroid membrane, the operator should rapidly prepare the neck and make a transverse full-thickness incision with a scalpel. A 4-cm incision should be extended down to the cricothyroid membrane. A hemostat or tracheostomy spreader is used to

Table 1 Trauma Scores

	Rate	Codes	Score
A. *Respiratory rate*	10–24	4	
Number of respirations in 15 sec;	25–35	3	
multiply by 4	≥36	2	
	1–9	1	
	0	0	A. ____
B. *Respiratory effort*			
Retractive—Use of accessory muscles or	Normal	1	
intercostal retraction	Retractive/none	0	B. ____
C. *Systolic blood pressure*	≤90	4	
Systolic cuff pressure—either arm	70–89	3	
auscultate or palpate	50–69	2	
	0–49	1	
No carotid pulse	0	0	C. ____
D. *Capillary refill*			
Normal—Forehead or lip mucosa color refill in 2 sec	Normal	2	
Delayed—More than 2 sec capillary refill	Delayed	1	
None—No capillary refill	None	0	D. ____
D. *Glasgow Coma Scale*	Total GCS		
1. *Eye opening*	Points	Score	
Spontaneous ____ 4	14–15	5	
To voice ____ 3	11–13	4	
To pain ____ 2	8–10	3	
None ____ 1	5–7	2	
2. *Verbal response*	3–4	1	E. ____
Oriented ____ 5			
Confused ____ 4			
Inappropriate words ____ 3			
Incomprehensible sounds ____ 2			
None ____ 1			
3. *Motor response*			
Obeys commands ____ 6			
Localizes pain ____ 5			
Withdraw (pain) ____ 4			
Flexion (pain) ____ 3			
Extension (pain) ____ 2			
None ____ 1			
Total GCS points (1 + 2 + 3) _____	(Total points A + B + D + C) *Trauma Score*_____		

stretch the incision and an endotracheal tube (No. 6 or larger) or tracheostomy placed. Once in place, the tube should be securely fastened with sutures and tracheostomy tape to avoid dislodgement when the patient is moved.

BREATHING

Once the airway is established, breathing (ventilation) via a bag is initiated with 100 percent oxygen. If hyperventilation is desired, mechanical ventilation at a ventilatory rate of 12 to 14 breaths per minute and a tidal volume of 12 to 15 cc per kilogram should be initiated. If the patient is breathing spontaneously at all, an intermittent mandatory ventilation circuit with pressure support should be used. Tension pneumothorax should be suspected if breath sounds are diminished or absent, the chest is hyperresonant, there is evidence of chest trauma, or the trachea is deviated in the presence of hypotension. If there is no time for radiologic confirmation, a 14- to 16-gauge Jelco-type catheter over needle should be placed anteriorly into the second or third interspace at the midclavicular line with a large syringe attached. If air is withdrawn, the catheter should be left in place until adequate tube thoracostomy can be performed.

Other potential life-threatening ventilatory problems are flail chest with a large contusion, aspiration secondary to decreased consciousness, and open pneumothorax. In the case of the latter an occlusive dressing should be placed. Simultaneously, a tube thoracostomy should be performed at a distant site. If the chest tube cannot be placed, then an occlusive dressing should be applied with the knowledge that this may create a tension pneumothorax that can be relieved by removing the dressing.

CIRCULATION

The presence of a pulse in the adult implies that a blood pressure is greater than 70 mm Hg; in a child, greater than 60 mm Hg. Electrocardiographic monitoring and the blood pressure readings by a cuff or automatic or pneumatic pressure should be obtained as soon as possible. Obvious massive bleeding should be controlled with pressure and not with clamps. Damage to vessels must be minimized to allow surgical repair.

The use of Trendelenburg position to improve circulation may be helpful, especially in spinal shock to offset peripheral vasodilation. The primary etiology for hypotension in the traumatized individual is hemorrhage. Therefore, treatment consists of arresting the hemorrhage and repleting lost fluid. The Vietnam experience demonstrated that the initial replacement fluid for hemorrhagic shock should be crystalloid, preferably Ringer's lactate. Normal saline is a reasonable second choice; however, it is more acidic (pH of 5.0 to 5.5) and can cause a hyperchloremic acidosis in large amounts. Recently the use of hypertonic saline (5 percent) to restore blood pressure in traumatized patients using smaller volumes has been studied. Plasma products are unnecessary and may be harmful if given faster than the recommended rate of 10 ml per minute. Blood should be administered for all major trauma involving blood loss of more than 20 percent or when ongoing blood loss is unavoidable (Table 2). The "three-to-one" rule is a guideline for replacing each 100 ml of blood with 300 ml of crystalloid to compensate for extravascular volume loss and equilibration. If the patient is unable to maintain hemodynamic stability after 3 to 4 L of crystalloid, then blood should be started. Type specific blood is preferred; however, O-negative blood can be given for women, whereas men can receive O-positive, if type-specific blood is not immediately available. Once an individual has received 10 U or two blood volumes of O blood, this should be continued because of the potential for transfusion reaction. All crystalloid fluids should be warmed to prevent hypothermia. Crystalloids can be warmed to 40° in a microwave, while large-volume transfusion should be given via a commercial blood warmer.

Two peripheral intravenous lines should be started in the upper extremities. Pouiseuille's law establishes resistance as indirectly proportional to the radius to the fourth power. This means that a 14-gauge catheter can deliver fluid much more effectively than an 18- or 20-gauge. Furthermore, stopcocks should be avoided because they have only an 18-gauge hole at the connector. If possible, large-bore trauma tubing should be used to allow maximal flow in the system.

The use of central venous access in resuscitation has been controversial because of the possibilities of pneumothorax, arterial puncture, and catheter misplacement. Therefore, the use of saphenous or femoral vein cutdowns still has a place, especially in children. However, the modified Seldinger technique with a No. 7 or 8.5 French Swan-Ganz catheter introducer is relatively safe in experienced hands and allows easy central vascular access with a large-bore cannula. The combination of a large-bore catheter and tubing permits 1 L of lactated Ringer's solution to be infused in less than 3 minutes. These lines are also useful if autotransfusion is needed in the operating room. Because the large central line is potentially dangerous, good blood return must be present prior to use and a chest film for position obtained immediately. The line itself should be discontinued within 24 hours.

An adjunctive measure for circulatory support is the pneumatic antishock garment (PASG) or military antishock trousers (MAST). MAST can elevate blood pressure and appear to be effective splints and decrease blood loss in pelvic fractures, but their effect on survival is controversial. MAST are contraindicated in congestive heart failure, may increase bleeding in thoracic hemorrhage and ruptured diaphragm, and may increase intracranial pressure in head injury. They should be removed as soon as possible after intravenous access is established by slowly deflating the compartments (abdomen first) and following the blood pressure. A fall of 5 to 10 mm Hg should halt deflation until resuscitation is adequate. Prolonged use of MAST has been associated with skin necrosis and compartment syndromes.

Vasopressors and vasodilators have no place in the management of the hypovolemic shocked patient. Although they may raise the blood pressure, catecholamines decrease tissue perfusion and cause further damage to hypoxic tissues. Most catecholamines also increase myocardial oxygen demand at a time when the heart may be hypoxic. Pressors can be useful for the treatment of shock secondary to myocardial contusion or spinal shock with uncontrolled peripheral vasodilatation.

Patients who arrive in full arrest from blunt trauma are invariably dead and do not respond to cardiopulmonary resuscitation (CPR), although occasionally 2 to 3 percent of resuscitative thoracotomies have been successful in multiply injured patients. The procedure is best applied to patients who have arrested en route or in the emergency department following penetrating chest trauma.

Table 2 Class of Hemorrhage for a 70-kg Man

	Class I	Class II	Class III	Class IV
Blood loss (ml)	Up to 750	750–1500	1500–2000	>2000
(%BV)	<15%	15–30%	30–40%	>40%
Pulse rate	<100	>100	>120	>140
Blood pressure	Normal	Normal	Decreased	Decreased
Respiratory rate	<20	<30	<35	>35
Urine output (ml/hr)	>30	<30	<30	Negligible
Fluid replacement (3:1 rule)	Crystalloid	Crystalloid	Crystalloid + blood	Crystalloid + blood

NEUROLOGIC CARE

The immediate treatment of central nervous system (CNS) injury is to avoid secondary insults from hypoxia and hypotension. This often means intubation to protect the airway and reasonable fluid resuscitation. Steroids have not proved to be useful in head injury and may cause hypoglycemia and increase infection rates. Mannitol (50 g over 30 minutes) may decrease cerebral edema but should be used only after restitution of adequate volume. Hyperventilation is of questionable long-term benefit but may help acutely to lower intracranial pressures. The use of hyperventilation requires careful monitoring to avoid overzealous increases in pH that shift the oxyhemoglobin association curve to the left and hinder the release of oxygen to the tissues.

SECONDARY SURVEY

Once the major systems have been primarily examined and resuscitative therapy begun, the clinician may then begin a more careful diagnostic work-up and follow this with definitive therapy. All abnormalities in trauma need to be explored or at least documented. Therefore, a uniform and thoughtful approach should be determined by the initial history and physical.

All patients with major blunt trauma require lateral cervical spine, a chest, and pelvic films as baseline data. A complete blood count, urinalysis and type and crossmatch are minimal laboratory tests, but an electrocardiogram, arterial blood gases, and chemistries also may be necessary. An intravenous pyelogram to determine the presence or absence of nephrograms and extravasation of dye is a relatively benign procedure and rapid if it can be done in the emergency suite.

Adjunctive to the abdominal examination is the peritoneal lavage, which is useful in patients with an equivocal abdominal examination, hypotension of unknown etiology, altered mental status, or stab wounds to the anterior abdomen. Recently computed tomography (CT) scans have been successfully employed in the place of lavage and have shown promise in the diagnosis of intra-abdominal trauma, especially in the pediatric age group.

SPECIFIC ORGANS

Cardiac contusion should be suspected in any multiple-trauma patients with chest injuries. The diagnosis consists of a combination of electrocardiographic changes, history, and two-dimensional echocardiogram or radionucleotide angiography. The use of creatine phosphokinase isoenzymes is rarely helpful. Treatment includes continuous monitoring, adequate oxygenation, and occasional use of catecholamines. Intra-aortic balloon pumping has been successfully attempted on several patients requiring surgery with severe contusion. Contusion is not a contraindication to immediate definitive surgical intervention.

The attitudes of trauma surgeons toward intra-abdominal blunt injury have changed over the past 10 years. It is now accepted practice to observe children with suspected or known hemoperitoneum who are hemodynamically stable from either a small liver laceration or splenic trauma. Likewise, there has been a slower move to observation as treatment for some liver and spleen lacerations in adults.

The treatment of long bone fractures, especially of the femur and tibia, has likewise changed over the past 10 years. Several studies of polytrauma patients have demonstrated that immediate open reduction and fixation of long bone fractures enabled patients to be mobilized almost immediately and lowers the incidence of pneumonia and skin complications. Present practice is to perform open reduction of these fractures within the first 48 to 72 hours of admission as soon as the patient is stabilized and other life-threatening injuries are addressed. Infection rates have been very low, and morbidity has decreased significantly compared with prolonged traction in bed.

Finally, the treatment of chest trauma in the multi-injured patient has likewise undergone a change. Many patients with flail chest and pulmonary contusion can be managed conservatively without intubation. If ventilatory support can be avoided, then morbidity and mortality appear to be significantly lower. Therefore, patients with flail chest and contusion are intubated only if (1) they are hypoxic on oxygen, (2) ventilation is compromised with increasing PCO_2 and increasing respiratory distress, (3) intubation is required for other reasons such as hyperventilation or operation, and (4) they cannot cooperate with chest physical therapy. To avoid intubation, a vigorous program of pulmonary toilet including nasotracheal suctioning and adequate pain control must be offered. Epidural morphine or Marcaine has been very effective in alleviating the pain and allowing the patients to ventilate despite the presence of flail chest or multiple fractured ribs.

ANTIBIOTIC THERAPY

Gunshot wounds that enter the peritoneum injure intra-abdominal contents 70 to 90 percent of the time and therefore require resuscitation and immediate laparotomy. Antibiotics have been useful in the management of these wounds. Because colon injury is the most devastating bowel injury, broad-spectrum antibiotics with anaerobic as well as gram-negative aerobic coverage should be used. No study has ever demonstrated the efficacy of aminoglycosides in the initial treatment of penetrating abdominal wounds, and they are to be avoided when possible. Maximum efficacy of an antibiotic regimen is enhanced by its use preoperatively and, therefore, antibiotics and tetanus antitoxin should be administered early in the treatment of the multiply injured patient. Second- and third-generation antibiotics penetrate even uninjured blood-brain barriers and should be useful for grossly contaminated head wounds. Although older studies have shown the combination of first-generation cephalosporins and aminoglycosides is the treatment of choice for severe open fractures, the use of first- and third-generation cephalosporins should be sufficient in the majority of cases. Newer antibiotics with gram-positive and gram-negative coverage may also be useful in the treatment of open fractures. The use of first-generation cephalosporins is advocated to prevent empyema when chest tubes are placed in the emergency room for evacuation of hemopneumothorax.

SUGGESTED READING

American College of Surgeons. Advances in trauma life support course. Chicago: American College of Surgeons, 1989.
Mattox K, Moore EE, Feliciano DV, eds. Trauma. Norwalk CT: Apple and Lang, 1988.

BURN MANAGEMENT

ROBERT DEMLING, M.D.

Burn injuries remain a leading cause of mortality and severe long-term dysfunction, especially in the child and young adult patient population. The incidence of severe burns remains highest in the 18- to 30-year old age group, with males predominating.

Many advances have been made in burn management that have resulted in a marked decrease in mortality, especially in the young age population. Burns involving 70 to 80 percent of body surface used to be 100 percent fatal. Now the mortality rate is reported to be less than 50 percent in many centers. The major advances have been in two areas. The first is the rapid removal of burn tissue prior to infection and wound closure, using temporary skin substitutes, as well as available skin. The second advance has been in the area of critical care management, which allows the patient to avoid major organ failure during the excision and healing period. It is now well established that treatment of organ failure in the presence of remaining burn tissue is extremely difficult, in view of the fact that the organ failure will be perpetuated by the inflammation and infection in the wound. In addition, a persistent immune-deficient state leads to a high risk of continued nosocomial infections. Multi-system organ failure in the burn patient has a mortality of nearly 100 percent, compared with 50 to 70 percent in the nonburn patient. Elderly burn patients are particularly vulnerable to organ failure, and mortality in the elderly has not decreased nearly to the same degree as mortality in the younger patient, with the major problem being the limited cardiopulmonary reserve required to cope with the burn-induced stress response.

The importance of critical care management is emphasized by the fact that the leading cause of death in burn patients is now respiratory failure, replacing burn wound sepsis. Pulmonary problems, of course, are particularly common after smoke inhalation, markedly increasing mortality rates in the burn and inhalation group.

Because of the importance of preventing complications in order to optimize survival and take advantage of the new developments in wound management, a clear understanding of burn-induced disease is essential. Postburn problems occurring over the time course of injury are remarkably predictable, and this predictability can be used to avoid major problems before they evolve.

The simplest and most accurate way to clarify the postburn pathophysiology is to divide the postburn period into three very well-defined periods: resuscitation period (0 to 36 hours), postresuscitation period (2 to 5 days), and inflammation-infection period (6 days to wound closure).

Treatment among these phases changes dramatically, as does the patient's physiology.

RESUSCITATION PERIOD

There are three key components of management: airway and pulmonary support, cardiovascular support, and wound management.

Pulmonary Problems

Airway and lung dysfunction are of particular concern early after burn, not because they are most evident at this time, but rather because early preventive measures need to be initiated to avoid subsequent life-threatening problems. Lung and airway problems are most evident in patients who have also suffered a smoke inhalation injury, but airway problems can also readily develop in the absence of smoke exposure, if there are full-thickness burns to face and neck.

Smoke inhalation injury complex can be divided into phases, based not on the time of the injury, but rather on the timing of manifestation of the injury (Table 1).

Table 1 Onset of Symptoms from Smoke Inhalation Injury

Process	Onset of Symptoms
Hypoxia injury from low inspired oxygen in the fire	Immediate
Carbon monoxide, cyanide	Immediate
Upper airway impairment from heat and chemicals	Delayed for 6 to 18 hours
Lower airway injury from chemicals in smoke	Delayed for hours to days

Carbon monoxide and cyanide toxicity will be evident on admission. The major difficulty in making the diagnosis is the misinterpretation of symptoms, which usually fit a host of other disease processes, in particular central nervous system (CNS)–induced impairments such as alcohol, drug abuse, and head injury. A high index of suspicion is mandatory. Clues to the diagnosis of carbon monoxide toxicity include a *measured* oxygen saturation of hemoglobin lower than predicted by the oxygen tension and an unexplained increased anion gap metabolic acidosis. Verification is done by obtaining a carboxyhemoglobin level (normal less than 5 percent). The value will often underestimate the initial magnitude of the carbon monoxide toxicity, as invariably initial emergency care responders will have begun to displace the carbon monoxide with oxygen provided at scene. Continued oxygen administration (90 to 100 percent) is required. Cyanide is more difficult to treat pharmacologically because levels are not readily available. Restoration and maintenance of perfusion will allow the cyanide to be metabolized. Treatment with sodium nitrate can be initiated if high cyanide levels are evident.

Upper airway injury from heat and chemicals in smoke can be detected simply by direct laryngoscopy, looking for a reddened mucosa. However, the degree of injury and risk of subsequent edema cannot be accurately predicted. In the absence of a burn, the injury can often be treated without intubation. A burn injury, however, markedly compounds the edema process, especially with the infusion of large amounts of fluids.

Most importantly, a deep facial burn will lead to massive facial edema over the next 12 to 18 hours, making it extremely difficult to intubate a patient later, if necessary. Therefore, early *elective* intubation is indicated with deep facial burns and any evidence of an airway injury. Intubation is often indicated with deep facial burns alone (Fig. 1). The latter would certainly be the case if a large body burn is also present, necessitating excision and grafting beginning the next day. Intubation for the operation the next day will be extremely difficult, if not impossible, with the massive facial swelling that will develop over the next 24 hours.

The pulmonary response to a chemical burn to the lower airway is initially bronchorrhea, bronchoconstriction, and marked ventilation-to-perfusion mismatch. Endotracheal intubation is often indicated for access to secretions and for positive pressure ventilatory support. The increase in airway pressures from mechanical support is a particular problem in a patient with a large burn because of the concomitant state of hypovolemic shock. It is virtually impossible to "fill up the tank" in these patients and, therefore, ideal matching of ventilator set-

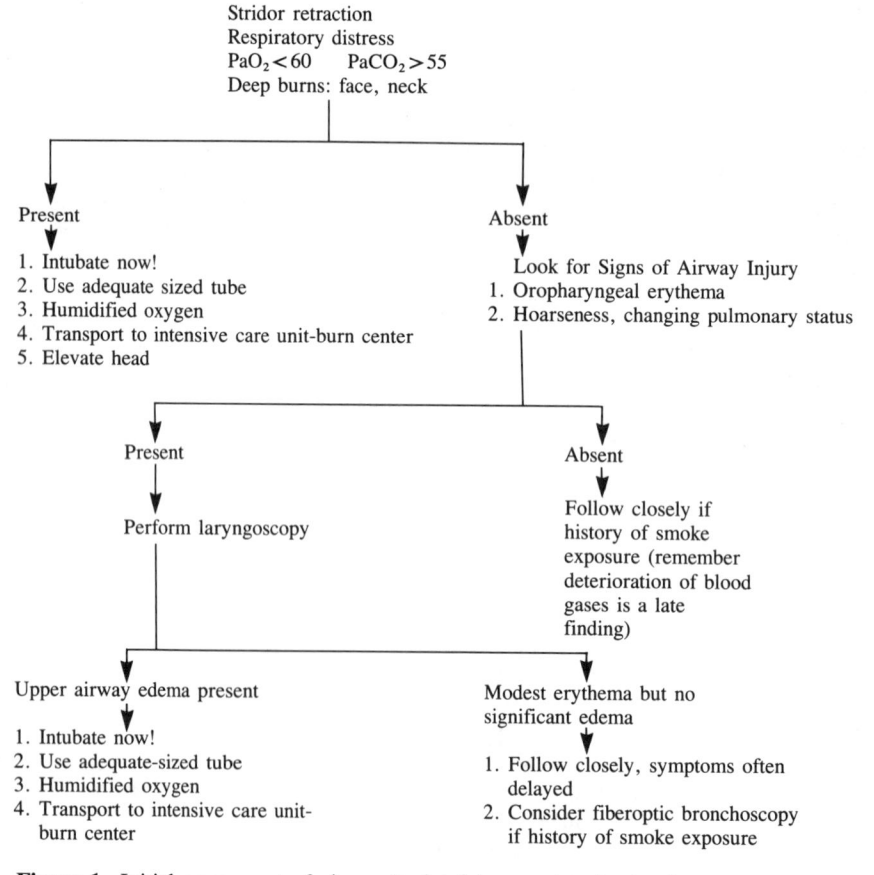

Stridor retraction
Respiratory distress
$PaO_2 < 60$ $PaCO_2 > 55$
Deep burns: face, neck

Present
1. Intubate now!
2. Use adequate sized tube
3. Humidified oxygen
4. Transport to intensive care unit-burn center
5. Elevate head

Absent
Look for Signs of Airway Injury
1. Oropharyngeal erythema
2. Hoarseness, changing pulmonary status

Present
Perform laryngoscopy

Absent
Follow closely if history of smoke exposure (remember deterioration of blood gases is a late finding)

Upper airway edema present
1. Intubate now!
2. Use adequate-sized tube
3. Humidified oxygen
4. Transport to intensive care unit–burn center

Modest erythema but no significant edema
1. Follow closely, symptoms often delayed
2. Consider fiberoptic bronchoscopy if history of smoke exposure

Figure 1 Initial assessment of airway (to intulate or not to intubate).

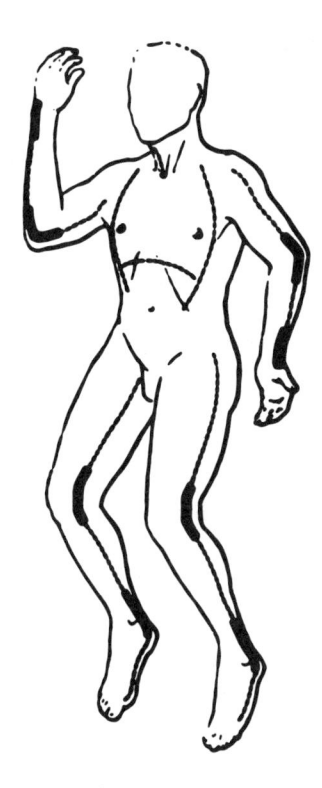

Figure 2 Preferred sites of escharotomy.

tings and positive end-expiratory pressure (PEEP) for example, with the status of perfusion is particularly difficult.

Pulmonary dysfunction can also occur with deep burns to the chest wall, producing a restrictive defect and necessitating chest wall escharotomy (Fig. 2). It is often difficult to distinguish the pulmonary effects of a stiff chest wall from those of a progressive airway edema.

Cardiovascular Support

The massive fluid losses from a skin burn are the result of three processes. The first is the alteration in vascular permeability as a result of heat and vasoactive mediators in burn tissue, leading to a loss of plasma into burn tissue. The second is a marked increase in negative interstitial forces, either increased osmotic pressure or a negative interstitial pressure, both of which markedly accentuate the initial fluid shifts. It is well documented that the initial plasma volume loss exceeds that from increased permeability alone. Both an increase in interstitial osmolarity from released cellular electrolytes (mainly sodium) and decreased interstitial pressure of over 100 mm Hg negative have been reported. The third source of volume loss is a fluid shift into nonburn interstitium as a result of burn-induced hypoproteinemia. A component of decreased cardiac contractility is seen in large burns (Fig. 3).

Fluid resuscitation to restore perfusion is guided by formulas to at least estimated needs, but after the initial decision as to the type and rate of fluids, subsequent replacement is dictated by ongoing assessment of perfusion. Isotonic crystalloid is the initial fluid of choice. The first 24-hour fluid need is often estimated from the formula:

$$\text{fluid need} = 4 \text{ cc fluid} \times \text{percent body surface burn} \times \text{kg body weight}$$

One-half is given in the first 8 hours. Since the fluid loss is ongoing and the ratio of loss also dependent on the ratio of fluid infusion, it becomes very easy to begin to "chase one's tail." The parameters of adequacy of perfusion become the key elements. In a young patient, a pulse rate of 120 or less, a systolic blood pressure of 100 mm Hg, or mean blood pressure of approximately 85 mm Hg, a urine output of 0.5 ml per kilogram per hour, and a decreasing base deficit are currently used parameters. The risks of infection and thrombotic complications usually preclude the routine use of pulmonary artery catheters. Lactated Ringer's solution is the initial fluid. Protein or nonprotein colloids can be initiated at about 6 hours postburn, if perfusion is inadequate with crystalloid alone. More crystalloid than 4 cc per kilogram per percent burn is often not the answer. The fluids should be infused at a constant rate, rather than bolused, since the latter maneuver simply increases the rate of plasma loss into the burn tissue, as the capillaries of the burned tissue leak for days postburn.

Renal and splanchnic blood flow are more selectively decreased and antidiuretic hormones, such as aldoster-

Decreased preload	Increased afterload	Decreased contractility
Loss of plasma into burn tissue	Increased systemic vascular resistance due to circulating vasoconstrictors	Mostly with large third-degree burns
Positive-pressure ventilation effects on cardiac output		
Loss of water into nonburn tissue and space		

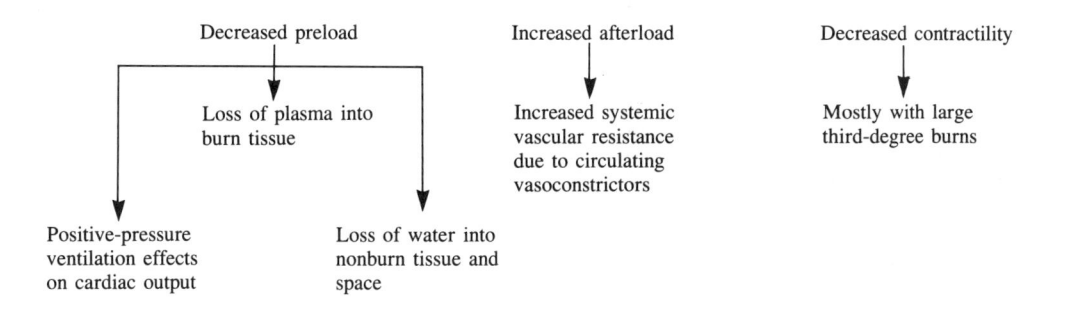

Figure 3 Postburn decreased oxygen delivery to tissues.

one, are increased. Low-dose dopamine is very useful to help restore blood flow and decrease the aldosterone effect and to prevent one from excessively pushing fluids to maintain urine output when all other aspects of perfusion appear adequate.

Wound Management

Assessing the size and depth of the wound is the next priority, and the subsequent operative management is best determined in the early resuscitation period, since the ideal time for excision is prior to the onset of wound inflammation and systemic hypermetabolism (Fig. 4).

The specific management of the wound and the choice of topical antibiotics will not be covered in this chapter. However, it is important to point out that heat loss is a major problem and a warm environment is mandatory for patients with large burns to avoid severe hypothermia. Since glucose stores are used up very early, there are few energy reserves available to counteract the low body temperature by added heat production.

POSTRESUSCITATION PERIOD

In general, this period is the ideal time to initiate aggressive wound excision and closure. In order to do so, the patient must be hemodynamically stable, which means that an optimal initial resuscitation is required. Hypovolemia or excessive massive edema further impairing the chest wall compliance will markedly increase operative risks. It is also important to recognize that this "grace period" is short-lived and that once wound colonization, inflammation, and profound hypermetabolism develop, operative risks again escalate. To optimize cardiopulmonary function, an understanding of the physiologic changes during this period is necessary.

Pulmonary Support

In the presence of smoke inhalation, this period is one of continuing problems with small airway plugging from secretions and resulting increased shunt. In addition, airway edema is still present, resulting in increased resistance, which often requires the need for PEEP. Nosocomial pneumonia is usually not a high risk factor at this time but becomes a major problem toward the end of the first week, as oropharyngeal colonization develops. Fluid shifts back into the circulation from tissue edema can lead to hypervolemia, which can, of course, aggravate the lung problem. However, as fragile as the lung may be at this point, the marked increase in carbon dioxide production and infection risks that will occur in the subsequent weeks is worse.

Of extreme importance is that the operative procedures be kept short, i.e., less than 2 hours, and optimal pulmonary support be provided. Early initiation of systemic antibiotics with signs of bacterial lung infection is also critical, since local lung defenses have been substantially diminished with the airway's mucosal injury. However, prophylactic antibiotics for this purpose are contraindicated.

Cardiovascular Support

This period is characterized by major fluid shifts in both directions, as well as by a progressive decrease in red cell mass in large burns. There are continued losses of plasma into burn tissue in deep burns and from the wound surface in superficial burns. The higher the capillary pressure, the greater the losses. In addition, there is a marked and continued evaporative water loss from the wound surface. Losses per hour can be estimated from the formula:

$$\text{cc/hr loss} = (25 + \% \text{ body surface burn}) \times M^2 \text{ surface area}$$

Fluid gains include resorbing edema. Much of the edema fluid is sequestered in poorly perfused tissues, so that resorption will be slow at first, particularly for third-degree burns. Resorption is much more rapid with second-degree burns, where some blood flow is preserved (Fig. 5).

Red cell injury from heat and oxidants, as evidenced by membrane lipid peroxidation, results in a rapid clearance of injured cells by the reticuloendothelial system. In addition, red cell production is markedly impaired, comparable to that seen with any severe chronic disease. One hypothesis is that the bone marrow stem cells are being diverted into formation of inflammatory cells, markedly diminishing the precursor cells available for hematopoiesis.

Monitoring volume by the same perfusion parameters as during resuscitation will be misleading. When wound inflammation develops, heart rate increases, reflecting a hyperdynamic state and not necessarily hypovolemia. In addition, as the solute byproducts of injured cells are cleared by the kidney, an osmotic diuresis can develop. Urine output may appear excellent, but unless specific gravity is checked, a misinterpretation of the value may occur. A high specific gravity, as is commonly present, and a high urine output may indicate the need for more rather than less fluid.

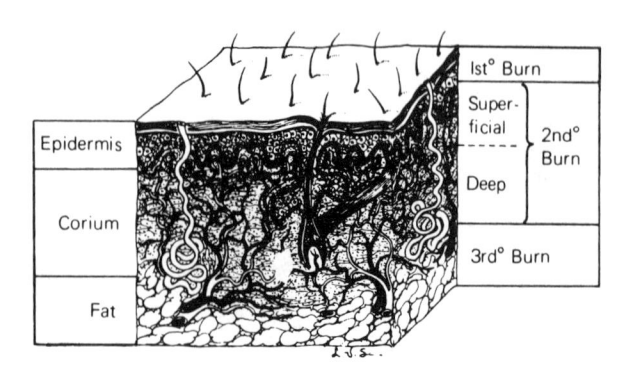

Figure 4 Assessment of the size and depth of burns.

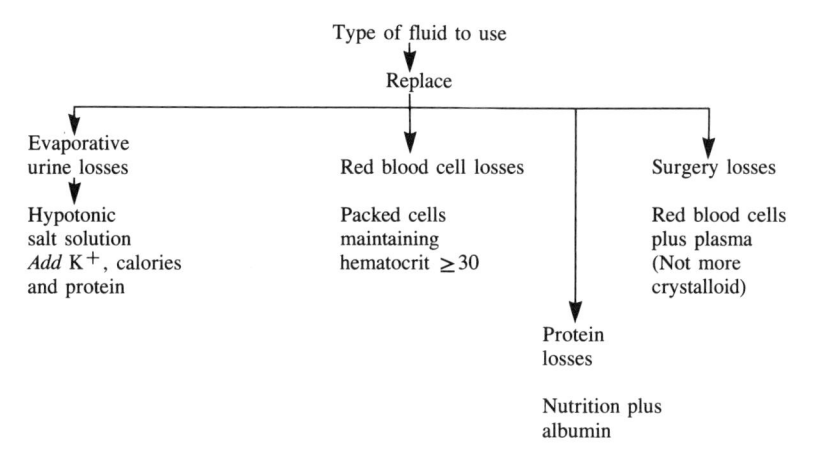

```
                    Type of fluid to use
                           ↓
                        Replace
        ┌──────────────────┼──────────────────┐
        ↓                  ↓                  ↓
  Evaporative        Red blood cell      Surgery losses
  urine losses         losses
        ↓                  ↓                  ↓
   Hypotonic          Packed cells      Red blood cells
  salt solution       maintaining         plus plasma
  Add K⁺, calories    hematocrit ≥ 30     (Not more
  and protein                             crystalloid)
                           ↓
                       Protein
                        losses
                           ↓
                    Nutrition plus
                       albumin
```

Fluids of choice
1. Use low salt-glucose containing
2. Add increased amounts potassium
3. Add nutrients: glucose, amino acids, lipid
4. Maintain albumina bove 2.5 g/dl
5. Maintain adequate red blood cell mass (hematocrit ≥ 30)

Figure 5 Fluid replacement for burn patients.

The fluids used during this time should also contain nutrients and be hypotonic in terms of salt content to replace water loss and restore nutrients. Protein colloid and red cells are needed to replace ongoing losses.

Wound Management

In addition to twice-daily use of topical antibiotics, excision of burn tissue and skin closure is performed during this period. A consumptive coagulopathy is often present on the second and third days, and coagulation factors and platelets are often needed, at least with the first excision. Operation time must be kept short, i.e., less than 2 hours, and the operating room environment must be kept as warm as the ICU or burn unit environment. Blood loss can be substantial, but for the same area excised in the first 3 to 4 days, it is less than half that seen with excisions after one week, when wound hypervascularity develops. Since the wounds are invariably colonized with organisms, usually *Staphylococcus aureus*, perioperative antibiotic coverage is indicated. A first-generation cephalosporin is usually adequate.

INFLAMMATION-INFECTION PERIOD

The hypermetabolic response to injury begins at about 4 to 5 days and peaks at about 7 to 10 days. The process does not require infection, but of course, infection is also a major complication in burn patients. Unfortunately, it is extremely difficult to distinguish burn inflammation–induced hypermetabolism from an infection-induced process.

This period is by far the most difficult management period, taxing the decision-making skills of even the most experienced burn expert.

Pulmonary Support

The smoke-injured lung remains prone to pneumonia for weeks after injury until the mucociliary border is restored. Nosocomial pneumonia is, therefore, a major problem during this period. In addition, the marked increase in metabolic rate results in a concomitant increase in carbon dioxide production, increasing the work of breathing. The addition of the increased carbon dioxide production onto a lung already injured can result in a rapid deterioration, especially as fatigue develops. The combined need for vigorous pulmonary toilet and increased minute ventilation often requires partial ventilatory assist, at least until pulmonary inflammation resolves. Recognition of these increased demands is particularly important in the operating room and during transport, to avoid severe hypercarbia.

Sepsis or inflammation-induced adult respiratory distress syndrome (ARDS) is also a prominent problem during this period.

Cardiovascular Support

Maintaining adequate fluid replacement for evaporative water loss and for blood and plasma loss from debridements is required. The hyperthermic response to inflammation with or without infection will further accentuate the evaporative losses at a rate of 8 to 10 percent per degree increase in body temperature.

Cardiac output is often more than double normal in order to supply the necessary increased oxygen demands. In addition, blood flow to burn tissue is increased two- to threefold above normal. Elderly patients with limited cardiac reserve will often develop myocardial dysfunction as work load exceeds functional ability. The need for inotropic support is much more common during this period than during the initial resuscitation.

Metabolic Support

Maintenance of adequate nutrition is critical during this period, as the severe hypermetabolism and catabolism initiated by inflammation will result in a severe loss of muscle mass and impaired wound healing if not aggressively managed. The ideal route, of course, is the gastrointestinal tract. Some parenteral nutrition may also be required, but this can usually be given in the form of a peripheral vein solution in view of the increased water requirements of the burn patient (Fig. 6).

Infection Control

Nosocomial infection is particularly prevalent during this period, in view of the combination of an immunosuppressed host and bacterial colonization. The burn wound is best managed by topical antibiotics and aggressive excision prior to this phase. Systemic antibiotics for the burn wound are only indicated if there is evidence of an invasive burn infection diagnosed by burn wound biopsy or for perioperative management.

Vascular catheter sepsis is a major problem that can only be controlled by frequent rotation of lines (i.e., every 4 days) and by removal of monitoring lines (i.e., arterial lines) as soon as possible. Nosocomial pneumonia is a particularly common problem in the burn- and inhalation-injury patient. Since the entire tracheobronchial tree is usually injured, multiple areas of the lung may develop a pneumonia if early treatment is not initiated. An increase in the quantity and purulence of sputum and increased white cells and bacteria on Gram's stain of a deep sputum sample is sufficient evidence to initiate antibiotic therapy.

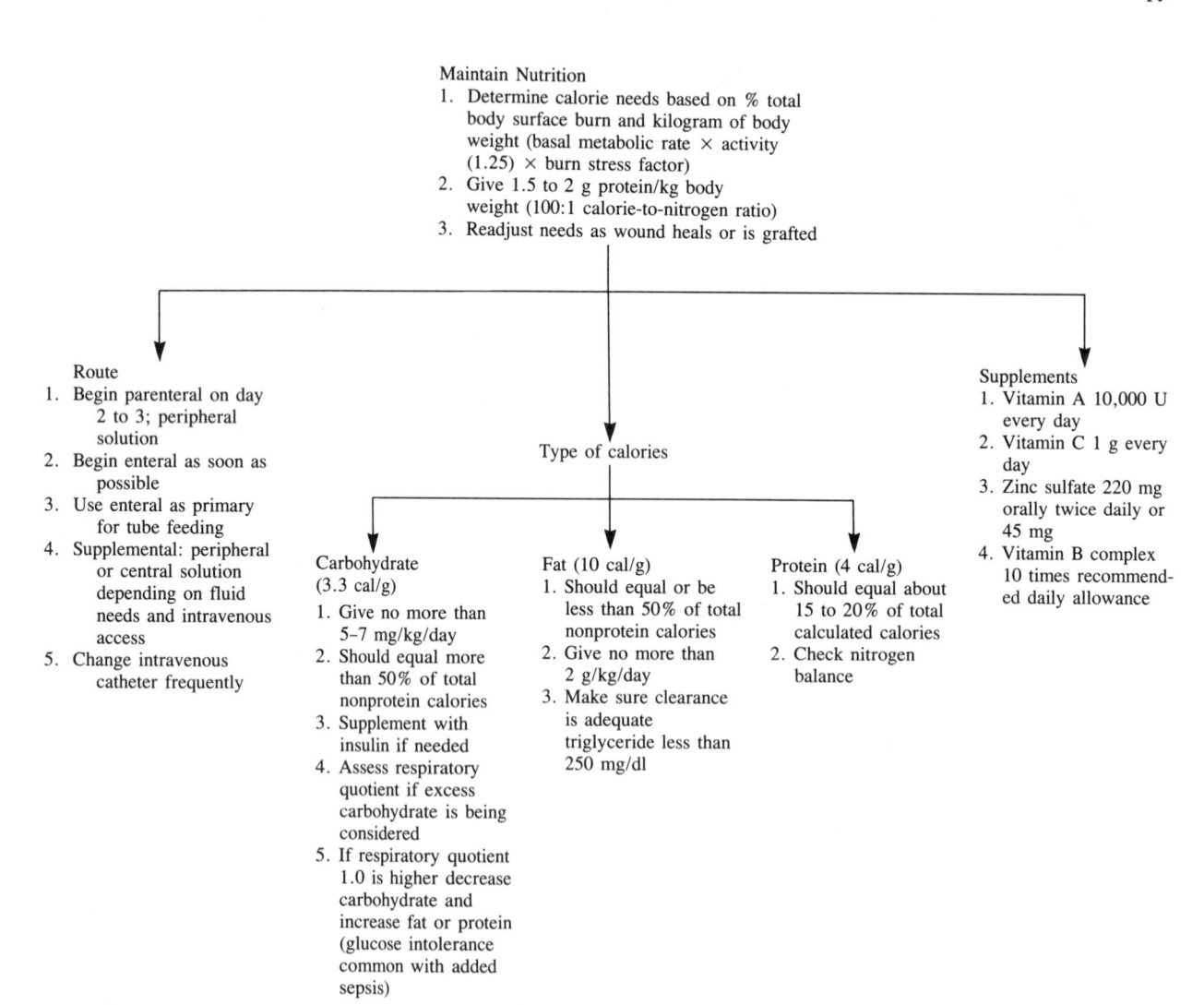

Maintain Nutrition
1. Determine calorie needs based on % total body surface burn and kilogram of body weight (basal metabolic rate × activity (1.25) × burn stress factor)
2. Give 1.5 to 2 g protein/kg body weight (100:1 calorie-to-nitrogen ratio)
3. Readjust needs as wound heals or is grafted

Route
1. Begin parenteral on day 2 to 3; peripheral solution
2. Begin enteral as soon as possible
3. Use enteral as primary for tube feeding
4. Supplemental: peripheral or central solution depending on fluid needs and intravenous access
5. Change intravenous catheter frequently

Type of calories

Carbohydrate (3.3 cal/g)
1. Give no more than 5–7 mg/kg/day
2. Should equal more than 50% of total nonprotein calories
3. Supplement with insulin if needed
4. Assess respiratory quotient if excess carbohydrate is being considered
5. If respiratory quotient 1.0 is higher decrease carbohydrate and increase fat or protein (glucose intolerance common with added sepsis)

Fat (10 cal/g)
1. Should equal or be less than 50% of total nonprotein calories
2. Give no more than 2 g/kg/day
3. Make sure clearance is adequate triglyceride less than 250 mg/dl

Protein (4 cal/g)
1. Should equal about 15 to 20% of total calculated calories
2. Check nitrogen balance

Supplements
1. Vitamin A 10,000 U every day
2. Vitamin C 1 g every day
3. Zinc sulfate 220 mg orally twice daily or 45 mg
4. Vitamin B complex 10 times recommended daily allowance

Figure 6 Metabolic support for burn patients.

Wound Management

Gentle daily debridement is the appropriate management during this period of burn not yet excised. A granulation tissue bed will then develop, which is more resistant to infection and which will be used for the appropriate bed for a skin graft. Aggressive surgical debridement of infected tissue, although sometimes necessary, frequently leads to postoperative bacteremia and hemodynamic instability, which must be anticipated.

REHABILITATION

Exercise routines, including active and passive range of motion of all burned and nonburned areas, are necessary, beginning shortly after admission, to avoid permanent loss of function in burned joints. This activity must be considered a high priority in daily management, as many losses in function cannot be regained.

SUGGESTED READING

Demling RH. Burn management. In: Wilmore D, ed. Pre and postoperative care. New York: Scientific American, 1988.

THE NEAR-DROWNING VICTIM

DOUGLAS L. MALLORY, M.D.

EPIDEMIOLOGY

Near-drowning is a tragic event that presents unique challenges to the intensivist. There were approximately 7,000 drownings per year in 1971, which decreased to 5,000 in 1984 despite huge increases in the number of potential victims at risk. This salutary reduction is attributable to careful epidemiologic studies that have been effectively translated into preventive as well as interventional measures through public health, education, and legislative efforts. Concomitant clinical and basic scientific studies have improved in on-site, emergency room, and intensive care measures and probably contributed to improving outcomes as well.

Nonetheless, major public health and critical care challenges remain, including better elucidation of pathophysiologic events, improved clinical trials regarding controversial management options, and improved public understanding and compliance with known and emerging water safety information.

PATHOPHYSIOLOGY

Animal studies have delineated the probable pathophysiologic sequence of events for near-drowning victims. Panic, struggle, hyperventilation and/or breath-holding, water ingestion, vomiting, violent coughing, involuntary gasping (90 percent), or laryngospasm (10 percent) is followed by hypoxic sequelae of unconsciousness, convulsive movements, and irreversible brain damage or death. It is important to realize that the major lethal factor is hypoxic brain damage.

Human survivors of the acute episode experience a wide spectrum of immediate and delayed complications consequent to both the unique features of each near-drowning, as well as individual variability. The most consistent and important pathophysiologic events include metabolic acidosis; pulmonary problems including rapidly-resolving alveolar flooding, adult respiratory distress syndrome (ARDS), and aspiration lung injury (acidic and/or infectious); minor or major electrolyte disorders; hypoglycemia; acute renal failure; and most importantly, cerebral sequelae varying from complete normalcy to highly variable diffuse or focal syndromes.

CLINICAL PRESENTATION

The intensivist will usually see patients following resuscitation at the scene of the accident as well as evaluation and stabilization in the emergency room. Victims are conveniently classified by Simcock's method according to their condition at the time of rescue and emergency department evaluation, as well as by specific initial diagnostic problems, including (in approximate order of decreasing prevalence): metabolic or a mixed acidosis; pulmonary problems including transient initial alveolar flooding, shunting, decreased compliance, and bronchospasm; hypotension (usually due to intravascular hypovolemia); electrolyte abnormalities including elevations of sodium and chloride for salt-water victims; neurologic deficits; associated conditions such as traumatic injuries plus substance abuse or overdose; as well as hypothermia.

EVALUATION AND MANAGEMENT

Initial rescue and resuscitation at the scene and in the emergency room should follow the "Standards and Guidelines for Cardiopulmonary Resuscitation (CPR) and Emergency Cardiac Care (ECC)" and will not be discussed further here.

Admission and Initial Management Guidelines According to Simcock's Classification

1. *Patients who were unable to save themselves, and with no "inhalation" (i.e., aspiration) of water:* Admit to a hospital general ward for at least 24 hours and observe for pulmonary or cerebral edema. It is questionable whether further testing is cost-effective in light of the low frequency of substantial abnormalities, although the physician should consider obtaining arterial blood gases, hemoglobin, blood glucose, serum urea and serum electrolytes, and a chest film.
2. *Patients with "inhalation" (i.e., aspiration of water) and adequate ventilation in the emergency department:* Admit to an intensive care unit, since respiratory distress frequently develops.
3. *Patients with "inhalation" (i.e., aspiration of water) and inadequate ventilation:* Admit to an intensive care unit for continuous pressure mask (CPAP) ventilation, or intubation and mechanical ventilation.
4. *Patients with cardiorespiratory arrest:* Continue advanced cardiac life support measures in an intensive care unit until improvement occurs, or fails to occur despite optimization of temperature, right atrial filling pressure, and resuscitation measures. For patients with somatic viability and Glasgow coma scores of 3, institute appropriate brain death examinations not less than 12 hours apart, and consider management for potential organ donation.

All unresponsive patients must receive an immediate and thorough evaluation of unconsciousness including a triage neurologic examination, computerized tomogram (CT) of the head, arterial blood gas, serum glucose and electrolytes, complete blood count, and drug screens. As soon as these tests have been initiated, the patient should be given a standard idiopathic coma "cocktail," including intravenous administration of 100 mg of thiamine, 50 cc of 50 percent glucose, as well as 2 mg of naloxone (Narcan) if there is a clinical suspicion or physical evidence of narcotic overdose.

All adolescent or older patients should have a blood alcohol level, as well as a screen for abused substances, which together are related to half of near-drownings.

Management of Specific Conditions

Central Nervous System Support

Hypoxic damage is the major morbid or lethal event. The intensivist can do little to reverse severe damage though attention to maintenance of oxygenation will prevent further brain hypoxia. One should assure a reasonable mean arterial pressure of at least 60 mm Hg, or not less than a 25 percent reduction from the reasonably estimated preaccident mean arterial pressure for hypertensive patients. Hypertension consisting of a mean arterial pressure of greater than 120 mm Hg should be avoided except in patients known to have been severely hypertensive before near-drowning, and hypertension should certainly not be induced. Transiently popular brain "resuscitation" measures—including intracerebral monitoring, steroids, hypothermia, and empiric hyperventilation—have not been supported in subsequent randomized clinical trials and are not recommended.

Hypothermia

This is usually mild (i.e., core temperature greater than 34 °C), and therapy with a heated blanket or bed pad and warmed intravenous fluids will suffice. Hypothermia may rarely be severe and will require heated humidified ventilation, peritoneal dialysis, thoracotomy for irrigation of the heart with warm fluids, or extracorporeal partial bypass as discussed further in the chapter on "Hypothermia and Hyperthermia."

Physical manipulations of hypothermic patients may induce ventricular fibrillation, including endotracheal intubation, Swan-Ganz catheter insertion, or pacemaker placement; however, such measures should be instituted based on usual indications. Ventricular fibrillation can usually be successfully treated when the core temperature exceeds 29 °C. Metabolism of most drugs will be unpredictably reduced; hence caution with maintenance infusions and frequent use of serum levels are appropriate.

Pulmonary Sequelae

Initial alveolar flooding is managed by frequent suctioning. Bronchospasm is usually transient and responds to two 90-μg albuterol inhalations every 4 hours. Continuous positive airway pressure is administered by either close-fitting mask (for patients who can tolerate it) or PEEP by endotracheal tube, for usual respiratory failure indications as elaborated in the chapter "Adult Respiratory Distress Syndrome." It is not known whether simple interventions such as incentive spirometry or blow bottles are effective for victims of near-drowning, although they can be tried and continued if there is evidence of benefit from symptoms or mixed venous oxygen saturation.

Hypotension

A central venous pressure (CVP) line should be inserted in patients who fail to show rapid respiratory improvement, require PEEP, remain hypotensive despite vigorous volume resuscitation, or who become oliguric despite aggressive volume challenges. If the CVP indicates that volume resuscitation has been adequate (i.e., is 8 to 12 cm H_2O) and the preceding conditions persist or require vasopressor or inotropic support, the CVP should be converted to a flotation-tipped pulmonary artery (Swan-Ganz) catheter. Since this possibility exists for all unstable near-drowning victims, the preferred site for CVP insertion is the right internal jugular vein, followed by right subclavian or left internal jugular sites and, only if these are unobtainable, the femoral vein.

Acidosis

Metabolic or mixed acidosis is usually transient and responds to optimization of intravascular volume and oxygenation. Severe metabolic acidosis with pH less than 7.2 is best managed by induction of a compensatory iatrogenic respiratory alkalosis rather than bicarbonate therapy, until general supportive measures alleviate anaerobic metabolism.

Prophylactic Measures

For patients who remain in the ICU, standard nursing measures such as turning every 2 hours and airway management are needed. In addition, stress ulcer prophylaxis with a histamine$_2$-receptor blocker or sucralfate, and deep venous thrombosis prophylaxis with sequential compression stockings or minidose heparin should be instituted for most patients who are free of contraindications for specific prophylactic regimens. Although Simcock recommends prophylactic antibiotics (ampicillin or trimethoprim-sulfamethoxazole), I do not, except in cases where brackish or filthy water has been aspirated.

General Recommendations

The arterial oxygen saturation should be maintained at greater than 90 percent, the pH between 7.3 and 7.6 and PaCO$_2$ between 25 and 35 mm Hg. The intravenous fluid of choice is a balanced crystalloid solution, initially without dextrose or potassium, either of which can be added if abnormally low during surveillance testing. Hypervolemia should be judiciously avoided.

Seizures may be subclinical; therefore prolonged coma must be evaluated by electroencephalography, in addition to the immediate measures discussed under "Admission and Initial Management Guidelines." Phenytoin prophylaxis of seizures—including a loading dose of 1 g by pump-controlled intravenous piggyback administration at a rate not to exceed 50 mg per minute (i.e., administer over at least 20 minutes)—is probably desirable after resuscitation. Measures with experimental promise but unproven clinical benefit are not encouraged except in controlled clinical trials, including calcium-channel blockers, prostaglandin inhibitors, free radical inhibition, and hemodilution.

Associated Injuries and Conditions

For salt-water victims, serum sodium and chloride are expected to rise. Although these patients usually return to normal without specific treatment, occasionally severe hypernatremia (serum sodium greater than 160) or hyperchloremic acidosis (serum chloride greater than 115, with pH less than 7.2) require aggressive diuresis, intravenous fluid adjustment, and consideration of dialysis. Electrolyte changes are usually negligible for fresh-water victims. Critically dangerous elevations of magnesium and calcium occur in Dead Sea near-drowning victims, for which hemodialysis may be lifesaving.

Multiple trauma—particularly closed-head, cervical spine, and musculoskeletal injuries, as well as alcohol and substance abuse—are common in nearly drowned patients, may be clinically occult, and therefore require appropriate consideration or evaluation.

COMPLICATIONS AND LONG-TERM MANAGEMENT

Standard brain injury management includes aggressive prevention of decubitus ulcers and attention to expeditious removal of invasive appliances, particularly bladder catheters, central lines, nasal tubes, and the endotracheal tube. Nutrition is maintained with a high-protein solution, by the enteral route whenever feasible.

Late pulmonary complications include the adult respiratory distress syndrome (ARDS), aspiration pneumonia, near-drowning-related pneumonia (specifically with *Francisella philomiragia* [formerly *Yersinia philomiragia*] or *Legionella pneumophilia*), atelectasis, and pulmonary edema. Patients with good initial arteriolar-alveolar gradients and chest radiographs may show critical worsening due to any of these possibilities during 24 hours following admission, and hence require close observation. Delayed gastrointestinal complications may occur following ingestion of pathogens.

"Secondary" Drowning

"Secondary" drowning is a controversial term referring to the phenomenon of recurrent respiratory failure 6 to 24 hours following successful initial resuscitation. Secondary drowning is indistinguishable from ARDS and the related differential diagnostic conditions that must be excluded and should be managed as such, with particular attention to evaluation of treatable pathogens and specific pulmonary disorders.

OUTCOME AND PROGNOSIS

Neurologic outcome can be excellent for adults who have been immersed in *cold* water for up to 40 minutes. For the four groups described under "Admission and Initial Management Recommendations" above, the prognosis is as in Table 1. Neurologic outcome was normal for

Table 1 Number of Survivors by Simcock's Classification*

Group	Number of Patients	Survivors
1	53	53
2	50	49
3	8	6
4	10	1

*Republished with permission from Simcock AD. Treatment of near drowning: a review of 130 cases. Anaesthesia 1986; 41:643.

all survivors in Simcock's series. Other series report less favorable neurologic outcomes. It is not clear whether near-drowning survivors have a better prognosis than the unfortunate 50 percent of cardiac resuscitation survivors who sustain permanent neurologic impairment.

SUGGESTED READING

Modell JH. Treatment of near-drowning: is there a role for H.Y.P.E.R. therapy? Crit Care Med 1986; 14:593–595.
Pearn J. The management of near drowning. Br Med J 1985; 291:1447–1452.
Simcock AD. Treatment of near drowning: a review of 130 cases. Anaesthesia 1986; 41:643–648.
Standards and guidelines for cardiopulmonary resuscitation (CPR) and emergency cardiac care (ECC). JAMA 1986; 255:2905–3104.
Zell SC, Kurtz KJ. Severe exposure hypothermia: a resuscitation protocol. Ann Emerg Med 1985; 14:339–345.

APPROACH TO TOXICOLOGY

JERROLD B. LEIKIN, M.D.
PAUL K. HANASHIRO, M.D.

Peter Mere Latham (1789–1875) is credited with the statement, "Poisons and medicines are oftentimes the same substance given with different intents." While this remark was penned in a bygone era, it is probably more true today than it was then. For confirmation of this fact, one can open any clinical pharmacology textbook (or even the *Physician's Desk Reference*) and see therapeutics that can lead to specific toxic syndromes or abuse when used with varying intents or dosage. In this way, there are few fields in medicine that demand such immediate, decisive, and definitive treatment strategy with as small an information base as in the area of toxicologic emergencies. Despite the potential for the wide range of clinical presentations due to a virtually unlimited amount of toxins, less than 0.05 percent of all poison exposures called into a Poison Control Center result in death. While this statistic may be somewhat misleading due to a biased population sample, it is still evident that if one follows a consistent treatment algorithm of the poisoned patient, the outcome will be favorable in a vast majority of cases.

This general treatment plan is not unlike general treatment plans taught in advanced cardiac life support (ACLS) or advanced trauma life support (ATLS) courses. In this manner, the initial approach to the poisoned patient should be essentially similar in every case, irrespective of the toxin ingested, just as the initial approach to the trauma patient is the same irrespective of the mechanism of injury. This approach, which can be termed as routine poison management, essentially includes the following aspects:

1. Stabilization: ABCs (airway, breathing, circulation).
2. History, physical examination leading toward the identification of class of toxin (toxic syndrome recognition).
3. Prevention of absorption (decontamination).
4. Specific antidote, if available.
5. Removal of absorbed toxin (enhancing excretion).
6. Support and monitoring for adverse effects.

STABILIZATION OF THE PATIENT

While the evaluation of the patient's airway, breathing and circulatory status has been discussed in a previous chapter, certain concepts must be considered when approaching the toxic patient. For example, the treating physician must remember that the most common cause of airway obstruction in the unconscious patient is passive obstruction by the tongue. In this way, the neck lift with jaw thrust may be the first maneuver performed by the physician on the unconscious poisoned patient followed by endotracheal intubation. Indications for endotracheal intubation in the poisoned patient include (1) protection of the airway in the obtunded or comatose patient with a depressed or absent gag reflex to prevent aspiration during gastric lavage, (2) controlled ventilation in patients who demonstrate respiratory depression or failure, (3) removal of secretions in patients who develop pulmonary edema secondary to a toxic substance, and (4) institution of positive end-expiratory pressure therapy (PEEP) for those patients who are at risk for developing adult respiratory distress syndrome (ARDS). A chest film is required to note the position of the endotracheal tube.

Following evaluation of airway and breathing, the circulatory status needs to be assessed. Hypotension in the toxic patient must be addressed as quickly as possible in order to avoid the sequelae of shock. While hypotension in this group of patients may arise from a variety of mechanisms (ranging from decreased cardiac output due to myocardial depression; to venous pooling; to decreased peripheral resistance or to hemorrhage), the initial treatment is essentially the same: intravenous fluid administration. A fluid challenge of 100 to 200 ml of a crystalloid solution is often given at this time while urine output is monitored (0.5 to 1 ml per kilogram per hour).

At this time, if the patient's mental status is altered or if hypotension exists, four essentially innocuous drugs are administered for a combination of diagnostic and therapeutic reasons:

1. 50 g of dextrose intravenously to reverse the effects of drug-induced hypoglycemia: This can be especially effective in those patients with limited glycogen stores (i.e., neonates and patients with cirrhosis). While caution should exist with regard to extravasation of this hyperosmolar solution (causing Volkmann's contractures), the adverse metabolic effects are minimal and easily controlled.
2. 50 to 100 mg of intravenous thiamine to prevent Wernicke's encephalopathy: Groups at risk for this complication include the chronic alcoholic patient, malnourished individuals (including those on weight-reduction programs), septic individuals, and patients on hemodialysis.
3. Naloxone, a specific opiate antagonist: Initial dosage should be 2.0 mg in adult patients preferably by the intravenous route, although intramuscular, subcutaneous, and intratracheal routes may also be utilized. It should be noted that some semisynthetic opiates (such as meperidine or propoxyphene) may require higher initial doses for reversal, so that a total dose of 6 to 10 mg is not unusual (Table 1).

    If the patient responds to a bolus dose and then relapses to a lethargic or comatose state, a naloxone drip can be considered. This can be accomplished by administering two-thirds of the bolus dose that revives the patient per hour or injecting 4 mg of naloxone in one liter of crystalloid solution and administering at a rate of 100 cc per hour (0.4 mg per hour).
4. Oxygen, utilized in 100 percent concentration: While oxygen is antidotal for carbon monoxide intoxication, the only minor relative toxic contraindication is in paraquat intoxication (in that it can promote pulmonary fibrosis).

Table 1 Agents for Which Naloxone Has Been Shown to be Effective

Effectiveness Well Established
 Alphaprodine
 Anileridine
 Apomorphine-induced emesis
 Butorphanol
 Codeine
 Cyclazocine
 Diphenoxylate
 Fentanyl
 Heroin
 Hydromorphine
 Levallorphan
 Levorphanol
 Meperidine
 Methadone
 Morphine
 Nalbuphine
 Nalorphine
 Opium
 Oxymorphone
 Pentazocine
 Propoxyphene

Effectiveness Questionable
 Alcohol
 Diazepam
 Clonidine
 Valproic Acid
 Captopril
 Guanabenz
 Guanfacine

*Adapted from Bryson PD, ed. Comprehensive review in toxicology. 2nd ed. Rockville, MD: Aspen, 1989; *and* Rumack BH, Spoerke DS, eds. Poisindex information system. Denver: Micromedex, 1990.

HISTORY AND PHYSICAL EXAMINATION

While the history and physical examination is the cornerstone of clinical patient management, it takes on special meaning with regard to the toxic patient. While taking a history may be a more direct method of the determination of the toxin, quite often it is not reliable. Information obtained may prove minimal in some cases and could be considered partial or inaccurate in suicide gestures and addicts. A quick physical examination often leads to important clues about the nature of the toxin. These clues can be specific symptom complexes associated with certain toxins and can be referred to as "toxidromes."

Sensorium. Determine whether the patient is comatose, stuporous, lethargic, or alert.

Behavior and Hallucinations. Often the hallucinatory pattern of the patient can be specific for certain drugs. For example, with atropine the patient experiences lilliputian hallucinations; with cocaine, there is a simple visual hallucinatory pattern with objects appearing in the periphery of vision; with phencyclidine, complex hallucinations are often indistinguishable clinically from a paranoid psychosis; and with LSD, the patient experiences a combination of illusions, hallucinations, and pseudohallucinations.

Motor Signs. Tremors, hypo- and hyper-reflexes, and even the nature of seizures can be useful diagnostic tools. Like hallucinations, seizures caused by specific toxins can exhibit certain specific properties. For example, strychnine is unique in that it can cause generalized seizures while the patient is alert. This can be referred to as a spinal seizure. Other drug-induced seizures will respond only to specific antidotal therapies and not to conventional antiseizure medication. Examples of this property include antichlolinergic-induced seizures, which respond to physostigmine, and isoniazid-induced seizures, which respond to pyridoxine. Additionally, theophylline-induced seizures rarely respond to phenytoin and often only to multidrug therapy.

Vital Signs. Sympathomimetics and anticholinergics essentially cause an increase in all of the vital signs parameters. This is particularly true for cocaine intoxication, where it has been noted that hyperthermia may be a particularly ominous sign for mortality. Additionally, organophosphates, opiates, barbiturates, and clonidine toxicities result in hypothermia, respiratory depression, and bradycardia.

Ocular Findings. This can be divided into two categories: pupillary size and reactivity, and demonstration of nystagmus.

Pupillary Signs. Both atropine and cocaine can result in mydriasis, but in cocaine intoxication the pupils will respond to light, whereas with anticholinergics the pupils will not. Agents that contribute to miosis include organophosphate insecticides, narcotics, bromide, clonidine, and nicotine. Phencyclidine has been known to cause either mydriasis or miosis.

Nystagmus. Alcohols are probably the most common etiology of horizontal nystagmus, although lithium, carbamazepine, solvents, meprobamate, quinine, and primidone can also result in horizontal nystagmus. Phencyclidine can cause a combination of vertical, horizontal, and even rotary nystagmus, as can phenytoin and sedative-hypnotics.

In addition to these physical signs, odors emanating from the patient may also provide important directions in management. For example, a garlic odor is often caused by arsenicals, phosphorus compounds, and organophosphates.

Radiographs can be of some utility in toxic exposure analysis. Factors that influence radiodensity include molecular weight, atomic number, relative contrast to surrounding tissues, and compactness of the form of drug. It should be pointed out that this is not a reliable method for evaluating toxic exposure and should be utilized in only specific cases. These cases include evaluation of heavy metal exposure (including leaded paint chips), concretion formation of drugs (such as aspirin, meprobamate, iron, and theophylline), and the body packing/stuffing phenomenon.

The clinical laboratory evaluation includes the evaluation of the "three gaps of toxicology": anion gap, osmolar gap, and oxygen saturation gap. What these "gaps" have in common is that a substance is accounting for a difference between calculated and measured determination. Drugs known to cause these gaps are listed in Table 2.

PREVENTION OF ABSORPTION

Toxic substances can enter the body through the derma, ocular, pulmonary, parenteral, and gastrointestinal routes. The basic principle of decontamination involves appropriate copious irrigation of the toxic substance relatable to the route of exposure. For example, with ocular exposure, this can be done with normal saline for 30 to 40 minutes through a Morgan therapeutic lens. With alkali exposures, the pH should be checked until the runoff of the solution is either neutral or slightly acidic. Skin decontamination involves removal of the toxin with nonabrasive soap. This should be especially considered for organophosphates, methylene chloride, dioxin, radiation, hydrocarbons, and herbicide exposures. Separate drainage areas should be obtained for the contaminated runoff.

Since more than 80 percent of incidents of accidental poisoning in children occur through the gastrointestinal

Table 2 Drugs and Toxins Causing "Three Gaps of Toxicology"

Anion Gap (greater than 12 mEq/L)
  Nonacidotic
    Carbenicillin
    Sodium salts
  Metabolic Acidosis

Methanol	Carbon monoxide	Phenformin (off the market)
Toluene	Hydrogen sulfide	Ibuprofen (ingestion >300 mg/kg)
Vacor	Isoniazid	Nalidixic acid
Ethylene glycol	Iron	Propylene glycol
Paraldehyde	Cyanide	Papaverine
Ethanol	Salicylates	Tetracycline (outdated)
Acetaminophen (ingestion of greater than 75 to 100 g)	Strychnine	Iodine Phenylbutazone Formaldehyde Sorbitol (IV)

Osomolar Gap (by Freezing-Point Depression, gap is greater than 10 mOsm)
  Methanol   Mannitol
  Ethanol   Sorbitol
  Ethylene glycol   Glycerol
  Isopranol (acetone)   Hypermagnesemia (greater than 9.5 mEq/L)
  Iodine (questionable)

Oxygen Saturation Gap (Greater than 5% difference between measured and calculated value)
  Carbon monoxide
  Hydrogen sulfide (possible)
  Methemoglobin
  Cyanide (questionable)

tract, a thorough knowledge of gastric decontamination is essential. Essentially, there are three modes of gastric decontamination, of which two are physical removal (emesis and gastric lavage). Activated charcoal associated with a cathartic is the third mode for preventing absorption.

Emesis. Emesis by means of syrup of ipecac (a derivative of the plant alkaloid emetine) has been one of the standards of gastric decontamination. Utilized at a dose of 30 ml accompanied with 16 oz of fluid for adults (repeated in 20 minutes if no emesis), 15 ml in children 1 to 12 years of age accompanied with 8 oz of fluid, or 10 ml in infants 6 to 12 months of age with 4 oz of fluid, it is virtually 100 percent effective in producing emesis. However, it is apparent that a 100 percent rate of emesis is not equatable to a 100 percent rate of removal of toxin. In the best of circumstances, only about a 30 to 40 percent removal rate can be achieved within 1 to 2 hours postingestion, although significantly higher removal rates can be achieved if emesis is obtained within 30 minutes postingestion. For this reason, while ipecac may be quite useful for home use (when administered in consultation with the appropriate health professional), its use as a method of gastric decontamination in the hospital setting is decreasing.

Gastric Lavage. Gastric lavage through a 28- to 40-French Ewald tube is the second mode of physical removal of the ingested toxin. With the patient in the left lateral decubitus position, feet elevated 15 degrees, approximately 200 to 300 ml of saline is lavaged per run (10 to 15 ml per kilogram in children), with an additional 1 to 2 L used for irrigation after clearing. As with ipecac, an approximate 30 to 40 percent removal rate can be achieved. The contraindications to both of these methods are ingestion of caustic material, hydrocarbons, hemorrhagic diathesis, and seizures. Patients with altered mental status should never be given ipecac, and lavage should only be considered with the presence of a cuffed endotracheal tube if the gag reflex is not present. The use of salt water, detergents, apomorphine, copper sulfate, and physical induction of emesis should be confined to the medical history books.

Activated Charcoal. The use of activated charcoal has had a resurgence over the past 10 years, with several studies comparing it favorably to the other forms of physical gastric decontamination. As an inert, nontoxic adsorbent with a surface area as high as 300 m^2 per gram, it is quite effective in binding high molecular weight compounds due to intermolecular attractions (van der Waals forces). The dose of activated charcoal is 1 gram per kilogram, and it can be instilled through a Ewald tube. While children may not want to drink activated charcoal because it is black and gritty, mixing it with juice may bring a higher acceptance rate. Tablets of activated charcoal should not be utilized for gastric decontamination.

Activated charcoal is usually administered in conjunction with a cathartic to facilitate evacuation of the toxic substance. Cathartics most often administered are magnesium sulfate (15 to 20 g in a 10 percent solution), magnesium citrate (200 to 300 ml), sodium sulfate or sorbitol (100 to 150 ml in a 70 percent solution, or 1 to 2 ml per kilogram in pediatric patients). Cathartics should not be utilized in the presence of ileus. Additionally, recent reports of hypermagnesemia in the setting of magnesium-containing cathartic administration with renal insufficiency, and diarrhea with emesis associated with increasing amounts of sorbitol, indicate that cathartics are not a benign medication.

Whole bowel irrigation with the use of GoLYTELY has been advocated for certain intoxications, but it can be quite impractical and is not recommended for routine use.

ANTIDOTES

One can use as a definition of an antidote that of any drug that increases the median lethal dose (LD$_{50}$) of a toxin. While certain drugs may modify symptoms produced by a toxin (i.e., beta-blockers reducing heart rate in cocaine intoxication) only a relatively few toxins have specific antidotes. Table 3 lists some of these antidotes that are commonly utilized.

ENHANCEMENT OF ELIMINATION

It was only until recently that this aspect of poison management has received more than cursory attention in practice and in the literature. The standard practice for enhancement of elimination consisted primarily of forced diuresis in order to excrete the toxin.

However, the past 10-years' experience has produced a radical change in the approach to this and therefore a more focused methodology to eliminating absorbed toxins. Essentially, there are three methods by which absorbed toxins may be eliminated: recurrent adsorption with multiple dosings of activated charcoal, use of forced diuresis in combination with possible alkalinization of the urine, and use of dialysis or charcoal hemoperfusion.

Recently, multiple dosing of activated charcoal ("pulse dosing") has been advocated as a method for removal of absorbed drug. This procedure has been demonstrated to be efficacious in drugs that re-enter the gastrointestinal tract through enterohepatic circulation (i.e., digitoxin, carbamazepine, glutethimide) and with drugs that diffuse from the systemic circulation into the gastrointestinal tract due to formation of a concentration gradient (the "infinite sink" hypothesis). Essentially this can be thought of as "gastric dialysis." The toxins by which this method appears to be most efficacious are those with low volume of distribution (less than 1.0 L per kilogram), uncharged, lipophilic, low protein-binding and undergo enterohepatic circulation (although the latter property is not essential). Note that these are the same criteria required for a toxin to be removed by hemoperfusion.

Despite these above limitations, multiple dosing of activated charcoal is utilized quite often. The literature has demonstrated that only chlorpropamide clearance is not enhanced and the data on imipramine, phenytoin, and salicylates are somewhat equivocal due primarily to their high protein-binding.

Text continues on page 326

Table 3 Poison Control Center Antidote Chart*

Antidote	Poison/Drug	Indications	Dosage	Comments
Acetylcysteine (Mucomyst)	Acetaminophen	1. Unknown quantity ingested and <24 hours has elapsed since the time of ingestion or unable to obtain serum acetaminophen levels within 12 hours of ingestion. 2. Greater than 7.5 g of acetaminophen acutely ingested. 3. Serum acetaminophen level greater than 140 μg/ml at 4 hours post ingestion. 4. Ingested dose >140 mg/kg.	Dilute to 5% solution with carbonated beverage, fruit juice or water, administer orally *Loading:* 140 mg/kg one dose *Maintenance:* 70 mg/kg for 17 doses, starting 4 hours after the loading dose and given every 4 hours thereafter unless assay reveals a nontoxic serum level.	SGOT, SGPT, bilirubin, prothrombin time, creatinine, BUN, blood sugar, and electrolytes should be obtained daily if a toxic serum acetaminophen level has been determined *Note:* Activated charcoal has been shown to absorb acetylcysteine in vitro and may do so in patients. Serum acetaminophen levels may not peak until 4 hours postingestion, and therefore serum levels should not be drawn earlier.
Amyl nitrate, sodium nitrate, sodium thiosulfate (Cyanide Antidote Package)	Cyanide	Begin treatment at the first sign of toxicity if exposure is known or strongly suspected.	Break ampule of amyl nitrate and allow patient to inhale for 15 sec., then take away for 15 sec.; use a fresh ampule every 3 min. Continue until injection of sodium nitrate 300 mg can be injected at 2.5–5 ml/min. Then immediately inject 12.5 g of 25% sodium thiosulfate, slow IV.	If symptoms return, treatment may be repeated at half the normal dosages. For pediatric dosing see package insert. Do NOT use methylene blue to reduce elevated methemoglobin levels. Oxygen therapy may be useful when combined with sodium thiosulfate therapy.
Atropine	Organophosphate and carbamate insecticides	Myoclonic seizures, severe hallucations, weakness, arrhythmias, excessive salivation, involuntary urination and defecation.	*Adult:* 2 mg IV *Child:* 0.05 mg/kg IV Repeat dosage every 10 min. until patient is atropinized (normal pulse, diluted pupils, absence of rates dry mouth)	Caution should be used in patients with narrow angle glaucoma, cardiovascular disease, or pregnancy. Plasma and erythrocyte cholinesterase levels will be depressed from normal. Atropine should only be used when indicated otherwise use may result in anticholinergic poisoning.
	Digoxin	Bradyarrhythmias, heart block.	*Adult:* 0.6 mg/dose IV. *Child:* 10–30 μg/kg/dose up to 0.4 mg/dose IV.	
Calcium EDTA (Calcium disodium versenate)	Lead	Symptomatic patients or asymptomatic children with blood levels >50 μg/dl.	50–75 mg/kg/day deep IM or slow IV infusion in 3 to 6 divided doses for up to 5 days.	If urine flow is not established, hemodialysis must accompany calcium EDTA dosing. In most cases, the IM route is preferred.
Calcium gluconate	Hydrofluoric acid	Calcium gluconate gel 2.5% for dermal exposures of HF of <20% conc. SC injections of calcium gluconate for dermal exposures of HF in >20% conc. or failure to respond to calcium gluconate gel.	Massage 2.5% gel into exposed area for 15 min. Infiltrate each square centimeter of exposed area with 0.5 ml of 10% calcium gluconate SC using a 30 gauge needle.	Injections of calcium gluconate should not be used in digital area. With exposures to dilute concentrations of HF, symptoms may take several hours to develop. Calcium gluconate gel is not currently available. Contact your regional poison control center for compounding instructions.

Table 3 Continued

Antidote	Poison/Drug	Indications	Dosage	Comments
Deferoxamine (Desferal)	Iron	SI level exceeds TIBC. SI >350 μg/dl and TIBC is unavailable Inability to obtain SI in a reasonable time and patient is symptomatic.	*Mild Symptoms:* 90 mg/kg IM up to 1 g every 48 hours. *Symptoms:* 10–15 mg/kg/hr IV, not to exceed 6 g in 24 hours.	Passing of Vin Rosè-colored urine indicates free iron was present. Therapy should be discontinued when urine returns to normal color. Monitor for hypotension, especially when giving deferoxamine IV.
Digoxin immune fab (Ovine) (Digibind)	Digoxin	Life-threatening cardiac arrhythmias progressive bradyarrythmias, 2nd- or 3rd-degree heart block unresponsive to atropine, serum digitoxin level >10 mg/ml or potassium levels >5 mEq/L.	Multiply serum digitoxin concentration by 5.6 and multiply the result by the patient's weight in kilograms, divide this by 1,000 and divide the result by 0.6. This gives the dose in number of vials to use. For other dosing methods, see package insert.	Monitor K levels, continuous ECG. *Note:* Digibind interferes with free serum digitoxin levels.
Dimercaprol (BAL in oil)	Arsenic, lead, mercury	Any symptoms due to arsenic exposure. All patients with symptoms or asymptomatic children with blood levels >70 μg/dl. Any symptoms due to mercury and patient unable to take D-penicillamine.	3–5 mg/kg/dose deep IM every 4 hours until GI symptoms subside and patient switched to D-penicillamine. 3–5 mg/kg/dose deep IM every 4 hours for 2 days then every 4–12 hours for up to 7 additional days. 3–5 mg/kg/dose deep IM every 4 hours for 48 hours, then 3 mg/kg/dose every 6 hours, then 3 mg/kg/dose every 12 hours for 7 more days.	Patients receiving dimercaprol should be monitored for hypertension, tachycardia, hyperpyrexia and urticana. Used in conjunction with calcium EDTA in lead poisoning.
Ethanol	Ethylene glycol or methanol	Ethylene glycol or methanol blood levels >20 mg/dl. Blood levels not readily available and suspected ingestion of toxic amounts. Any symptomatic patient with a history of ethylene glycol or methanol ingestion.	*Loading Dose:* 7.6–10 ml/kg IV ethanol in D5W over 1 hour. *Maintenance Dose:* 1.4 ml/kg/hr IV of 10% ethanol in D5W. Maintain blood ethanol level of 100-130 mg/dL.	Monitor blood glucose, especially in children, as ethanol may cause hypoglycemia. Do not use 5% ethanol in D_5W, as excessive amounts of fluid would be required to maintain adequate ethanol blood levels. If dialysis is performed, adjustment of ethanol dosing is required.
Naloxone (Narcan)	Opiates (e.g., heroin, morphine, codeine)	Coma or respiratory depression from unknown cause or from opiate overdose.	Give 0.4–2.0 mg IV bolus. Doses may be repeated if there is no response, up to 10 mg.	For prolonged intoxication, a continuous infusion may be used. See package insert for details.
D-penicillamine (Cuprimine)	Arsenic, lead, mercury	Following BAL therapy in symptomatic acutely poisoned patients. Asymptomatic patients with excess lead burden. Patient symptomatic from mercury exposure or excessive levels.	100 mg/kg/day up to 2 g in 4 divided doses for 5 days. 1–2 g/day in 4 divided doses for 5 days. *Adult:* 250 mg PO four times daily. *Child:* 100 mg/kg/day up to 1 g daily in 4 divided doses. Given for 3–10 days.	Possible contraindication for patients with penicillin allergy. Monitor heavy metal levels daily in severely poisoned patients. Monitor CBC and renal function in patients receiving chronic D-penicillian therapy. Dosages given are for short-term acute therapy only.

Table continues on the following page

Table 3 *Continued*

Antidote	Poison/Drug	Indications	Dosage	Comments
Physostigmine salicylate (Antilirium)	Atrophy and anticholinergic agents, cyclic antidepressants	Myoclonic seizures, hypertension, severe arrhythmias, halucinations. Refractory seizures or arrhythmias unresponsive to conventional therapies.	*Adult:* 0.5–2 mg slow IV push. *Child:* 0.5 mg slow IV slow push. Repeat as requires for life threatening symptoms. Same as above	Dramatic reversal of anticholinergic symptoms after IV use. Should not be used just to keep patient awake. *Contraindications:* asthma, gangrene, physostigmine use in cyclic antidepressant-induced cardiac toxicity is controversial. *Extreme* caution is advised — should be considered only in the presence of marked anticholinergic symptoms.
Pralidoxime (2-Pam, Protopam)	Organophosphate Insecticides	An adjunct to atropine therapy for treatment of profound muscle weakness, respiratory depression, muscle twitching.	*Adult:* 2 g IV at 0.5 g/min. or infused in 250 ml N.S. over 30 min. *Child:* 25–50 mg/kg in 250 ml saline over 30 min.	Most effective when used in initial 24–36 hours after the exposure. Dosage may be repeated in 1 hour followed by every 8 hours if indicated.
Pyridoxine (Vitamin B_6)	Isoniazid	Unknown overdose or ingested amount >80 mg/kg.	Pyridoxine IV in the amount of INH ingested or 5 g if amount is unknown given over 30–60 minutes.	Cumulative dose of pyridoxine is arbitrarily limited to 40 g in adults and 20 g in children.
Vitamin K_1/Phytonadione	Warfarin	Large acute ingestion of warfarin rodenticides. Chronic exposure or greater than normal prothrombin time.	*Adult:* 10 mg IM *Child:* 1–5 mg IM With severe toxicity, vitamin K_1 may be given IV.	Vitamin K therapy is contraindicated for patients with prosthetic heart valves unless toxicity is life-threatening.
Antivenin (cortalidae) polyvalent (equine origin)	Pit viper bites (rattlesnakes, cottonmouths, copperheads)	Mild, moderate or severe symptoms and history of envenomation by a pit viper. *Mild:* Local swelling (progressive) pain, no systemic systems. *Moderate:* Ecchymosis and swelling beyond the bite site, some systemic symptoms and/or lab changes. *Severe:* Profound edema involving entire extremity, cyanosis, serious systemic involvement, significant lab changes.	*Mild:* 3–5 vials of antivenin in 250–500 ml of N.S. *Moderate:* 6–10 vials of antivenin in 500 ml of N.S. *Severe:* Minimum of 10 vials in 500 to 1,000 ml of N.S. Administer over 4–6 hours. Additional antivenin should be given on the basis of clinical response and continuing assessment of severity of the poisoning.	Draw blood for type and cross-match, hematocrit, BUN, electrolytes, CBC, platelets, coagulation profile. DO NOT administer heparin for possible allergic reaction. A tetanus shot should also be given.

CBC = complete blood count; D_5W = 5 percent dextrose in water; EDTA = ethylenediaminetetra-acetic acid; HF =c hydrofluoric acid; INH = isoniazide; N.S. = normal saline; SI = serum iron.
*Published with permission from the Rush Poison Control Center, Rush-Presbyterian-St. Luke's Medical Center, Chicago, IL.

Overall, substantial decreases in half-life in the range of 40 to 60 percent have been demonstrated with various compounds. Although the reduction in half-life is impressive for many toxins, it should be noted that the sole case-control study utilizing multiple dosing of activated charcoal failed to demonstrate any clinical improvement in 10 patients with barbiturate toxicity.

The usual dosage of activated charcoal is 1 g per kilogram as the initial dose, followed by 0.5 g per kilogram every 2 to 4 hours. Cathartics should not be administered more than once daily.

The practice of blindly overloading the toxic patient with intravenous fluids to promote diuresis has not been supported in the literature and carries with it the risk of pulmonary edema, hyponatremia, and increased intracranial pressure. The use of this modality (with or without ion trapping) should be limited to certain specific drugs (Table 4). Alkalinization can be achieved by administration of 44 to 88 mEq of sodium bicarbonate per liter to titrate a urine pH of 7.5. The practice of acidifying the urine should be discouraged in that it can produce metabolic acidosis and promote renal failure in the presence of rhabdomyolysis.

Hemodialysis can be utilized to increase clearance with certain drugs (see Table 4). It is especially effective in correcting metabolic acidosis induced by certain toxins such as salicylates. Drugs in which hemodialysis is required at an early stage include methanol and ethylene glycol.

Charcoal hemoperfusion can increase clearances of toxins that are absorbed by an absorbent. Unlike hemodialysis, drug clearance through hemoperfusion is less de-

Table 4 Methods of Enhancement of Elimination

Agent	Multiple Dosing Activated Charcoal	Forced Saline Diuresis	Alkaline Diuresis	Hemodialysis	Hemoperfusion
Amitriptyline	X				X
Amphetamine				X	
Amoxapine	X				
Arsenic					
Baclofen	X (?)				
Benzodiazepines	X (?)				
Boric acid					
Bromides		X		X	
Camphor					X
Carbamazepine	X				
Carbon tetrachloride					X (?)
Carisoprodol				X	
Chloral Hydrate				X	X
Chlordecone	X				
Chromium		X		X	
Cimetidine		X (?)		X	
Dapsone	X				
Digitoxin	X				X
Digoxin	X				X
Ethanol				X	
Ethchlorvynol					X
Ethylene glycol				X	
Fluoride			X	X	
Glutethimide	X				X (?)
Isoniazid		X (?)			
Isopropanol				X	
Lindane					X
Lithium		X		X	
Maprotiline	X				
Meprobamate	X				
Methanol				X	
Methaqualone					X
Methotrexate	X			X	X
Methyprylon	X			X	X
Nadolol	X				
Nortriptyline	X				
Paraquat					X
Phencyclidine	X				
Phenobarbital	X		X	X	X
Phenylbutazone	X				
Phenytoin	X (?)				
Primidone			X		
Procainamide				X	
Quinidine				X	
Salicylates	X			X	
Strychnine				X	
Theophylline	X			X	X
2, 4-D: chlorophenoxyacetic acid			X		

Table 5 Criteria for Admission of the Poisoned Patient to ICU

Respiratory depression (PCO$_2$ > 45 mm Hg)
Emergency intubation
Seizures
Cardiac Arrhythmia
Hypotension (systolic blood pressure < 80 mm Hg)
Unresponsiveness to verbal stimuli
Second- or third-degree atrioventricular block
Emergent dialysis or hemoperfusion
Increasing metabolic acidosis
Tricyclic or phenothiazine overdose manifesting anticholinergic signs, neurologic abnormality, *or* QRS duration > 0.12 second
Administration of pralidoxime in organophosphate toxicity
Pulmonary edema induced by drugs or toxic inhalation (ARDS)
Drug-induced hypothermia or hyperthermia including neuroleptic malignant syndrome
Hyperkalemia secondary to digitalis overdose
Body packers and stuffers
Concretions secondary to drugs
Emergent surgical intervention
Antivenom administration in *Crotalidae* envenomation.

*Adapted from Kulling P, Persson H. Role of the intensive care unit in the management of the poisoned patient. Med Toxicol 1986; 1: 375–386; *and* Brett AS, Rothschild N, Gray R, Perry R, Perry M. Predicting the clinical course in intentional drug overdose: implication for use of the intensive care unit. Arch Intern Med 1987; 147: 133–137; *and* Callaham M. Admission criteria for tricyclic antidepressant ingestion. West J Med 1982; 137: 425–429.

pendent on water solubility. Complications of hemoperfusion include thrombocytopenia, hypotension, hypocalcemia, and infection.

SUPPORT AND MONITORING FOR ADVERSE EFFECTS

This aspect of poison management is the least studied. The usual disposition of the admitted poisoned patient is an intensive care unit bed or cardiac monitored bed to evaluate the late sequelae of the toxic agent. However, the practice of admitting the poisoned patient routinely to the intensive care unit is being questioned. A recent retrospective study identified eight clinical risk factors that predicted ICU interventions: (1) arterial carbon dioxide pressure greater than or equal to 45 Hg mm, (2) need for emergency intubation, (3) seizures, (4) cardiac arrhythmia, (5) QRS duration greater than or equal to 0.12 seconds, (6) systolic blood pressure less than 80 mm Hg, (7) second- or third-degree atrioventricular block, and (8) unresponsiveness to verbal stimuli. If a toxic patient did not exhibit any of these characteristics, no ICU interventions (such as intubation, antiseizure therapy, intravenous vasopressors, antiarrhythmics, and dialysis or hemoperfusion) were performed.

Additionally, other risk factors that should be considered for ICU admission include (1) need for emergent hemodialysis or hemoperfusion, (2) increasing metabolic acidosis, and (3) any tricyclic or phenothiazine overdose manifesting anticholinergic signs of cardiac abnormalities. While many drugs (such as ibuprofen) will manifest their toxicity within 4 hours after ingestion, tricyclic overdoses are renowned for their incidence of delayed complications. It has been noted that most of these patients exhibited cardiac or neurologic abnormality prior to the delayed arrhythmia, Table 5 lists criteria for ICU admission.

SUGGESTED READING

Brett AS, Rothschild N, Gray R, Perry M. Predicting the clinical course in intentional drug overdose: implications for use of the intensive care unit. Arch Intern Med 1987; 147:133–137.
Bryson PD, ed. Comprehensive review in toxicology. 2nd ed. Rockville, MD: Aspen Publications, 1989.
Callaham M. Admission criteria for tricyclic antidepressant ingestion. West J Med 1982; 137:425–429.
Ellenhorn MJ, Barcelous DG, eds. Medical toxicology: diagnosis and treatment of human poisoning. New York: 1988.
Goldfrank LR, ed. Toxicologic emergencies. Norwalk, CT: Appleton-Century-Crofts, 1986.
Kulling P, Persson H. Role of the intensive care unit in the management of the poisoned patient. Med Toxicol 1986; 1:375–386.
Noji EK, Kelen EK, eds. Manual of toxicologic emergencies. Chicago: Year Book Medical Publishers, 1989.
Rumack BH, Spoerke DS, eds. Poisindex information system. Denver: Micromedex, Inc., edition expires 2/28/90.

HYPOTHERMIA AND HYPERTHERMIA

J. CHRISTOPHER FARMER, M.D.

Clinically significant hypothermia and hyperthermia result from acute and chronic imbalance between heat generation and heat dissipation. They are generally underrecognized conditions but nevertheless significant contributors to ICU patient morbidity and mortality. Baseline function of virtually every organ system may be impaired by either condition.

At rest, most heat is produced by energy-consuming processes of the viscera. However, with exertion, most heat is produced by skeletal muscle metabolic activity. In contrast, body heat is dissipated through conduction, convection, and/or evaporation. These processes are accomplished via sweating and cutaneous vasoreactivity. Advanced age, a variety of chronic diseases and medications, and climatic extremes adversely affect the efficiency of these normal physiologic occurrences as heat-dissipating or heat-conserving mechanisms. Advanced age also blunts normal perception and responsiveness to abnormal body temperature (e.g., shivering or voluntarily seeking a more favorable climate). Tables 1 and 2 provide a comprehensive listing of those conditions associated with accidental hypothermia and hyperthermia.

ACCIDENTAL HYPOTHERMIA

Environmental cold injury is generally considered as peripheral (frostbite) or systemic (hypothermia). Frostbite involves actual freezing of soft tissues exposed to ambient temperatures less than 0°C (32°F). Hypothermia is defined as a core body temperature of less than 35°C (95°F). Primary therapy focuses on the return of body temperature to normal. All other supportive and resuscitative therapeutic measures for hypothermia should continue until core body temperature is again normal, otherwise irreversible death may be falsely assumed.

Aggressiveness of therapy required for hypothermia is to some extent contingent on its severity. Patients with

Table 1 Conditions Associated with Accidental Hypothermia

Intact Thermoregulation
Environmental Exposure
 Outdoor activities/exhaustion
 Cold water immersion
 Inadequate indoor heating

Endocrine/Metabolic Disorders
 Hypothyroidism
 Panhypopituitarism
 Hypoglycemia
 Anorexia nervosa/malnutrition
 Hypoadrenalism

Loss of Dermal Integrity
 Burns
 Erythroderma
 Ichthyosis
 Psoriasis

Impaired Thermoregulation
Central Regulatory Failure
 Hypothalamic infarction
 Massive stroke
 Subarachnoid hemorrhage
 Head trauma
 CNS tumor
 Wernicke's encephalopathy
 Shapiro's syndrome
 Carbon monoxide poisoning
 Drugs (ethanol, phenothiazines, barbiturates, anesthetics)
 Uremia

Peripheral/Other Regulatory Disorders
 Spinal cord transection
 Advanced age
 Diabetes mellitus
 Sepsis

Table 2 Conditions Associated with Heat Stroke Syndrome

Exertional
 Extraordinary ambient temperatures/high humidity levels
 Lack of physical conditioning
 Lack of acclimatization

Nonexertional
 Extraordinary ambient temperatures/high humidity levels
 Advanced age
 Chronic diseases
  Alcoholism
  Congestive heart failure
  Renal insufficiency
  Diabetes mellitus
  Chronic obstructive pulmonary disease
  Dyshidrosis
  Previous episode of heatstroke
  Schizophrenia
  Morbid obesity
  Thyrotoxicosis
  Hypokalemia

 Drugs
  Diuretics
  Phenothiazines
  Antiparkinsonian agents
  Anticholinergic agents
  Beta-blockers
  Tricyclic antidepressants
  Amphetamines
  Butyrophenones

mild hypothermia have a core temperature between 32 and 35°C (90 and 95°F). These patients are stiff but still shivering. Level of consciousness varies from mild confusion to stupor. Vital signs are generally normal to increased but may become subnormal as the core temperature drops still further. In most instances, passive external warming techniques (e.g., wrapping the patients in an insulating blanket and allowing their own endogenous heat-generating mechanisms to rewarm them) are sufficient. Systemic complications are uncommon; the majority of these patients recover uneventfully when hypothermia is the only problem.

Moderate hypothermia is defined by a core body temperature ranging from 28 to 32°C (82 to 90°F). These patients are typically obtunded to frankly comatose, hypotensive, and rigid. Shivering is notably absent. Supportive therapy must aggressively focus on "the ABCs." Airway protective reflexes are often impaired, so aspiration of gastric contents is a very common complication. Therefore, early intubation is recommended.

Volume resuscitation must be individualized; however, significant intravascular volume depletion is common. As hypothermia develops, basal metabolic rate (BMR) will decrease, and renal tubular reabsorption of free water also decreases. In addition, cold-induced cutaneous vasoconstriction leads to increased capacitance blood vessel volume, and therefore decreased antidiuretic hormone (ADH) secretion. Ultimately, both of these processes lead to intravascular volume depletion. Normal saline should be used preferentially to lactated Ringer's solution for volume repletion; the liver has a decreased capacity to metabolize lactate to bicarbonate while cold. To aid rewarming efforts, these fluids can be safely heated to 45°C (113°F) prior to administration.

Myocardial compliance decreases variably but progressively as the heart cools, thus requiring higher cardiac filling pressures to maintain adequate cardiac output. Myocardial stimulant and vasoactive drugs, as well as excessive patient handling, should generally be avoided as these maneuvers may precipitate spontaneous ventricular fibrillation. Temporary transvenous pacemakers for bradydysrhythmias and pulmonary artery catheters for volume management are potentially equally hazardous. When ventricular fibrillation does develop, subsequent attempts to restore a perfusing cardiac rhythm are generally unsuccessful until the core temperature exceeds 30°C (86°F). Bretylium tosylate is considered the drug of choice for modulating the ventricular fibrillatory threshold. The usual dose is a bolus of 5 to 10 mg per kilogram, which may be repeated, followed by a continuous infusion of 2 to 4 mg per minute.

Efforts to rewarm moderately hypothermic victims must be more aggressive. Active external warming techniques such as warm (not hot) water immersion tanks or heating blankets should be considered. Intravascular volume repletion remains paramount. Throughout history one can find well-described accounts of intravascular volume-depleted patients who were actively rewarmed only to vasodilate, develop hemodynamic instability, and die. Invasive core rewarming techniques may also be considered for those patients who are more compromised by hypothermia. These methods include partial cardiopulmonary bypass; thoracotomy with mediastinal lavage; peritoneal, gastric, or rectal lavage; and mechanical ventilation with warm, humidified air. Of these, partial cardiopulmonary bypass and thoracotomy with mediastinal lavage are the most calorically efficient. Interestingly, invasive core rewarming methods shorten time required for CPR and other resuscitative measures but do not offer improved survival over less aggressive active external rewarming techniques.

Severe hypothermia is considered present at core body temperatures less than 28°C (82°F). These patients usually lack any demonstrable cortical, brain-stem, or spinal reflex function. Pulselessness is very common and is usually related to ventricular fibrillation, asystole, or a nonperfused agonal rhythm. In other words, these patients appear to be dead. Let me emphasize again that the clinical determination that a patient is dead cannot be reliably made until core temperature exceeds at least 32°C (90°F). In my opinion, if it is available, one should go straight to partial cardiopulmonary bypass for these patients. Despite the lack of supporting clinical data, this seems to be the best choice for rewarming, while also providing a more effective adjunct to cardiopulmonary circulation. Early rewarming of a patient may be associated with an initial decrease in measured core temperature, or so-called afterdrop. This reflects the return of cold, acidotic blood from the periphery to the core as vasodilatation occurs with extremity rewarming.

As suggested, aspiration of gastric contents is a common complication in hypothermic patients. However, empiric administration of broad-spectrum antibiotics in anticipation of this problem has not proved beneficial. These drugs should be reserved for patients with clinical aspiration pneumonitis. Gastric erosions with gastrointestinal hemorrhage is a very common ICU complication in this patient population. These patients should routinely receive some form of acceptable stress ulcer prophylaxis.

Alcoholism is the most commonly associated disorder with hypothermia in the United States. As such, intravenous thiamine should be routinely administered, especially before any glucose-containing solutions that might precipitate Wernicke's syndrome. Conversely, the bedside clinician should also resist the urge to treat hyperglycemia with insulin while a patient remains hypothermic. Subcutaneous insulin will be poorly absorbed, but more importantly, insulin does not work well in a hypothermic milieu. As rewarming occurs, the patient given insulin may develop sustained, dangerous hypoglycemia.

Steroids should not be routinely used, but instead should be reserved for patients with suspected or probable adrenocortical insufficiency. Intravenous L-thyroxine may also be considered but is generally not recommended for patients unless they are strongly suspected as having myxedema. Pancreatitis may also develop in the hypothermic patient after rewarming. Conservative therapy with bowel rest and nasogastric suction are usually sufficient. Therapy for frostbite should be delayed until renewed exposure to the cold after rewarming is assured.

HYPERTHERMIA

Heat stroke is defined by a core body temperature exceeding 41.1°C (106°F), or alternatively as a syndrome where core temperature exceeds 40.6°C (105°F), along with anhidrosis, altered sensorium, or both. Heat stroke is traditionally considered as either exertional or nonexertional (classic heat stroke). Exertional heat stroke is usually seen in otherwise healthy young adults who overexert themselves in extraordinarily hot weather, or in hot, humid environments to which they are not acclimatized. These individuals start out with intact thermoregulation; unfortunately, endogenous heat production and heat absorption exceed overall heat dissipation, resulting in net heat gain. In contrast, classic heat stroke develops nonexertionally in elderly or debilitated patients with impaired thermoregulatory mechanisms.

Primary therapy for heat stroke centers on the rapid return of body temperature to normal. Survival is most directly related to duration of hyperpyrexia rather than degree of hyperpyrexia. A variety of methods have been devised to cool patients. Active external cooling methods are quite effective. Invasive techniques such as gastric or intraperitoneal lavage can be used but really offer little additional advantage. Examples of active external cooling include immersion in an ice-water bath or other evaporative methods such as wetting down a patient with tepid or cool water while blowing a fan across the torso. Either method is effective; however, placing a critically ill, intubated patient connected to a cardiac monitor in an ice bath may not be feasible. Shivering during cooling is associated with additional heat generation and may impede overall efforts to cool the patient. Chlorpromazine given in doses of 10 to 50 mg every 6 hours may help prevent shivering. Efforts to cool a hyperthermic patient should be terminated when the core body temperature falls to 38 to 39 °C (100.4 to 102.2 °F). Core temperature will continue to drop an additional 1 to 2 °C.

Dehydration and intravascular volume depletion are more commonly seen with exertional heat stroke. In contrast, chronically ill, debilitated patients who develop classic heat stroke have an unpredictable intravascular volume status. Therefore, volume repletion must be individualized. Hypotension, regardless of the clinical presence of vasodilatation, may still represent cardiac pump failure and not relative intravascular volume depletion. Extreme hyperpyrexia is directly toxic to myocytes, even in young healthy individuals without underlying heart disease. If any doubt as to the adequacy of myocardial performance exists, a pulmonary artery catheter should be inserted to guide subsequent fluid therapy. Isoproterenol has been traditionally considered the inotrope of choice for use in these patients. It does not cause peripheral alpha-receptor stimulation, which may impede heat loss. However, life-threatening ventricular ectopy often coexists in these patients and may be exacerbated by isoproterenol. Dobutamine is probably a better choice for the patient with refractory cardiac pump failure.

For patients with exertional heat stroke, a variety of significant electrolyte disorders are associated with excessive sweating and may require specific therapy. These include hyponatremia, hypokalemia, hypomagnesemia, hypocalcemia, and hypophosphatemia. Hypokalemia may lead to decreased sweat production and cutaneous vasoconstriction, thus impairing further heat dissipation. Renal hypoperfusion from dehydration may be reflected as increased BUN and creatinine values. Severe metabolic acidosis from lactate accumulation is the rule. Treatment with bicarbonate should be reserved for patients with a serum pH less than 7.1 to 7.0.

When rhabdomyolysis develops, it is usually associated with exertional heat stroke and can be devastating. Acute renal failure develops six times more frequently in these patients. Hyperuricemia, myoglobinuria, and renal hypoperfusion appear causal. The most immediate threat to survival for patients with rhabdomyolysis is generally hyperkalemia. Emergency administration of intravenous insulin, 50 percent dextrose water, sodium bicarbonate, and calcium should be implemented when electrocardiographic changes of hyperkalemia or increasing ventricular ectopy are present. Otherwise calcium should not be given, even when significant hypocalcemia is present, as it may potentiate existing muscle injury. Ultimately, acute hemodialysis may be required for adequate modulation of these metabolic processes. Appropriate volume resuscitation is also crucial during the acute phases of rhabdomyolysis. Finally, patients who develop rhabdomyolysis following overexertion are at risk for a compartment syndrome. This generally occurs in the lower extremities during initial volume repletion, which then results in myoedema and increased intracompartmental pressures. Fasciotomy is generally required to relieve neurovascular compromise.

Generalized seizures are common with either form of heat stoke. Therapy should always ensure adequate airway protection to avert aspiration of gastric contents. Intravenous benzodiazepines are considered first-line therapy for seizures. Cerebral edema and increased intracranial pressure may be clinically associated with these seizures. Not surprisingly, their presence portends a much poorer outcome. Mechanical ventilation with hyperventilation, intravenous dehydrating agents (e.g., mannitol), and judiciously limiting the use of intravenous crystalloids should also be considered.

MALIGNANT HYPERTHERMIA

Malignant hyperthermia and the neuroleptic malignant syndrome are hypothesized to be similar conditions that result from abnormal skeletal muscle membrane-

Table 3 Drugs Associated with Malignant Hyperthermia and the Neuroleptic Malignant Syndrome

Malignant Hyperthermia
  Volatile anesthetics
    Halothane
    Enflurane
    Methoxyflurane
    Isoflurane
    Sevoflurane
  Depolarizing muscle relaxants
    Succinylcholine
    Decamethonium

Neuroleptic Malignant Syndrome
  Phenothiazines
    Fluphenazine
    Chlorpromazine
    Levomepromazine
    Thioridazine
    Trimeprazine
    Trifluoperazine
    Prochlorperazine
  Butyrophenones
    Haloperidol
    Bromoperidol
  Thioxanthenes
    Thiothinexe
  Dibenzoxepines
    Loxapine
  Dopamine-depleting drugs
    Alphamethyltyrosine
    Tetrabenazine
  Withdrawal of dopamine agonists
    Levodopa
    Levodopa/carbidopa
    Amantadine

calcium ion interactions. Both conditions are probably associated with a familial predisposition. They can be precipitated by a variety of psychotropic and anesthetic drugs. Table 3 provides a listing of these agents. These syndromes are characterized by profound, catastrophic elevations in core body temperature, along with extreme total body muscular rigidity. It is this muscular rigidity that results in such overwhelming and rapid temperature elevations. Maximum temperature elevations are generally less with the neuroleptic malignant syndrome.

Therapy for patients with malignant hyperthermia is three-pronged. First, the clinician should be suspicious of early muscle rigidity associated with the use of these inhaled anesthetic agents and depolarizing drugs. Trismus is frequently the earliest indicator. Their use should be aborted at this time. Once muscle rigidity becomes prominent, however, rapid temperature elevations quickly follow. Therefore, sodium dantrolene should be administered to reverse this process. The recommended dose is 2 mg per kilogram intravenously. This may be repeated every 5 minutes to a total dose of 10 mg per kilogram. Further dosing has been associated with hepatic toxicity. Intubation and mechanical ventilation are usually necessary to ensure adequate gas exchange. Finally, evaporative cooling techniques described previously are useful therapeutic adjuncts.

When the neuroleptic malignant syndrome is considered, the suspected inciting drug should be discontinued. The return of the patient to his or her baseline may not occur for 5 to 7 days. Sodium dantrolene may also help these patients resolve their muscular rigidity, although the definitive supportive data for its use with this syndrome are lacking. Bromocriptine and amantadine have also been used for treatment of the neuroleptic malignant syndrome with variable success.

Rhabdomyolysis may occur with either condition, and can be life-threatening. Vigorous volume resuscitation as well as emergency therapy for hyperkalemia may be required. Acute renal failure may also develop. Disseminated intravascular coagulation (DIC) is very common but will rarely require specific therapy.

SUGGESTED READING

Gronert GA. Malignant hyperthermia. Anesthesiology 1980; 53:395–423.

Guze BH, Baxter LR. Neuroleptic malignant syndrome. N Engl J Med 1985; 313:163–166.

Ledingham IMcA, Mone JG. Treatment of accidental hypothermia: a prospective clinical study. Br Med J 1980; 280:1102–1105.

Knochel JP. Environmental heat illness: an eclectic review. Arch Intern Med 1974; 133:841–864.

PSYCHIATRIC AND ETHICAL ISSUES

PSYCHIATRIC PROBLEMS

DAVID A. BARON, M.S.Ed., D.O.
DAVID R. RUBINOW, M.D.

Behavioral disturbances that present in a critical care unit (CCU) are often the product of several factors, including the medical illness, its treatment, the personality style and coping mechanisms of the patient, and the patient's vulnerability to psychiatric illness. The contribution of each of these factors must be adequately assessed in all cases in order to generate a sensible, effective therapeutic regimen. A psychiatric disorder is defined on the basis of disturbances in cognition, affect, mood, or behavior; there is no presumption about etiology. All psychiatric syndromes may represent a manifestation of organic dysfunction secondary to a variety of known or undiagnosed conditions including hypoxia, vascular/degenerative disease, infection, neoplasm, and endocrine/metabolic dysregulation. The toxic effects of medications, particularly in association with the general medical compromise of the acutely ill, may also precipitate behavioral disturbances. Thus, with any sudden change in behavior, one should exhaustively consider all possible organic sources of behavioral dysfunction *before* inferring the existence of a primary psychiatric disorder. Compendia of medications and medical disorders associated with psychiatric symptoms can be consulted if one is unfamiliar with potential sources of psychiatric dysfunction.

The generic and personal stressors encountered in the CCU interact with pre-existing personality styles and coping mechanisms to produce "illness behavior." Certainly, immobilization, pain, and disturbed sleep are all capable of initiating or contributing to behavioral alteration, perceptual distortion, or clouding of consciousness. Additionally, the meaning of an illness to a patient as well as the dependency imposed by the CCU may powerfully determine behavior. For example, patients for whom careful control of their environment is important will often experience acute anxiety during their illness as a result of suddenly feeling completely out of control. The mere presence of extensive monitoring devices constantly reminds patients of their dilemma and can serve as a continual source of stress. Disruptive noncompliant behavior under these circumstances may be a maladaptive attempt by patients to diminish anxiety by showing that they are in charge. The personal meaning of critical illness may also contribute to patients' behavioral response. For example, patients recovering from an acute myocardial infarction often struggle for the first time with the reality of their mortality, contemplate limitations and loss that they anticipate will be conferred by their "new condition," and may predict their prognosis on the basis of their experience with others with a "similar" illness. Finally, in addition to the protean forms of "illness behavior," psychiatric syndromes that occur during hospitalization may represent the re-emergence of an underlying psychiatric disorder or the de nova appearance of a primary psychiatric disorder. All CCU patients with a prior history of psychiatric illness should be considered at risk for re-emergence of psychiatric symptoms while in the unit.

As in all clinical medicine, effective psychiatric treatment begins with a thorough diagnostic assessment. In order to disentangle the effects of organic dysfunction, toxicity, environmental stressors, personality style, and psychiatric vulnerability, this assessment should include the following: a description of current mood, behavioral, and cognitive difficulties (both patient-reported and staff-observed); a review of current laboratory values and medications; past personal psychiatric history (including any treatments) and substance abuse history; and a mental status examination. While the need for acute psychopharmacologic intervention may preclude a complete diagnostic work-up, the physician's familiarity with relevant details of the patient's history will enhance the likelihood of selection of an effective treatment. Often preliminary effective therapeutic interventions will include active solicitation of the patient's questions and concerns and provision of appropriate information about the current illness or injury and anticipated treatment strategies. If the patient feels the physician welcomes rather than eschews questions and concerns, many potential problems will be presented sooner, solved more easily, and require far less time and effort to resolve.

The psychiatric problems most likely to be encountered in critical care patients include the following: anxiety (as a symptom or syndrome), depression (as a symptom or syndrome), anger (toward self, family, or staff), behavioral management problems, delirium, sleep disturbances, and pain. The following sections will describe the pharmacologic and nonpharmacologic treatment of these problems. A comprehensive diagnostic assessment will be presumed to have occurred prior to initiation of treatment. Psychiatric syndromes (e.g., depression) may require different treatment from that indicated for the individual symptoms (e.g., sadness) that constitute the syndrome. Therefore, the clinician needs to determine whether he or she is attempting to treat symptom or syndromal dysfunction. Also, treatment in the context of the CCU may differ from ongoing, outpatient management regarding choice of medication and dose. The potential adverse effects of long term-maintenance therapy are of minimal concern in this setting.

DEPRESSION

Symptoms of sadness in the critical care unit will most commonly present in the context of major depressions or demoralization syndromes. Obviously the diagnosis of depression in the CCU is complicated by the ubiquitous occurrence of the neurovegetative disturbances—sleep disorder, appetite disorder, and alteration in energy levels—that are customarily an integral part of the diagnosis. These "symptoms" could all be a normal response to the CCU environment. Therefore, the syndrome is usually diagnosed on the basis of the distinctness of the mood disturbance, its similarity to prior depressions (if any have occurred), and the pervasiveness and severity of symptoms. Feelings such as hopelessness, helplessness, guilt, and impaired self-esteem, when present, strongly suggest the diagnosis of a major depressive disorder.

When treating depression in the CCU, one should employ nonpharmacologic strategies first to allow additional time for assessment and to avoid, if possible, undesirable side effects of these medications. Educate the patient about depression: that it is an illness, that it influences the patient's perceptions, and that it is treatable. Describe symptoms that can be alleviated (disturbed sleep, appetite, energy) and available treatment options. The patient should be asked about specific questions or concerns. Many patients must be given permission to state their fears, a process that can very effectively establish a trusting therapeutic relationship, which itself may significantly reduce emotional symptoms. If antidepressant therapy is initiated, the patient should be informed about expected therapeutic effects (e.g., improved mood and sleep) and side effects (e.g., dry mouth) likely to be experienced. The therapeutic latency (several days to several weeks, depending upon the medication selection) should be estimated so that the patient learns what to expect. If present, the patient's pessimism regarding the likelihood of the efficacy of antidepressants should be acknowledged and described for the patient as a symptom of a treatable depression.

Pharmacologic treatments potentially effective for treating depression include tricyclic and nontricyclic antidepressants, psychostimulants and, for patients with anxiety associated with depression, a benzodiazepine, alprazolam.

Several factors should be considered when choosing an antidepressant medication in the CCU setting. In general, familiarity with and confidence in the compound along with a thorough knowledge of side effect profiles should guide selection of an antidepressant. The most commonly prescribed medications for treating depression are the tricyclic antidepressants (TCAs). Although many different TCAs are marketed, these drugs tend to be more similar to each other than different in their overall effectiveness, despite the claims of pharmaceutical representatives. The biggest differences are in their side-effect profiles. All (with the possible exception of protriptyline) have sedative effects and possess anticholinergic activity to some degree and thus may produce dry mouth, blurred vision, urinary retention, constipation, and a slowing of cardiac conduction (a quinidine-like effect). Patients on TCAs, particularly the elderly, who are concomitantly treated with other compounds possessing anticholinergic properties are at increased risk for developing an anticholinergic psychosis. Although anticholinergic-induced urinary retention can be a serious complication, its relevance for CCU patients is diminished by their catheterization. Desipramine is the least anticholinergic of the tricyclics and may be the drug of choice for patients on other anticholinergic compounds or with a history of prior severe side effects when taking medications with anticholinergic properties. The most serious potential side effects of TCAs are related to the cardiovascular system. TCAs are not contraindicated in patients with arrhythmias and may decrease ventricular ectopy; however, they increase cardiac conduction time (increased H-V interval) and, therefore, may exacerbate heart block. Of particular importance in the CCU setting, intravenous epinephrine and norepinephrine will display a markedly enhanced pressor response when used in combination with TCAs. The mechanism for this interaction is not known. Of the TCAs, nortriptyline is the least likely to cause postural hypotension, a potential concern at the time of increasing patient mobilization. It is worth noting that the side effects of the antidepressants can be exploited, as when one selects a sedating antidepressant or uses doxepin, a powerful histamine (H_1 and H_2) blocker, to obviate the need for concomitant antihistamines (e.g., cimetidine).

A typical starting dose of TCAs in the CCU setting is 50 to 75 mg per day with an increase of 25 or 50 mg every other day. We generally employ desipramine in CCU patients in order to avoid adverse anticholinergic side effects. The emergence of significant side effects (e.g., excessive dry mouth or blurred vision) can be used as indications for slowing the rapidity of dosing increases. Therapeutic doses are usually in the range of 100 to 300 mg per day but vary with individual compounds. Measures of serum levels of the TCAs are available and can be used to ensure adequate absorption in nonresponders. We find, in general, little use for serum TCA levels in the CCU. Tricyclics have a full therapeutic latency of up to 3 weeks. However, our experience is that patients generally report some symptomatic relief (e.g., improved sleep, increased energy, improved appetite) within 7 to 10 days.

For patients unable to take medications by mouth, amitriptyline and imipramine are available for intramuscular use. For severely depressed patients, amitriptyline can be administered intravenously, 10 mg per 100 cc of normal saline infused over 1 hour at bedtime. The dose can be increased 5 to 10 mg per day. (Intravenous amitriptyline has been reported to approach the efficacy of ECT.) Imipramine can be started at 50 mg intramuscularly twice a day and increased 25 mg every other day. Again, side effects or improvement of the target symptoms of dysphoria, sleep disorder, and appetite disorder should be used to titrate dosing increments.

Stimulant drugs, like d-amphetamine and methylphenidate, have been reported to be effective in the treatment of depression in medically ill depressed patients. Unlike the TCAs, the antidepressant effect can occur in the first 24 to 48 hours of therapy. Because of this rapid onset of antidepressant action, lack of significant side effects in most patients, and possible persistent antidepressant effect after only a short (2 to 3 weeks) course of treatment, psychostimulants may offer several advantages over tricyclics in the treatment of depressed CCU patients. However, psychostimulants can precipitate nervousness, insomnia, and anorexia and are contraindicated in patients with glaucoma. These compounds exacerbate cardiac arrhythmias and tachycardia and obviously should be used with caution in patients experiencing these problems. Methylphenidate should be started at 5 to 10 mg in the morning. Nonresponders can be increased up to 30 to 40 mg per day, given in divided doses (usually twice a day).

Recent clinical trials have shown alprazolam, a triazolobenzodiazepine, to have short-term antidepressant action. Although a reasonable choice for the acutely depressed patient with anxiety, its long-term efficacy for depression remains unproved.

Although not commonly employed, electroconvulsive therapy (ECT) can be lifesaving in severely depressed suicidal patients or in patients unable to tolerate antidepressant medications. Six to twelve treatments may be given at the bedside in the CCU on an every-other-day regimen. When used properly, ECT is a safe and effective procedure.

For patients experiencing demoralization and not major depression, effective nonpharmacotherapeutic interventions include the following: illness education, provision for opportunity to express concerns, and, where appropriate, reassurance. False reassurance by the medical staff may damage the therapeutic relationship, an otherwise powerful tool when properly employed. Demoralization differs from depression by the absence of anhedonia and the presence of reactivity (i.e., demoralized patients will respond dramatically to the news that their illness has been cured and they've won the lottery; the depressed patient will not show any positive response to the same news).

We do not advocate the use of pharmacotherapy for the treatment of demoralization. In addition to being ineffective, further demoralization is likely following an unsuccessful drug trial.

ANXIETY

Symptoms of restlessness, difficulty falling asleep, and excessive worry and fear are ubiquitous in patients in the CCU. These symptoms can manifest feelings of anxiety or may be part of an anxiety syndrome. In contrast to the isolated symptom of sadness for which we do not recommend pharmacologic intervention, the isolated symptom of anxiety may warrant symptomatic treatment with benzodiazepines, depending upon the degree of distress experienced and the potential adverse consequences of unmodulated anxiety. In the CCU, the most common psychiatric disorders manifesting anxiety symptoms include the following: generalized anxiety disorder, panic attacks, and organic brain syndromes.

Generalized Anxiety Disorder. This disorder (GAD) is characterized by unrealistic or excessive anxiety and worry, motor tension (trembling, feeling shaky, muscle tension, restlessness), autonomic hyperactivity (shortness of breath, palpitations, sweating, dry mouth, nausea), hypervigilance (feeling on edge, exaggerated startle response), difficulty with concentration, irritability, and difficulty falling asleep. GAD is not likely to present for the first time in CCU patients; patients with this disorder will have a history of chronic, severe anxiety preceding their acute medical problem. It is not unusual for any patient to develop anxious symptoms while being treated in a CCU setting, particularly those on mechanical respirators and in the first day or two immediately following a myocardial infarction. Both patients with GAD as well as patients who develop acute anxious symptoms in the context of the CCU are best treated with benzodiazepines and emotional support. Clarification, explanation, and reassurance by the clinician are effective nonpharmacologic interventions and necessary adjuncts to pharmacotherapy.

Of the available antianxiety agents, the benzodiazepines are generally the safest and most effective. Unlike barbiturates, they do not induce hepatic microenzymes, which will alter the pharmacokinetics of other concurrent medications. Benzodiazepines can offer symptomatic relief of anxiety within 30 minutes to 2 hours. We recommend the use of shorter-acting agents (lorazepam, alprazolam, or oxazepam) to avoid accumulation of active metabolites that can lead to excess sedation. Shorter-acting compounds do not produce active metabolites, are easily handled by the liver via glucuronide conjugation, and can be used in patients with advanced cirrhosis. Additionally, unlike other benzodiazepines, the plasma levels of oxazepam and lorazepam are not elevated by concomitant use of cimetidine. Appropriate daily doses are 0.75 to 3 mg of alprazolam, 3 to 6 mg of lorazepam, or 30 to 60 mg of oxazepam. Alprazolam and lorazepam have a metabolic half-life of approximately 12 hours and a therapeutic duration of about 8 hours. They should be given three times a day. Oxazepam has an 8-hour metabolic half-life with a 4- to 6-hour therapeutic effect and should be administered four times a day. Lorazepam is available for intramuscular or intravenous administration, with a metabolic half-life similar to that following oral administration. The dosing is equivalent to that used orally, the peak drug concentration being reached in 2 hours. These drugs are extremely safe, sedation being the most common side effect. Dosage increases can be titrated against patient sedation. Patients requiring 2 weeks or less of benzodiazepine therapy should nonetheless have medications slowly tapered over 3 to 5 days (decrease the dose 20 to 30 percent per day) to avoid the emergence of rebound or withdrawal anxiety.

Panic Attacks. Panic attacks are characterized by a symptom cluster similar to that experienced during acute myocardial infarction. Dyspnea, dizziness, palpitations, trembling, chest discomfort, and a fear of dying or going crazy are the most common clinical complaints. Panic attacks are usually very short in duration (minutes) but very frightening to the patients. Although some investigators believe that single episodes of panic are manifestations of pre-existing panic disorder that can be identified through careful history taking, we have, nonetheless, seen panic attacks in CCU patients from whom we have been unable to elicit a history of antecedent anxiety disorder. These panic attacks can occur with hypoxia but are most commonly seen in association with attempts to wean patients from mechanical ventilators and center around the patient's concern that he will suffocate (even if adequately oxygenated). While relaxation and hypnotic techniques frequently may be helpful in patients with intense anxiety, the sense of the patient being weaned from a ventilator that he is unable to breathe slowly and deeply often renders these techniques ineffective. Therefore, prompt pharmacotherapeutic intervention may be required. For rapid relief of acute panic and anxious symptoms, 1 or 2 mg sublingually or 2 mg (or .04 mg per kilogram) of intravenous lorazepam has demonstrated clinical effectiveness. Alprazolam is also effective in the treatment of panic attacks and will usually require an initial dose of 1 mg.

Organic Brain Syndrome. Delirium will commonly present with symptoms of anxiety and agitation. The existence of delirium as a source of anxiety or agitation can best be determined by the associated presence of fluctuating levels of consciousness, distractibility, and altered mental status findings, all indications of an organic brain syndrome. In addition to agitation and anxiety, a delirium will commonly manifest itself in the form of disruptive behavior. For example, delirious agitated CCU patients will frequently attempt to pull out intravenous lines, pacing wires, nasogastric tubes, or monitoring leads, thereby requiring rapid treatment intervention. Geriatric patients are at particular risk for the development of delirium with their increased prevalence of pre-existing (albeit often mild) organ brain syndrome and increased metabolic vulnerability to endogenous (e.g., azotemia) or exogenous (e.g., medications such as cimetidine or lidocaine) toxins.

Although psychosocial measures will not correct the physical disturbances responsible for the delirium, they may provide dramatic relief of symptoms, particularly when used to augment pharmacotherapy. Adequate lighting, frequent orientation of the patient to where they are and why they are in the CCU, clocks, calendars, pictures from home, and frequent visits from family members and friends are all effective in reducing agitation and confusion. (In our experience with interleukin-2–induced organic brain syndrome arising in the context of treatment for cancer, patients on whom emergency psychiatric consultations were called and who had family members available to stay with them did not require neuroleptics, in contrast to those patients who had no significant others present.) Low doses of neuroleptics are effective in treating the extreme agitation commonly seen in these patients. Haloperidol, 0.5 to 2 mg intramuscularly, is our drug of choice. Haloperidol can be administered as an oral concentrate (5 mg) in patients able to cooperate or, when necessary, as an intravenous (0.5 to 2 mg) preparation. Although not FDA-approved, intravenous administration offers a number of therapeutic advantages for acute delirium with agitation, including improved and more rapid drug absorption, less pain, and, reportedly, decreased incidence of extrapyramidal side effects. Intravenous lines should be flushed with 2 mg of normal saline prior to administration of haloperidol, as haloperidol may precipitate with heparin in the intravenous line. The patient's behavior should be evaluated every 15 minutes until stable, and the drug dose should be titrated against behavioral agitation every 30 minutes. Once behaviorally stable, vital signs should be monitored at 30-minute intervals for 2 to 3 hours. Conversion to oral medication can be accomplished by administering orally half of the total amount of parenteral medication necessary to control behaviors over a 24-hour period. Neuroleptics used for a week or less can be rapidly tapered to complete withdrawal in 2 to 3 days with little likelihood of adverse reactions. Although reports suggest the efficacy of a combination of neuroleptic and lorazepam in the treatment of organic brain syndrome associated agitation, we recommend caution with the use of benzodiazepines in this context because of the possible precipitation of paradoxical behavioral disinhibition.

ANGER

The overt manifestation of anger in the CCU may take the form of behavioral management problems (e.g., noncompliance), verbal or physically abusive or disruptive behavior, or demands to leave against medical advice. One must, of course, rule out organic brain syndromes and withdrawal as sources of disruptive behavior in the CCU. In some instances, however, angry, maladaptive behavior results from conflicts about dependency and the emotional experience of loss of control. For these latter patients, several therapeutic strategies can be employed. First, the patient should be encouraged to articulate concerns, thereby decreasing the need for their behavioral expression. Significant reduction in a patient's anxiety may accompany empathic understanding of frustration coupled with reassurance about the physician's commitment to do whatever is necessary to promote the patient's welfare. Second, anxiety about loss of control can be further diminished by allowing the patient to make decisions (even trivial) about some element of care. Third, firm limit-setting may be a necessary therapeutic adjunct if the patient's behavior is disruptive.

While we do not recommend pharmacologic treatment for anger, if the associated behavior is potentially dangerous to the patient or staff, rapid treatment with neuroleptics (haloperidol) and/or physical restraints should be instituted.

PAIN

Pain is a subjective experience that reflects a patient's emotional state as well as the severity of the nociceptive stimulus. Thus, the meaning of pain to the patient may dramatically alter the patient's pain-related behavior. A minor discomfort that the patient believes represents impending relapse or disease progression may be accompanied by great anxiety and frequent complaints. In patients in whom adequate control of pain appears difficult, the physician should both reassure the patient that the pain can be managed and ask if the patient is worried about pain. Failure to solicit this information may lead to inappropriate conclusions or interventions. An unfortunately common concern of physicians treating pain is the risk of inducing an iatrogenic addiction to narcotic analgesics. Physicians should dismiss any pre-existing notions about the need to prevent addiction (a rare occurrence when treating pain), which otherwise result in the failure to provide adequate analgesia. In our experience, almost all consultations surrounding the question of addiction stem from the attempt to treat patients with inadequate doses and/or schedules of analgesics and the fear on the physician's part that he or she is being manipulated. When patients are not given analgesics frequently enough (e.g., meperidine every 4 to 6 hours when its analgesic half-life is 3 hours), their pain returns and increases even after they receive their next dose. They therefore become anxious about the absence of pain control, which intensifies the painful experience. If patients have to ask for the analgesic, they feel more out of control and experience the not-so-subtle opprobrium of the staff ("It is not time for your analgesic, Mr. Jones!"). If, instead, the patient is prescribed analgesics on a reverse "as-needed" schedule (in which patients are offered analgesics at fixed intervals and can refuse them, rather than having to request them), they are removed from a dependent, helpless position. This serves to provide some measure of control and, after several doses, allows the patient to feel less anxious, rendering analgesia more effective. The patient almost invariably will then refuse one of the offered doses, reassuring the staff that the patient, indeed, is not an addict. The best way to diminish anxiety around pain is to provide adequate analgesia.

DYSSOMNIAS

Although frequently time-limited and self-remitting, sleep disturbances in the CCU may be of sufficient severity to require therapeutic intervention. Effective management requires a consideration of the multifactorial causes of dyssomnias. In the CCU, sleep disturbance may be a symptom of underlying psychiatric disorder (anxiety, depression, or delirium), be secondary to symptoms or treatment of a medical illness, or result from environmental factors such as uncomfortable beds, noisy medical devices, or frequent awakenings for monitoring or medication delivery.

Patients with upper airway obstruction, cardiac arrhythmias, hypertension, or pain not infrequently experience sleep disturbances. In our experience, inadequate night-time analgesia is one of the most common causes of sleep difficulties in the CCU setting. The appropriate therapeutic intervention in these situations is to correct the underlying medical abnormality (where possible) and afford adequate pain relief.

Prior to initiating sedative-hypnotics, the clinician should review the nursing notes concerning sleeping patterns and amount of daytime sleep. It is remarkable how many patients complain of difficulty sleeping at night despite napping 2 to 3 hours during the daytime.

In choosing an appropriate hypnotic, we do not recommend the use of barbiturate or barbiturate-like compounds such as chloral derivatives, glutethimide, methaqualone, or ethchlorvinyl. These compounds induce hepatic microenzymes, thus altering the kinetics of other drugs, and as a group have a low therapeutic index. As a class, the benzodiazepines are as effective as barbiturates, safer, and have substantially fewer adverse side effects. The key factors to consider when choosing a benzodiazepine to be used as a hypnotic is the rapidity and duration of action and the route of metabolism. The best hypnotics are those with a rapid absorption rate. Oxazepam, 15 to 30 mg orally 1 hour before bedtime, with its rapid absorption and short duration (thereby avoiding daytime sedation or cognitive impairment), is our hypnotic of first choice. Flurazepam, a popular hypnotic, has an acceptable half-life of 9 to 10 hours but is metabolized in the liver, producing an active metabolite, desalkyl flurazepam, which has a half-life of 50 to 100 hours. Like oxazepam, triazolam and lorazepam are not metabolized by the liver, have no known active metabolites, have short half-lives (3 to 5 hours for triazolam and 8 to 12 hours for lorazepam), and have a rapid rate of elimination. Triazolam, although effective, may produce disorientation or disequilibrium in patients the following day. Lorazepam is available for intramuscular or intravenous usage in patients unable to take oral medications. We do not recommend hypnotic use beyond 1 to 2 weeks, as the likelihood of dependency and rebound insomnia will increase. This temporary condition can be modulated by gradually tapering the dose over 2 to 4 days. The importance of maintaining adequate sleep time should not be underestimated.

SUGGESTED READING

Cavenar JO, et al. Psychiatry. Vol.3: consultation-liaison psychiatry and behavioral medicine. New York: Basic Press, 1986.

Guggenheim FG, Weiner MF. Manual of psychiatric consultation and emergency care. Northvale, NJ: Aronson, 1984.

Hackett TP, Cassem NH. Massachusetts General Hospital handbook of general hospital psychiatry. 2nd ed. Chicago: Year Book Medical Publishers, 1987.

ETHICAL ISSUES

ALISON WICHMAN, M.D.
KATHLEEN MARIE DIXON, Ph.D.

Critical care presents health care providers, patients, and policy makers with some of the most challenging problems in medicine. The supply of ethical issues seems inexhaustible. Each new advance in medical technology and standard of care comes at the price of painful questions about appropriate use. The critical care unit has become an arena for such basic questions as: How do we offer humane care and what is death? We cannot hope to provide final resolutions to these problems here, but we offer insights derived from our experience and share considered moral judgments. We hope this will give practical guidance and encourage critical reflection.

Three questions will be considered in this chapter. How is the process of informed consent best applied in critical care medicine? What ethical standards ought to be used when making decisions to withhold and/or withdraw life-sustaining treatment? How should physicians respond to the controversies concerning brain death?

INFORMED CONSENT

The Ethical Foundations of Informed Consent

Two related ethical principles are embodied in the requirement to obtain consent for medical care. The first is the principle of respect for persons. This ethical norm requires us to recognize persons' intrinsic value and to act in ways consistent with this value. It prohibits us from treating persons, including ourselves, as mere means to ends. We demonstrate our respect for persons when we recognize the integrity of interpersonal boundaries. The second and related ethical principle is the principle of autonomy. This principle asserts that autonomous persons ought to be free to perform whatever self-regarding actions they wish, even if they involve serious risk to themselves or if others consider the choice foolish. This ethical principle requires physicians to honor competent patients' treatment decisions.

The concept of informed consent would be of limited value if we failed to acknowledge the realities and demands of critical care medicine. While some critical care patients are truly autonomous, many are either cognitively incapacitated or require urgent care. Thus there is a wide range in patients' capacities to make medical decisions. When patients are nonautonomous or suffer significantly diminished autonomy, we demonstrate our respect by taking appropriate measures to protect them from harm. We attempt to supplement limited decision-making capacity, trying to maximize self-determination while protecting patients from serious and enduring harm.

Elements of Informed Decision-Making

Although "informed consent" is an established term in medical, ethical, and legal spheres, we prefer to use "informed decision-making." It more accurately describes a process that leads either to a valid consent or valid refusal. Informed decision-making has four elements: disclosure of information, cognitive capacity, comprehension, and voluntariness. If patients are to make informed treatment decisions, they must be able to evaluate available options knowledgeably. Consequently, they are entitled to information about the inherent and potential risks of the proposed treatments, a description of alternatives to the proposed treatment, the benefits that can reasonably be expected from each option, and results of failure to obtain treatment. Disclosure of information is a necessary but not a sufficient condition for informed decision-making. Patients must be capable of understanding the information. If patients' cognitive functioning does not permit them to process and apply the information, the provision of that data is futile. Minimal requirements for decision-making capacity include the abilities to understand clear and simply phrased explanations of medical treatments and to communicate a choice. Further, patients must reach a decision in the absence of coercion or substantial control by others. Although serious illness and the demands of intensive care may limit a patient's options, health care providers should make every effort to enhance patients' potential for autonomous choices. This requires the judicious use of sedative medications. Physicians will have to balance the obligation to relieve pain and anxiety with their obligation to elicit patient participation in medical decision-making.

The Application of Informed Consent to Critical Care

Medically effective, ethically acceptable critical care cannot be achieved by rote application of consent practices borrowed from other medical settings. Because of the realities of the critical care setting, all parties to treatment decisions may experience significant limitations to thorough deliberation and analysis. Health care providers may fasten on narrow notions of patient benefit and aggressively pursue isolated tasks that respond to a particular disease or problem but leave the patient's ultimate status unchanged. Patients may overemphasize immediate goals and needs and fail to assess their own long-range interests. Patients' decision-making may be clouded by strong emotional influences related to serious illness. Family members may face painful conflicts of interest as they consider limitation of treatment or long-term care plans. They may be unsure of, or deeply divided over, appropriate limitations to medical care.

Many obstacles associated with decision-making in critical care medicine can be overcome by the use of an interdisciplinary team approach. Inclusion of primary physicians, nurses, social workers, chaplains, and ethicists permits us to enhance our view of available options. Patients or surrogate decision-makers stand at the center of this expanded treatment community. Candid interdisciplinary discussions of medical, psychosocial, and ethical aspects of treatment decisions empower patients or surrogate decision-makers.

Because the critical care setting often requires rapid decision-making, hospitals should set up procedures for emergency bioethical consultation. These services could be utilized when a full interdisciplinary team approach is not possible.

Advance Directives: Living Will and Durable Power of Attorney

Advance directives could guide critical care physicians and families in end-of-life decision-making. There are two types of advance directives: treatment directives (e.g., living wills) and proxy or surrogate directives. A treatment directive is a written statement that indicates the kinds of medical care that a patient would or would not want in specific medical circumstances. These preferences are intended to prevail when a patient loses decision-making capacity.

While these documents reveal the patient's most general wishes, they may be too vague to give critical care physicians much specific advice. The value of a living will is a function of the quality and type of information contained in the document. Unfortunately, few patients express their views of a minimally adequate quality of life in precise cognitive parameters. The guidance offered by living wills and their value as guarantors of patients' wishes would be enhanced if these directives were formulated with the assistance of the patient's primary care physician. Critical care physicians can explain the potential merit of these documents. They can offer seminars to primary care physicians that would provide additional data on subtle care distinctions that should be incorporated into living wills.

A proxy or surrogate directive is a document that identifies the individual who is to assume decision-making authority for an incompetent patient. A durable power of attorney (DPA) is one type of proxy directive. Although a DPA is usually held by a family member, it may name as proxy a friend, lover, or other individual who is familiar with the patient's moral or religious commitments.

Proxies' decisions should be based on one of two standards of reasoning. The preferred standard, "substituted judgment," requires the proxy to adopt the pattern of deliberation and value scheme that the patient would utilize if he or she were capable of making the decision. The "best interest" standard is adopted when available information does not allow the proxy to arrive at a patient-authentic choice. This standard directs the proxy to select the course of action that maximizes patient benefit. Proxies should include such factors as relief of suffering, preservation or restoration of functioning, and quality as well as extent of life sustained.

WITHHOLDING OR WITHDRAWING LIFE-SUSTAINING TREATMENT

Decisions to forego (withhold or withdraw) life-sustaining treatments raise some of the most frequent and complex problems in acute care medicine. A long tradition of medical ethics acknowledges that a proper goal of medicine is to preserve life and to promote patient well-being. A dilemma emerges when the duty to promote patient well-being—presumably by preserving or extending life—conflicts with the duty not to harm the patient. Extending life is usually but not always a desirable goal. If the patient's life would be full of pain and suffering, he or she may prefer to forego treatment even though it means an earlier death. In the clinical setting, some of the most difficult problems arise over how we ought to resolve conflicts in competing duties to respect persons, promote well-being, and avoid harm to patients. There are a number of standards, some with rich philosophical and religious traditions, which have been used to resolve such conflicts. Among these are the distinctions between ordinary and extraordinary, between act and omission, and between benefit and burden. In making a distinction between ordinary and extraordinary forms of treatment, some argue that there is an obligation to offer ordinary treatments but no obligation to offer or continue extraordinary ones. The problem with this distinction is that "ordinary" can mean several things: technologically unsophisticated, easy to administer, readily available, or minimally invasive. Because of the ambiguous and controversial nature of this distinction, it should not be used in decision-making. With regard to the act-versus-omission distinction, some argue that it is more ethically problematic to withdraw a treatment than not to initiate it. This distinction continues to be heavily debated and offers no consistent ethical justification for medical decision-making. In our view the essential concern is not with the debate over acting (withdrawing) or failing to act (withholding) but whether our decisions show sufficient regard for the patient's values, preferences, expectations, and needs as well as the prevailing medical, professional, and legal standards.

The best standard to apply in decision-making about foregoing life-sustaining treatments is the benefit-versus-burden standard. This standard requires the evaluation of the benefit and burdens of each treatment being considered and often reveals rich and complex meanings. Benefit, for example, has both medical and nonmedical connotations. In the context of health, benefit means either improvement in the patient's condition, cure of the patient's disease, or a lessening of the patient's pain and suffering. There are also nonmedical benefits. These benefits are measured by subjective patient standards and reflect the patient's assessment of his or her quality of life. The patient's or surrogate's perceived benefits may be quite independent of the medical benefits. For example, discharging a medically marginal patient from a hospital to home might be less desirable from the standpoint of monitoring his or her disease but may allow the patient to spend more time with loved ones, thereby improving well-being. A "burden" usually implies that which increases pain, suffering, or debilitation without any benefit to health or the patient's self-perceived quality of life.

A number of groups have provided ethical guidance on the benefit-burden criterion for foregoing life-sustaining treatments, including, among others, The President's Commission for the Study of Ethical Problems in Medicine and Biomedical Research, and the Hastings Center Project on Termination of Treatment and Care of the Dying. The developing medical, legal, and ethical consensus in the United States affirms that as in other medical decisions, decisions to forego life-sustaining treatment rest with capable patients in a context of shared decision-making with families and health care professionals. The decision-making process should promote patient autonomy, helping patients to make decisions that reflect their personal values while preserving professional values essential to the ethical integrity of medical practice.

When medical benefit clearly outweighs the burden, it is obligatory to give the treatment unless a cognitively capable patient refuses. If the patient is incompetent and the appointed surrogate or family member refuses treatment that has clear and substantial medical benefit, the physician should err on the side of preserving life until a clear justification for the refusal is identified. Consultation with the institutional ethics committee or other multidisciplinary group may be appropriate.

When the burden of a medical treatment outweighs its benefit—for example, performing cardiopulmonary resuscitation in a person whose death is imminent—it is ethically permissible to forego the treatment. The physician has the duty to inform the patient, if capacitated, or the appropriate decision-maker, of the medical futility of the treatment(s) under consideration. Informing patients or surrogate decision-makers of the futility of treatment is required in the context of shared decision-making. If the patient or surrogate decision-maker demands medically futile treatment, the physician should respectfully disagree and make all attempts to resolve the conflict. Although physicians are not obligated to provide clearly futile medical treatment, disagreements should be taken seriously since there may be nonmedical or psychological benefits which, in rare instances, justify continuation of treatment. Attempts should be made through whatever hospital consultative procedures exist for resolving such substantive disagreements.

An important part of any dialogue on foregoing treatment includes a frank discussion of the ethical standards and values held by patients, families, surrogate decision-makers, and members of the health care team. Health care professionals have an obligation to respect the considered choices of the patient or the patient's surrogate. However, when the patient or surrogate chooses a course of action that violates the health care provider's strongly held personal, ethical, or religious commitments, health care providers should discuss this problem with the patient or surrogate. If a resolution is not possible, it may be necessary to transfer the care of the patient to another equally qualified professional.

All decisions to forego treatment make references to values and personal preferences. Even when the benefit-burden standard is used to justify ethical decisions, it is important to consider other factors including the strong symbolic significance attributed to certain treatments such as mechanical ventilators and artificially supplied hydration and nutrition. The symbolic significance of these treatments emanates from our basic human desires to provide comfort and sustenance to other people. Nevertheless, decisions to forego these treatments should be made in the same manner as other medical decisions, taking into consideration the patient's diagnosis, prognosis, benefits and burdens of the treatment, and the preferences of the patient and family. Once a decision is medically and ethically justifiable, attention should be paid to ethical aspects of the implementation. Our experience with decisions to discontinue mechanical ventilation and nutrition/hydration has taught us the importance of clear communication with the patient, the family, and health care team about the process of withdrawing the instituted therapy. Concerns that the patient may suffer, experience dyspnea, gasp for air, or experience thirst when hydration is withdrawn should be honestly discussed. If the patient is able to participate in the decision, his or her preference should be elicited especially concerning attitudes toward sedation. Some patients want to be sedated as little as possible after extubation unless they experience discomfort, so that they can spend their remaining time interacting with their families.

Other patients facing withdrawal of mechanical ventilation may want deep sedation before the withdrawal to avoid any discomfort. If relieving the patient's dyspnea or discomfort requires sedation to the point of unconsciousness, it is ethically obligatory to provide such sedation with the patient's or surrogate's consent. Hospital policies concerning withdrawing and withholding life-sustaining treatment should address not only when it is permissible to forego treatment but also should provide guidelines on how to alleviate pain and suffering when foregoing treatments, including mechanical ventilation. Policies should provide guidelines for ethical decision-making and ethical implementation of the decisions. When decisions to withdraw nutrition and hydration are made, careful attention to family support, comfort, and nursing measures should continue. The family and health care team should be aware that the dying process following withdrawal of artificially supplied nutrition and hydration may be days to weeks. Decisions to withdraw artificial nutrition and hydration should be reviewed with the institutional ethics committee since some jurisdictions may have legal restrictions on foregoing nutrition/hydration which may need to be taken into account.

BRAIN DEATH

Critical distinctions must be made between technical issues involved in a declaration of death and ethical questions that reflect our attempts to understand the nature and significance of death. Philosophical concepts of death provide a formal conceptual structure for understanding death. They tell us what death is. Methodologic criteria for determining death describe tests and measurements that should be applied to diagnose death. Some of the language used to discuss death has added to public confusion, feeding ancient fears of false-positive results. Families wonder whether their loved ones are truly and completely dead. Terms like "brain death" and "heart death" are unfortunate because they misdirect attention. We should not focus on the destruction of particular cells, organs, or organ systems, but on the death of the individual. The terms "brain death" and "heart death" make it easy to avoid analysis of the radical alteration that occurs in the individual as a whole.

Distinctions between declarations of death and decisions to forego treatments to dying persons must be upheld. We cannot afford to become involved in arbitrary attempts to redefine death. It may seem easier to declare death than to deal with the difficult questions of whether and under what circumstances individuals should be allowed to die. Artificial characterizations of death can be considered a from of self-deception and spoil our efforts to present a coherent scientific perspective to families. Our language may reveal our confusion, suggesting that patients died twice—once when death was declared and a second time when support equipment was removed.

Two Concepts of Death

Public thought and professional practice reveal two concepts of death. One philosophical concept defines death as the irreversible loss of integrated organic functioning. We are all familiar with the traditional criteria associated with this concept: irreversible cessation of cardiopulmonary function. When cardiopulmonary function is maintained by mechanical means and when patients have suffered irreversible loss of all brain function, physicians can employ whole-brain criteria in accordance with medical standards and state uniform death statutes.

The second philosophical concept defines death as the irrevocable loss of what is essential to a person. The methodologic criteria associated with this concept assess either cerebral or cortical function. Application of these criteria would allow declarations of death to be made on patients in persistent vegetative state. Although these criteria have not been incorporated into any uniform death act, many philosophers and clinicians advocate adoption of these standards. They believe that whole-brain criteria are excessive and that the philosophical concept of death as irreversible loss of integrated organic functioning is inadequate because it fails to define death in terms of loss of unique human characteristics.

There are two forms of the concept of death as the irreversible loss of what is essential to a person. One asserts that death is the permanent loss of the capacity for personhood. The other states that death is the irreversible loss of one's status as a particular person. Effective implementation of these definitions presupposes genuine comprehension of the legal, moral, and social category of "person." These insights would also have to be expressed in uniform statutes. We have been mired for years in a fruitless debate about prerequisites for personhood. No professional or public consensus has emerged, and we seem to have made little progress in our attempt to grapple with this extraordinarily complex notion. This fact alone makes legislation and subsequent professional implementation of these concepts of death impractical.

Additional difficulties limit the value of these concepts of death. If what is of interest in death is the loss of a particular and unique person, difficulties will arise when we try to determine which metaphysical, biologic, or psychological factors constitute the relevant notion of identity. We might be placed in the awkward position of arguing that a person's continued life is dependent on the longevity of a specific perception of the self.

Three possible options confront those who wish to apply a philosophical concept of death as the irreversible loss of what is essential to a person. They can employ morally indefensible, species-based definitions of personhood. They can make use of minimal prerequisites of personhood and argue that sentience and consciousness are necessary conditions for personhood. These may not, as proponents intend, focus attention on the activities of the cerebral cortex. If death is defined as the irreversible loss of consciousness or sentience, then areas of anatomic interest will have to be broadened to include the thalamic reticular system.

A third option, which is gaining prominence, uses a cognitively demanding concept of personhood. Some definitions require that individuals recognize themselves as independent entities whose actions are consciously determined by long-range goals. Others demand that they be rational members of a moral community. Some of the cognitively impaired could not meet these strict standards of personhood. If we define death as the irreversible loss of what is essential to a person and these individuals have no capacity to engage in the necessary functions, they would be declared dead. Such an approach is unacceptable because it denies them moral standing and treats them as property to be exploited.

Critical care physicians play a crucial role in the evolution of criteria of death. Many families initially confront "brain death" in an emergency or intensive care unit. Critical care physicians may be the first to offer the family a definition or explanation of the significance of this classification. It is imperative, therefore, that critical care physicians have complete and accurate information about whole brain criteria of death. They need to assuage families' fears of false-positive declarations of death, discussing the foundation and reliability of these standards. Critical care physicians can work with other clinical specialists and researchers to ensure that criteria of death reflect our growing achievements in neurology. Our methods for determining death must keep pace with advancing technology. Only then will our philosophical concepts of death be appropriately employed.

SUGGESTED READING

Hastings Center. Guidelines on the termination of life-sustaining treatment and the care of the dying. Bloomington and Indianapolis: Indiana University Press, 1987.

President's Commission for the Study of Ethical Problems in Medicine and Biomedical and Behavioral Research. Deciding to forego life-sustaining treatment. Washington DC: Government Printing Office, 1983.

President's Commission for the Study of Ethical Problems in Medicine and Biomedical and Behavioral Research. Defining death: medical, legal, and ethical issues in the determination of death. Washington DC: Government Printing Office, 1981.

Youngner SJ, Allen M, Bartlett ET, et al. Psychological and ethical implications of organ retrieval. N Engl J Med 1985; 313:321–324.

Youngner SJ, Landefeld S, Coulton C, et al. "Brain death" and organ retrieval: a cross-sectional survey of knowledge and concepts among health professionals. JAMA 1989; 261:2205–2210.

INDEX

A
Abdominal trauma, 310
Acetaminophen poisoning, 324
Acetazolamide, diuretic action of, 82
Acetylcysteine, in acetaminophen poisoning, 324
Acid-base balance, in cardiopulmonary resuscitation, 2, 23
Acidity, gastric, reduction of, 186
Acidosis
  diabetic ketoacidosis, 302-304
  metabolic, 21
    in near-drowning victims, 319
  respiratory, 22
Acquired immunodeficiency syndrome
  mycoses in, systemic, 231
  Pneumocystis carinii pneumonia in, 218
Actinomycosis, of larynx, 195
Adrenal insufficiency, 305-306
AIDS. *See* Acquired immunodeficiency syndrome
Airway
  anatomy of, 5
  dysfunction in burns, 311-313
  management of
    bronchoscopy in, 16
    in cardiopulmonary resuscitation, 1
    in intracranial pressure increase, 250
    in trauma, 307-308
  obstruction in upper tract, 193-197
    allergic and immunologic causes of, 197
    in bronchospasm, 180-185
    foreign bodies in, 196
    in infections, 193-195
    management of, 197
    in trauma, 196-197
    in tumors, 195-196
Albumin infusions, 295
Albuterol
  in bronchospasm, 181
  in obstructive lung disease, 177
Alcohol
  in ethylene glycol or methanol poisoning, 325
  in prevention of infections, 211
Alkalosis
  metabolic, 21-22
  respiratory, 22
Allergic reactions, upper airway in, 197
Alprazolam, in depression, 335
Alteplase, in myocardial infarction, 119
Alveolar hypoventilation, 188-191
Amiloride, diuretic action of, 83-84
Amin Aid feeding solution, 265, 266
Amino acid solutions, 267
Aminophylline
  in acute respiratory failure, 164
  in anaphylaxis, 61
  in bronchospasm, 182-183
  in obstructive lung disease, 178
Amiodarone
  in arrhythmias with hypertrophic cardiomyopathy, 137
  in ventricular arrhythmias, 106
Amitriptyline, in depression, 334-335
d-Amphetamine in depression, 335

Amphotericin B, 224-226, 230-231
  flucytosine with, 229
  resistance to, 231
Amrinone
  in heart failure, congestive, 95
  in dilated cardiomyopathy, 134
  in valvular regurgitation, acute, 143
Amylase levels in pancreatitis, 276
Analgesia
  in endotracheal intubation, 9
  in myocardial infarction, 116-117
Anaphylactoid reactions, 58-59
Anaphylaxis, 58-62
  assessment of patient in, 59-60
  initial management of, 60-61
  therapy for persistent symptoms in, 61-62
Anesthetic agents in endotracheal intubation, 10
Anger, manifestations of, 336
Angina pectoris
  in hypertrophic cardiomyopathy, 138
  postinfarction, 121
  unstable, 112-115
    aspirin and heparin in, 112-114
    beta-blockers in, 113-114
    calcium antagonists in, 113
    coronary angiography in, 114
    coronary artery bypass surgery in, 114-115
    intra-aortic balloon counterpulsation in, 114
    nitroglycerin in, intravenous, 113
    percutaneous transluminal coronary angioplasty in, 114
    thrombolytic therapy in, 114
Angioedema, hereditary, 197
Angiography
  coronary, in unstable angina pectoris, 114
  in gastrointestinal hemorrhage
    lower tract, 286
    upper tract, 280, 281
Angioplasty
  coronary, in myocardial infarction, 121
  percutaneous transluminal, in unstable angina pectoris, 114
Angiotensin-converting enzyme inhibitors in heart failure, 90-91
  in dilated cardiomyopathy, 134
Anistreplase, in myocardial infarction, 120
Antacids, 186
Antibiotics, 219-224
  in aspiration of stomach contents, 187-188
  broad-spectrum empiric therapy with, 220
  in bronchospasm, 184
  monitoring of serum levels, 222-223
  new agents, 223-224
  in obstructive lung disease, 179
  pharmacokinetics in critically ill patients, 221
  in pneumonia, 172, 173-174
  in respiratory failure, acute, 164
  restricted use of, and prevention of infections, 212-213
  in septic shock, 64-65
  single versus combination drug regimens, 221
  toxicities and drug interactions, 221-222

in trauma, 310-311
Anticholinergic agents in bronchospasm, 184
Anticoagulants
  in dilated cardiomyopathy, 135
  postoperative, in cardiac surgery, 153
  in prevention of pulmonary embolism recurrence, 123-124
Anticonvulsant agents, 247-249
  in intracranial pressure increase, 235-236
Antidepressants, tricyclic, 334
Antidiuretic hormone secretion, inappropriate, in Guillain-Barré syndrome, 245
Antidotes used in poisonings, 323, 324-326
Antifungal therapy, 224-231
Antihistamines in anaphylaxis, 62
Antiseptic agents, 211-212
Antishock garments or trousers, 309
Anxiety disorders, 335-336
Aorta
  balloon counterpulsation
    in angina pectoris, unstable, 114
    in cardiogenic shock, 57-58, 149-150
    in dilated cardiomyopathy, 134
    in valvular regurgitation, acute, 145
  dissection of, 158
  echocardiography in, 40
  trauma of, 161
Aortic valve regurgitation
  acute, 142-145
  chronic, 146
Aortoenteric fistula, 283
Aprazolam, in anxiety disorders, 335
Arrhythmias
  atrial
    and digitalis in heart failure, 80
    fibrillation, 99-100
    flutter, 99
    in myocarditis, treatment of, 130
    tachycardia, 100-101
  atrioventricular junctional tachycardia, nonparoxysmal, 101
  cardiac arrest in, 2-4
  defibrillation in, 1, 106
  in dilated cardiomyopathy, 135
  echocardiography in, 42
  in hypertrophic cardiomyopathy, 137-138
  postoperative, in cardiac surgery, 150-151
  in septic shock, 67
  sick sinus syndrome, 98-99
  sinus tachycardia, 97-98
  supraventricular, 97-102
  torsades de pointes, 102, 107-108
  in trauma of heart and great vessels, 159
  in valvular regurgitation, acute, 144-145
  ventricular, 102-108
    amiodarone in, 106
    beta-blocker drugs in, 104-105
    bretylium tosylate in, 104
    cardioversion and defibrillation in, 106
    catheter ablation in, 106
    disopyramide in, 105
    encainide hydrochloride in, 106
    fibrillation, 108
    flecainide in, 105-106
    lidocaine in, 103
    mexiletine in, 105

343

Index

Arrhythmias (*Continued*)
  in myocardial infarction, 118
  in myocarditis, 129–130
  pacing therapy in, 106
  phenytoin in, 104
  premature contractions, 107
  procainamide in, 103–104
  quinidine in, 105
  surgery in, 106
  tachycardia, 107
  tocainide in, 105
  Wolff-Parkinson-White syndrome, 101–102
Arsenic poisoning, 325
Arterial blood gases, analysis of, 20–24
Arytenoid cartilage, 5
Ascites
  echocardiography in, 42
  in liver failure, 273
Aspergillosis
  pulmonary, 230
  treatment of, 228
Aspirations
  of foreign bodies, 196
    bronchoscopy in, 16
  pneumonia in, 171, 185
    in acute respiratory failure, 164
  of stomach contents, 185–188
    initial approach in, 186
    intubation and suctioning in, 187
    prevention of, 185–186
Aspirin
  in angina pectoris, unstable, 112–113
  in myocardial infarction, 117
  postoperative, in cardiac surgery, 153
Asthma, bronchospasm management in, 180–185
Asystole, cardiac arrest in, 3–4
Atelectasis, bronchoscopy in, 16
Atenolol in myocardial infarction, 118
Atracurium in endotracheal intubation, 11
Atrial arrhythmias. *See* Arrhythmias, atrial
Atrial pressure measurements
  echocardiography in, 41
  pulmonary artery catheter in, 49
Atrioventricular block, 108–111
  first-degree, 108
  His bundle recording in, 110
  in myocardial infarction, 109–110
  second-degree, 108
  third-degree, 108–109
  transvenous pacing in, temporary, 110–111
Atrioventricular dissociation, 109
Atrioventricular junctional tachycardia, nonparoxysmal, 101
Atropine in insecticide poisoning, 324
Azathioprine in myocarditis, 130

B

Balloon counterpulsation, intra-aortic. *See* Aorta, balloon counterpulsation
Barbiturates
  in coma induction
    in intracranial pressure increase, 236
    in seizures, 247–248
  high-dose, in intracranial pressure increase, 251
Benzodiazepines
  in anxiety disorders, 335
  as hypnotics, 337
  in seizures, 247
Beta-adrenergic agonists
  in bronchospasm, 181–182
  in obstructive lung disease, 177
Beta-adrenergic blocking agents. *See* Beta-blocker drugs
Beta-blocker drugs
  in angina pectoris, unstable, 113–114
  in myocardial infarction, 117–118
  in restrictive cardiomyopathy, 141
  in tachycardia with hypertrophic cardiomyopathy, 137
  in ventricular arrhythmias, 104–105
Bicarbonate therapy
  in cardiopulmonary resuscitation, 2
  in diabetic ketoacidosis, 304
Bitolterol in bronchospasm, 181–182
Blastomycosis
  of larynx, 195
  treatment of, 228
Blood gases, arterial, analysis of, 20–24
Blood transfusions, 292–296. *See also* Transfusions
Brain
  cerebral perfusion pressure, 250
  edema of, 249
    in liver failure, 273
  organic brain syndrome, 336
Brain death, 340–341
Bretylium tosylate in ventricular arrhythmias, 104
Bronchitis, chronic, 176–180
Bronchodilators
  in aspiration of stomach contents, 187
  in obstructive lung disease, 177
Bronchoscopy, 16–20
  in aspiration of stomach contents, 187
  complications of, 19–20
  contraindications to, 19, 20
  indications for, 16–17
  repeat procedures in, 18–19
  technique in, 17–18
Bronchospasm, 180–185
  aminophylline in, 182–183
  antibiotics in, 184
  anticholinergic agents in, 184
  beta-adrenergic agonists in, 181–182
  corticosteroids in, 183–184
  fluid therapy in, 184
  mechanical ventilation in, 184–185
  severe refractory, 185
Bumetanide, diuretic action of, 83
Bundle branch block, 109
Burns, 311–317
  cardiovascular support in, 313–314
  fluid replacement in, 313, 314–315
  inflammation-infection period in, 315–317
  postresuscitation period in, 314–315
  pulmonary problems in, 311–313
  resuscitation period in, 311–314
  wound management in, 314
Bypass surgery
  cardiopulmonary, hematologic effects of, 152–153
  coronary artery, in unstable angina pectoris, 114–115

C

Calcium
  channel blockers
    in acute tubular necrosis, 254
    in angina pectoris, unstable, 113
    in heart failure, congestive, 90
    in hypertensive emergencies, 157
    in hypertrophic cardiomyopathy, 138
    in restrictive cardiomyopathy, 141
  hypercalcemia
    in cancer patients, 297
    severe, 261–262
  hypocalcemia, severe, 262
  nutritional requirements, 269
Calcium EDTA, in lead poisoning, 324
Calcium gluconate, in hydrofluoric acid poisoning, 324
Calorie intake, determination of, 268
Calorimetry, indirect, 264
Cancer, 296–301
  cardiac complications of, 298
  colonic, hemorrhage in, 287
  gastrointestinal complications of, 299
  hematologic complications of, 299–300
  interleukin-2 in, toxicity of, 300–301
  of larynx, 196
  metabolic complications of, 297–298
  neurologic complications of, 299
  pulmonary complications of, 298–299
  tumor-lysis syndrome in, 297
Candidiasis
  refractory disseminated, 230
  treatment of, 228
Capnography, 24, 31
Captopril, in congestive heart failure, 90–91
  in dilated cardiomyopathy, 134
Carbon dioxide tension, arterial
  elevated, 23
  noninvasive techniques for monitoring of, 24
Cardiogenic shock, 54–58
Cardiomyopathy
  dilated, 131–135
    arrhythmias in, 135
    diagnosis of, 132–133
    etiology of, 131
    heart failure in, 133–135
    shock in, 134
  hypertrophic, 136–139
    asymptomatic, 139
    consequences of, 137–139
    pathophysiology of, 136–137
  restrictive, 139–141
    medical management of, 140–141
Cardiopulmonary resuscitation, 1–4
  acid-base balance in, 2, 23
  chest compression in, 1–2
  defibrillation in, 1
  drug therapy in, 2
  management of specific arrhythmias in, 2–4
  open chest massage in, 4
  pediatric, 4
  postresuscitation care in, 4
Cardioversion in ventricular arrhythmias, 106
Cerebral perfusion pressure, 250
Cerebrospinal fluid leaks, in head trauma, 234
Charcoal, activated, 323, 326
Chest
  compression in cardiopulmonary resuscitation, 1–2
  pain in hypertrophic cardiomyopathy, 138
  physiotherapy in obstructive lung disease, 179
  trauma of, 310
Chlorhexidine in prevention of infections, 211
Chlorthalidone, diuretic action of, 83
Chromium, dietary recommendations, 269
Cimetidine in reduction of gastric acidity, 186
Circulatory support
  assist devices in heart failure with dilated cardiomyopathy, 134
  in trauma, 308–309
Coagulation
  disorders of, 290–291
  disseminated intravascular, 291
    in cancer patients, 299–300
Cocaine as local anesthetic in nasal intubation, 10
Coccidioidomycosis, treatment of, 228
Colonoscopy in lower gastrointestinal hemorrhage, 286
Coma, 236–240
  barbiturate
    in intracranial pressure increase, 236
    in seizures, 247–249
  diabetic, 302–304
  diffuse or multifocal causes of, 238
  in herniation syndromes, 237–238
  localization of causes in, 237

Coma (*Continued*)
  management of, 238–239
  prognosis of, 239
  traumatic, 239
  vegetative state in, 239–240
Compleat Modified feeding solution, 265
Consciousness, disorders of, 236
Consent for therapy, informed, 338–339
Copper, dietary recommendations, 269
Coronary arteries
  angiography in unstable angina pectoris, 114
  angioplasty
    in myocardial infarction, 121
    percutaneous transluminal, in unstable angina pectoris, 114
  bypass surgery of, in unstable angina pectoris, 114–115
Corticosteroid therapy
  in adrenal insufficiency, 305
  in anaphylaxis, 61
  in aspiration of stomach contents, 187
  in bronchospasm, 183–184
  in intracranial pressure increase, 251
  in obstructive lung disease, 178
  in pericarditis, 128
  in radiation pneumonitis, 202–203
  in respiratory failure, acute, 164
  in septic shock, 66
Cricoid cartilage, 5
Cricothyrotomy
  in obstruction of upper airway, 197
  in trauma, 307–308
Croup, 194
Cryoprecipitate transfusions, 294–295
Cryptococcosis, treatment of, 228
Cyanide poisoning, 324
Cyclosporine in myocarditis, 130

D

Death
  concepts of, 341
  definition of, 240, 340–341
  neurologic criteria for, 240–243
  sudden, in hypertrophic cardiomyopathy, 138
Deferoxamine, in iron poisoning, 325
Defibrillation in ventricular arrhythmias, 106
  in cardiopulmonary resuscitation, 1
Delirium, 336
Depression, 334–335
Desipramine, in depression, 334
Dextrose solutions, 267
Diabetes mellitus, 302–304
Dialysis
  in acute renal failure, 255–256
  in poisonings, 327
Diazepam
  in endotracheal intubation, 9–10
  in myocardial infarction, 116
Diazoxide in hypertensive emergencies, 156
Diet. *See* Nutrition
Digitalis
  in heart failure, congestive, 78–81, 95
  in dilated cardiomyopathy, 133
  in obstructive lung disease, 179
  pharmacology of, 78–79
  poisoning from, 324, 325
  in valvular regurgitation, acute, 144
Digoxin immune fab, 325
Diltiazem
  in angina pectoris, unstable, 113
  in hypertrophic cardiomyopathy, 138
Dimercaprol in poisonings, 325
Diphenylhydantoin. *See* Phenytoin
Diphtheria, 195
Disinfectants, chemical, 211–212
Disopyramide
  in hypertrophic cardiomyopathy, 138–139
  in ventricular arrhythmias, 105

Dissociation
  atrioventricular, 109
  electromechanical, cardiac arrest in, 3
Diuretics
  in acute tubular necrosis, 254
  in cardiogenic shock, 57
  classification of, 82–84
  in heart failure, congestive, 81–87
    in dilated cardiomyopathy, 133
    in elderly patients, 84–86
  in intracranial pressure increase, 251
  in obstructive lung disease, 179
  in poisonings, 326–327
  in restrictive cardiomyopathy, 140–141
  in valvular regurgitation, acute, 143, 144
Diverticula, lower gastrointestinal hemorrhage in, 286–287
Dobutamine
  in cardiogenic shock, 55
  in heart failure, congestive, 93–94
    in dilated cardiomyopathy, 134
  in valvular regurgitation, acute, 143
Dopamine
  in anaphylaxis, 61
  in cardiogenic shock, 55
    postoperative, 149
  in heart failure, congestive, 95
  in septic shock, 69
  in shock with dilated cardiomyopathy, 134
  in valvular regurgitation, acute, 143
Drowning, and near-drowning victims, 317–320
Drug-induced gaps of toxicology, 322
Dyspnea in hypertrophic cardiomyopathy, 137, 138

E

Echocardiography, 35–45
  in aortic dissection, 40
  in arrhythmias, 42
  in ascites or peripheral edema, 42
  in clots and tumors, 42
  definitive or serial evaluation in, 42–44
  in heart failure, congestive, 40
  in hypotension, 39
  M-mode, 35
  in myocardial infarction, 116
  in pericardial tamponade, 36
  in pericarditis, constrictive, 39
  prognostic information in, 45
  in prosthetic valve dysfunction, 41
  pulmonary artery pressure in, 41
  in pulmonary edema, 40
  technique of, 35–36
  transesophageal, 35
  in traumatic heart disease, 42
Eclampsia of pregnancy, 157
Edema
  of brain, 249
    in liver failure, 273
  peripheral, echocardiography in, 42
  pulmonary
    diuretics in, 81–82
    echocardiography in, 40
    neurogenic, 250
Elderly patients, diuretic therapy in congestive heart failure, 84–86
Electrocardiography in myocardial infarction, 116
Electroconvulsive therapy in depression, 335
Electrolyte disorders, 256–262
Electromechanical dissociation, cardiac arrest in, 3
Embolectomy, pulmonary, 126
Embolism, pulmonary, 123–126
  in acute respiratory failure, 164
  and anticoagulants in prevention of recurrence, 123–124

  echocardiography in, 42
  embolectomy in, 126
  prevention by interruption of venous system, 124–125
  thrombolytic therapy in, 125–126
Emesis induction in poisonings, 323
Emphysema, pulmonary, 176–180
Enalapril in congestive heart failure, 91
Encainide hydrochloride in ventricular arrhythmias, 106
Encephalopathy
  in cancer patients, 299
  in liver failure, 272–273
Endocarditis, infective
  prophylaxis in hypertrophic cardiomyopathy, 139
  valvular regurgitation with, 145
Endoscopy in upper gastrointestinal tract hemorrhage, 280, 281
Endotracheal intubation, 5–15
Enrich feeding solution, 265
Ensure feeding solution, 265
Enteral feeding, 264–266
  examples of products in, 265
Enterocolitis, neutropenic, in cancer patients, 299
Enzyme diagnosis of myocardial infarction, 116
Epidemics, nosocomial, 213–314
Epiglottis, 5
Epiglottitis, 193–194
Epinephrine
  in anaphylaxis, 60, 61
  in cardiopulmonary resuscitation, 2
  in heart failure, congestive, 96
  nebulized racemic, in laryngeal edema, 62
  in obstructive lung disease, 177
  in septic shock, 70
Esmolol
  in myocardial infarction, 118
  in ventricular arrhythmias, 104
Esophagus, varices of, 282–283
Ethacrynic acid, diuretic action of, 83
Ethical issues, 338–341
  in brain death, 340–341
  informed consent in, 338–339
  in withholding or withdrawing of life-sustaining treatments, 242–243, 339–340
Ethylene glycol or methanol poisoning, 325
Eye signs in poisonings, 322

F

Factor VIII concentrate, 295
Factor IX concentrate, 295
Fenoterol
  in bronchospasm, 181–182
  in obstructive lung disease, 177
Fentanyl in endotracheal intubation, 9
Fibrillation
  atrial, 99–100
    in dilated cardiomyopathy, 135
  ventricular, 108
    cardiac arrest in, 1, 2–3
Fistula, aortoenteric, 283
Flecainide in ventricular arrhythmias, 105–106
Florinef in adrenal insufficiency, 305
Fluconazole, 227, 230
Flucytosine, 226
  amphotericin B with, 229
Fluid therapy
  in anaphylaxis, 60–61
  in bronchospasm, 184
  in burns, 313, 314–315
  in cardiogenic shock, 55
  in diabetic ketoacidosis, 303
  in hemorrhagic shock, 72–73, 309
  in intracranial pressure increase, 234
  in septic shock, 68–69

Flurazepam, in sleep disturbances, 337
Flutter, atrial, 99
Foreign bodies, aspiration of, 196
　bronchoscopy in, 16
Fungus infections
　antifungal compounds in, 224–227
　of larynx, 195
　mucocutaneous, 227–228
　systemic, 228–230
　　in AIDS, 231
Furosemide
　in acute tubular necrosis, 254
　diuretic action of, 82–83
　in heart failure in dilated cardiomyopathy, 133
　in valvular regurgitation, acute, 143

G

Gas electrodes, transcutaneous, 24
Gases in arterial blood, analysis of, 20–24
Gastric lavage in poisonings, 323
Gastrointestinal complications in cancer patients, 299
Gastrointestinal hemorrhage
　in lower tract, 284–288
　　causes of, 284–285
　　clinical features of, 284
　　in diverticula, 286–287
　　management of, 285–286
　　in polyps and cancer, 287
　　in small bowel lesions, 287–288
　　in vascular malformations, 287
　in upper tract, 279–284
　　angiography in, 280, 281
　　in aortoenteric fistula, 283
　　bleeding in, severity of, 279
　　endoscopy in, 280, 281
　　in esophageal varices and portal hypertension, 282–283
　　in high-risk patients, 279–280
　　in Mallory-Weiss tear, 283
　　management of, 281–284
　　obscure, 283–284
　　rebleeding in, risk of, 280
　　in stress ulcerations, 283
　　surgery in, 281–282
Glanders, larynx in, 195
Glasgow Coma Scale, 239
Glucose
　hypoglycemia in liver failure, 274
　ratio to fat in parenteral nutrition, 268
　serum levels in diabetic ketoacidosis, 302
Guillain-Barré syndrome, 243–245
　autonomic dysfunction in, 244–245
　deep venous thrombosis in, 245
　infections in, 245
　nutrition in, 245
　pain in, 245
　plasmapheresis in, 243–244
　respiratory control in, 244
　urine retention in, 245

H

Haloperidol in delirium, 336
Head trauma, 233–236
　cerebrospinal fluid leaks in, 234
　hematomas in, 233–234
　monitoring of intracranial pressure in, 234
　and treatment of increased intracranial pressure, 234–236
Heart
　angina pectoris, unstable, 112–115
　arrhythmias. See Arrhythmias
　artificial, 58
　cardiogenic shock, 54–58
　complications in cancer patients, 298
　echocardiography, 35–45
　myocardial infarction, 115–122

　prosthetic valve dysfunction, echocardiography in, 41
　radionuclide ventriculography, 45–47
　surgery of, postoperative care in, 147–154
　　cardiac care in, 147–151
　　in infections, 154
　　metabolic responses in, 153
　　neurologic function in, 153
　　in renal failure, 154
　　respiratory care in, 151–152
　tamponade, 74–77
　trauma, 158–161, 310
　　open-chest resuscitation in, 160
　　operative repair in, 160–161
　　shock in, 159
　valvular regurgitation
　　acute, 142–145
　　chronic, 145–147
　　tricuspid, echocardiography in, 41
　ventricular assist devices, 58
Heart block
　atrioventricular, 108–111
　bundle branch, 109
Heart failure
　in cancer patients, 298
　digitalis in, 78–81, 95
　　circulatory effects of, 79–80
　　contraindications to, 80–81
　　indications for, 80
　　recent clinical trials of, 80
　in dilated cardiomyopathy, 133–135
　diuretic therapy in, 81–87
　　drug response and side effects in, 86–87
　　in elderly patients, 84–86
　　in pediatric patients, 86
　　sites of action in kidney, 82–84
　echocardiography in, 40
　inotropic agents in, 92–96
　　amrinone, 95
　　digitalis, 78–81, 95
　　dobutamine, 93–94
　　dopamine, 95
　　epinephrine, 96
　　norepinephrine, 95
　in myocardial infarction, 122
　in myocarditis, treatment of, 130
　nutritional support in, 271
　postoperative, in cardiac surgery, 150
　vasodilator therapy in, 87–92
　　angiotensin-converting enzyme inhibitors, 90–91
　　calcium channel blockers, 90
　　hydralazine, 89
　　indications for, 91–92
　　minoxidil, 90
　　nitrates, 88–89
　　prazosin, 90
Heat stroke, 330–331
Heimlich maneuver, 196
　modification of, 1
Hematoma
　epidural, 233–234
　intraparenchymal, in head trauma, 234
　subdural, 233
Hemodynamic monitoring, bedside, 47–53
Hemofiltration, continuous arteriovenous, in acute renal failure, 256
Hemoperfusion, charcoal, in poisonings, 327
Hemophilia, cryoprecipitate in, 294–295
Hemorrhage
　and exsanguination, in trauma of heart and great vessels, 159
　gastrointestinal
　　in liver failure, 273–274
　　in lower tract, 284–288
　　in upper tract, 279–284
　postoperative, in cardiac surgery, 152–153
　shock in, 70–74

Hemorrhagic disorders, management of, 289–291
Heparin
　in angina pectoris, unstable, 112–113
　coagulation disorders from, 291
　in myocardial infarction, 117
　in prevention of pulmonary embolism recurrence, 123–124
Hepatic Aid feeding solution, 265, 266
Hepatitis from transfusions, 295–296
Herniation syndromes, coma in, 237–238
His bundle recordings in atrioventricular block, 110
Histoplasmosis, treatment of, 228
Hydralazine in congestive heart failure, 89
　in dilated cardiomyopathy, 134
Hydrochlorothiazide, diuretic action of, 83
Hydrofluoric acid poisoning, 324
Hypercalcemia
　in cancer patients, 297
　severe, 261–262
Hypercapnia, 23, 31–33
Hyperkalemia, 256–257
Hypernatremia, 260
Hyperosmolar syndrome, 302–304
Hypertension
　in Guillain-Barré syndrome, 244–245
　portal, 282–283
Hypertensive emergencies, 155–157
　in eclampsia of pregnancy, 157
　immediate management of, 155–156
　initial management of, 156–157
　malignant-phase hypertension in, 157
Hyperthermia, 330–332
　malignant, 331–332
Hyperventilation in intracranial pressure increase, 250–251
Hypnotics
　in endotracheal intubation, 9–10
　in sleep disturbances, 337
Hypocalcemia, severe, 262
Hypoglycemia in liver failure, 274
Hypokalemia, 257–258
Hypomagnesemia in cancer patients, 298
Hyponatremia, 258–259
Hypophosphatemia
　in cancer patients, 297
　in diabetic ketoacidosis, 304
　severe, 260–261
Hypotension
　echocardiography in, 39
　in near-drowning victims, 318
Hypothermia, accidental, 329–330
　in near-drowning victims, 318
Hypoventilation, alveolar, 188–191
Hypovolemic shock, 70–74
　in trauma, 309
Hypoxemia, 23, 33
Hypoxia, in near-drowning victims, 318

I

Ibuprofen, in pericarditis, 127
Imidazole antifungal agents, 226–227
Imipramine in depression, 335
Immune globulin preparations, 295
Immunosuppressed host
　central nervous system infection in, 218–219
　infections in, 216
　pneumonia in, 174, 217–218
　septic shock in, 215–217
Immunosuppressive therapy
　in heart failure with dilated cardiomyopathy, 135
　in myocarditis, 130
Indapamide, diuretic action of, 83
Indomethacin in pericarditis, 127–128
Infarction, myocardial, 115–122
　atrioventricular block in, 109–110

Infarction, (Continued)
 cardiogenic shock in, 121
 complications of, 121–122
 diagnosis of, 115–116
 heart failure in, 122
 initial therapeutic approach to, 116–118
 pathophysiology of, 115
 and postinfarction angina, 121
 postoperative, in cardiac surgery, 150
 right ventricular, 121–122
 rupture of heart in, 122
 thrombolytic therapy in, 118–121
Infections
 airway obstruction in, 193–195
 antibiotics in, 219–224
 antifungal therapy in, 224–231
 in burns, 316
 in Guillain-Barré syndrome, 245
 in immunosuppressed host, 215–219
 in liver failure, 273
 nosocomial, 208–215
 pneumonia in, 173–174
 postoperative, in cardiac surgery, 154
 septic shock in, 64–70
Informed consent, 338–339
Inotropic agents
 in heart failure, 92–96
  in dilated cardiomyopathy, 134
  in valvular regurgitation, acute, 144
Insect stings, management of anaphylaxis in, 60–61
Insecticide poisoning, 324, 326
Insulin therapy in diabetic ketoacidosis, 303–304
Interleukin-2, toxicity of, 300–301
Intracranial pressure
 increased, 249–252
  in cancer patients, 299
  diagnostic studies in, 249–250
  hyperventilation in, 250–251
  physiologic considerations in, 250
  treatment of, 234–236, 250–252
 monitoring of, 234, 249
Intubation, endotracheal, 5–15
 and anatomy of airway, 5
 in aspiration of stomach contents, 187
 blind nasal technique in, 13–14
 equipment for, 5–9
  preparation of, 12–13
 fiberoptic laryngoscope in, 15
 and laryngoscopy technique, 13
 oral intubation in
  awake, 14–15
  two-person technique, 307
  unconscious, 15
 pharmacologic agents in, 9–11
 preparation in, 11–13
 rapid sequence approach in, 14
 securing of tube in, 15
 techniques for, 13–15
 in trauma, 307
 verification of tube position in, 15
  bronchoscopy in, 16
Iodine, dietary recommendations, 269
Ipratropium bromide
 in anaphylaxis, 62
 in bronchospasm, 184
Iron
 antidote for, 325
 nutritional requirements, 269
Isocal feeding solution, 265
Isoetharine
 in bronchospasm, 181–182
 in obstructive lung disease, 177
Isolation precautions for infected patients, 212, 213
Isoniazid poisoning, 326
Isoproterenol
 in bronchospasm, 181

in obstructive lung disease, 177
Isosorbide dinitrate in heart failure with dilated cardiomyopathy, 134
Itraconazole, 227, 230

K
Ketamine in endotracheal intubation, 10
Ketoacidosis, diabetic, 302–304
Ketoconazole, 226–227, 230
Kidney
 acute failure, 253–256
  in acute tubular necrosis, 253, 254–255
  dialysis in, 255–256
  continuous arteriovenous hemofiltration in, 256
  in liver failure, 274
  management of, 255–256
  nutritional support in, 270
  postoperative, in cardiac surgery, 154
 acute tubular necrosis, 253
  prevention and treatment of, 254–255
 sites of diuretic action in, 82–84
Kyphoscoliosis, alveolar hypoventilation in, 190–191

L
Labetalol in hypertensive emergencies, 157
Laryngitis, tuberculous, 194
Laryngoscopes, 5–8
 fiberoptic, for endotracheal intubation, 15
Laryngoscopy technique, 13
Laryngotracheobronchitis, acute, 194
Larynx, 5
Lasix in intracranial pressure increase, 235
Lavage, gastric, in poisonings, 323
Lead poisoning, 324, 325
Legionellosis, treatment of, 218
Leprosy, laryngeal, 195
Leukocyte transfusions, 294
Lidocaine
 in arrhythmias with acute valvular regurgitation, 144
 in endotracheal intubation, 10
 in ventricular arrhythmias, 103
Lipid emulsions, 267
Lisinopril in congestive heart failure, 91
Liver failure, 271–275
 acute, 272
 ascites in, 273
 cerebral edema in, 273
 chronic, 272
 coagulation disorders in, 290–291
 encephalopathy in, 272–273
 gastrointestinal hemorrhage in, 273–274
 hypoglycemia in, 274
 infections in, 273
 nutritional support in, 270–271
 renal failure with, 274
 transplantation in, 275
Living wills, 339
Lorazepam
 in anxiety disorders, 335
 in seizures, 247
 in sleep disturbances, 337
Lumbar puncture in intracranial pressure increase, 249
Lungs
 dysfunction in burns, 311–313
 obstructive disease, 176–180
  acute respiratory failure in, 176–177
  prevention of complications in, 179–180
  treatment of, 177–179
 pneumonia, 170–175
 radiation pneumonitis and fibrosis, 201–203

M
Magnacal feeding solution, 265
Magnesium
 hypomagnesemia in cancer patients, 298

nutritional requirements, 269
Magnesium sulfate in arrhythmias with acute valvular regurgitation, 144
Mallory-Weiss tears, 283
Manganese, dietary recommendations, 269
Mannitol
 in acute tubular necrosis, 254
 diuretic action of, 82
 in intracranial pressure increase, 235, 251
MCT oil, 265
Mechanical ventilation. See Ventilation, mechanical
Meningitis
 antibiotics in, 222
 in immunosuppressed host, 218–219
Mercury poisoning, 325
Metaproterenol
 in anaphylaxis, 61–62
 in bronchospasm, 181–182
 in obstructive lung disease, 177
Methylphenidate in depression, 335
Methylxanthines in acute respiratory failure, 164
Metolazone
 diuretic action of, 83
 in heart failure with dilated cardiomyopathy, 133
Metoprolol
 in angina pectoris, unstable, 113
 in myocardial infarction, 118
 in ventricular arrhythmias, 104
Mexiletine in ventricular arrhythmias, 105
Miconazole, 226, 229
Midazolam in endotracheal intubation, 10
Minoxidil in congestive heart failure, 90
Mitral valve regurgitation
 acute, 142, 143–145
 chronic, 145–146
Molybdenum, dietary recommendations, 269
Morphine
 in endotracheal intubation, 9
 in myocardial infarction, 116
Mucocutaneous fungal infections, 227–228
Muscle relaxants in endotracheal intubation, 10–11
Myocardial infarction, 115–122
Myocarditis
 diagnosis of, 129
 pericarditis with, 126–130
 treatment of, 129–130

N
Naloxone, 321, 325
Narcotic analgesics in endotracheal intubation, 9
Natamycin, 224
Near-drowning victims, 317–320
 acidosis in, 319
 hypotension in, 318
 hypothermia in, 318
 hypoxia in, 318
 initial management of, 318
 prophylactic measures in, 319
 pulmonary sequelae of, 318
Neurogenic pulmonary edema, 250
Neuroleptics in organic brain syndrome, 336
Neurologic criteria for death, 240–243
Neurologic disorders
 in cancer patients, 299
 coma, 236–240
 encephalopathy in liver failure, 272–273
 Guillain-Barré syndrome, 243–245
 head trauma, 233–236
 in immunosuppressed host, 218–219
 intracranial pressure increase, 249–252
 in poisonings, 321
 postoperative, in cardiac surgery, 153
 seizures, 246–249
 in trauma, 310

Neuromuscular blocking drugs, in endotracheal intubation, 10–11
Neuromuscular disease, alveolar hypoventilation in, 191
Nifedipine
  in acute tubular necrosis, 254
  in angina pectoris, unstable, 113
  in heart failure, congestive, 90
  in hypertensive emergencies, 157
  in hypertrophic cardiomyopathy, 138
Nitrate therapy in cyanide poisoning, 324
Nitrogen balance, 263
Nitroglycerin
  in heart failure, 88–89
  intravenous
    in myocardial infarction, 117
    in unstable angina pectoris, 113
  in valvular regurgitation, acute, 143
Nitroprusside
  in heart failure, 89
  in dilated cardiomyopathy, 133
  in valvular regurgitation, acute, 143
Norepinephrine
  in anaphylaxis, 61
  in cardiogenic shock, postoperative, 149
  in heart failure, 95
  in septic shock, 69–70
  in shock with dilated cardiomyopathy, 134
  in valvular regurgitation, acute, 143
Nortriptyline in depression, 334
Nosocomial infections, 208–215
  control measures in, 210–213
    chemical disinfectants and antiseptics in, 211–212
    handwashing in, 211
    isolation precautions in, 212, 213
    and precautions with invasive devices, 212
    restricted use of antibiotics in, 212–213
    selective antimicrobial decontamination in, 213
  epidemics in, 213–214
  epidemiology of, 208–210
  management of, 214–215
  pneumonia, 173–174
  profile in intensive care unit, 208, 209
  and protection of health care workers, 214
Nuclear scanning, 45–47
Nutrition, 262–271
  assessment of, 263–264
  in burns, 316
  calories in, 268
  enteral feeding in, 264–266
    examples of products in, 265
  glucose-to-fat ratio in, 268
  in Guillain-Barré syndrome, 245
  in heart failure, 271
  in hepatic failure, 270–271
  parenteral, 266–268
  protein in, 268–269
  in pulmonary failure, 271
  in renal failure, 270
  requirements in, 268–270
  in respiratory failure, acute, 164–165
  trace elements in, 269–270
  vitamins in, 270
  water and electrolytes in, 269
  in weaning from mechanical ventilation, 204
  withdrawal of, ethical issues in, 340
Nystagmus in poisonings, 322
Nystatin, 224–225

O

Obesity, hypoventilation in, 189–190
Ocular findings in poisonings, 322
Organophosphate insecticide poisonings, 324, 326
Osmolite feeding solution, 265

Oxazepam
  in anxiety disorders, 335
  in sleep disturbances, 337
Oximetry
  pulmonary artery, 24
  pulse, 30–31
Oxygen tension, arterial, 22–23
  noninvasive techniques for monitoring of, 24
Oxygen therapy
  in acute respiratory failure, 163
  in obstructive lung disease, 177
  toxicity of, 198–201
Oxygenation with mechanical ventilation. See Ventilation, mechanical

P

Pacing
  cardiac, in ventricular arrhythmias, 106
  phrenic nerve, in alveolar hypoventilation, 190
  transvenous, temporary, in atrioventricular block, 110–111
Pain
  In Guillain-Barré syndrome, 245
  psychiatric issues in, 337
Pancreatitis, acute, 273–278
  clinical features of, 276
  complications of, 277
  diagnosis of, 276–277
  etiology of, 275
  medical management of, 277–278
  prognosis of, 277
Pancuronium in endotracheal intubation, 11
Panic attacks, 336
Papilloma, laryngeal, 195–196
Paraldehyde in seizures, 247
Pediatric patients
  cardiopulmonary resuscitation, 4
  diuretic therapy in congestive heart failure, 86
PEEP therapy. See Ventilation, mechanical
D-Penicillamine in poisonings, 325
Pentobarbital coma
  in intracranial pressure increase, 236
  in seizures, 247–248
Pericardial effusions, cardiac tamponade in, 74–77
Pericardiocentesis, 76–77
Pericardiostomy in cardiac tamponade, 77
Pericarditis
  constrictive
    in cardiac tamponade, 77
    echocardiography in, 39
  diagnosis of, 127
  malignant, 129
  myocarditis with, 126–130
  in postcardiac injury syndrome, 129
  postoperative, in cardiac surgery, 150
  purulent, 129
  recurrences of, 128
  treatment of, 127–129
  tuberculous, 129
  uremic, 129
Phenobarbital in seizures, 247
Phenytoin
  in intracranial pressure increase, 236
  in seizures, 247
  in ventricular arrhythmias, 104
Phosphate levels in hypophosphatemia, 260–261
  in cancer patients, 297
  in diabetic ketoacidosis, 304
Phosphorus, dietary recommendations, 269
Phrenic nerve pacing, in alveolar hypoventilation, 190
Physiotherapy, chest, in obstructive lung disease, 179
Physostigmine salicylate in poisonings, 326

Pimaricin, 224
Plasma
  fresh frozen, 294
  protein fraction infusions, 295
Plasmapheresis in Guillain-Barré syndrome, 243–244
Platelets
  disorders of, 290
  transfusions of, 293–294
Plethysmography, respiratory inductance, 31
Pneumocystis carinii pneumonia, 218
Pneumonia, 170–175
  antibiotics in, 223
  aspiration, 171, 185
    in acute respiratory failure, 164
  atypical, 170, 171
  in cancer patients, 299
  in chronic lung disease, 174
  community-acquired, 170–173
  in immunocompromised patients, 174, 217–218
  initial therapy in, 172
  nosocomial 173–174
  potential complications of, 174–175
  typical, 170, 171
Pneumonitis, radiation-induced, 202–203
Pneumothorax in acute respiratory failure, 163–164
Poison management, 320–328. See also Toxicology
Polycose feeding solutions, 265
Polyene antifungal agents, 224–226
Polyneuritis, ascending, 243–245
Polyps, colonic, hemorrhage in, 287
Portal hypertension, 282–283
Positioning of patient in intracranial pressure increase, 234
Potassium
  hyperkalemia, 256–257
  hypokalemia, 257–258
  nutritional requirements, 269
  replacement therapy
    in cardiogenic shock, 57
    in diabetic ketoacidosis, 304
Povidone-iodine in prevention of infections, 211
Power of attorney, durable, 339
Pralidoxime in insecticide poisoning, 326
Prazosin in congestive heart failure, 90
Prednisone
  in heart failure with dilated cardiomyopathy, 135
  in myocarditis, 130
Pre-excitation syndrome, 101–102
Pregnancy, eclampsia in, 157
Premature ventricular contractions, 107
Procainamide
  in arrhythmias with acute valvular regurgitation, 144–145
  in ventricular arrhythmias, 103–104
Pro-Pac feeding solution, 265
Propranolol
  in angina pectoris, unstable, 113
  in arrhythmias with hypertrophic cardiomyopathy, 137
  in ventricular arrhythmias, 104
Prosthetic valve dysfunction, echocardiography in, 41
Protein
  dietary intake determination, 268–269
  plasma protein fraction infusions, 295
Psychiatric problems, 333–337
  anger, 336
  anxiety, 335–336
  depression, 334–335
  pain, 337
  sleep disturbances, 337
Psychogenic unresponsiveness, 238

Pulmocare feeding solution, 265, 266
Pulmonary artery
  catheter use, 47–53
    cardiac output measurements, 51
    central pressure measurements, 49
    choice of catheter in, 49
    complications of, 52–53
    indications for, 47–49
    insertion sites, 49
    limitations of, 50–51
    oxygen delivery measurements, 51–52
    in septic shock, 66–67
  oximetry, 24
  pressure estimation with echocardiography, 41
Pulmonary edema
  diuretics in, 81–82
  echocardiography in, 40
  neurogenic, 250
Pulmonary embolism, 123–126
Pulse oximetry, 30–31
Pulseless idioventricular rhythm, cardiac arrest in, 3–4
Pupillary signs in poisonings, 322
Pyridoxine in isoniazid poisoning, 326

Q

Quinidine in ventricular arrhythmias, 105

R

Radiation therapy
  fibrosis of lung from, 203
  in intracranial pressure increase, 251
  pneumonitis from, 202–203
Radionuclide scanning, 45–47
Ranitidine in reduction of gastric acidity, 186
Respiratory distress syndrome, adult, 165–170
  clinical course and outcome of, 166–167
  etiology of, 165–166
  mechanism of lung damage in, 167
  nutritional support in, 271
  positive end-expiratory pressure in, 167–169
Respiratory failure, acute, 162–165
  in cancer patients, 298–299
  impending, monitoring for, 31–33
  mechanical ventilation in. See Ventilation, mechanical
  methylxanthines in, 164
  in obstructive lung disease, 164, 176–180
  oxygen therapy in, 163
  pneumothorax in, 163–164
Respiratory function, bedside evaluation of, 30–34
  in impending respiratory failure, 31–33
  in mechanical ventilation, 33–34
  new technologies in, 30–31
  in weaning from mechanical ventilatory support, 34
Respiratory inductance plethysmography, 31
Respiratory muscle dysfunction, 191–192
Resuscitation, cardiopulmonary, 1–4

S

Sarcoid of larynx, 195
Scanning, nuclear, 45–47
Sedatives
  in endotracheal intubation, 9–10
  in intracranial pressure increase, 235
  in myocardial infarction, 116
Seizures, 246–249
  anticonvulsants in, 247–249
  diagnostic studies in, 246
  in head trauma, 235–236
  in heat stroke, 331
  in near-drowning victims, 319
  in poisonings, 321
  status epilepticus in, 248–249
Selenium, dietary recommendations, 269

Septic shock, 64–70
Shock
  anaphylactic, 58–62
  antishock garments or trousers, 305
  cardiogenic, 54–58, 121
    coronary angioplasty and bypass surgery in, 58
    intra-aortic balloon counterpulsation in, 57–58
    pharmacologic agents in, 55–57
    postoperative, in cardiac surgery, 149–150
    ventricular assist devices in, 58
  in dilated cardiomyopathy, 134
  distributive, 62–64
  hemorrhagic and hypovolemic, 70–74
    blood component therapy in, 73
    clinical features of, 70–72
    complications of, 74
    fluid therapy in, 72–73
    and re-evaluation after initial resuscitation, 73–74
    in trauma, 309
  septic, 64–70
    antibiotics in, 222
    cardiovascular support in, 67–70
    clinical features of, 64
    eradication of infection in, 64–66
    hemodynamic monitoring in, 66–67
    in immunosuppressed host, 215–217
    laboratory monitoring in, 67
    neutralization of toxins in, 64
    supportive care in, 66–70
    in trauma of heart and great vessels, 159
Sick sinus syndrome, 98–99
Sinus tachycardia, 97–98
Sleep disturbances, 337
Smoke inhalation injury, 311
Snake bites
  antivenin in, 326
  management of anaphylaxis in, 60
Sodium
  hypernatremia, 260
  hyponatremia, 258–259
  nutritional requirements, 269
Spironolactone, diuretic action of, 83–84
Status epilepticus, 248–249
Stomach contents, aspiration of, 185–188
Streptokinase therapy, 291
  in myocardial infarction, 119–120
  in pulmonary embolism, 125–126
Stress ulcers, gastrointestinal hemorrhage in, 283
Succinylcholine chloride, in endotracheal intubation, 10–11
Suctioning in aspiration of stomach contents, 187
Swan-Ganz catheter. See Pulmonary artery, catheter use
Syphilis of larynx, 194–195

T

Tachycardia
  atrial, 100–101
  atrioventricular junctional, nonparoxysmal, 101
  sinus, 97–98
  supraventricular, in hypertrophic cardiomyopathy, 137
  ventricular, 107
    cardiac arrest in, 1, 3
    in dilated cardiomyopathy, 135
Tamponade, cardiac, 74–77
  in cancer patients, 298
  clinical features of, 75
  definitive treatment of, 76–77
  echocardiography in, 36
  and effusive-constrictive pericarditis, 77
  pericardiocentesis in, 76–77

pericardiostomy in, 77
postoperative, in cardiac surgery, 150
supportive therapy in, 75–76
in trauma of heart and great vessels, 159
Technetium 99m pyrophosphate scans, myocardial, 46–47
Terbutaline
  in bronchospasm, 181–182
  in obstructive lung disease, 177
Thallium-201 scans, myocardial, 46
Theophylline
  in acute respiratory failure, 164
  in anaphylaxis, 61
  in obstructive lung disease, 178
Thiazide diuretics, 83
Thiopental sodium in endotracheal intubation, 9
Thiosulfate sodium in cyanide poisoning, 324
Thrombocytopenia, 290
Thrombolytic therapy, 291–292
  in angina pectoris, unstable, 114
  in myocardial infarction, 118–121
  in pulmonary embolism, 125–126
Thrombosis
  cardiac, echocardiography in, 42
  venous
    in Guillain-Barré syndrome, 245
    prevention of, 292
Tissue plasminogen activator (t-PA), 291–292
  in myocardial infarction, 119
  in pulmonary embolism, 125–126
Tocainide, in ventricular arrhythmias, 105
Torsades de pointes, 102, 107–108
Toxicology, 320–328
  antidotes in, 323, 324–326
  enhancement of elimination in, 323, 326–328
  physical examination in, 321–322
  prevention of absorption in, 322–323
  stabilization of patient in, 320–321
Trace elements, dietary recommendations, 269
Tracheal intubation, 5–15
Tracheotomy in obstruction of upper airway, 197
Transcutaneous gas electrodes, 24
Transfusions, 292–296
  adverse effects of, 295–296
  clotting factor concentrates in, 295
  cryoprecipitate in, 294–295
  fresh frozen plasma in, 294
  in hemorrhagic shock, 73
  immunoglobulin preparations in, 295
  leukocytes in, 294
  platelet counts in, 291
  platelets in, 293–294
  red cells in, 292
    frozen/deglycerolyzed, 293
    leukocyte-poor, 292–293
  whole blood in, 292
Transplantation
  of heart
    in heart failure with dilated cardiomyopathy, 134–135
    in restrictive cardiomyopathy, 141
  of liver, 275
Trauma
  abdominal, 310
  airway management in, 307–308
  antibiotic therapy in, 310–311
  bone fractures in, 310
  in burns, 311–317
  categorization scores in, 308
  of chest, 310
  of head, 233–236
  of heart and great vessels, 158–161, 310
  initial management of, 307–311
  neurologic care in, 310
  secondary survey in, 310
  of upper airway, 196–197

Triamterene, diuretic action of, 83–84
Triazolam, in sleep disturbances, 337
Triazole antifungal agents, 227
Tricuspid regurgitation, echocardiography in, 41
Tricyclic antidepressants, 334
Tuberculous conditions
    laryngitis, 194
    pericarditis, 129
Tubes, endotracheal, 8–9
Tumors
    laryngeal, 195–196
    malignant. *See* Cancer

U

Ulcers, stress, gastrointestinal hemorrhage in, 283
Ultrasonography. *See* Echocardiography
Urea nitrogen, urinary, 263
Urine retention, in Guillain-Barré syndrome, 245
Urokinase therapy, 291–292
    in myocardial infarction, 120
    in pulmonary embolism, 125–126

V

Vallecula, 5
Valvular regurgitation
    aortic and mitral
        acute, 142–145
        chronic, 145–147
    tricuspid, echocardiography in, 41
Varices, esophageal, 282–283
Vascular malformations, lower gastrointestinal hemorrhage in, 287
Vasodilator therapy
    in cardiogenic shock, 55
    in heart failure, congestive, 87–92
    in dilated cardiomyopathy, 133–134
    in restrictive cardiomyopathy, 141
Vecuronium in endotracheal intubation, 11
Vegetative state, 239–240
Vena cava
    interruption in prevention of pulmonary embolism, 124–125
    superior, syndrome in cancer patients, 298
Ventilation, mechanical, 24–30
    in acute respiratory failure, 163
    in adult respiratory distress syndrome, 167–169
    in alveolar hypoventilation, 189–191
    in aspiration of stomach contents, 187
    assist/control mode in, 26
    in bronchospasm, 184–185
    in cardiogenic shock, 57
    complications of, 29–30
    in Guillain-Barré syndrome, 244
    high-frequency, 25
    indications for, 25
    initiation of, 25–26
    intermittent mandatory, 26
        synchronized, 26
    in intracranial pressure increase, 235
    maintenance of, 27
    modes of, 26–27
    monitoring in, 28–29, 33–34
    in near-drowning, 318
    in obstructive lung disease, 179
    positive-pressure, 25
    positive end-expiratory pressure (PEEP) in, 27–28
    postoperative, in cardiac surgery, 151–152
    in trauma, 308
    types of ventilators in, 25
    weaning from, 203–207
        monitoring in, 34
    nutritional support in, 271
    in patients with pre-existent lung disease, 206–207
    in previously healthy patients with acute lung disease, 205–206
    withdrawal of, ethical issues in, 340
Ventricular arrhythmias, 102–108
Ventricular assist devices, 58
Ventricular drainage in intracranial pressure increase, 252
Ventriculography, radionuclide, 45–47
Verapamil
    in angina pectoris, unstable, 113
    in hypertrophic cardiomyopathy, 138
    in restrictive cardiomyopathy, 141
Vital HN feeding solution, 265
Vitamin B_6 in isoniazid poisoning, 326
Vitamin K
    deficiency of, 290
    in warfarin poisoning, 326
Vitamin requirements, nutritional, 269
Vivonex TEN feeding solution, 265
Vomiting induction in poisonings, 323

W

Warfarin
    antidote to, 326
    in prevention of pulmonary embolism recurrence, 124
Weaning from mechanical ventilation, 203–207
Wills, living, 339
Wolff-Parkinson-White syndrome, 101–102

Z

Zinc requirements, nutritional, 269
Zygomycosis, treatment of, 228